IFMBE Proceedings

AF848200

Volume 47

The International Federation for Medical and Biological Engineering, IFMBE, is a federation of national and transnational organizations representing internationally the interests of medical and biological engineering and sciences. The IFMBE is a non-profit organization fostering the creation, dissemination and application of medical and biological engineering knowledge and the management of technology for improved health and quality of life. Its activities include participation in the formulation of public policy and the dissemination of information through publications and forums. Within the field of medical, clinical, and biological engineering, IFMBE's aims are to encourage research and the application of knowledge, and to disseminate information and promote collaboration. The objectives of the IFMBE are scientific, technological, literary, and educational.

The IFMBE is a WHO accredited NGO covering the full range of biomedical and clinical engineering, healthcare, healthcare technology and management. It is representing through its 60 member societies some 120.000 professionals involved in the various issues of improved health and health care delivery.

More information about this series at http://www.springer.com/series/7403

Fong-Chin Su · Shyh-Hau Wang
Ming-Long Yeh
Editors

1st Global Conference on Biomedical Engineering & 9th Asian-Pacific Conference on Medical and Biological Engineering

October 9–12, 2014, Tainan, Taiwan

Springer

Editors
Fong-Chin Su
Department of Biomedical Engineering
National Cheng Kung University
Tainan
Taiwan

Ming-Long Yeh
Department of Biomedical Engineering
National Cheng Kung University
Tainan
Taiwan

Shyh-Hau Wang
Department of Computer Science and Information Engineering
National Cheng Kung University
Tainan
Taiwan

ISSN 1680-0737 ISSN 1433-9277 (electronic)
ISBN 978-3-319-12261-8 ISBN 978-3-319-12262-5 (eBook)
DOI 10.1007/978-3-319-12262-5

Library of Congress Control Number: 2014951226

Springer Cham Heidelberg New York Dordrecht London

The IFMBE Proceedings is an Official Publication of the International Federation for Medical and Biological Engineering (IFMBE)

Printed on acid-free paper

Springer is part of Springer Science+Business Media (www.springer.com)

Foreword

Welcome to the GCBME 2014 - APCMBE 2014

Biomedical engineering is such exciting field engineering, and it contributes so much to biomedical and engineering science! Modern biomedical engineering was born mid 20th century and since then it experienced tremendous growth. I would also like to mention that large contribution is expected from biomedical engineers in approaching and solving the big challenges of the 21st century, such as reverse-engineering the brain, advancement of health informatics or engineering new medicines, the challenges listed among fourteen challenges by the National Academy of Engineering of the USA. Today, we know so little about how the brain operates. However, by systematic engineering analysis and study we are able to gain more and more information on brain functions and organization and thus help people with serious physical disabilities, like deafness or blindness by designing appropriate devices, cochlear implants or artificial retina. Accurate information, from stages of their acquisition, processing, management to their use, enhances the quality of health care for each person individually, while shearing gathered information and extracting new knowledge out of it, health care is improved globally and from being mainly reactive, it becomes proactive, preventive and predictive.

In Asia, there is tremendous growth in medical and health awareness due to a significant increase in population's income and level of education. Augmented income boosted the healthcare sector and enabled its greater affordability, caused also significant increase in population in Asian countries which, in turn, raised the need for qualified biomedical professionals. In most countries of Asia, universities have included Biomedical Engineering, Bioengineering and Clinical Engineering as major educational studies. Only in Japan, according to a recent WHO survey, there are at least 22 universities with biomedical engineering education, and other countries in the regions also have their biomedical engineering educational institutions. Universities in the host country of this conference are well known of their successful collaboration with industries and on their innovative approach in engineering.

Everywhere in the world, employment of biomedical engineers has shown grow much higher than average for all engineering. The Bureau of Labor in the USA presented the ten-year forecasting of growth in engineering occupations through 2018, where biomedical engineers held the highest position in ranking with 72% of growth, and these numbers showed to be exactly the truth for 2012 and 2013. These forecast showed also a significant increase in jobs offering services to aging population and appropriate demand for medical devices and equipment designed for elderly by biomedical engineers. Along with the need for sophisticated medical equipment, concern for cost efficiency and effectiveness is present which again demands biomedical engineering knowledge and optimization.

GCBME 2014, the 1st Global Conference on Biomedical Engineering and APCMBE 2014, the 9th Asian-Pacific Conference on Medical and Biological Engineering, held at the National Cheng Kung University in Tainan from October 9 to 12, 2014, have a unique opportunity to gather the best biomedical engineering scientists from the Asia-Pacific region and, based on the experience of the Asia-Pacific Working Group of the International Federation for Medical and Biological Engineering (IFMBE), to offer a platform for a sustainable collaboration among scientists and Biomedical Engineering Societies in the forthcoming decades to be marked by biomedical engineering growing importance.

On behalf of the IFMBE and personally, I wish all participants of the Conference a successful meeting and a pleasant stay in Tainan.

Ratko Magjarević
President, IFMBE

Preface

The Global Conference on Biomedical Engineering 2014 (GCBME 2014) in conjunction with the 9th Asian-Pacific Conference on Medical and Biological Engineering (APCMBE 2014) is held on October 9–12, 2014 at National Cheng Kung University, Tainan, Taiwan. APCMBE 2014 is a triennial Asia Pacific Conference of the International Federation for Medical and Biological Engineering (IFMBE).

The general theme of GCBME 2014-APCMBE 2014 is "Biomedical Engineering Innovation-Transforming the Future". The conference program consists of opening, plenary, keynote, and invited lectures, symposia, workshops, invited sessions, oral and poster sessions, and exhibitions. Submissions to the GCBME 2014-APCMBE 2014 were numerous and resulted in about 500 poster and podium presentations. Only full-length papers are collected in the Conference Proceedings published in IFMBE Proceedings Series.

Frost & Sullivan predicts total Asia Pacific healthcare spending is expected to grow from USD1.34tn to USD2.2tn in 2018 at a CAGR 10.5% healthcare expenditure per capita. Ageing population in APAC drives the rising demand in medical device market. Biomedical engineering plays an important role in innovation of medical devices. Therefore, the major theme of GCBME 2014-APCMBE 2014 is "Medical Device Innovation". Several symposia, workshop and invited sessions are related to this special theme. In addition, Asia Pacific Innovation Competition on Medical Device Design is for the first time included to encourage students' medical innovation, especially in low-resource settings.

GCBME 2014-APCMBE 2014 is a conference with great opportunity for an exchange of ideas and knowledge of the latest research and developments in all areas within the field of biomedical engineering. It will strongly encourage the young generations to involve in rapidly growing bioengineering. More importantly, the continuing development of medical technology innovation will fit into tomorrow's healthcare needs.

Fong-Chin Su
Shyh-Hau Wang
Min-Long Yeh

Organising Committee

Organizing Committee

Honorary President	Ratko Magjarevic
Congress President	Fong-Chin Su
Co-President	Kang-Ping Lin
Secretary-General	Shyh-Hau Wang
Scientific Program Chair	Ming-Long Yeh
General Affairs Chair	Wen-Tai Chiu
Social Program Chair	Chia-Ching Wu
Treasurer Chair	Shyh-Hau Wang
Sponsorship Chair	Han-Sheng Chuang
Venue Activity Chair	Chih-Chung Huang
Registration Chair	Jin-Jia Hu

Promotion Committee

Jaw-Lin Wang	National Taiwan University
Woei-Chyn Chu	National Yang-Ming University
Yuh-Show Tsai	Chung Yuan Christian University
Jia-Jung Wang	I-Shou University
Pau-Choo Chung	National Cheng Kung University
Mei-Jung Chen	Ming Chuan University
Chen, Hsian-Min	Hungkuang University
Chou, Kuo-Feng	Yuanpei University
Xiaohon Weng	China Association for Science and Technology
Feng-Huei Lin	National Taiwan University
Jeng-Jiann Chiu	National Health Research Institutes
Hui-Hua Chiang	National Yang-Ming University
Hsin-Cheng Chiu	National Tsing Hua University

International Advisory Committee

Ratko Magjarević	University of Zagreb, Croatia
Herbert F. Voigt	Boston University, USA
James CH Goh	National University of Singapore, Singapore
Shankhar M. Krishnan	Wentworth Institute of Technology, USA
Marc Nyssen	Vrije Universiteit Brussel, Belgium
Andrel C. Linnenbank	Academisch Medisch Centrum, Netherland
Martha Lucía Zequera Díaz	Javeriana University, Colombia

Ákos Jobbágy	Budapest University of Technology and Economics (BME), Hungary
Makoto Kikuchi	National Defense Medical College, Japan
Jos AE Spaan	University of Amsterdam, Netherlands
Sun-I, Kim	OSONG Medical Innovation Foundation, South Korea
Mário Forjaz Secca	Universidade Nova de Lisboa, Portugal
Saide Jorge Calil	Universidade Estadual de Campinas, Brazil
Nicolas Pallikarakis	University of Patras, Greece
Olof Lindahl	Umeå Universitet, Sweden
Luis Kun	National Defense University, USA
Maria Siebes	University of Amsterdam, Netherlands
K. Kirk Shung	University of Southern California, USA
Edward R. Scully	Engineers Australia, Australia
Yubo FAN	Beihang University, Beijing
Yong-Ping Zheng	The Hong Kong Polytechnic University, Hong Kong
Ichiro Sakuma	The University of Tokyo, Japan
Kyung-Sun Kang	Seoul National University, South Korea
Nahrizul Adib Bin Kadri	Universiti Malaya, Malaysia
Biziya Enkhjargal	Mongolian University of Science and Technology
Toh Siew Lok	National University of Singapore, Singapore
James O. Wear	Akamai University, USA
Arthur F.T. Mak	The Chinese University of Hong Kong, Hong Kong
Nitish V. Thakor	The Johns Hopkins University School of Medicine, Baltimore, USA
Mark Pearcy	Queensland University of Technology, Australia
Vo Van Toi	Vietnam National Universities, Ho Chi Minh City, Vietnam

Editorial Boards

Table of Contents

Biomaterials and Tissue Engineering

Biomechanics and Computational Bioengineering

Biomedical Images and Signals

Biosensors

Medical Devices and Instrumentation

Neuroengineering and Rehabilitation Engineering

Special Topics

Erratum

Silanization of Silicone Elastomer with Zwitterionic Surface Modifier for Robust Biocompatibility

Shiou-Bang Yeh[1], Chien-Sheng Chen[3], Wen-Yih Chen[1,2], Chia-Yu Liu[1], and Chun-Jen Huang[1,2,*]

[1] Graduate Institute of Biomedical Engineering, National Central University, Jhong-Li, Taoyuan 320, Taiwan
[2] Department of Chemical and Material Engineering, National Central University, Jhong-Li, Taoyuan 320, Taiwan
[3] Graduate Institute of Systems Biology and Bioinformatics, National Central University, Jhong-Li, Taoyuan 320, Taiwan

Abstract—**Biofouling generally causes adverse effects to health, such as thrombosis, infection, and pathogenic calcification. Hydrophilic and charge-balanced surface is proved to provide an energy barrier serving as a strong repulsive force against the nonspecific absorption. Unfortunately, the state-of-art technology for silicone modification cannot provide a stable and effective coating for the long-term applications under complex conditions. In this study, we aim to modify the silicone surfaces with a zwitterionic surface ligand to resist nonspecific adsorption of protein, lipid and bacteria. We synthesized a silanized surface ligand conjugated with a head residue of zwitterionic sulfobetaine (SBSi) that bears positively charged quaternary amine and negatively charged sulfonate groups. The bacterial adhesion tests and protein fouling test revealed the excellent antifouling properties of modified silicones. For the real-world application, we modified commercially available silicone hydrogel contact lenses with developed zwitterionic ligands and showed their capability of anti-bacterial adhesion and anti protein fouling. In summary, the strategy of surface engineering in this work can be applied to not only contact lenses but other silicone-based medical devices in facile and effective fashion.**

Keywords— **Biocompatibility, anti-fouling, zwitterionic materials, contact lenses.**

I. Introduction

Silicone is widely used biomaterial in medical devices and catheters due to its non-sensitizing and non-irritating properties. As the silicone material exhibits hydrophobic characteristic, the non-specific adsorption of proteins, cells or bacteria occurs frequently and generally induces serious pathogenic problems to constrain their exploitation [1, 2]. A hydrophilic surface enables to strongly interact with water molecules to form a tightly bound water layer, which provides an energy barrier against the protein absorption. Based on that, the facile and widely used method to reduce protein fouling of silicones is to make the surface hydrophilic by oxidizing the surface using oxygen plasma or UV-ozone [3], or an oxidative wet chemical method [4]. These strategies can generate hydroxyl groups directly onto the silicone surface to increase surface hydrophilicity, and hence reduce nonspecific protein fouling events. However, silicone chains reconstruct and reorganize almost surface coatings [5, 6]. Therefore, these modifications often last only a few hours or sometimes a matter of minutes. This study aims to modify the surfaces of silicone materials with zwitterionic silane build block to increase surface wetting and effectively reduce bio-fouling under a physiological condition. We synthesized 3-(Dimethyl(3-(trimethoxysilyl)-propyl)ammonio)propane-1-sulfonate (sulfobetaine silane, SBSi) which bears positive charged quaternary amine and negative charged sulfonate groups [7]. We applied SBSi onto the silicone surfaces to develop a super hydrophilic and charge-balanced antifouling biointerface (Fig. 1). The fouling resistance of the modified PDMS elastomer was verified by exposing to bacterial, protein, and lipid solutions. The results revealed its excellent capability to repel the foulant adsorption, even after 30-day storage in ambient. The cytotoxicity test for SBSi was carried out by MTT assay. In addition, the modification strategy was applied to silicone hydrogel contact lenses to verify the applicability to the commercial products.

II. Results and Discussion

A. *Surface Characterization and Long-Term Stability*

The elemental composition of the SBSi-tailored PDMS was determined using XPS. XPS signatures originating from Si, C, O, N, and S atoms within the sample were measurable. The [N]/[S] atomic ratios derived from their XPS spectral area ratio were 0.94, which means approximately

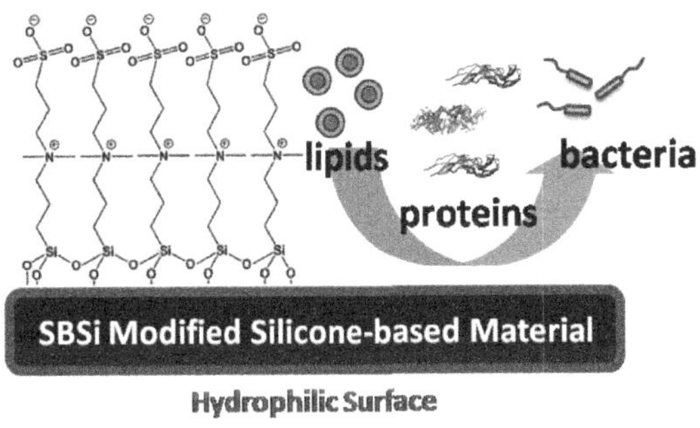

Fig. 1 Surface modification of PDMS with SBSi for antifouling properties.

I. Lackovic (ed.), *1st Global Conference on Biomedical Engineering & 9th Asian-Pacific Conference on Medical and Biological Engineering*, IFMBE Proceedings 47, DOI: 10.1007/978-3-319-12262-5_1

Table 1 Atomic percentage at listed binding energy (eV) of SBSi modified PDMS surface as determined by XPS

Atom	Si	C	O	N	S
Atomic percentage (%)	13.87	3.17	52.48	2.97	3.17

equal quantity for both elements (Table 1). As a result, the N and S spectra clearly indicate the presence of SB zwitterions on the PDMS sample. The surface energy was tested by static contact angle measurements. As shown in Fig. 2, the contact angles of the O_2-plasma treated PDMS significantly increased with time. This hydrophobic recovery was observed in previous research, attributed to the thermodynamically favorable rotation of the oxidized groups and the diffusion of low-molecular-weight chains from the bulk.[8-10] On the contrary, the SBSi-modified PDMS retained the hydrophilic property for more than 400 h. The slight increase in the contact angle should be the result of the disappearance of the unreacted oxidized groups on PDMS.

B. Resistance to Bacterial Adsorption

The fouling properties of SBSi-modified PDMS were verified by challenging with common biomaterial-associated pathogens, *P. aeruginosa* and *S. epidermidis,* and observed the adherent bacteria under a fluorescent microscope (Fig. 3). In order to compare the effectiveness of the SBSi adlayer, PDMS was partially modified with SBSi and incubated in bacterial solutions under a physiological condition. As shown in Fig. 3a and b, the SBSi-modified areas obviously have lower bacterial densities than bare ones. Moreover, Gram-positive *S. epidermidis* exhibited weaker adsorption capability than Gram-negative *P. aeruginosa.* We further quantified the adhered bacteria by using software ImageJ and determined the long-term fouling resistance of modified substrates. Fig. 3c indicates that O_2-plasma treated PDMS enables reducing adsorption of *S. epidermidis*, but exhibits a limited capability to *P. aeruginosa.* However, after 30-day

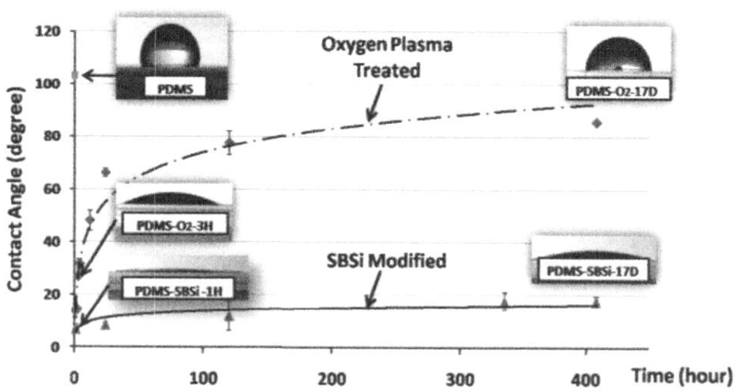

Fig. 2. Contact angle changes with time for SBSi-modified and O2-plasma treated PDMS samples.

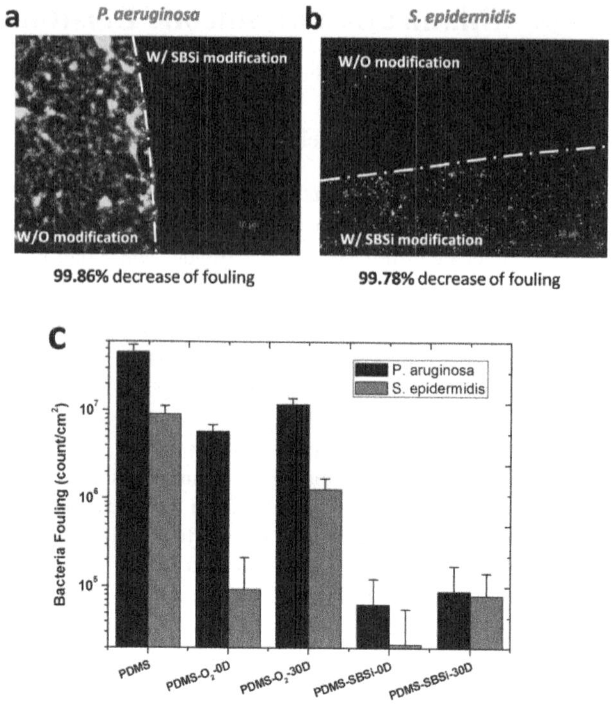

Fig. 3 P. aeruginosa (a) and S. epidermidis (b) adsorption on partially modified PDMS. The quantitative results of bacterial adsorption on PDMS samples with various treatments and aging time (c).

storage, the oxidized PDMS had reduced fouling resistance to both bacteria, which should be due to the hydrophobic recovery. [8-10] For the SBSi-modified PDMS, the reduction rate for *P. aeruginosa* and *S. epidermidis* were 99.86 % and 99.78 %, respectively, by using freshly prepared samples (PDMS-SBSi-0D). For the aged sample (PDMS-SBSi-30D), its capability to resist *P. aeruginosa* adsorption was comparable with the freshly prepared one, while slightly loss of resistance to *S. epidermidis.* Nevertheless, the overall fouling reduction rates of SBSi-modified PDMS reached over 90 % relative to bare samples.

The feasibility of SBSi for modification of commercial products was demonstrated with silicone hydrogel contact lenses (Fig. 4). Contact lenses become daily consumable of silicone-based medical device, on which the accumulation of bacteria and proteins from tear can cause protein denaturation, bacterial infection and conjunctivitis.[11] In this work, the surfaces of the contact lenses were tailored with SBSi as the procedure for PDMS modification described above. The contact lenses were brought to contact with the *P. aeruginosa* solution. As one can see, the number of adherent bacteria on SBSi-modified contact lens is much less than on unmodified one. This result reveals the potential of SBSi for industrial implementation.

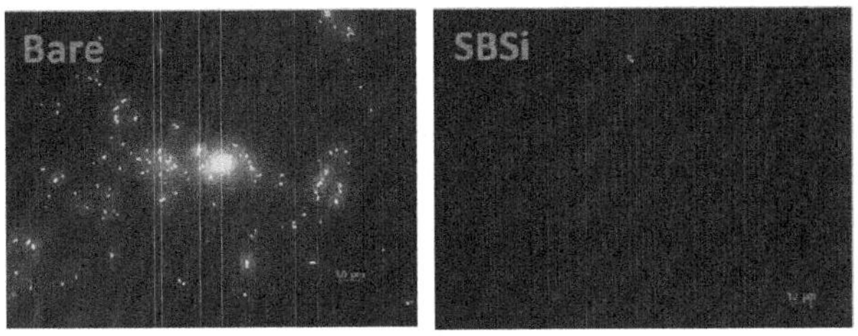

Fig. 4 SBSi modification for silicone hydrogel contact lenses.

C. Resistance to Protein and Lipid Fouling

BSA, mucin, lysozyme and lipids were used for investigating the antifouling properties of SBSi-PDMS by ELISA and fluorescence scanner. In the Fig. 5, the fouling levels on bare, oxidized and SBSi-modified PDMS samples were present. BSA is a standard protein that has been widely investigated in the field of biomaterials and has also been reported to adsorb on hydrophobic surfaces [12]. Many of reports have used BSA as a target to examine nonfouling property [13, 14]. Moreover, albumin is the most abundant protein in blood circulation, and easily to fouling on any medical devices which once contacted to blood to cause further biological interaction. Reduction of the albumin fouling level highlighted the potential of SBSi modified PDMS application in short/long-term blood contacting implants. The reduction rates of SBSi-modified PDMS were 98 % for BSA relative to unmodified sample (Fig. 5a). Fig. 5c and d show PDMS-SBSi resist 97 % and 49 % of mucin and lysozyme fouling level, respectively, relative to unmodified sample. Clearly, resistance of SBSi to biomolecules was shown, reflecting the function of superhydrophilic and

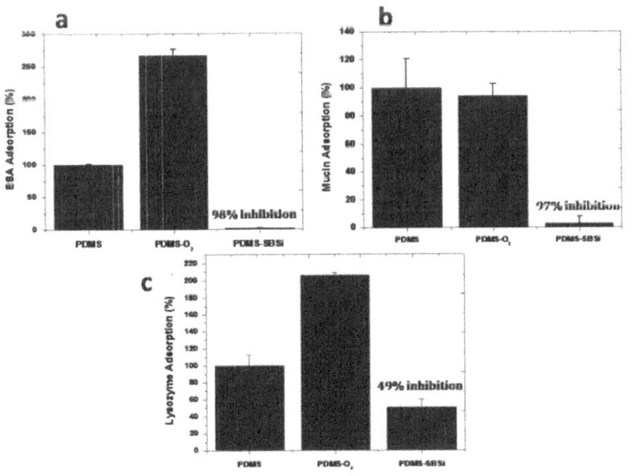

Fig. 5 ELISA measurements for (a) BSA, (b) mucin and (c) lysozyme on PDMS samples.

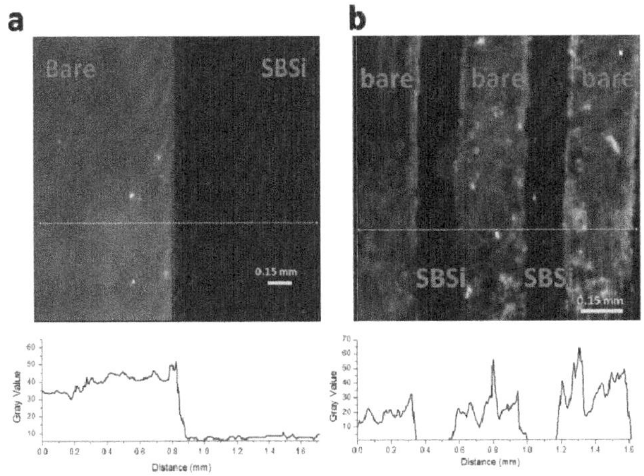

Fig. 6 Adsorption of SRB-encapsulated liposomes on SBSi-patterned PDMS.

charge-balanced properties of SB moieties. Interestingly, the fouling levels on O_2-plasma treated PDMS were higher than unmodified ones. This observation can be explained by increased surface roughness after irradiation, offering larger areas for adsorption [15]. The hydrophobic silicone elastomer is lipophilic, facilitating absorption of lipids and other nonpolar agents. Early study indicated that the silicone-containing heart valves failed in vivo due to significant dimensional swelling by absorption of lipids from blood.[16] Therefore, the adsorption of lipid on substrates was investigated by observing the fluorescence signals from SRB-encapsulated liposome (Fig. 6). The patterned surfaces were prepared by elastomeric stencils and microchannels as removable masks for the selective modification with SBSi as the methods present in previous publication.[17] The unprotected areas were oxidized by O_2-plasma irradiation, followed by contacting with the SBSi solution. After adsorption of SRB-encapsulated liposomes, the fluorescence images and the intensity profiles were recorded using fluorescence microscope. The clear edges in profiles between bare and SBSi modified surfaces indicate that the liposomes namely adsorbed on the unmodified areas for the samples patterned by both methods.

D. Cytotoxicity of SBSi

The concern of the cytotoxicity of SBSi may be arisen before introduction it to the in vivo test. SBSi and its precursors, 1,3-propanesultone and DMASi, were dissolved in the culture medium at concentrations ranging from 0.1 to 20 mM. After 16-h incubation, the viability of cells was determined by MTT assay. As shown in Fig. 7, the cytotoxicity of 1,3-propanesultone is very high, which is classified as a toxic and carcinogenic agent. On the contrary, the SBSi and

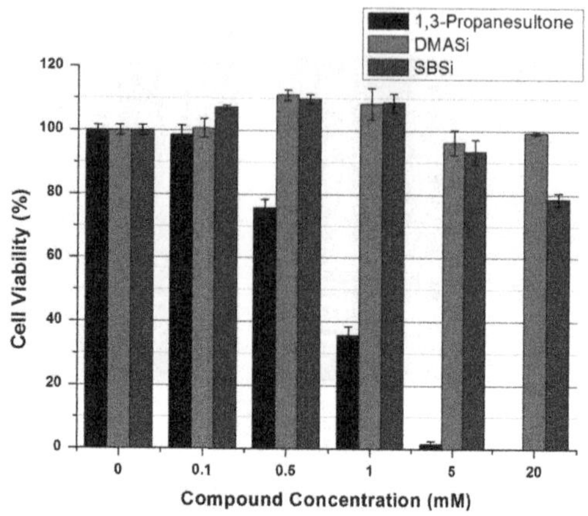

Fig. 7 MTT assay for the viability of cells after the incubation with compounds of SBSi, DMASi, 1,3-propanesultone.

DMASi have almost no cytotoxicity at a concentration below 5 mM. At a concentration of 25 mM, SBSi exhibits low cytotoxicity. However, as a thin layer coating, the concentration of SBSi in solution should be extremely low even if the leaching occurred. Consequently, the SBSi can be regarded as a very low cytotoxic and biocompatible material for potential uses in vivo.

III. CONCLUSION

In this study, a surface coating strategy for modification of silicones based on zwitterionic sulfobetain silane (SBSi) for robust biocompatibility was proposed. The coating was characterized using x-ray photoelectron spectroscopy and contact angle goniometer. The long-term stability of SBSi-modified PDMS was demonstrated by high surface wetting and excellent capability to resist bacterial adsorption, which should be results of suppressing the rotation of PDMS backbones and transport of low-molar-mass molecules by network crosslinking and superhydrophilicity of SBSi adlayers. Biomolecules, including bovine serum albumin, mucin, lysozyme and lipid, were effective repelled from the silicone by the SBSi coatings, rendering improved biocompatibility of silicone materials. The experiment for the cytotoxicity indicated that SBSi has very low cytotoxicity. Moreover, the applicability of SBSi for modification of commercial products was demonstrated by applying it on silicone hydrogel contact lenses. The improvement in the biocompatibility and stability of silicone-based medical devices with SBSi modification enables a wide range of applications, particularly implants for in vivo uses.

ACKNOWLEDGMENT

The authors thanks for the financial support from the National Science Council (NSC 101-2118-E-008-009; 102-2221-E-008-011).

REFERENCES

1. Belanger, M.C. and Y. Marois, J Biomed Mater Res, 2001. 58(5): p. 467-77.
2. Wong, I. and C.M. Ho, Microfluid Nanofluidics, 2009. 7(3): p. 291-306.
3. Olah, A., H. Hillborg, and G.J. Vancso, Applied Surface Science, 2005. 239(3-4): p. 410-423.
4. Bodas, D. and C. Khan-Malek, Microelectronic Engineering, 2006. 83(4-9): p. 1277-1279.
5. Delamarche, E., et al., Langmuir, 2003. 19(21): p. 8749-8758.
6. Hellmich, W., et al., Langmuir, 2005. 21(16): p. 7551-7557.
7. Litt, M. and T. Matsuda, Journal of Applied Polymer Science, 1975. 19(5): p. 1221-1225.
8. Chen, I.J. and E. Lindner, Langmuir, 2007. 23(6): p. 3118-3122.
9. Morra, M., et al., Journal of Colloid and Interface Science, 1990. 137(1): p. 11-24.
10. Hillborg, H. and U.W. Gedde, Polymer, 1998. 39(10): p. 1991-1998.
11. Rebeix, V., et al., Biomaterials, 2000. 21(12): p. 1197-1205.
12. Yu, Y., P.Q. Ying, and G. Jin, Chinese Chemical Letters, 2004. 15(12): p. 1465-1468.
13. Venault, A., et al., Journal of Membrane Science, 2012. 423: p. 53-64.
14. Lin, P., et al., Langmuir, 2014.
15. Owen, M.J. and P.J. Smith, Journal of Adhesion Science and Technology, 1994. 8(10): p. 1063-1075.
16. McHenry, M.M., et al., J. Thorac. Cardiovasc. Surg., 1970. 59(3): p. 413.
17. Tourovskaia, A., et al., Langmuir, 2003. 19(11): p. 4754-4764.

Author: Chun-Jen Huang , PhD
Institute: Graduate Institute of Biomedical Engineering, National Central University
Street: No.300, Jhongda Rd.
City: Jhongli City
Country: Taoyuan County 32001, Taiwan
Email: cjhuang@ncu.edu.tw

Development and Characterization of Magnetic Bioceramic Nanocrystals for Intracellular Hyperthermia

H.C. Wu[1], J.Y. Lin[1], S.Y Hsieh[2], T.W. Wang[2], and J.S. Sun[3]

[1] Department of Materials Engineering, Tatung University, Taipei, Taiwan
[2] Department of Materials Sciences and Engineering, National Tsing Hua University, Hsinchu, Taiwan
[3] National Taiwan University Hospital Hsin-Chu Branch, Department of Orthopedic Surgery, Hsinchu, Taiwan

Abstract— **Hyperthermia for the treatment of resistant tumors has been reported with promising results. Repeated treatment times and applicable for many kinds of cancers are the potential benefits of hyperthermia. Of note is that the success of intracellular hyperthermia is largely dependent on the development of an adequate heat mediator. In this work, we have successfully developed an intracellular hyperthermia system using magnetic hydroxyapatite (mHap) nanocrystals as a thermoseed. After surface modification, poly (ethylene glycol) (PEG) and hyaluronic acid (HA) modified mHap nanocrystals could not only be localized and accumulated in cancer cells, but also efficiently taken up by targeted tumor cells via HA receptor mediated endocytosis process. Furthermore, these Hap-based magnetic nanocrystals may also serve as a tracer for the diagnostic contrast agent under MRI and a drug delivery carrier for therapeutic applications in cancer therapy in vitro and in vivo.**

Keywords— **Magnetic nanocrystals, hyperthermia, surface modification.**

I. INTRODUCTION

Nowadays, superparamagnetic nanoparticles (SPNPs) can be attracted to and maintained at a precise location by an external magnet, have been of recent interest for numerous biomedical applications including cell sorting/ separation, drug targeting/ labeling, drug delivery, contrast agent for magnetic resonance imaging (MRI), heat mediator for hyperthermia, tissue repair for tissue engineering (TE), etc[2]. One of the most common SPNPs types is lunar halo-like structure. The central core contains magnetic substrate such as iron oxide nanoparticles (NPs), which is enveloped by outside shell polymeric materials for improving targeting and non-toxicity purposes[1].

Hydroxyapatite (Hap) not only has similar composition to the main mineral components in human bone tissue, but also a well-known biocompatible biomaterial for extensive bioengineering applications. It is a potential good candidate of ceramic-based, non-toxic material to provide magnetic property if doping with magnetic-elements for serving as a useful tool for diagnostic or therapeutic agents[4].

In this study, magnetic Hap with covalently conjugated PEG and HA is developed and characterized. We expect that this biocompatible, magnetic bioceramic-based nanocrystal can be internalized into tumor cells through ligand mediated endocytosis for the purpose of intracellular hyperthermia and anti-cancer therapeutic properties.

II. EXPERIMENT

The mHAP nanocrystals were prepared using controlled co-precipitation process as reported previously[3]. For preparation of HA-modified mHap crystals, the N-ethyl-N'-(3-dimethylaminopropyl) carbodiimide hydrochloride (EDC) and N-hydroxysuccinimide (NHS) were added into hyaluronic acid (HA) in 0.1M MES buffer. PEG-modified mHap crystals were added into the previous mixture, treated with ultrasound for 10 min and stirred for 24 hours. After the reaction, the composites were collected through magnetic separation and were washed by deionized water for several times. The products were dried and preserved at vacuum conditions. The physicochemical properties of nanocrystals were analyzed using transmission electron microscope (TEM), Fourier transform infrared spectroscopy (FTIR), vibrating sample magnetometer (VSM) and inductively coupled plasma mass spectrometry (ICP-MS). The heating experiments in AC magnetic field were performed by frequency induction heating apparatus at room temperature under aqueous culture medium solution. Cell viability was determined through lactic dehydrogenase assay (LDH).

III. RESULTS

From the TEM images (Fig. 1), the size and morphology of the individual mHap nanocrystal was rod-like shape around 100 nm in length and 25 nm in width. The small sphere particles (less than 10 nm) of magnetite were adhered surrounding the surface of spindle Hap nanocrystal. According to the XRD spectrum, the developed mHap was suggested to maintain intact Hap lattice. Therefore, iron oxide NPs were getting heterogeneous nucleation growth and accommodated in the interstitial spaces.

I. Lackovic (ed.), *1st Global Conference on Biomedical Engineering & 9th Asian-Pacific Conference on Medical and Biological Engineering*, IFMBE Proceedings 47, DOI: 10.1007/978-3-319-12262-5_2

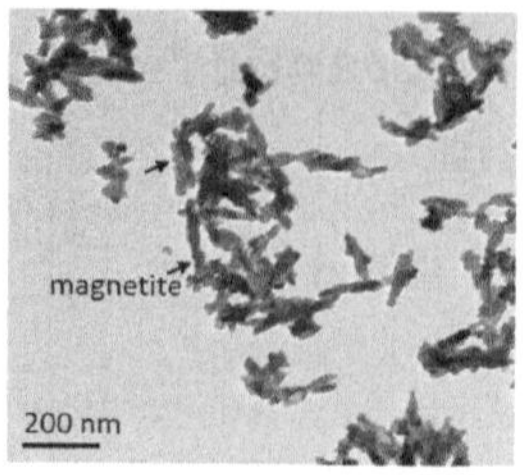

Fig. 1 TEM images of mHap-HA.

The magnetization curves were used to illustrate the magnetism of mHap (Table. 1). No noticeable coercivity or remanence was observed in the magnetic hysteresis loop for all of the three samples. This experimental evidence showed that the mHap nanocrystals possessed superparamagnetic property.

Table 1 The summary of saturation magnetization of nanocrystals

Samples	Ms (emu/g)
mHap	33.4
mHap-HA	28.3

The heat generating ability of synthesized magnetic nanocrystals in water was measured and recorded for different samples at 0.5 mg/mL concentrations (Table. 2). The results showed the increase of the delta-delta T was accompanied with the increase of treatment time and crystal concentration. These results suggest mHap could be utilized as heat mediator for hyperthermia.

Table 2 The heat generation ability of nanocrystals

Samples (5 min)	$\Delta\Delta$T
mHap	7.7
mHap-HA	5.4

The LDH assay was used to evaluate the cytotoxicity of modified mHap (Fig. 2). Compared to the control spontaneous release group, there was no noticeable cytotoxic effect of nanocrystals under the tested concentrations from 0.01 to 0.5 mg/mL. It is indicated that the mHap nanocrystals did not have significant influence on cell viability.

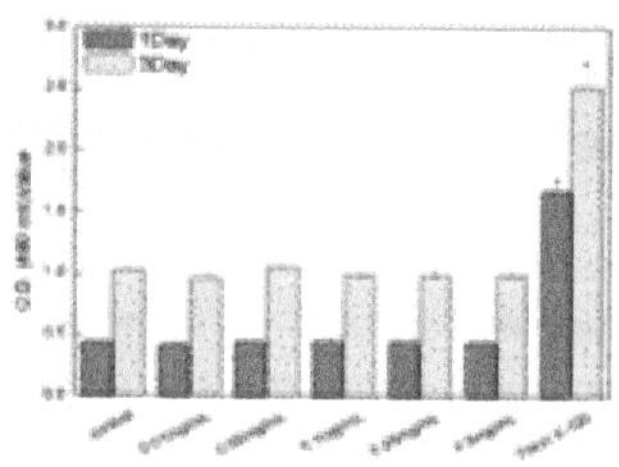

Fig. 2 Optical density readings for the LDH assay after coclulture with 3T3 cells for 1 and 3 day with mHap-HA. (one-way ANOVA, mean ± SD, n = 5, *p < 0.05: significantly different)..

The cell uptake of transfection nanocomplex was also observed by TEM (Fig. 3). The results showed internalized mHap nanoparticles and these nanoparticles were enclosed in intracellular vacuole. Some of the particles outside of the cells were attached to the cell membrane and the characteristic concave shape could be identified. The vehicles containing numerous NPs located in close to the nucleus could be seen at 24 and 48 hours post-transfection. This study revealed that agglomerated nanoparticles were internalized by cells through endocytosis.

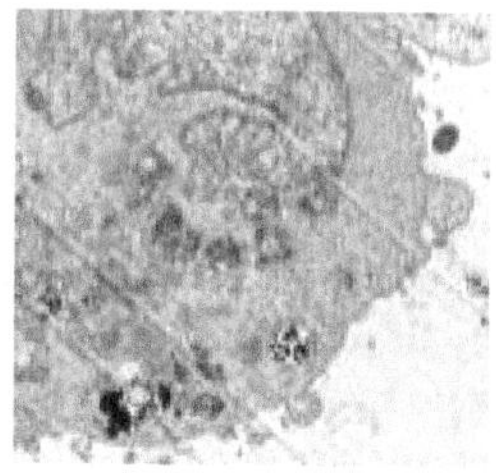

Fig. 3 TEM images of MDA-MB-231 cells co-cultured and treated with mHap-HA for 4 hours

IV. CONCLUSIONS

The spacer arms of PEG and targeting moieties of HA were successfully immobilized onto the surface of mHap. The HA modified mHap nanocrystals mediated low cytotoxicity and could generate heat as heat mediator for hyperthermia. The modified mHap nanocrystals can be specifically recognized and targeted to HA receptor overexpression breast cancer cells. In conclusion, the developed PEG- and HA- modified mHap nanocrystals could not only be localized and targeted to cancer cells, but also generated heat by applied external magnetic field for hyperthermia therapeutic applications in cancer therapy.

ACKNOWLEDGMENT

The authors thank F.-H. Lin, National Taiwan University for discussion on the subject of cancerous cell biology, and also acknowledge the financial support of the National Science Council, Taiwan (NSC-102-2221-E-036-002-MY3), National Taiwan University Hospital Hsin-Chu Branch (HCH103-019) and Tatung University (B103-T02-018).

CONFLICT OF INTEREST

The authors declare that they have no conflict of interest.

REFERENCES

1. Gao J, Gu H, Xu B (2009) Multifunctional magnetic nanoparticles: design, synthesis, and biomedical applications Acc Chem Res 42: 1097-107
2. Mornet S, Vasseur S, Grasset F et al. (2004) Magnetic nanoparticle design for medical diagnosis and therapy Journal of Materials Chemistry 14: 2161-75
3. Wu H C, Wang T W, Bohn M C et al. (2010) Novel Magnetic Hydroxyapatite Nanoparticles as Non-Viral Vectors for the Glial Cell Line-Derived Neurotrophic Factor Gene Advanced Functional Materials 20: 67-77
4. Wu H C, Wang T W, Sun J S, et al. (2007) A novel biomagnetic nanoparticle based on hydroxyapatite Nanotechnology 18: 165601

The Research of Ascorbic Acid-Loaded Gelatin Nanoparticles and Cell Uptake Studies with NCTC Clone 929 Cell Line

Meng Hsuan Lin, Yi Ling Hsieh, Hsian Chih Chen, Wei Chen Liao, Yu Ting Lo, Yi Jhih Chiou, Yun ju Chuang, and Pei Ru Chen*

Department of Biomedical Engineering, Ming Chuan University, Taoyuan, Taiwan

Abstract— **One of the reason caused the production of scar is the excessive sediment or the overtime precipitation during the wounds healing. So far amount all the medical supplies, hydrocolloid dressings which used to repair the burn wounds and the normal trauma are bass on promotion of wound healing. Nevertheless there are no medical supplies combine hydrocolloid dressings with anti-pigmentation drugs; therefor our research has focused on preparing gelatin nanoparticle. First, prepared different size of particles by controlling the parameters. Second, loaded various concentrations of ascorbic acid into particles, analyzed the drug entrapment efficiency and the rate of drug release. Last, co-culture nanoparticle with fibroblast, research the effect of nanoparticle on the fibroblast, in order to prepare a successful anti pigmentation gelatin nanoparticle. Under distinct condition, particle size 150nm ~ 300nm of gelatin nanoparticle could be prepared, furthermore the effective concentration of ascorbic acid 0.3%~10% is successfully completed and the drug-loaded nanoparticles are able to extend the life-span of the fibroblast.**

Keywords— **Gelatin, Nanoparticle, Ascorbic acid.**

I. INTRODUCTION

Skins cover all over the body, it not only protect body from invasion of harmful substance and physical, chemical injure, but also prevent the loss of the water, electrolyte and any other benefic matter.

When the skins got injured and produce the wounds, the repair could classify into three steps, first, inflammation, the white blood cell gather and devour the slough, then secreted the heal-promote excretions, in this step, wounds turn red and tumescent maintain three or more days, granulation tissue grow subsequently, the white blood cell function more effective, last, the wounds become scarred, collagenous fiber regularly arrange and the complete healing required for a long time.

Ascorbic acid is an efficient antioxidant in the organism which Reduced ascorbic peroxidase substrate oxidation capacity.

The research's purpose is producing a hydro-colloid dressings combine anti- pigmentation drugs in order to exert the whitening effect successfully.

* Corresponding author.

II. MATERIALS AND METHODS

A. *Materials*

Gelatin type A from porcine skin (Bloom 175) was used as the carrier polymer; glutaraldehyde solution (25 %), trypsin and ascorbic acid (99.7 %) were all purchased from Sigma-Aldrich. Acetone analytical grade (99.5 %) were products of Shimakyu. Milli-Q water (conductivity 18.2 mΩ) was obtained with Milli-Q system.

B. *Preparation of Gelatin Nanoparticles*

a) Method A

Gelatin nanoparticles were formulated according to the double desolvation approach by Coester et al. in 2000[1] with modifications. The following primary preparation procedure: dissolve 1.25g of type-A gelatin into 25 mL milli-q water under 50°C. The first desolvation step is commence by the addition of 25 mL acetone. After sedimentation for a certain time, the supernatant which consist of some desolvated gelatin as well as gelatin in solution has to be removed. Then the sediment is once more dissolving by adding 25 mL Milli-Q water under 50°C, gelatin nanoparticles are formed during the second desolvation step by adding 50 mL acetone slowly under stirring. After period of time, glutaraldehyde grade II (25%) are added to the solution to crosslink the nanoparticles. Last, remove the acetone by using vacuum air pump for 24 hours.

b) Method B

Gelatin nanoparticles were formulated according to the double desolvation approach by Manoj Maha et al. in 2008[2] with modifications. The following primary preparation procedure: dissolve 200mg of type-A gelatin into 10 mL milli-q water under 40°C. The first desolvation step is commence by the addition of 10 mL acetone. After sedimentation for a certain time, the supernatant which consist of some desolvated gelatin as well as gelatin in solution has to be removed. Then the sediment is once more dissolving by adding 10 mL Milli-Q water under 50°C, gelatin nanoparticles are formed during the second desolvation step by adding 30 mL acetone slowly under stirring. After period

I. Lackovic (ed.), *1st Global Conference on Biomedical Engineering & 9th Asian-Pacific Conference on Medical and Biological Engineering*,
IFMBE Proceedings 47, DOI: 10.1007/978-3-319-12262-5_3

of time, glutaraldehyde grade II (25%) are added to the solution to crosslink the nanoparticles. Last, remove the acetone by using vacuum air pump for 24 hours.

C. *Formulation of Ascorbic Acid-Loaded Gelatin Nanoparticles*

The required volume of stock drug solution was added after the first step of desolvation. Then the second desolvation was then executed by adding drop wise acetone. Next, glutaraldehyde grade II (25%) are added to the solution to crosslink the nanoparticles and stirring for 12 hours. Last, remove the acetone by using vacuum air pump for 24 hours.

D. *Evaluation of Ascorbic Acid Loading into Gelatin Nanoparticles*

Base on the research by Kenneth Ofokansi et al in 2010. [3] The ascorbic acid-loaded nanoparticles was centrifuged at 16,000g for 20 min and the ultraviolet light intensity of the supernatant measured to obtain the amount of ascorbic acid bound to the surface of the particles. The sediment was finally dispersed in 5 ml of trypsin solution (0.4 mg/ml) and stirring until a clear solution was obtained which indicated a complete digestion of the gelatin nanoparticles and release of all ascorbic acid entrapped in the core of the particles. The loading capacity of ascorbic acid was calculated from the obtained values.

E. *Cell Culture*

NCTC clone 929 cell line (Fibroblast) was used for the cell uptake studies. The fibroblast was thaw from the liquid nitrogen.

a) Culture

Place culture vessels in a laminar flow hood along with the culture medium components which have been pre-warmed to 37°C. Aspirate medium and wash cells twice with PBS before adding the new medium.

b) Subculture

Place culture vessels in a laminar flow hood along with the culture medium components which have been pre-warmed to 37°C. Aspirate medium and wash cells twice with PBS. Add Trypsin to disaggregate the cells. Incubate culture vessels at 37°C and monitor cell detachment under the microscope. After cells detach, add medium to stop trypsinization and to disperse the cells. Transfer cells to two sterile culture vessels.

F. *In vitro Cell Uptakes Studies*

Fibroblast were cultured in 10ml dish at 37 °C in an atmosphere of 5% CO2, 95% air and 95% relative humidity using medium supplemented with 10% fetal bovine serum and 10% ascorbic acid-loaded nanoparticle as the culture medium. The culture medium was replaced every 48 hours. The proceeding sustained for 96 hours. At definite intervals of time, observe the fibroblast under the microscope.

III. RESULTS

A. *Preparation of Gelatin Nanoparticles*

Several key formulation parameters were investigated and optimized which according to the exhaustive research by Verleg Dr. Hut et al in 2006 [4]. The adjustment of the pH was adjusted to 3.0.and the volume of glutaraldehyde grade II (25%) was also been adjusted. In this research, nanoparticles were analyzed with particle size analyzer. The studies were focus on the size of nanoparticles.

Table 1 Characteristics of the method A gelatin nanoparticles

Mean size(nm)	Polydispersity
494.7 nm	0.146
619.4 nm	0.242
785.2 nm	0.279
1093 nm	0.239
977.9 nm	0.216
1111 nm	0.105

Table 2 Characteristics of the method B gelatin nanoparticles

Mean size(nm)	Polydispersity
235.0 nm	0.210
198.9 nm	0.267
206.3 nm	0.353
314.3 nm	0.198
181.3 nm	0.164
301.3 nm	0.207

According to the results, the preparation of gelatin nanoparticles were not quite stable, the reason caused might be the temperature in the second step of desolvation and the stirring speed of the stirrer. Therefore, we will attempt to figure out the effect of the parameter and successfully prepare the gelatin nanoparticle.

B. *Formulation of Ascorbic Acid-Loaded Gelatin Nanoparticles*

The pH of the gelatin nanoparticles was adjusted to 2.1~2.6 is because of the adding of the ascorbic acid.

Table 3 Characteristics of the method A ascorbic acid-loaded gelatin nanoparticles

Mean size(nm)	Polydispersity
1093 nm	0.239

Table 4 Characteristics of the method B ascorbic acid-loaded gelatin nanoparticles

Mean size(nm)	Polydispersity
61.38 nm	0.540
80.22 nm	0.584

C. Evaluation of Ascorbic acid Loading into Gelatin Nanoparticles

According to the result of the Preparation of the gelatin nanoparticles, we select the method B of the preparation to continue the study. To analyze the entrapment efficiency of ascorbic acid-loaded nanoparticles, the standard curve should be drawn. The Absorbances of ascorbic acid were analyzed with Enzyme-Linked ImmunoSorbent Assay.

Table 4 Absorbance of ascorbic acid

Concentration of ascorbic acid	Absorbance
0.5% of ascorbic acid	0.061014
1.0% of ascorbic acid	0.062893
2.0% of ascorbic acid	0.072633
4.0% of ascorbic acid	0.089121
8.0% of ascorbic acid	0.122279

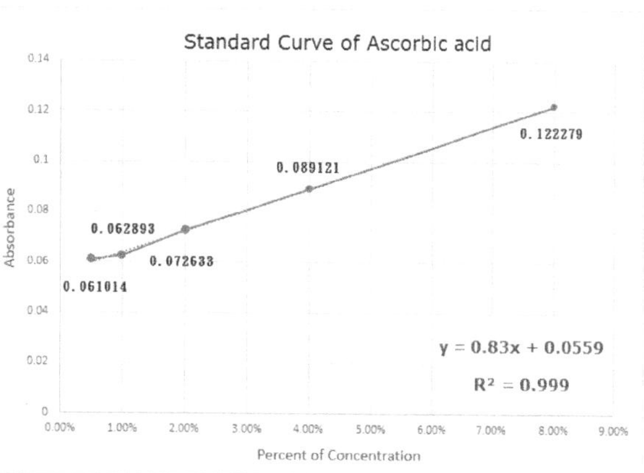

Fig. 1 Standard curve of ascorbic acid

D. Cell Culture

In order to continue the cell uptake studies, the cell culture must be preceded. The medium was changed every two days and the subculture was execute every four or five days, cause the growth rate was very.

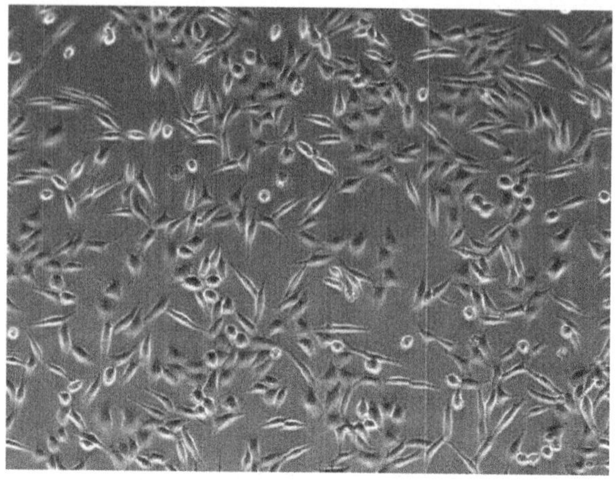

Fig. 2 Cell culture: the fourth day of fibroblast

IV. DISCUSSION

A. The results of the particles size are not stable; the following factor might be the most influencing.

a) The temperature before the first desolvation
b) The sedimentation time
c) The stirring speed
d) The temperature before the second desolvation
e) The volume of the acetone
d) The volume of the glutaraldehyde

B. Acetone deficiency bring about the increasing of the particles size.

C. Increasing the concentration of glutaraldehyde did not show any significant effect on the particle size of the nanoparticles.

D. The absorbances of ascorbic acid were the average of 100 measurements. Though the errors are existing, the coefficients of correlation are approach to 1.

V. CONCLUSIONS

For now, the gelatin nanoparticles can stably prepare by two step desolvation.

The particles size 150~300nm of gelatin could be prepared and each parameter of the preparation bring about enormous influence.

The two different method lead to various particles size. Both of the method could coutinue the research of the formulation of ascorbic acid-Loaded gelatin nanoparticles. However we choose the method B as our formulation of the experiment for cell uptake studies.

The remainder of the research shall carry on.

ACKNOWLEDGMENT

Although the research has just begin for a while, we thanks to all the member of the team for spending time studying the research and working diligently, without their help and support, our research must not carry out smoothly, and to my adviser, we are grateful for her altruistic tutoring, she always guide us enthusiastically and correctly, and last we thanks to the professor Zeng for assisting our research. Altogether, there are more people that I should be appreciate with, hereon, I have expressed the depth of my gratitude to everyone who takes part in.

CONFLICT OF INTEREST

The authors declare that they have no conflict of interest.

REFERENCES

1. Coester CJ, Langer K, Von Briesen H, Kreuter J. et al (2000) Gelatin nanoparticles by two step desolvation—a new preparation method, surface modifications and cell uptake. J Microencapsul. ;17 (2):187–93.
2. Manoj Nahar, MPharm, Dinesh Mishra, MPharm, Vaibhav Dubey, MPharm, Narendra Kumar Jain et al (2008) Development, characterization, and toxicity evaluation of amphotericin B–loaded gelatin nanoparticles. Nanomedicine: Nanotechnology, Biology, and Medicine 4 (2008) 252–261
3. Kenneth Ofokansi, Gerhard Winter, Gert Fricker, Conrad Coester et al (2010) Matrix-loaded biodegradable gelatin nano-particles as new approach to improve drug loading and delivery. European Journal of Pharmaceutics and Biopharmaceutics Vol-ume 76, Issue 1.
4. Verlag Dr. Hut, Munich et al (2006) Gelatin Nanoparticles as Delivery System for Nucleotide-Based Drugs. Published www.dr.hut-verlag.de, ISBN: 3-89963-451-9
5. Shirzad Azarmi, Yuan Huang, Hua Chen, Steve McQuarrie, Douglas Abrams, Wilson Roa, Warren H. Finlay, Gerald G. Miller, Raimar Löbenberg et al (2006) Optimization of a two-step desolvation method for preparing gelatin nanoparticles and cell uptake studies in 143B osteosarcoma cancer cells, J Pharm Pharmaceut Sci (www.cspscanada.org) 9(1):124-132.
6. Noble Kuntworbe and Raida Al-Kassas et al (2012) Design and In Vitro Haemolytic Evaluation of Cryptolepine Hydrochloride-Loaded Gelatine Nanoparticles as a Novel Approach for the Treatment of Malaria , AAPS PharmSciTech, Vol. 13, No. 2, June 2012 DOI: 10.1208/s12249-012-9775-6.

Author: Meng Hsuan Lin
Institute: Department of Biomedical Engineering, Ming Chuan University
Street: No.5, Deming Rd.
City: Taoyuan
Country: Taiwan
Email: wexs9361414@yahoo.com.tw

Effect of Contrast Medium Encapsulated in Liposome on Lesion Diagnosis and Contrast Medium Induced Nephropathy

Yu-Cheng Chang[1], Pei-Hsuan Lu[1], Gi-Da Lee[2], and Kuo-Chih Liao[1,*]

[1] Graduate Institute of Biomedical Engineering, National Chung-Hsing University

[2] Department of Radiology, Taichung Veterans General Hospital

Abstract— **Liposome is by far the most successful drug delivery vesicle commercialized for clinical use, and can fundamentally modify the performance and clearance of encapsulated drug. The encapsulation of contrast medium of computed tomography in liposome could improve the lesion screening efficiency by EPR effect of liposome, and prevent the incidence of contrast medium induced nephropathy by shielding of liposome.**

Keywords— **liposome encapsulation, computed tomography, contrast medium, lesion malignancy screening, contrast medium induced nephropathy.**

I. INTRODUCTION

Nanoparticles (NP, such as liposome, dextran, dendrimer, other polymer……) have been extensively investigated as conventional iodinated contrast medium (CM) carrier for improving in vivo circulation time and passively targeting liver and spleen lesion detection [1-4]. For general lesion malignancy prediction, the passive enhanced permeation and retention (EFR effect, enhanced permeation from leaky neovascular vessel to tumor than normal peripheral blood vessel with smaller pore, and limited development of lymphatic drainage in tumor tissue) associated with liposome in malignant tumor could improve the diagnosis outcome of dynamic computed tomography with iodinated CM encapsulated. The Encapsulation can also prevent the renal cells/tissue from direct exposure to contrast medium and the corresponding chemical or physical damages [5].

II. MATERIAL AND METHOD

A. Preparation of CM Encapsulated Liposome

Long circulation liposomes (DPPC : SoyPC : Chol : DSPE-PEG2k = 54 : 27 : 16 : 6) were fabricated by thin film hydration with iobitridol (Xenetix, Guerbert, France) and extrusion method, then purified by either size exclusive gel filtration with sephadex G-75 or dialysis if necessary. The size distribution of the resulting liposomes was measured by dynamic laser scattering. The stability of liposomes was monitored with self-quench fluorescein solution encapsulated, and was calculated by the time-dependent release percentage detected fluorescence increase (eliminating self-quench by dilution of released fluorescein) with the following equation:

$$\text{release}(\text{t}, \%) = \frac{fluorescence_t - fluorescence_{t_0}}{fluorescence_{N-OG} - fluorescence_{t_0}}$$

B. In Vitro Cell Viability and Apoptosis Study

MDCK cells were seeded on 24-well plate to reach 70% confluence, and then treated with mixture of DMEM medium and iobitrodol or saline (same osmolarity as iobitridol) or column chromatography purified iobitridol encapsulated liposome (distributed in saline with the same osmolarity as iobitridol) in the volume ratio, 1:1, for 24 hours. Cell viability was detected by MTT (3-[4,5-Dimethylthiazol-2-yl]-2,5-diphenyltetrazolium bromide) assay with spectrophotometer (Synergy Mx , BioTeK). Cell apoptosis was quantified by annexin-V-FITC/PI assay with Flow Cytometry (Cytomics TM FC500 flow cytometry, Beckman Coulter).

C. In Vivo Lesion Diagnosis and Contrast Medium Bio-distribution

NU/NU mice, implanted with both malignant (MDA-MB 231) and benign (matrigel TM) xenografts, were administrated with iobitridol, or partially encapsulated iobitridol in liposome (dried lipid film, 10mg or 20mg, was rehydrated by iobitridol) intravenously as a bolus through the tail vein at the dosage of 1mg iodine / g. Dynamic CT imaging was acquired with Philips BR64 (Andover, MA, USA).

III. RESULT AND DISCUSSION

A. Properties of CM Encapsulated Liposome

CM encapsulated liposomes were with 113 ± 17.8 nm diameters. About 55% liposomes maintained integrity in rat

* Corresponding author.

I. Lackovic (ed.), *1st Global Conference on Biomedical Engineering & 9th Asian-Pacific Conference on Medical and Biological Engineering*, IFMBE Proceedings 47, DOI: 10.1007/978-3-319-12262-5_4

plasma or cell culture medium (with 10% FBS) between 3-24 hours (180-1440 minutes) at 37°C.

B. In Vivo Lesion Screening with/without Liposome

CM/liposome increased the peak malignant implant enhancement (with partial CM, 35%, encapsulation in liposome) by 2 folds (of enhancement by CM without liposome encapsulation). However, the maximal enhancement contrast of malignancy ($SI_{malignant}/SI_{benign}$) of CM/liposome group was 471.3 at 24 hours post administration, compared to merely 2.36 at 20 minutes of CM group (Fig. 1).

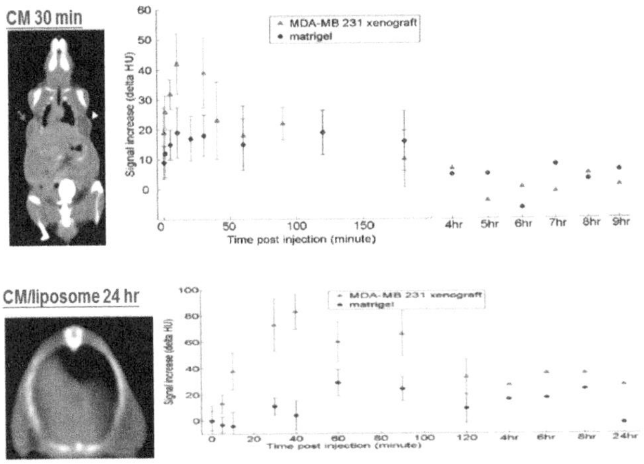

Fig. 1 Cell damage caused by CM (24 hours treatment)

C. In Vitro CIN Prevention with Liposome Encapsulation

The preliminary results indicated that CM concentrations, which were larger than 18mg/ml, caused statistically significant cell damage as shown in Fig. 2. It was also found that chemical effect of CM caused more significant damage than physical effect (under saline with similar osmolality) as shown in Fig. 3.

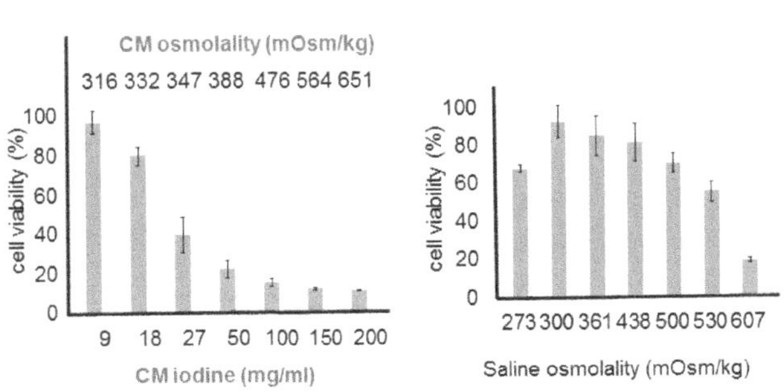

Fig. 2 Cell damage caused by CM (24 hours treatment)

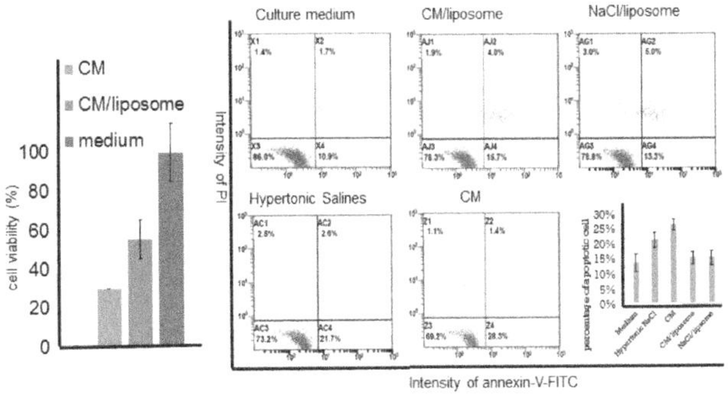

Fig. 3 Prevention CM caused damage in vitro (8 hours treatment)

D. In Vivo CM/Liposome Biodistribution

CM/liposome reduced 56-76% CM accumulation concentration in kidney between 30-300 min, and resulted in narrower harmful dosage (>18mg/ml) of CM distribution by 41-61% between 10-90 min.

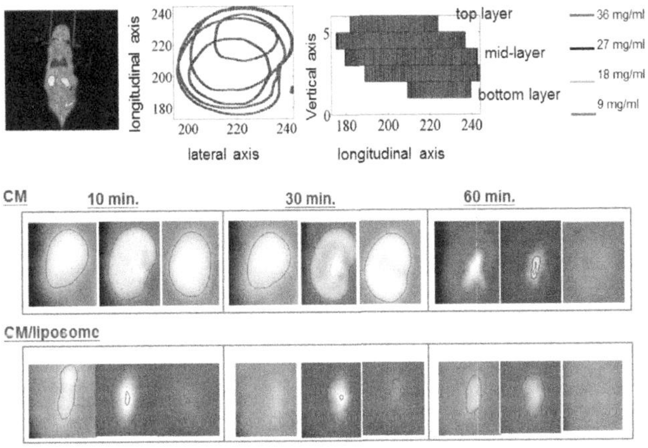

Fig. 4 Reduced accumulation of CM in kidney with liposome encapsulation

IV. Conclusions

The encapsulation of iobitridol in liposome could significantly enhance the contrast of malignant lesion and reduce CM accumulation in kidney from xenograft study. It also restored the renal cell viability and reduced cell apoptosis from cell culture studies.

Conflict of Interest

The authors declare that they have no conflict of interest.

REFERENCES

[1] W. Krause, Delivery of diagnostic agents in computed tomography, Adv Drug Deliv Rev., 37:159-173, 1999.

[2] Lee N, Choi SH, Hyeon T. Nano-sized CT contrast agents. Adv Mater. 2013 May 21;25(19):2641-60. doi: 10.1002/adma.201300081.

[3] Shilo M, Reuveni T, Motiei M, Popovtzer R. Nanoparticles as computed tomography contrast agents: current status and future perspectives. Nanomedicine (Lond). 2012 Feb;7(2):257-69. doi: 10.2217/nnm.11.190.

[4] Leander P, Höglund P, Børseth A, Kloster Y, Berg A. A new liposomal liver-specific contrast agent for CT: first human phase-I clinical trial assessing efficacy and safety. Eur Radiol. 2001;11(4):698-704.

[5] Gi-Da Lee, Jyn-Wen Chai, Jiunn-Wang Liao, Li-Che Hu, Pei-Hsuan Lu, Kuo-Chih Liao. Prevention of contrast medium induced nephropathy by liposome encapsulation. International Journal of Bioscience Biochemistry and Bioinformatics, 3, 562-565, 2013.

Single Functionalized of Different Size Nanoparticles Effect

Hsin-An Chen[1], Walter H. Chang[1,2,*], and Cheng-An J. Lin[1,2,*]

[1] Center of Biomedical Technology, Chung Yuan Christian University, Chung Li, Taiwan
[2] Department of Biomedical Engineering, Chung Yuan Christian University, Chung Li, Taiwan

Abstract— **Nanomaterials is one of the areas most highly concerned about medical technology nowadays.Such as metal nanoparticles,nanorods,and so on.**

Functionalized nanoparticles can be used as cancer probes, drug carriers to help us to investigate more research about biotechnology.

In this study,we synthesize different size metal nanoparticles and conjugate with Amine-Polyethylene glycol-Biotin (NH_2-PEG-Biotin) to functionalize it. We can control the number of NH_2-PEG-Biotin on the surface of nanoparticles successfully.

We believe the interaction of different size nanoparticles and different numbers of NH_2-PEG-Biotin can improve the area for biomedical application.

Keywords— **nanoparticles,amine-polyethylene glycol-biotin.**

I. INTRODUCTION

The importance of nanoparticles for areas ranging from contrast agents of electrons microscopy,chemical and biological sensors, drug carrier, cancer target.

Biological molecules have been immobilized on polymer matrices and inorganic supports through a variety of techniques that includes physical adsorption, electrostatic binding,specific recognition, and covalent coupling.[1]

II. METHODS

A. Gold Nanoparticles Synthesis

Materials: Gold(III) Chloride 99%,5g, ACROS, Tetrabu tylammoniumborohydrid(TBAB), 10g, Aldrich, Didodecyldimethylammonium bromide(DDAB),50g,Fluka, Decanoic acid,250g,Alfa, $HAuCl_4$,5g,ACROS,Oleylamine, 1L,ACROS,Toluene,4L,J.T.Baker.

6nm AuNPs: We added 2.5 ml Decanoic acid solution (17.2 mg Decanoic acid/1 ml toluene) as stabilizer in the via, and added 1 ml TBAB solution (25 mg TBAB / 1 ml 100mM DDAB solution in Toluene) as reduction. DDAB is used as surfactants in this synthesis, and added 0.8 ml $AuCl_3$ solution (7.5 mg Gold(III) Chloride 99% / 1ml 100mM DDAB solution) as precursor. Stirred 24 hours , and 6nm AuNPs was synthesized.[2]

15 nm AuNPs: 15 nm Au nanoparticles were obtained by quickly injecting a solution of 50 mg (0.15 mmol) of $HAuCl_4$ in 1.0 g (3.7 mmol, 1.2 ml) of oleylamine (technical quality, Acros) and 1.0 ml of toluene into a boiling solution of 1.7 g (6.4 mmol, 2.9 ml) of oleylamine in 7.5 ml of toluene. Over the course of 5-10 min, the color of the reaction mixture changes to bright yellow and then gradually to deep red. Heating was stopped after 2 hours.[3]

Phase tansfer: We addad methanol appropriately when the particle color changed from deep red to deep brown. Centrifuge 3000 r.p.m. , 5mins . Drying in vacuo yielded the product as a black solid, which could be readily redissolved in organic solvents.We added 0.8 M polymer appropriately and mixed with nanoparticles to transfer water phase. We used concentrated under reduced pressure machine to dry out organic solvent and redissolved in the water.[4]

III. RESULT

A. Gold Nanopartlces Properties

When an author or the institution of the author has a relationship, financial or otherwise, with individuals or organizations that could influence the author's work inappropriately, a conflict of interest may exist. Examples of potential conflicts of interest may include but are not limited to academic, personal, or political relationships; employment; consultancies.

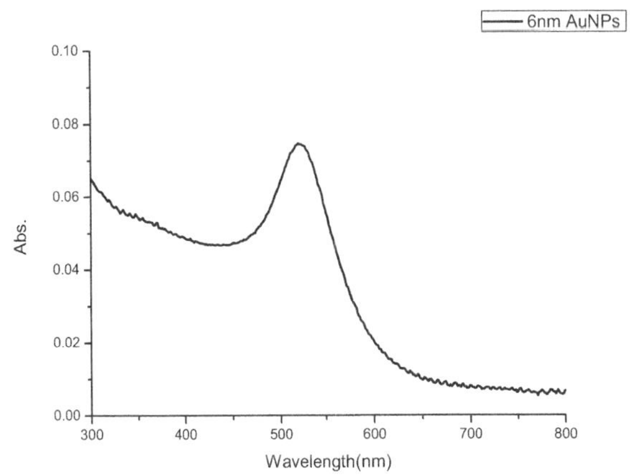

Fig. 1 Absorbtion of 6 nm gold nanoparticles

* Corresponding authors.

I. Lackovic (ed.), *1st Global Conference on Biomedical Engineering & 9th Asian-Pacific Conference on Medical and Biological Engineering*, IFMBE Proceedings 47, DOI: 10.1007/978-3-319-12262-5_5

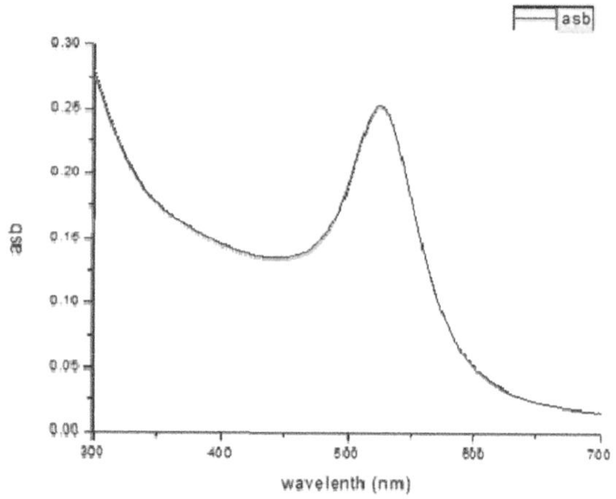

Fig. 2 Absorbtion of 15 nm gold nanoparticles

B. Gel Picture of 6nm Particles Conjugate with NH_2-PEG-Biotin

Patients have a right to privacy that should not be infringed without informed consent. Identifying information, including patients' names, initials, or hospital numbers, should not be published in written descriptions, photographs, and pedigrees unless the information is essential for scientific purposes and the patient (or parent or guardian) gives written informed consent for publication. Informed consent for this purpose requires that a patient who is identifiable be shown the manuscript to be published. Authors should identify Individuals who provide writing assistance and disclose the funding source for this assistance.

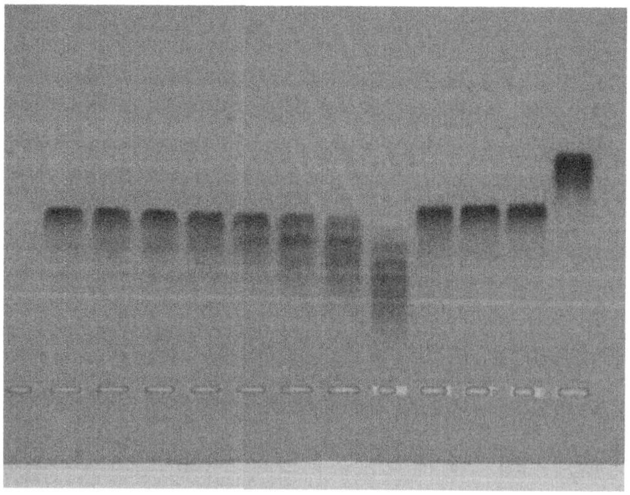

Fig. 3 15nm AuNPs conjugate with 10K-mPEG

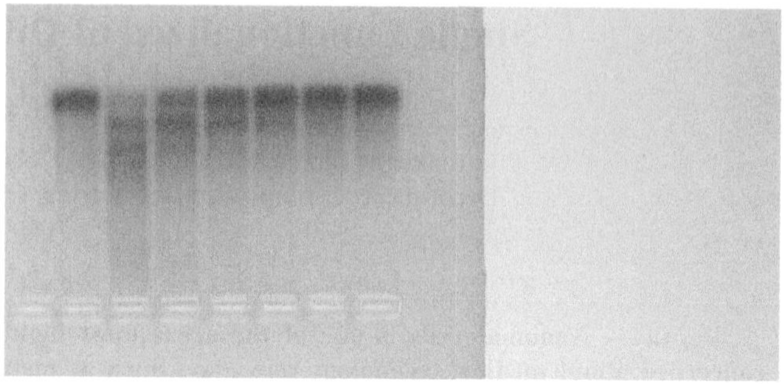

Fig. 4 6 nm AuNPs conjugate with 5K-mPEG

C. Statement of Human and Animal Rights

When reporting experiments on human subjects, authors should indicate whether the procedures followed were in accordance with the ethical standards of the responsible committee on human experimentation (institutional and national) and with the Helsinki Declaration of 1975, as revised in 2000 and 2008. If doubt exists whether the research was conducted in accordance with the Helsinki Declaration, the authors must explain the rationale for their approach, and demonstrate that the institutional review body explicitly approved the doubtful aspects of the study. When reporting experiments on animals, authors should be asked to indicate whether the institutional and national guide for the care and use of laboratory animals was followed.

IV. CONCLUSIONS

This study presents a simple, clear validation method to compare the efficiency of different sizes of nanoparticles for grafting functional groups and biomolecules.

We believe that this research will have a greater breakthrough for the field of nanotechnology and nanomedicine.

ACKNOWLEDGMENT

This research was supported by Chung Yuan Christian University and the Ministry of Science and Technology (MOST) of Taiwan under grant number: NSC 102-2622-E-033-010-CC3, 102-2221-E-033-007-MY3, 101-2628-E-033-001-MY3, 102-2627-M-033-001

CONFLICT OF INTEREST

The authors declare that they have no conflict of interest.

REFERENCES

1. Katz, E. and I. Willner, *Integrated nanoparticle-biomolecule hybrid systems: synthesis, properties, and applications.* Angew Chem Int Ed Engl, 2004. **43**(45): p. 6042-108.
2. Jana, N.R. and X. Peng, *Single-phase and gram-scale routes toward nearly monodisperse Au and other noble metal nanocrystals.* J Am Chem Soc, 2003. **125**(47): p. 14280-1.
3. Hiramatsu, H. and F.E. Osterloh, *A simple large-scale synthesis of nearly monodisperse gold and silver nanoparticles with adjustable sizes and with exchangeable surfactants.* Chemistry of Materials, 2004. **16**(13): p. 2509-2511.
4. Lin, C.A., et al., *Design of an amphiphilic polymer for nanoparticle coating and functionalization.* Small, 2008. **4**(3): p. 334-41.

Author: Chen-An J Lin
Institute: Chung Yuan Christian University
Street: 200, Chung Pei Rd.
City: Chung Li
Country: Taiwan
Email: chengan_lin@cycu.edu.tw

Dark-Field Hyperspectral System for Monitoring the Nanoparticles Interaction with the Cells

Chun-Wei Wang[1], Wei-Che Huang[1], Zih-Yun Huang[2], Yi-Ting Lin[2], Walter H. Chang[2,3*], and Cheng-An J. Lin[2,3*]

[1] Master Program in Nanotechnology, Chung Yuan Christian University, Taiwan
[2] Department of Biomedical Engineering, Chung Yuan Christian University, Taiwan
[3] Center of Biomedical Technology, Chung Yuan Christian University, Chung-Li, Taiwan
whchang@cycu.edu.tw, chengan_lin@cycu.edu.tw

Abstract— **Nanomaterials are commonly used in biomedical research, mostly in cancer diagnosis and therapy. In this study, we used dark-field hyperspectral systems to investigate nanomaterials for the biological interaction of the opsonized or pegylated nanomaterials. Gold nanoparticles have good biocompatibility and exhibit strong light scattering behavior under the dark-field microscope. Those properties make it feasible to study the interaction between the surface functionalized nanomaterials and cellular micro-environments multidimensionally.**

Keywords— **Nano Medicine, Opsonin, PEGylation, Rayleigh Scattering, Hyperspectrum, Endocytosis.**

I. INTRODUCTION

These nanomaterial are transported through the blood, in which there are many Opsonin proteins[1]. Opsonin proteins are adsorbed on the foreign objects that allows monocytes or macrophages to be identified that results to phagocytosis. On the contrary, polyethylene glycol modified nanoparticle can reduce opsonin protein adsorption, thus causes hard identification of the immune system[2]. In this study, the opsonized with pegylated interaction surface with respect to the organism was investigated. Gold nanomaterials have good biological and optical properties, and so is the choice of material. J774A.1 macrophages were cultured and the interactions with gold nanomaterials were observed under the dark field microscopy.

II. MATERIALS AND METHODS

A. Nanoparticle. Gold Nanoparticles(20/40/60/80nm, 50OD, BBISolution)

B. Conjugate PEGylation. In this study, Optional Both ends A thiol group, respectively (-SH) and methyl (-CH3) of the polyethylene glycol molecule (mPEG5000-SH) for the gold nanoparticles (AuNPs) surface modification, by the formation of a thiol group and the gold nanoparticles Gold sulfur bond (Au-S) of properties, so the formation of self-assembled PEG-modified gold nanoparticles on the surface.

C. Cell Culture .The murine macrophage J774A.1 cell line was purchased from Bioresource Collection and Research Center. The cells were cultured in Dulbecco's modified Eagle medium (DMEM) supplemented with 10% fetal bovine serum, 2 mM L-glutamine, and 50 units/mL penicillin in an incubator at 37 °C, 5% CO2, and 95% relative humidity. Cells to be imaged under dark-field microscopy were grown on glass coverslides

D. Monitoring Nanoparticle Uptake. A glass slide containing adherent macrophages was covered with AuNPs (60nm, BBISolutions) in DMEM and incubated for 30 min at 37 °C. Then the cells were washed with pre-warmed PBS buffer, and the gold colloid solution in DMEM was replaced by culture medium. Subsequently the cells were cultured for another hour in nanoparticle-free culture medium and were observed under dark field microscopy.

III. RESULT

A. General Nanoparticles Scattered light. In the dark-field microscope and issued a strongly localized scattering spectroscopy of size dependent. (Fig1) Namely 40nm 60nm 80nm, and then retrieve the scattered light of different sizes (Fig2).

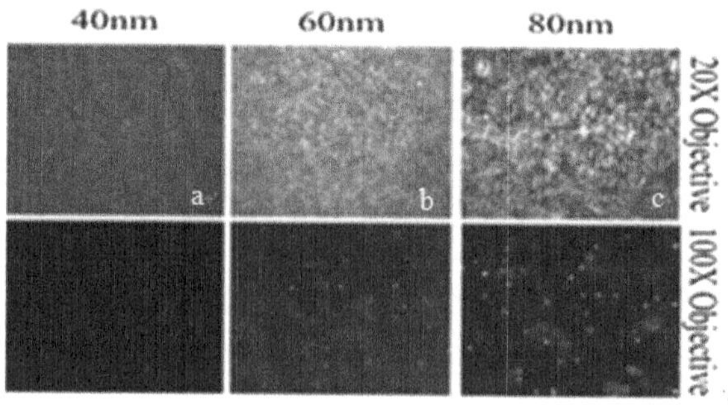

Fig. 1. Different nanoparticle size under dark-field a)40nm 、 b)60nm 、 c)80nm

* Corresponding authors.

I. Lackovic (ed.), *1st Global Conference on Biomedical Engineering & 9th Asian-Pacific Conference on Medical and Biological Engineering*, IFMBE Proceedings 47, DOI: 10.1007/978-3-319-12262-5_6

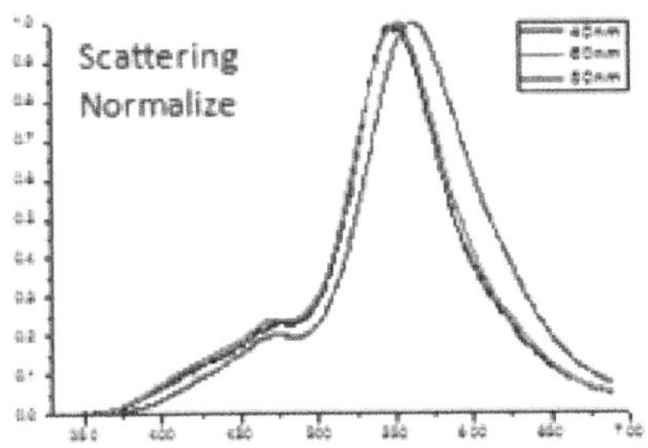

Fig. 2 Scattered light of different nanoparticle size: 40nm (black)、60nm (red)、80nm (blue).

B. Nanoparticles with Cell Interaction. Dark-field was used to observe macrophages and the case of co-culture 60nm nanoparticles (Fig3) Macrophages can be seen to exhibit translucence under dark-field, and light scattering of organisms are weaker, with gold nanoparticles show a strong contrast, With the increase of time, be involved in macrophage nanoparticles scattered light produced a change (Fig4).

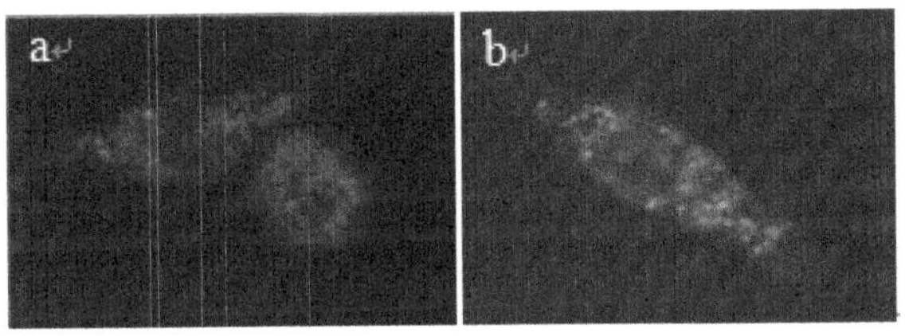

Fig. 3 Macrophages in the dark field image a) contain nanoparticles b) nanoparticles of 60nm and incubated for 1 hour

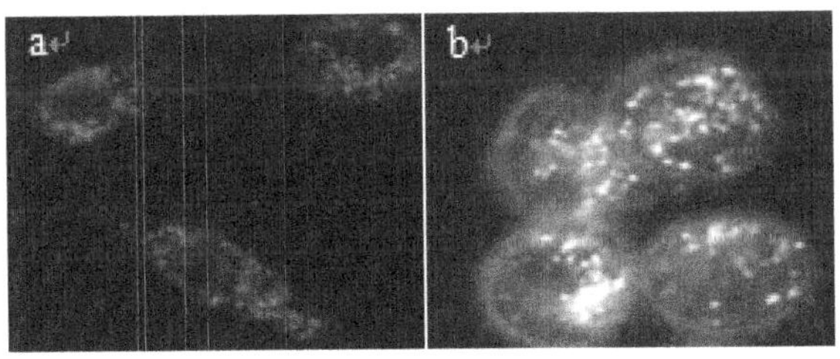

Fig. 4 Macrophages In Different Time with Nanoparticles Co-culture Image. A) 1 hour co-culture. B) 24 hours of culture

C. Different Concentration of Polyethylene glycol-modified impact. Gold nanoparticles modified by PEG are indeed an effective way to escape identification of macrophages (Fig5). Conjugation of gold nanoparticles with PEG can reach up to nine hours.

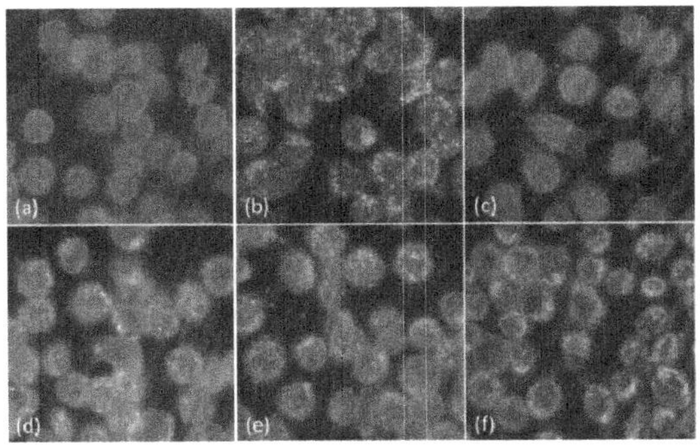

Fig. 5 Macrophages with different concentrations of PEG-modified gold nanoparticles 60nm culture darkfield image after 9 hours。(a) Without any AuNPs (b) 0μM (c) 1.2μM (d) 0.3μM (e) 0.15μM (f) 0.075μM Concentration of PEG。

D. Use Hyperspectral system. Retrieve hyperspectral Spectral change into the cells after the nanoparticles of different size with dark-field hyperspectral systems captures nanoparticles into the cell before and after Scattered light,(Fig6) Can Observed has red shift after gold nanoparticles entering the cell.

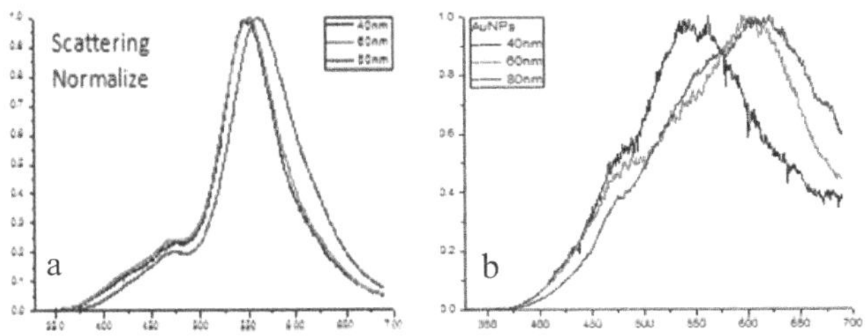

Fig. 6. Use Hyperspectral system captured different sizes nanoparticles into cells before and after the scattered light a) Before entering the cell Scattered light nanoparticles of different sizes.b) After entering the cell Scattered light nanoparticles of different sizes.

IV. CONCLUSIONS

Gold nanoparticles with good optical characteristics corresponding to the scattered light are emitted in the dark field system. We used this property to capture changes in the scattered light of nanoparticles before and after it is present in the cells by using hyperspectral imaging. The spectrum interception of the scattered light before entering the cell can be found in the partial scattered light similar to yellow-green light. However, after phagocytosis the formation of gold nanocluster results to a red shift[3]. Gold nanoparticles without PEG modification was observed to cause the macrophages to have a higher intake corresponding to the light scattering that was produced.

When the surface of gold nanoparticles are modified by PEG, which is confirmed under the dark field, it was founded that there is a complete inhibition of macrophage intake due to the good camouflage phenomena of the PEG modified gold nanoparticles. Preliminary results indicate that, when the amount of PEG was reduced, the uptake of macrophages increased. The gold nanoparticles were co-cultured with the cells and was observed to have a significant change in the scattered light. On the contrary, gold nanoparticles with PEG was observed to have less changes in the scattered light. When PEG was reduced, the light scattered was founded to have greater change. Through microfluidic observation, real-time interaction between the gold nanoparticles and macrophages can be observed up to ninety minutes. When a significant change in the focal length of the microscope was done, it was observed that some particles may be stacked on top of the cell membrane. With real-time recording, it can be observed for a very short time the macrophage uptake of the gold nanoparticles and interactions.[4]

ACKNOWLEDGMENT

This research was supported by Chung Yuan Christian University and the Ministry of Science and Technology (MOST) of Taiwan under grant number: NSC 102-2622-E-033-010-CC3, 102-2221-E-033-007-MY3, 101-2628-E-033-001-MY3, 102-2627-M-033-001.

CONFLICT OF INTEREST

The authors declare that there is no conflict of interest.

REFERENCES

1. Shruti R Saptarshi et al. (2013)Interaction of nanoparticles with proteins: relationto bio-reactivity of the nanoparticle. Journal of Nanobiotechnology 2013, 11:26
2. Abu Lila, A. S et al. (2013) Use of polyglycerol (PG), instead of polyethylene glycol (PEG), prevents induction of the accelerated blood clearance phenomenon against long-circulating liposomes upon repeated administration, International Journal of Pharmaceuticsa. vol.456,235-242
3. Hongyun Wang, Linxi Wu, (2012)Scavenger Receptor Mediated Endocytosis of Silver Nanoparticles into J774A.1 Macrophages Is Heterogeneous, Journal of ACS NANO VOL. 6 ' NO. 8 ' 7122–7132
4. Arnida et al. (2011) Geometry and surface characteristics of gold nanoparticles influence theirbiodistribution and uptake by macrophages , European Journal of Pharmaceutics and Biopharmaceutics , 77 417–423

Author: C. W. Wang
Institute: Master Program in Nanotechnology
Street: Chung Yuan Christian University
City: Taoyuan
Country: Taiwan
Email: yeye1022@yahoo.com.tw

Sulfur-Containing Natural Zwitterionic Amino Acids and Derivative on Gold: Study on Physicochemical and Anti-fouling Properties

Sz-Hau Chu[1], Chia-Yu Liu[1], Ying-Chih Chang[3], and Chun-Jen Huang[1,2,*]

[1] Graduate Institute of Biomedical Engineering, National Central University, Jhong-Li, Taoyuan 320, Taiwan
[2] Chemical & Materials Engineering Department, National Central University, Jhong-Li, Taoyuan 320, Taiwan
[3] Genomics Research Center, Academia Sinica, 128, Sec 2 Academic Road, Taipei 115, Taiwan

Abstract— **Many researchers have found that the stability of SAMs is an issue for long-term biomedical applications. The surface functional group is not stable under ambient conditions. To address this problem, we use cysteine, natural sulfur-containing zwitterionic compounds, and cysteine betaine which is the derivative of cycteine, with quaternary ammonium group at its terminal end, to decorate Au substrate by using the chemisorbing properties of the thiol group. By adding various different additives into the solution of alkanethiols during SAM formation to eliminate unbound thiol and to prevent the degradation processes of alkanethiol SAMs, we can decrease the film thickness and increase the wettability. Furthermore, we also compared their physical and chemical properties of amino acids SAMs on Au that were stored under different conditions for various lengths of time. Based on the above, our study aims to investigate the influence of different SAMs condition and chemical structure for anti-fouling properties. Contact angle analysis indicated that after degradation, the photooxidation sample decreased relative to that of the freshly prepared SAMs. X-ray photoelectron spectroscopy (XPS) not only used to detect the chemical elements of SAMs on Au substrates, but also detect the changes in the chemical state of the surface oxidized atoms. The bacterial adhesion tests revealed the excellent anti-fouling properties of zwitterionic amino acids SAMs. And adopt MTT assay to assessing cell viability.**

Keywords— **self assembled monolayers, amino acids, zwitterionic materials, stability, anti-fouling.**

I. Introduction

Surface modification in biomaterials is of tremendous importance in determining their biocompatibility and applicability. Enormous efforts were devoted to develop toolkits for engineering surfaces, with an attempt to meet desirable interfacial properties, such as roughness, wettability, free energy and chemical functionality [1-3]. In order to achieve this purpose, the spontaneously self-assembling surface ligands into an orderly packed monolayer at interfaces have attracted substantial attentions due to their unique properties, such as the ease of preparation and the potential to functionalize/pattern the nanostructure for different surface physicochemical properties [4].The most studied and best understood system among many ligands are the alkanethiol on Au(111) surfaces, which take advantage of the environmental inertness of gold substrate, the high affinity of the sulfur-gold bonding and the strong van der Waals forces between long carbon chains [4-5].

However, numerous researchers have investigated the stability of functional groups on Au substrate. Particularly, desorption of thiol groups to sulfonate groups has been reported [6-7]. In addition, Shyue et al. revealed that the amino groups were oxidized to nitroso groups [8], indicating that amine-modified Au surfaces are not stable in ambient environments.

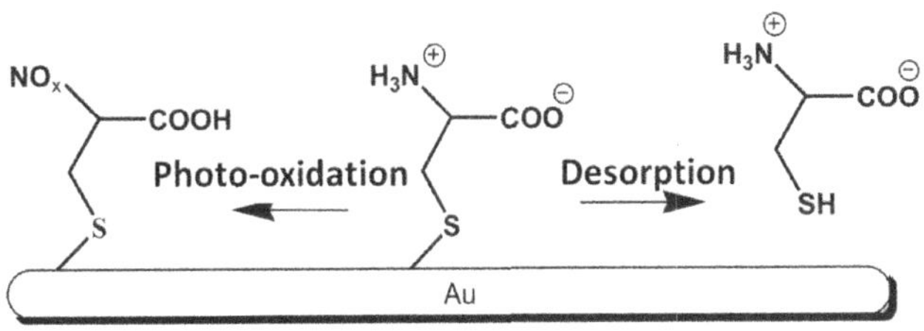

Fig. 1 Schematic diagram of photo-oxidation of amine-terminated SAMs & degradation of alkanethiol on Au surfaces.

Amino acids should have good biocompatibility and hemocompatibility because they are the basic components of protein which is required by human nutrition. As a natural zwitterion, cysteine has a carboxyl (-COOH), an amino (-NH_2), and a thiol functional group. The presence of one sulfur atom in cysteine makes it possible to modify Au substrate by covalent bond. On the other hand, we can also prevent the oxidation of amino groups via replacing it by quaternary ammonium group.

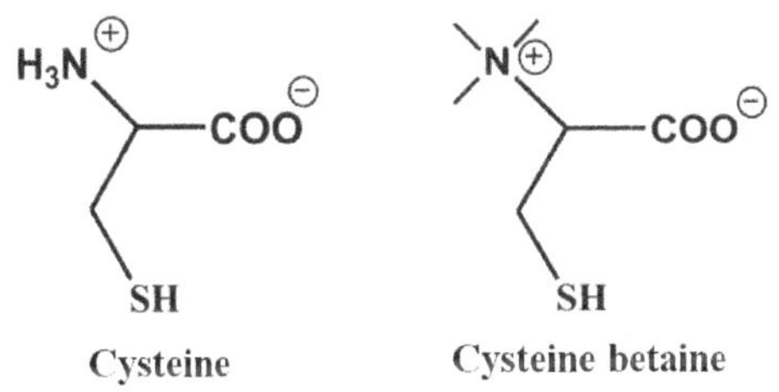

Fig. 2 The chemical structure of cysteine and cysteine betaine.

* Corresponding author.

I. Lackovic (ed.), *1st Global Conference on Biomedical Engineering & 9th Asian-Pacific Conference on Medical and Biological Engineering*,
IFMBE Proceedings 47, DOI: 10.1007/978-3-319-12262-5_7

In this study, X-ray photoelectron spectroscopy (XPS) was utilized to identify the elemental composition of SAMs. The surface wetting was measured using a contact angle goniometer. For the bacterial adsorption, gram positive (Staphylococcus epidermidis) and negative (Pseudomonas aeruginosa), the common bacterial pathogens of humans, was used to test the antifouling properties of amino acids SAMs surface. MTT cytotoxicity assays were performed to evaluate biocompatibility by 3T3 cells cell viability.

II. EXPERIMENTAL SECTION

1. Preparation of SAMs by natural organosulfur compounds.
2. Contact angle measurements.
3. XPS for element analysis on surfaces.
4. Bacteria anti-fouling tests.
5. Cytotoxicity (MTT assay).

III. RESULTS AND DISCUSSION

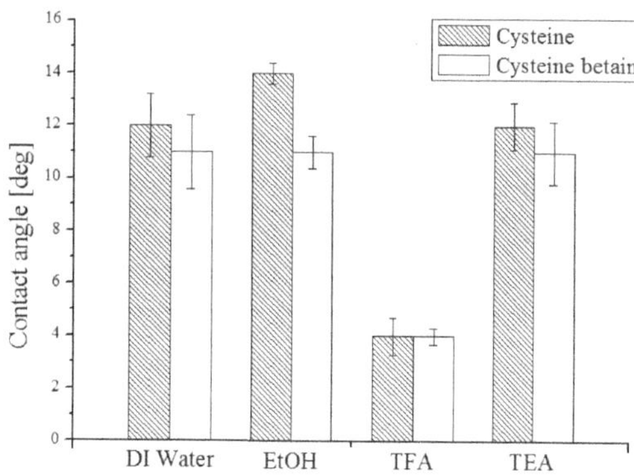

Fig. 3 Contact angle measurements for various additives into the DI H_2O of cysteine and cysteine betaine during SAM formation on Au substrate.

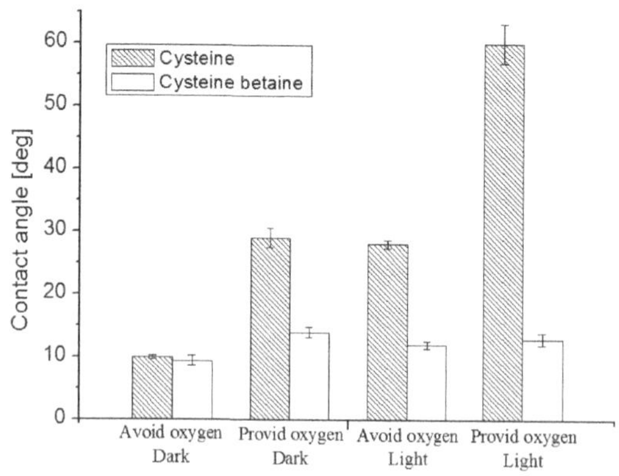

Fig. 4 Contact angle of cysteine and cysteine betaine modified on Au substrate after 12 hours photo-induced oxidization.

In Fig 1, the surface wetting tests for SAMs show that films prepared by adding a small amount TFA exhibited super-hydrophilicity (contact angles of θ=~5°) due to their complete coverage and strong hydration via ionic solvation and hydrogen bonding.

The methods for studying the oxidation of the amine functional group in 12 hours photo-induced oxidization experiment are shown in Fig 2. By isolating the SAM from either light or air, the oxidation is suppressed and the surface properties are preserved in Cysteine betaine SAMs. In other words, the shelf life of the amine-modified gold substrates is prolonged.

Table 1 XPS for Element Analysis on Surfaces

Sample	Atomic Concentration (%)				N/S ratio Theoretical	N/S ratio Experimental
	C1s	N1s	O1s	S2p		
Cysteine	15.66	2.72	19.48	2.84	1	0.95
Cysteine betaine	13.27	3.30	15.17	3.06	1	1.07

The atomic concentrations of different elements detected at the organosulfur-modified surfaces are shown in table 1. The experimental ratio of N and S is the area ratio of the N 1s and S 2p in the XPS spectra; the theoretical ratio of N and S is calculated by a stoichiometric ratio of SAMs on surfaces.

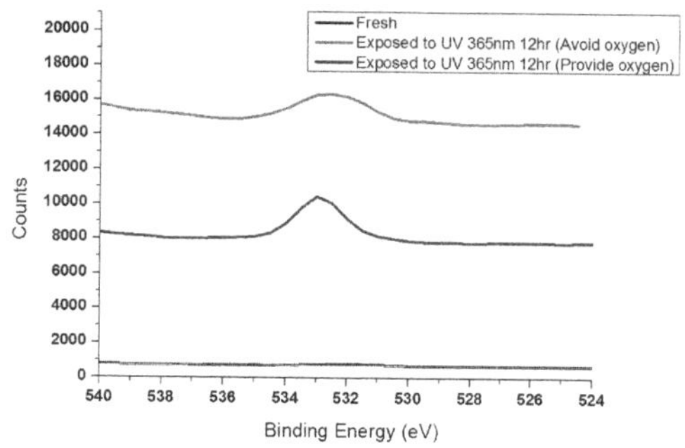

Fig. 5 XPS spectra of cysteine betaine SAMs stored in different environments for 12 hours

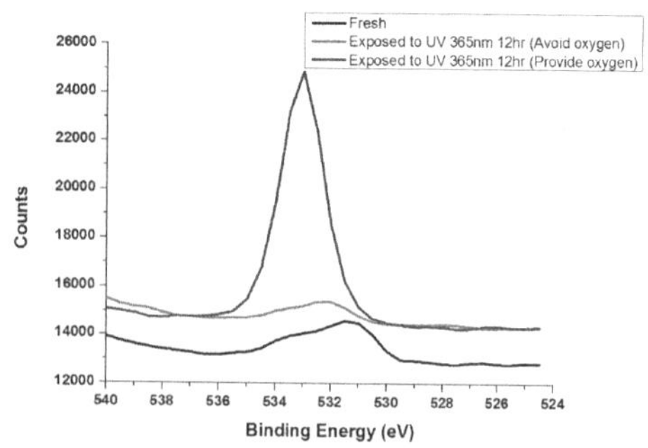

Fig. 6 XPS spectra of cysteine SAMs stored in different environments for 12 hours.

In X-ray photoelectron spectroscopy (XPS), the O1s increases significantly in Cysteine SAMs on Au substrate stored in 12 hours photo-induced oxidization environments (Fig 5-6). These results are consistent with previous study, which reveals that surface element of S and N is partially oxidized [8].

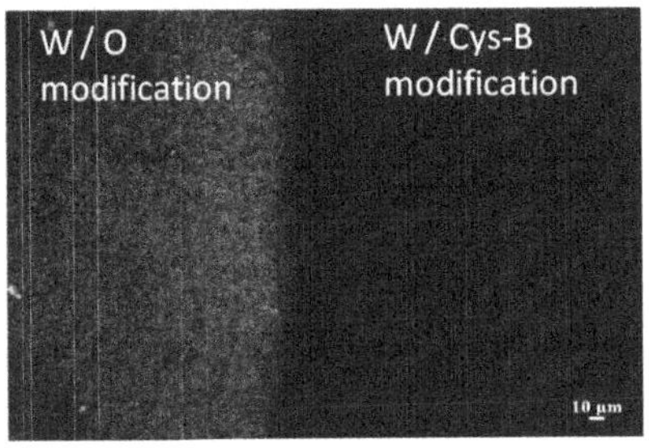

Fig. 7 P.aeruginosa (gram-) fouling on cysteine betaine patterned Au surface.

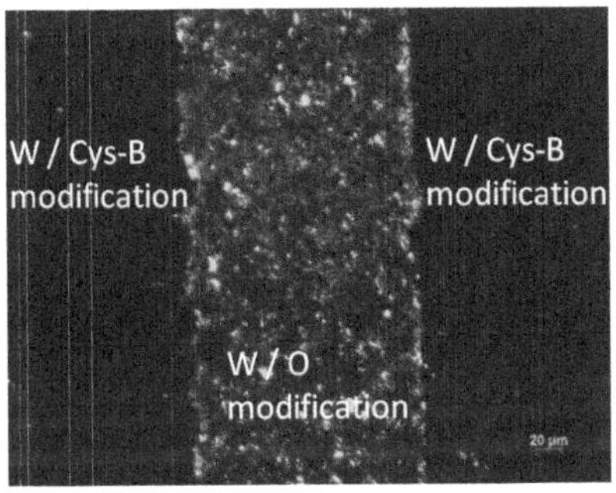

Fig. 8 S.epidermidis (gram+) fouling on cysteine betaine patterned Au surface.

There is an absence of attached bacteria in the treated section after exposure to P.aeruginosa (Fig 7.) and S.epidermidis (Fig 8.) for 3 hours, while bacteria are readily attached to the unmodified portion of the substrate. These results reveal the excellent performance of the modified surfaces to resist bacterial adhesion/biofilm formation.

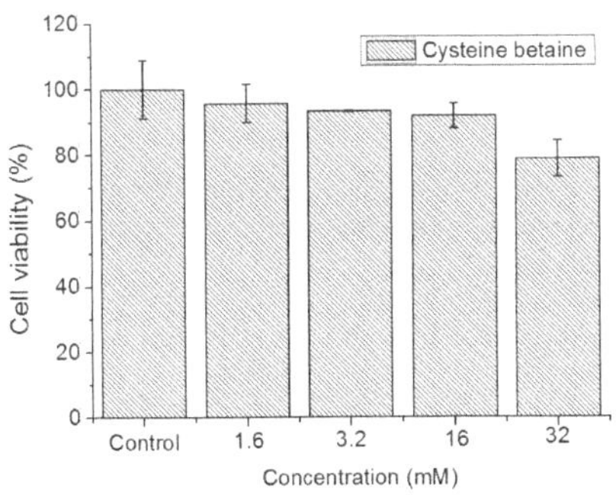

Fig. 9 The cell viability of 3T3 cells in MTT assay

The cytotoxicity was investigated by measuring the viability of 3T3 fibroblasts as a function of the concentration of cysteine betaine (Fig 9). MTT assay showed no obvious cytotoxicity on 3T3 fibroblast cells.

IV. CONCLUSIONS

By adding a small amount TFA into the DI H_2O of cysteine and cysteine betaine SAM formation, the formation of interplane hydrogen bonds between the terminal groups of bound thiolate on the surface and free thiols in the bulk is disrupted. Our study demonstrates that SAMs prepared in this method have better hydrophilic property than those prepared by adding other additives.

In addition, by changing the structure of cystine to cystine betaine, we can efficiently prevent the oxidation of nitrogen and maintain the well-known nonfouling ability of zwitterionic simultaneously. Furthermore, due to the non-toxic characteristic of these compounds, the medical application will be extensive, especially in the field of medical implants.

REFERENCES

1. Raynor JE, Capadona JR, Collard DM, Petrie TA, Garcia AJ. Polymer brushes and self-assembled monolayers: Versatile platforms to control cell adhesion to biomaterials (Review). Biointerphases. 2009;4:FA3-FA16.
2. Vasita R, Shanmugam K, Katti DS. Improved biomaterials for tissue engineering applications: Surface modification of polymers. Curr Top Med Chem. 2008;8:341-53.
3. Chen SF, Li LY, Zhao C, Zheng J. Surface hydration: Principles and applications toward low-fouling/nonfouling biomaterials. Polymer. 2010;51:5283-93
4. Love JC, Estroff LA, Kriebel JK, Nuzzo RG, Whitesides GM. Self-assembled monolayers of thiolates on metals as a form of nanotechnology. Chem Rev. 2005;105:1103-69.
5. Kondoh H, Kodama C, Nozoye H. Structure-dependent change of desorption species from n-alkanethiol monolayers adsorbed on Au(111): Desorption of thiolate radicals from low-density structures. J PhysChem B. 1998;102:2310-2.
6. Rieley, H.; Kendall, G. K.; Zemicael, F. W.; Smith, T. L.; Yang,S. H. X-ray Studies of Self-Assembled Monolayers on Coinage Metals. 1. Alignment and Photooxidation in 1,8-Octanedithiol and 1-Octanethiol on Au. Langmuir 1998, 14, 5147.
7. Scott, J. R.; Baker, L. S.; Everett, W. R.; Wilkins, C. L.; Fritsch, I. Laser desorption fourier transform mass spectrometry exchange studies of air-oxidized alkanethiol self-assembled monolayers on gold. Chem. 1997, 69, 2636
8. Szu-Hsian Lee,Wei-Chun Lin,Che-Hung Kuo,Manuel Karakachian,Yu-Chin Lin,Bang-Ying Yu,Jing-Jong Shyue. Photooxidation of Amine-Terminated Self-Assembled Monolayers on Gold. J. Phys. Chem. C 2010, 114, 10512–10519.

Novel Bio-inspired Zwitterion Dopamine Molecule for Anti-biofouling and Photocleavable Properties

Lin-Chuan Wang[1] and Chun-Jen Huang[1,2,*]

[1] Graduate Institute of Biomedical Engineering, National Central University, Jhong-Li, Taoyuan 320, Taiwan
[2] Department of Chemical and Material Engineering, National Central University, Jhong-Li, Taoyuan 320, Taiwan

Abstract— **Use of synthetic biomaterials as blood-contacting devices typically accompanies considerable nonspecific adsorption of proteins, cells and bacteria. These may eventually induce adverse pathogenic problems in clinic practices, such as thrombosis and biomaterials-associated infection. An effective surface coating for medical devices has been pursued to repel nonspecific adsorption from surfaces. In this study, bio-inspired adhesive dopamine conjugated with zwitterionic sulfobetaine moieties (SB-DA) was developed for anti-biofouling properties. The molecules can anchor onto various substrates via catechol groups to form a stable thin film. The results indicated that the formation of self-assembled monolayers (SAMs) was strongly dependent on the pH values in preparation, which correlates to the oxidization and reduction (redox) of catechol groups in dopamine molecules. The Other mussel-inspired catecholic zwitterionic nitro-sulfobetaine moieties (SB-nDA) assembly possessing antifouling and photocleavable characters for spatiotemporal tailoring of interfacial properties and controlling bio-adsorption. X-ray photoelectron spectroscopy (XPS) was used to analyze the bonding mechanism, accounting for distinct wetting and fouling levels from contact angle and quartz crystal microbalance with dissipation (QCM-D) measurements. The thickness simulation from XPS and ellipsometry showed about 1.1 nm for intact SB-DA films and 1.03 nm for intact SB-nDA. In addition, the bacterial test indicated the excellent resistance of films against *P. aeruginosa*. This work provides not only new surface chemistry but the new route for surface modification. Currently, SB-DA is applied onto various materials with different dimensions as a new generation of self-assembling biomaterials for a wide spectrum of applications then SB-nDA for potential applications in light-guided targeting and releasing of drug delivery and molecular imaging.**

Keywords— **zwitterionic, anti-biofouling, self-assembled monolayers, photocleavable, spatiotemporal tailoring.**

I. INTRODUCTION

A newly emerging class of charged materials, named zwitterionic materials, permits effective biofouling repellence, long-term durability, and environmental stability [1]. The promising achievements provoke the development of methodologies based on zwitterionic materials for surface engineering. Recently, increased numbers of assemblies carrying a variety of functional groups have been developed, and thereby constitute a toolkit for manipulating surface properties at a molecular level. A mussel-inspired adhesive chemistry based on catecholic derivatives has attracted wide-spread interest [2]. These researches carried out bio-inert interfaces via either the "graft-from" or "graft-to" strategies based on catecholic chemistry, showing the potency of thin films strongly depends on the grafting density of adhesive groups. However, the adhesion mechanism of catechol groups remains poorly understood [3].

In this work, we report our systematic investigations on the binding mechanism of zwitterionic sulfonbetaine dopamine (SB-DA) in response to pH transition and develop a modification strategy allowing formation of compact and stable antifouling SB-DA SAMs. zwitterionic nitro sulfobetaine moieties (SB-nDA) assembly possessing antifouling and photocleavable characters for spatiotemporal tailoring of interfacial properties and controlling bio-adsorption.

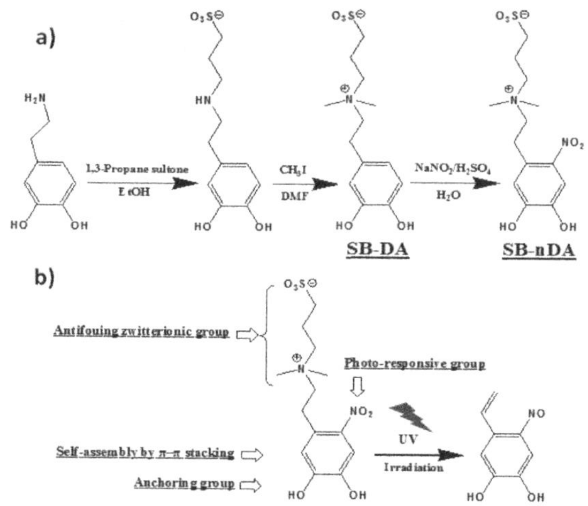

Scheme 1 (a) Synthetic route and chemical structures of SB-DA and SB-nDA. (b) Functions and photochemical mechanism of SB-nDA.

II. EXPERIMENTAL PROCEDURES

A. Preparation of SAMs by Zwitterion Dopamine Molecule

A metallic substrate was prepared by deposition of titanium onto a 20 mm × 20 mm glass slide in a high-vacuum thermal evaporator. A 50-nm thick layer of titanium was

[*] Corresponding author.

I. Lackovic (ed.), *1st Global Conference on Biomedical Engineering & 9th Asian-Pacific Conference on Medical and Biological Engineering*, IFMBE Proceedings 47, DOI: 10.1007/978-3-319-12262-5_8

formed and oxidized in ambient to have a layer of oxide. The TiO_2 substrates were cleaned by thoroughly washing with 1% SDS detergent, deionized water, and absolute ethanol, followed by drying in a stream of nitrogen. The substrates were exposed to O_2 plasma in a plasma cleaner (PDC-32G, Harrick Plasma, NY) for 10 min in order to remove final trace of organic contaminations on the surface. Buffers were prepared by titrating PBS with hydrochloric acid (pH 3, pH 4, pH 6) and Tris buffer (pH 8).The cleaned TiO_2 substrates were immersed in solutions (pH 3, pH 4, pH 6, pH 8) containing SB-DA molecules at a concentration of 2 mg ml^{-1} for 15 h at room temperature. In the pH transition approach, the substrates were subsequently transferred to a pH 8 buffer and incubated for 20 min. Afterwards they were washed with copious deionized water and dried in a stream of nitrogen for further measurements.

III. RESULTS AND DISCUSSION

A. Elemental Composition and Chemical State of Thin Films by Using XPS

As shown in Fig. 1a, N peak components with BE at 402.5 eV appear in the XPS N 1s core-level spectra for both samples. The peak components are associated with the quaternary ammonium cations (-$\underline{N}(CH_3)_3^+$) [4]. The S 2p doublets at the BEs of 167.0 and 168.2 eV are attributed to sulfonate C-$\underline{S}O_3^-$ species in the side chains of SB-DA(Fig. 1b). In Fig. 1c, the C 1s spectra with four peaks were assigned to CHx-/C-NH2, C-O/C-N+/C-SO3-, C=O and $\pi \rightarrow \pi^*$ species at BEs of 284.4, 285.6, 287.7 and 292.4 eV, respectively [5]. The O 1s region is fit with two peaks assigned to Ti-O_2, and C-$\underline{O}$-H/C-$\underline{O}$-Ti/Ti-$\underline{O}$H species at BEs of 530.3 and 531.6 eV, respectively. In Figure 1d, the fraction of C-O-H/C-O-Ti/Ti-OH species for the sample of SB-DA(3-8) (f = 52.1 %) is lower than that of SB-DA(3) (f = 68.8 %). According to the proposed binding mechanism in previous literature[6] the DA derivatives bind to TiO_2 surfaces by condensation between surface hydroxyl groups (i.e. Ti-OH) and catecholic hydroxyl groups (i.e. C-OH), forming C-O-Ti. Therefore, the decrease in the fraction of the peak at 531.6 eV observed in this work by XPS can be viewed as the formation of SB-DA molecular bonding with TiO2.Besides, the thickness of the SB-DA(3-8) film was estimated using XPS and ellipsometry. The XPS with the angle resolved technique and the ultrathin-film analysis built into Multipak provided a thickness of 1.12 nm that is comparable with that from the ellipsometry measurement as 1.25 nm.

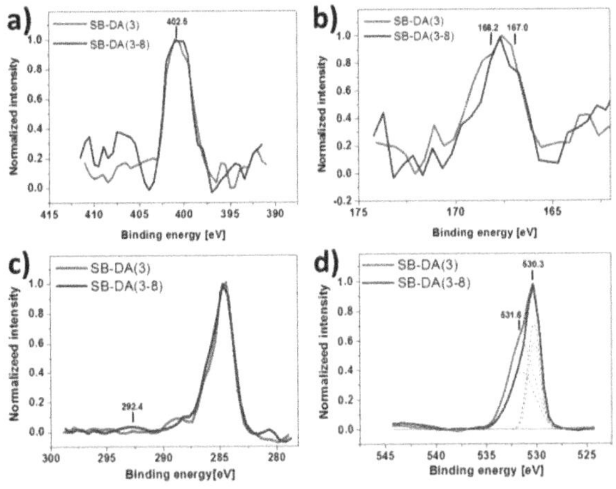

Fig. 1 XPS spectra of N 1s (a), S 2p (b), C 1s (c), and O 1s (d) for samples of SB-DA(3) and SB-DA(3-8).

B. Antifouling Properties of SB-DA SAMs

The antifouling properties of the SB-DA SAMs were demonstrated in protein and bacterial adsorption tests. For the protein fouling experiment, the QCM-D sensor was employed to monitor the increased surface mass on modified surfaces. Herein, based on aforementioned assumption, we examined the effectiveness of the pH transition approach for the formation of the SB-DA SAM and, thereby, the SAMs were prepared at distinct pH values from 3 to 8, followed by rinsing with the buffer at pH 8. The modified QCM-D chips were mounted on the sensors. After the base line was established in PBS, the protein solution containing BSA at a concentration of 1mg mL^{-1} in PBS was flowed over the surface for 15 min, then PBS washing for 20 min. Interestingly, the changes in ΔF attributable to protein adsorption increased with decrease in the initial pH value (Fig. 2a). The fouling resistance of SB-DA(8) is insignificant to the bare TiO_2 surface. The increased mass on the chip is well related to the change in frequency of the oscillating crystal through Sauerbrey relationship. The calculated surface mass of adsorbed BSA as a function of the initial pH is showed in Fig. 2b. The surface mass of the protein fouling on the SAM of SB-DA(3-8) (10.6 ± 2.5 ng cm^{-2}) was reduced by 97 % relative to that on the bare TiO_2 surface (310.5 ng cm^{-2}). Therefore, the antifouling capability of the SB-DA SAM prepared by the pH transition approach as demonstrated here has achieved an extent that is nearly compatible with established thiol-based systems to effectively repel the nonspecific adsorption.

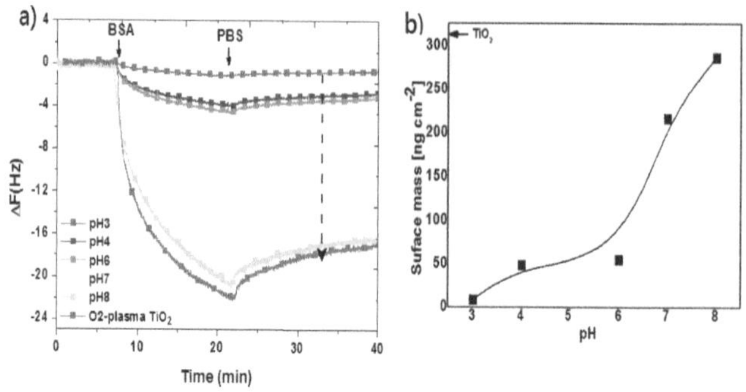

Fig. 2 QCM-D studies for the BSA adsorption on SB-DA SAMs prepared at the initial pH values of 3-8. The real-time kinetics of BSA adsorption are shown in the changes of resonance frequency (a). The calculated surface mass through Sauerbrey relationship as a function of the initial pH values is present (b)

As one can see in Fig. 3a, b, the numbers of adhered bacteria on samples of SB-DA(3-8) for *P. aeruginosa* and *S. epidermidis* are obviously lower than the other samples. The reductions in bacterial adsorption for *P. aeruginosa* and *S. epidermidis* reach 96.9 and 97.4 % relative to bare TiO_2 surfaces. For the SB-DA(8) sample, the numbers of adhered bacteria are significant higher than SB-DA(3-8), which can be the result of the insufficient coverage of SB-DA due to fast oxidation of catecholic hydroxyl groups at a high pH as discussion above. A convincing evidence showing the antifouling property of SB-DA(3-8) was present in Figure 3c, in which the surface was patterned with SB-DA(3-8) for the adsorption of *P. aeruginosa*. Clearly, the bacteria are favorable to attach onto the untreated TiO_2 surface, while only few cells are observed on SB-DA(3-8).

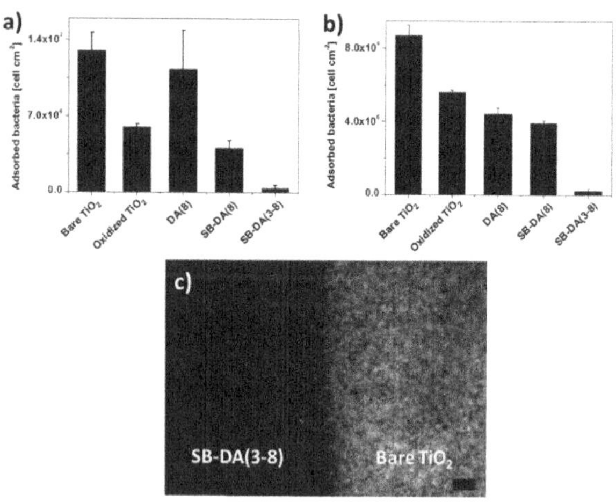

Fig. 3 The bacterial adsorption tests for *P. aeruginosa* (a) and *S. epidermidis* (b) on samples. Patterned TiO_2 surface with SB-DA(3-8) was incubated with *P. aeruginosa* solution and imaged under fluorescence microscope after washing (c).

C. Biofouling Resistance of SB-nDA SAMs

Moreover, the SB-nDA substrate was temporally exposed to UV in the time-resolved QCM-D sensor equipped with a quartz window on the flow cell. The sample was initially treated with a BSA solution for 14.5 min and, afterwards, the UV light source was turned on to in-situ trigger the photo-cleavage. As a result in Fig.4, the protein adsorption level after UV exposure is obviously higher than that before and increases 89.8 %.

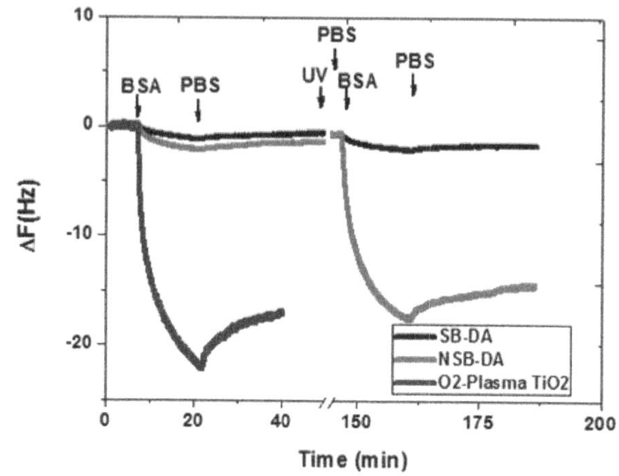

Fig. 4 QCM-D studies for the BSA adsorption on SB-DA SAMs (black), SB-nDA SAMs (red) and O_2-Plasma TiO_2. and dissipation (b).

The photo-responsive property of SB-nDA was carried out by UV irradiation at a laboratorial ambient environment. Firstly, the SB-DA and SB-nDA samples were exposed to UV light for 120 min, followed by washing with PBS. The samples were incubated with bacterial solutions as described above. Two representative strains of common pathogenic bacteria were used to contact with samples, which are the *P. aeruginosa* and *S. epidermidis*. The bacterial solutions were incubated with samples at 37°C for 2 h. After washing with PBS and dye staining, the samples were observed and quantified under a fluorescence microscopy. One can see in Fig. 5 where the bacterial adsorption levels on SB-nDA were significantly increased 95.7 % and 96.5 % for *P. aeruginosa* and *S. epidermidis* bacteria, respectively, while SB-DA remained its antifouling properties after UV light treatment. This should be namely attributed to the photo-cleavable property of SB-nDA to remove the SB moiety to become the vinyl group upon UV irradiation as illustrated in Scheme 1. More strikingly, the UV light spatially exposure to SB-nDA SAMs and afterwards to bring to contact with the bacterial solution in Fig. 5. The bacteria clearly appeared on the areas subjecting UV irradiation, while the shielded one preserved its intact antifouling function. Herein, we prepared the TiO_2 samples modified with SB-DA and SB-nDA SAMs as well as untreated substrates to compare their capability to repel protein and bacterial adsorption. Samples of SB-DA and SB-nDA expressed comparable capability to reduce the adsorption of both bacteria. With SB-DA, the adsorption were reduced 96.9 % and 97.4 %, respectively, with SB-nDA with respect to un-modified TiO_2. These results reflect the unique characters of SB moiety that possesses strong interaction with water and charge-balance to eliminate electrostatic interaction .

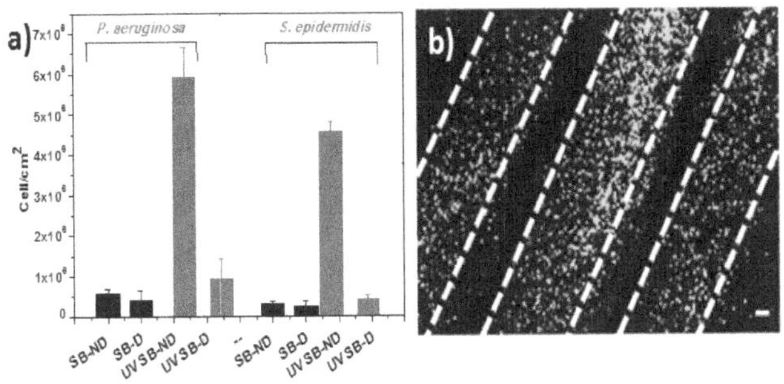

Fig. 5 The bacterial adsorption tests for *P. aeruginosa* and *S. epidermidis* on samples with UV light treatment (red) (a). Patterned TiO2 surface with SB-nDA(3-8) was inc bated with *P. aeruginosa* solution and imaged under fluorescence microscope after washing (b)

IV. CONCLUSIONS

We have shown that bio-inspired zwitterionic SB-DA enables to form a stable and fully-covered self-assembled monolayer (SAM) through the pH transition approach for effective antifouling property. The redox reaction of catecholic hydroxyl groups serves an important role in molecular assembly on TiO_2 surfaces. The results indicate that the SB-DA adsorbs on surfaces via hydrogen bonding with oxidized TiO_2 surface at low pH in the initial stage.The bonding of adsorbed SB-DA likely converts to bidentate bonds with the TiO_2 surface by the replacement of surface hydroxyl groups by deprotonated catecholic hydroxyl groups, leading to high coverage and stability of the SB-DA layer. More strikingly, owing to the charge-balance and hydrophilicity of SB moieties, the SAM was demonstrated to be capable to resist BSA and bacteria adsorption under a physiological condition.

Other hand we have developed a new zwitterionic SB-nDA assembly with integrated characters of simultaneous self-assembling, antifouling, and photo-cleavable properties. The formation of SAMs of SB-nDA was confirmed by contact angle, ellipsometry, and XPS measurements, showing the highly compact film can be established via a pH transition approach. In addition, the fouling resistance of SB-nDA against protein and bacterial adsorption was demonstrated to be employed as a biocompatible surface coating. More importantly, the spatiotemporal control over the bio-adsorption via UV light exposure with SB-nDA was verified and may be applied to nano-carriers for selective uptake by target cells for potential applications in molecular imaging and drug delivery.

ACKNOWLEDGMENT

The authors sincerely appreciate the financial support from the Ministry of Science and Technology of Taiwan (NSC 102-2221-E-008-011-) and Prof. Jeng-Kuei Chang from NCU for the electrochemical measurements.

REFERENCES

1. Chen, S.F., et al., *Surface hydration: Principles and applications toward low-fouling/nonfouling biomaterials*. Polymer, 2010. **51**(23): p. 5283-5293.
2. Lee, H., et al., *Mussel-inspired surface chemistry for multifunctional coatings*. Science, 2007. **318**(5849): p. 426-430.
3. Ye, Q., F. Zhou, and W.M. Liu, *Bioinspired catecholic chemistry for surface modification*. Chemical Society Reviews, 2011. **40**(7): p. 4244-4258.
4. Yang, W.J., et al., *Stainless steel surfaces with thiol-terminated hyperbranched polymers for functionalization via thiol-based chemistry*. Polymer Chemistry, 2013. **4**(10). p. 3105-3115.
5. Moulder, J.F.S., W .F.; Sobol, P. E.; Bomben, K. D. , *Handbook of x-ray photoelectron spectroscopy*. 1992, Boca Raton.
6. Malisova, B., et al., *Poly(ethylene glycol) Adlayers Immobilized to Metal Oxide Substrates Through Catechol Derivatives: Influence of Assembly Conditions on Formation and Stability*. Langmuir, 2010. **26**(6). p. 4018-4026.

Author: Chun-Jen Huang , PhD
Institute: Graduate Institute of Biomedical Engineering, National Central University
Street: No.300, Jhongda Rd.
City: Jhongli City
Country: Taoyuan County 32001, Taiwan
Email: cjhuang@ncu.edu.tw

Preparation of HA-Mineralized CS/PLA Composites Nanofiber GBR Mats

Yu-Ru Lee, Shu-Juan Fu, and Chi-Chang Lin*

Department of Chemical and Materials Engineering, Tunghai University, Taichung, Taiwan

Abstract— **In this work, a composited guided bone regeneration (GBR) membrane made of hydroxyapatite (HA) mineralized on electrospun chitosan (CS)-coated poly (lactic acid) (PLA) nanofiber mat was prepared and compared in terms of mineralization characteristics. Fabrication parameters of CS-co-PLA nanofibers and mineralized of calcium phosphate crystals were discussed in details. Fourier transform infrared spectroscopy (FTIR) showed a compositions of CS/PLA mixture and X-ray diffraction results further indicated that the composition of the deposited mineral was a mixture of dicalcium phosphate dehydrates and apatite. These results indicated the HA crystals can be simple mineralized on CS/PLA nanofiber mat which provides notonly better geometric properties but also biological functions for GBR application.**

Keywords— **chitosan, poly (lactic acid), electrospinning, guided bone regeneration, mineralization.**

I. INTRODUCTION

Because of the excellent biological properties, such as biodegradability, nontoxicity, antibacterial ability and biocompatibility, chitosan (CS) composite electrospun membrane has been known as promising material in many biomedical fields from skin to bone or cartilage [1]. However, the scaling-up of CS nanofiber fabrication by electrospinning is problematic and challenging. Due to its polyelectrolyte nature, CS cannot be continuously spun as droplets persistently [2]. Neat CS electrospun membrane has some other significant shortcomings such as poor mechanical strength, especially in vitro, chitosan hydrolysis might happen under the conditions of water or tissue fluid. To solve these problems, blending CS with some water-soluble polymers was available to make CS electrospinnable. As reported in the previous literature, poly(ethylene oxide) (PEO) and poly(vinyl alcohol) (PVA) were the most commonly employed to help the fabrication of chitosan-based nanofibers [3] and for the applications of tissue engineering scaffolds and wound healing dressings [4].

II. EXPERIMENTS AND RESULTS

A. Preparation and Characterization of Chitosan Derivative (SDS-CS)

A detail process was displayed as flowchart shown in Fig. 1. Briefly, chitosan (0.8 g) was dissolved in 50 mL 2 wt% acetic acid solution. Excess SDS (4.14 g) was dissolved in 50 mL distilled water. The above mixed solution was constantly stirred into homogeneous solution for 4 h at 25 ◦ C. SDS-CS was precipitated from the mixed solution, then was collected by high-speed centrifugation and washed with deionized water. Finally, the white powder SDS-CS was obtained from freeze-drying.

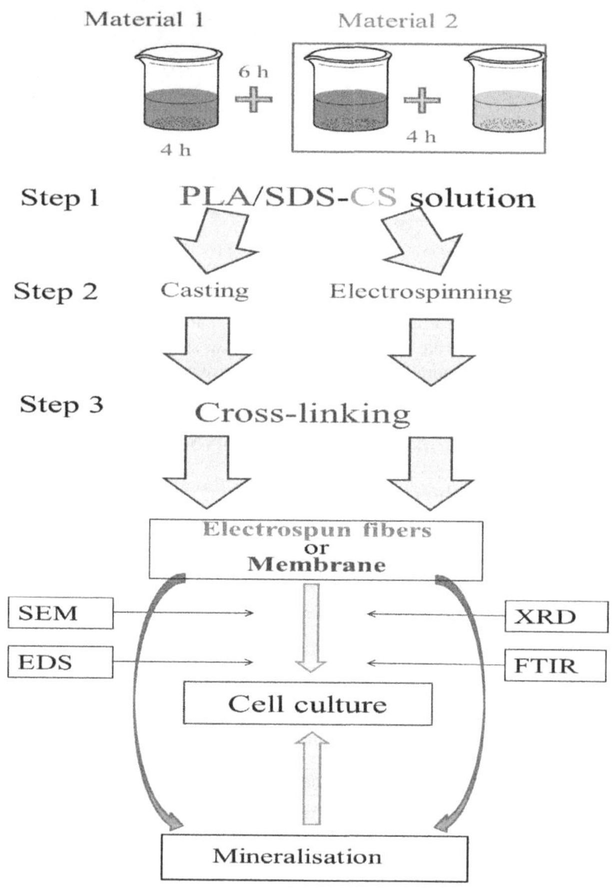

Fig. 1 Experimental flowchart

B. Preparation of Homogeneous Solution and Electrospinning

PLA and SDS-CS were dissolved in dichloromethane (DCM) and dimethyl sulfoxide (DMSO), respectively. The prepared two transparent solutions were than further mixed under different weight ratios. (PLA/SDS-CS = 80/20; 75/25; 60/40. Here the PLA only solution was marked

* Corresponding author.

I. Lackovic (ed.), *1st Global Conference on Biomedical Engineering & 9th Asian-Pacific Conference on Medical and Biological Engineering*,
IFMBE Proceedings 47, DOI: 10.1007/978-3-319-12262-5_9

as PLA/SDS-CS = 100/0 for the comparison). The electrospinning PLA/SDS-CS solution was prepared with the total concentration of 3%.

The electrospinning was performed at room temperature. The above mixed solution was placed into a plastic syringe (10 mL) equipped with a single nozzle. The electrospinning conditions were set as follows: The solution was supplied by a syringe pump which maintained at a constant feed rate of 0.5 ml/h. The positive electrode of a high voltage (25 kV) power supply was applied between the syringe tip and collector. An aluminum foil was used as the collector, tip-to-collector distance was fixed at 15 cm. The nanofibrous membranes were collected on the surface of aluminum foil and dried at room temperature in vacuum for 24 h.

C. Analysis of Chitosan-Bland Polymer

The morphology of electrospun nanofibers and the fibers diameter were significantly influenced by the composition of electrospinning solution [5]. The SEM micrographs and diameter distributions of electrospun PLA/SDS-CS nanofibers with different weight ratios from 80/20 to 60/40 were shown in Fig. 2. With SDS-CS increasing, it was difficult to form continuous nanofibers, the nanofibers might show a large number of beaded structure. It could be seen that the uniform ultrafine electrospun PLA/SDS-CS nanofibers had smooth and homogeneous morphology. With the increasing proportion of CS, the average diameter of the nanofibers gradually decreased. Generally, it was known that CS was a polyelectrolyte and electrospinning of polymers with higher polarity provided nanofibers with smaller diameters. Additionally, the influence of CS with lower weight could be explained by strong mobility. In this case, the PLA/SDS-CS solution was stretched into thinner fibers with smaller diameters than neat PLA nanofiber.

Fourier transform infrared spectroscopy (FTIR) data manifested very important information about the intermolecular and intramolecular interactions in polymers. Figure 3 displayed the FTIR spectra of neat electrospun PLA fibers and PLA/SDS-CS blend fibers with different weight ratios, neat CS and SDS modified CS powder. Compared with CS, the infra-red data of SDS modified CS showed the characteristic peaks at 1226 cm^{-1} ($RO-SO_3$ – stretch) and 818 cm^{-1} (S–O stretch). The absorption bands at 2800–3000 cm^{-1} (CH_2 stretch) significantly increased due to the existence of SDS. The result suggested SDS has been coupled onto the amino group of CS. The broad band at around 3400 cm^{-1} could be obviously observed (NH_2 and OH stretches). The coupling effect of NH_3^+ and SO_3^- broadened the shape of the peak, but no peak position change was observed.

Figure 4 showed the EDS analysis results of casted thin film (A1, A2) and the electrospun fiber mats (B1, B2). Carbon atomic ration increased from 40% to 55% while chitosan content rose from 20% to 25%. Moreover, both casted thin film and electrospun fiber mat represents the similar results as results sowed.

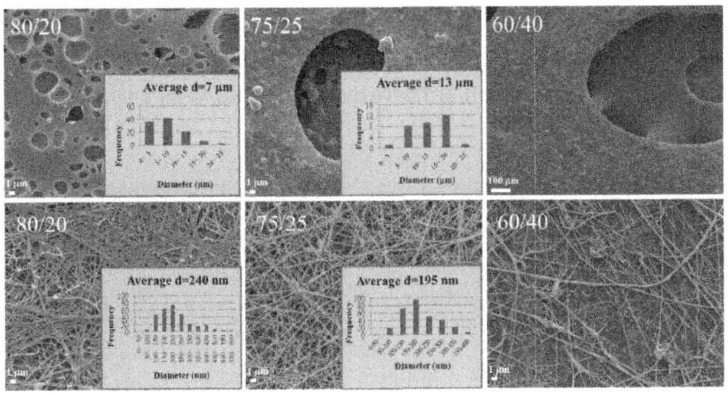

Fig. 2 SEM of casted film and electrospun fibers mat.

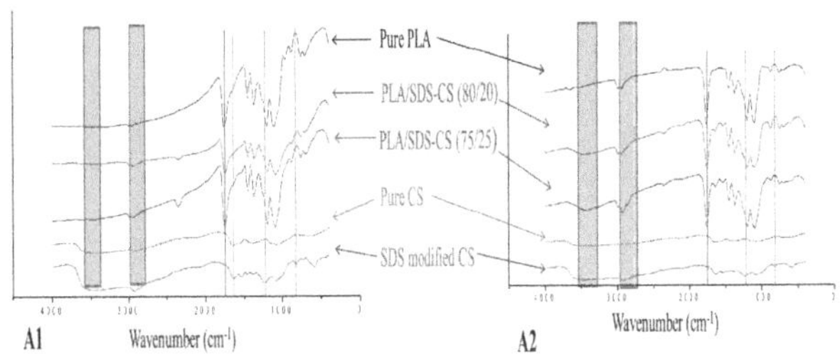

Fig. 3 IR spectrum of casted thin film (A1) and the electrospun fiber mats (A2).

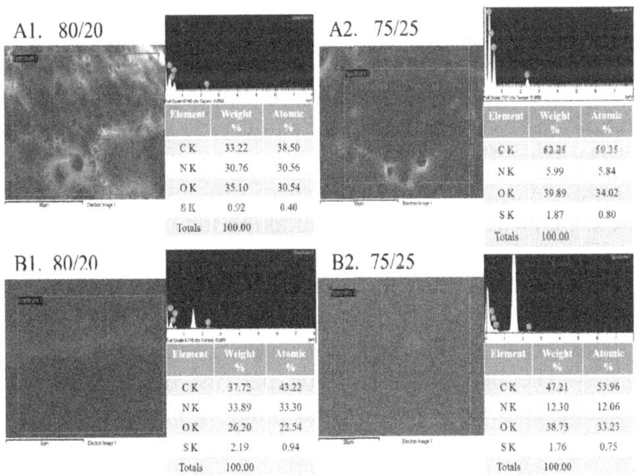

Fig. 4 EDS of casted thin film (A1, A2) and the electrospun fiber mats (B1, B2).

D. Analysis of Mineralized Membrane

SEM images showed the surface morphology of HA mineralized electrospun nanofiber mat which immersed in self-designed double diffusion chamber for 24 and 48 h. As shown in Fig. 5, the electrospun fiber mat was fully covered by mineralized HA crystalline with highly uniformity. By using EDXA analysis, calcium phosphate crystals represent in the apatite form and these crystals was precipitated on the surface and also within in the interior pore region of membrane. Moreover, the Ca/P ratio of apatite crystals increased from 1.9 to 2.7 when mineralization time was prolonged up to 48 h.

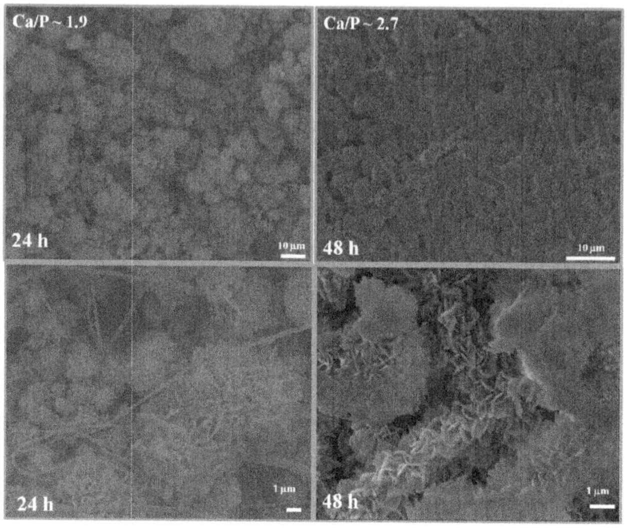

Fig. 5 SEM images of various mineralization time (24 and 48 h). Button figures represents an enlarge images.

Wide-angle X-ray diffraction was utilized to reveal the crystalline structure of electrospun nanofibers. Figure 6 illustrated XRD patterns of PLA nanofibers, SDS-CS and PLA/SDS-CS nanofibers with different polymer weight ratios. Here SDS-CS was a semi-crystal polymer and its XRD patterns exhibited a sharp diffraction peaks at the 2θ angle of 6.5 ° and 20.5°. The sharp diffraction peaks might be explained that SDS existing along the molecular chains to form crystal structure. Increasing the ratio of arranged molecular chains led to increase the polymer crystallinity. For PLA nanofibers,

XRD pattern showed only broad diffraction peak at 17.5°. The obtained diffraction patterns of PLA/SDS-CS nanofibers with various weight ratios exhibited almost the similar pattern as SDS-CS powder, however, but the position of the characteristic peaks changed to 15 ° and 20 °, which might cause by the influence of amorphous structure within the PLA.

The X-ray diffractograms of mineralized membrane within 48 h of immersion time is shown in Fig. 7. All the patterns look similar and show a strong reflection with a broad peak around 31 (2θ), which the hydroxyapatite formed on chitosan matrix is in apatite structure and no other calcium phosphate phases such as tricalcium phosphate was observed. The broader peak is due to the nano-crystalline of the nature apatite and a noise level exists in the diffraction data caused by the present of amorphous layer in the prepared polymer. The broad peak at 2 θ of 31° is defined by lattice planes (211), (112) and (300) of hydroxyapatite [6].

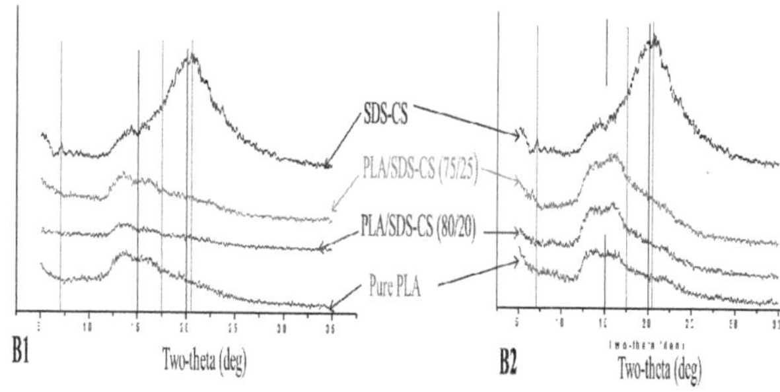

Fig. 6 XRD pattern of prepared casted thin film (B1) and electrospun fiber (B2).

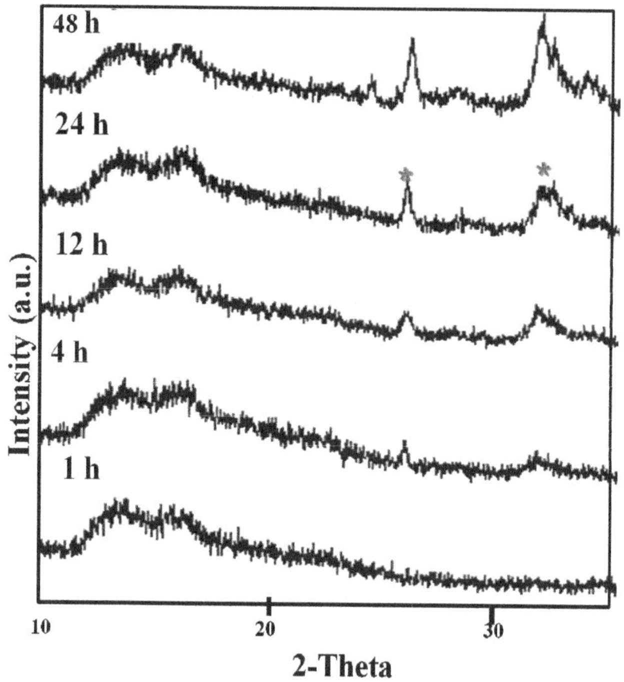

Fig. 7 Effect of mineralization time on XRD patterns.

III. CONCLUSIONS

The chitosan-blended PLA nanofiber mat is successfully prepared by using electrospun technology. Mineralized crystals with apatite structure are precipitated on both surface and inner connection pores of nanofiber mats via direct SBF immersion. Ca/P ration increased from 1.9 to 2.7 while immersion time up to 48 h. The HA mineralized electrospun CS/PLA nanofiber mat was successful prepared by combination of simple SBF immersion and electro-spinning technology.

ACKNOWLEDGMENT

This work is supported by the THU project of Global Research & Education on Environment and Society (GREEnS 001) and NSC project (101-2320-B-029-001).

CONFLICT OF INTEREST

The authors declare that they have no conflict of interest.

REFERENCES

1. Alves, N. M., & Mano, J. F. (2008). Chitosan derivatives obtained by chemical modifications for biomedical and environmental applications. International Journal of Biological Macromolecules, 43:401–414.
2. Muzzarelli, R. A. A. (2011). Biomedical exploitation of chitin and chitosan via mechano-chemical disassembly, electrospinning, dissolution in imidazolium ionic liquids, and supercritical drying. Marine Drugs, 9:1510–1533.
3. Jia, Y. T., Gong, J., Gu, X. H., Kim, H. Y., Dong, J., & Shen, X. Y. (2007). Fabrication and characterization of poly(vinyl alcohol)/chitosan blend nanofibers produced by electrospinning method. Carbohydrate Polymers, 67:403–409.
4. Zhou, Y., Yang, D., Chen, X., Xu, Q., Lu, F., & Nie, J. (2008). Electrospun water-soluble carboxyethyl chitosan/poly(vinyl alcohol) nanofibrous membrane as potential wound dressing for skin regeneration. Biomacromolecules, 9:349–354.
5. Spasova, M., Manolova, N., Paneva, D., & Rashkov, I. (2006). Perspectives on: Criteria for complex evaluation of the morphology and alignment of electrospun polymer nanofibers. Journal of Bioactive and Compatible Polymers, 21,465–479.
6. Sivakumar M, Manjubala I, Rao KP. Preparation, characterization and in vitro release of gentamicin from coralline hydroxyapatite–chitosan composite microspheres. Carb Polym 2002;49:281–8.

Author: Chi-Chang Lin
Institute: Tunghai University
Street: No.1727, Sec.4, Taiwan Boulevard
City: Taichung
Country: Taiwan
Email: chichang31@thu.edu.tw

Multi-walled Carbon Nanotubes and Chitosan Film Promote Nerve Regeneration by Releasing Nerve Growth Factor

Wei Chen Liao, Cheng Rung Yang, Meng Hsuan Lin, Yu Ting Lo, Yi Jhih Chiou, Yi Ling Hsieh, Mei Jung Chen, and Pei Ru Chen*

Department of Biomedical Engineering, Ming Chuan University, Taoyuan, Taiwan

Abstract— **The purpose of this study was to develop kinds of multi-walled carbon nanotubes (MWCNT)-based materials, which could replace current autografts for neuron regeneration. The alternative MWCNT films was developed by encapsulated chitosan. To evaluate the characteristics of MWCNT films after modification, the measurements of electrical conductivity, contact angle and the degree of degradation were carried out. Two kinds of chitosan film preparation were designed, one was the dish film and the other was microscope slide film. The microscope slide film was exterior, however, the dish film was wrinkling. Comparing the thickness by micrometer caliper, the thickness of the dish film was 0.1950 to 0.0425 mm, and the microscope slide film was 0.0584 to 0.0109 mm. This result indicated the microscope slide film was more suitable for the following experiment because of less error value. The contact angle of the chitosan film was measured between 60~90 deg, it indicated the film was more hydrophobic. In order to achieve better biocompatibility, adding MWCNT significantly increased hydrophilicity of chitosan film.**

Keywords— **Carbon nanotubes, chitosan, NGF.**

I. INTRODUCTION

Nerve damage is quite common the clinical problem which is caused by physical trauma, infection, traffic accidents, sports injuries, stroke, aging and genetic diseases. With damage of the central nervous system (CNS), message transduction will be affected and functional impairment resulted. Therefore, repairing the damaged neuron is one of the most important way to treat those patients with neuron injury.

To avoid rejection by immune system, traditional surgery for nerve repair usually uses autografts harvested from a remote site where minor sensory loss can be tolerated. Such treatment makes the best neurological recovery, but it still has lots of disadvantages, such as rare sources, repeated surgical interventions, multiple scars, hematoma, infection and painful neuroma formation. Recent studies, have disclosed some alternative materials for nerve repair. Among them, carbon nanotubes are kinds of new synthetic materials with properties of high strength, semiconductivity and stability, thus they have been wildly used in nerve repair. Nerve cells proliferation could be enhanced by electrical stimulation, so the carbon nanotubes are best to be made into encapsulated materials.It is possible to create a tunnel in the materials so that electric current can pass through to stimulate nerve regeneration, then improve functional recovery.

The purpose of this study was trying to develop a new multi-walled carbon nanotubes (MWCNT) with high activity and hydrophilic property. This modified materials of carbon nanotubes will be able to trap active compounds which are helpful for nerve repair. More studies such as biocompatibility should be carried out in the future.

II. MATERIALS AND METHODS

A. *Materials*

Chitosan from crab shells (C3646-100G), NaCl (S5886), CNT(687804), 99.9% acetic acid(9012-76-4), Poly-L-Lysine(P4707) were purchased from Sigma-Aldrich. NaHCO3 (3506-01), Na2HPO4 (3828-01), KH2PO4 (3246-01), EDTA (8991-01) and KCl (4001-01) were purchased from J.T. Baker (America).

B. *Preparation of Purified CNTs*

MWCNTs was purified by mixed strong acid with sulfuric acid and nitric acid which proportion is 3:2 under 100 ° C for 3 hours. After acid treatment method we repeatedly washed MWCNTs with milli-Q water by vacuum air pump until that pH value reached to neutral (pH = 7) and put it in the oven to dry for 24 hours. That obtained high purity MWCNTs[1].

C. *Preparation of Chitosan Film*

The primary preparation procedure of 3.5wt% solution of chitosan were as follows. Both 3.5 g of chitosan and 1.2 ml of 0.2 M acetate were dissolved into 100 ml of milli-Q water under 50°C for 24 hours. Based on dry-wet process, take different milliliters of chitosan solution on a dish and a microscope slide, placed in ventilated place for 24 hours until the solvent has evaporated. The sample was then placed in oven of 50 ° C for 24 hours. The films were soaked into a solution of 1 M NaOH for 24 hours and washed with a large amount of milli-Q water repeatedly

* Corresponding author.

I. Lackovic (ed.), *1st Global Conference on Biomedical Engineering & 9th Asian-Pacific Conference on Medical and Biological Engineering*, IFMBE Proceedings 47, DOI: 10.1007/978-3-319-12262-5_10

more than twice to remove the residual NaOH. The films were immersed in phosphate buffer solutions until that pH value reached to neutral (pH = 7), then put into the auto dry cabinet.

D. Preparation of MWCNTs with Chitosan Film

The primary preparation procedure of 3.5wt% solution of chitosan with MWCNTs was as follows. All the 3.5 g of chitosan, 1.2 ml of 0.2 M acetate and different grams of MWCNTs were dissolved into 100 ml of milli-Q water under 50°C for 24 hours. Based on dry-wet process, different milliliters solution of chitosan was took on a dish and a microscope slide. These sample were placed in ventilated place for 24 hours until the solvent has evaporated, then were transferred in oven of 50 ° C for 24 hours. The films were soaked into a solution of 1M NaOH for 24 hours, then washed with a large amount of milli-Q water repeatedly at least twice to remove the residual NaOH. The films were immersed in phosphate buffer solutions until that pH value reached to neutral (pH = 7), then put into the auto dry cabinet.

E. Characteristics of MWCNTs and Chitosan Film

Contact Angle Meter was used to detect the properties of MWCNTs and chitosan film. To identify the material as hydrophilicity or hydrophobe, the contact angle was measured when water dropping on the material. The contact angle was calculated as follows [2]:

$$(2 * (\frac{3*\text{volume}*\sin D^3}{\pi*[(1-\cos D)^2*(2+\cos D)]})^{\frac{1}{3}})$$

F. Dispersion Test

The MWCNTs have been uniformly dispersed state after modification. The original and modified MWCNTs were placed in separate glass bottles containing milli-Q water and stood on a stable platform for observation.

III. RESULTS

A. Preparation of Chitosan Film

Two kinds of chitosan film preparation were created in this study that one was the dish film and the other was microscope slide film.

Table 1 Characteristics of Chitosan dish Film

Liquid volume (ml)	Thickness(mm)
5	0.1112
4	0.0900
3	0.0537
2	0.0425
1	No films formed

Table 2 Characteristics of Microscope Slide Film

Liquid volume (ml)	Thickness(mm)
5	0.0584
4	0.0559
3	0.0509
2	0.0500
1	0.0109

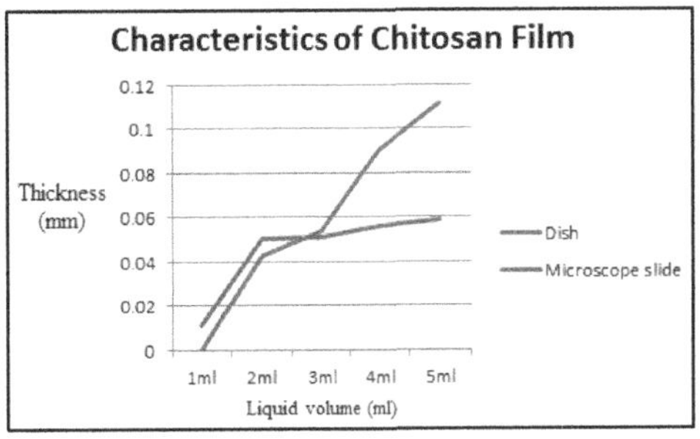

Fig. 1 Characteristics of Chitosan Film

The microscope slide film was exterior, however, the dish film was wrinkling. Comparing the thickness by micrometer caliper, the thickness of the dish film was within range of 0.1112 to 0.0425 mm, and the thickness of the microscope slide film was within range of 0.0584 to 0.0109 mm, The result indicated that the microscope slide film was more suitable for the following biocompatible experiment because the less error value.

B. Contact Angle Analysis

Measuring the contact angle of the chitosan film was in the range within 60~90 deg. That indicated the film had been more hydrophobic. Adding MWCNT significantly made chitosan film more hydrophilicity. It effectively improved the biocompatibility characteristics of chitosan film.

Table 3 Contact Angle Analysis of Dish Film

Liquid volume (ml)	Angle (deg)
5	62.785
4	67.610
3	82.179
2	90.723
1	No film formed

Table 4 Contact Angle Analysis of Microscope Slide Film

Liquid volume (ml)	Angle (deg)
5	93.114
4	95.882
3	67.380
2	68.611
1	77.359

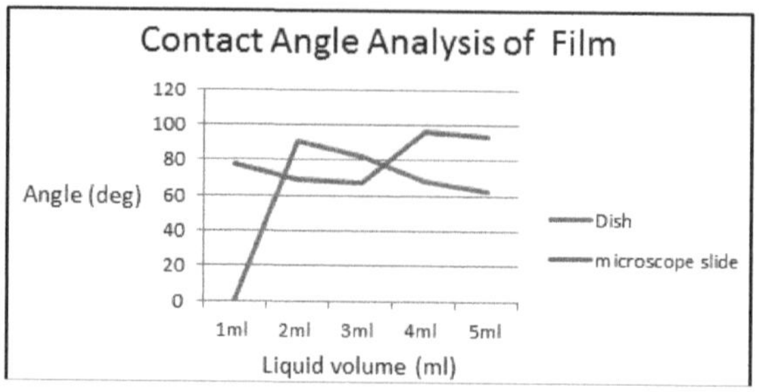

Fig. 2 Characteristics of Chitosan Film

C. *Dispersion Test*

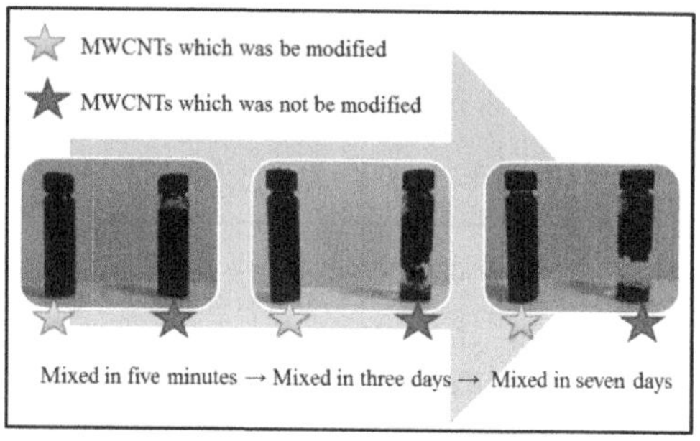

Fig. 3 Dispersion Test

Fig. 3 shows the respective results of dispersion test. Chitosan film modified with MWCNT was obviously not disperse over time. It proved that MWCNTs after acid treatment was successful.

IV. DISCUSSION

Considering the biocompatibility and functions of CNTs, scientists modified CNTs after various manufacture to increase their hydrophilic properties. Thus many compounds such as lipids, DNA and peptides can be adsorbed to the CNTs' surface. If a loner time attachment is desired, the nanotubes may instead of CNTs to covalently link to. Incubating nanotubes with strong oxidizing agents, like nitric acid, is most often used to add carboxyl groups to the ends of the tubes. Other groups are able to be added following. Many modification were carried out previous[3,4].

The new materials designed in this study were for neuron regeneration. Compounds able to promote neuron growth are of interest, such as nerve growth factor (NGF). In our preliminary study, the new materials were less cytotoxicity and were a good base to attach NGF (data not shown). Similar study was carried out by Matsumoto et al. in 2007[5]. However, many relative studies are going on to increase the value of the new materials created form this study.

V. CONCLUSIONS

Currently, the preparation of the film and the MWCNT has been completed. The film was further examined the surface properties then modified with NGF. Then several biocompatible tests will be carried out recently.

CONFLICT OF INTEREST

The authors declare that they have no conflict of interest.

REFERENCES

1. Yubing Wang,Zafar Iqbal and Somenath Mitra. Rapidly functionalized, water-dispersed carbon nanotubes at high concentration.J Am Chem Soc. 2006 Jan 11;128(1):95-99.
2. Bo Cang Chio. Chitosan and multi-walled carbon nanotube film with repair of nerve cell . Ming Chuan University.
3. Bekyarova, E.; Haddon, RC.; Parpura, V. Biofunctionalization of carbon nanotubes. In: Kumar, CSSR., editor. Biofunctionalization of nanomaterials (nanotechnologies for the life sciences). Vol.1. Wiley; 2005.
4. . Bekyarova E, Ni Y, Malarkey EB, Montana V, McWilliams JL, Haddon RC, Parpura V. Applications of carbon nanotubes in biotechnology and biomedicine. J Biomed Nanotechnol 2005;1:3–17
5. Matsumoto K, Sato C, Naka Y, Kitazawa A, Whitby RL, Shimizu N. Neurite outgrowths of neurons with neurotrophin-coated carbon nanotubes. J Biosci Bioeng 2007;103:216–220.

Author: Wei Chen Liao
Institute: Department of Biomedical Engineering, Ming Chuan University
Street: No.5, Deming Rd.
City: Taoyuan
Country: Taiwan
Email: 00670671@mail.mcu.edu.com.tw

Novel Zwitterionic Nanocomposite Hydrogel as Effective Chronic Wound Healing Dressings

Kang-Ting Huang[1] and Chun-Jen Huang[1,2,*]

[1] Graduate Institute of Biomedical Engineering, National Central University, Jhong-Li, Taoyuan 320, Taiwan
[2] Chemical & Materials Engineering Department, National Central University, Jhong-Li, Taoyuan 320, Taiwan

Abstract— **We have synthesized and characterized a novel zwitterionic nanocomposite hydrogel as effective chronic wound healing dressings. The hydrogel is composited of non-fouling zwitterionic polymer as a major composition, plus small quantity of nano-sized clay for improved mechanical strength and in-situ formation silver nanoparticles for anti-microbial function. The novel zwitterionic nanocomposite hydrogel possesses unique features, including 1. biocmpatibility; 2. high water content; 3. anti-biofouling properties; 4. strong durability; 5. suppression of bacterial growth; 6. controlled release of Ag ions. These features allow developed formulation becoming extraordinary chronic wound dressing for clinical applications.The hydrogel was fabricated via a "one-pot synthesis" approach and the physicochemical properties were characterized detail. Moreover, the antifouling properties of hydrogels were evaluated in contact with a protein and bacterial solutions.**

Keywords— **Zwitterionic hydrogel, chronic wound healing dressings, silver nanoparticles, antifouing properties.**

I. INTRODUCTION

The management for the chronic wounds, such as pressure sore, diabetic foot wound and vein/arterial ulceration wound, is a critical issue and remains great challenge in the medical care. They exist long healing time (>12 weeks) and persistent wound infection. So far, the commercial wound dressing products on the market are insufficient for rapid and scar-less healing at reasonable cost with minimal inconvenience to the patient. Generally, the ideal wound dressings should provide a warm moist environment, removal of excess exudate and prevention of harmful bacteria into the wound. Besides, the anti-fouling properties of dressings are realized of importance in healing, especially during frequent change of dressing in clinical practices. Currently, a new emerging class of polymeric biomaterials, called zwitterionic polymers, has attracted a great deal attention due to its superhydrophilic and charge-balanced characteristics, which are primary factors for antifouling materials. These zwitterionic materials have been used for resisting biofouling of proteins, cells and bacteria, showing their excellent and advantageous capabilities over traditional poly(ethylene glycol) (PEG).The hydrogel based wound healing dressing can effectively retain hydration of micro-environment for injured wound and promote the healing process. Besides to nonfouling properties, the zwitterionic hydrogels were recognized as the best materials to adsorb and storage water. The achievement has not been accomplished by other types of hydrophilic materials. However, the weak mechanical strength of hydrogel typically is unfavorable for the practical operation for clinical uses. Meanwhile, although the non-sticking properties of zwitterionic hydrogels, the bacteria from patients or environment could not be removed from the surfaces of materials without external forces, such as flowing stream. The adherent bacteria may cluster together and eventually result in the formation of biofilms. Therefore, in this study, we will combine the unique characteristics of the raw materials, i.e. zwitterionic polymer, nano-clay and Ag nanoparticles, together to develop novel zwitterionic nanocomposites for wound dressing, which possess strongly hydrated, non-sticking, mechanically durable and anti-microbial properties for the treatment of chronic wound healing.

II. MATERIALS AND METHODS

A. Materials

The zwitterionic sulfobetaine monomers used here were N,N-dimethyl(acrylamidopropyl) ammonium propanesulfonate(SBAA).2-Hydroxyethyl methacrylate (HEMA) (97%)was purchased from Acros organics.Oxygen dissolved in the purified water was removed by bubbling with nitrogen gas for more than 3 hours prior to use.The SBAA monomer was synthesized in a manner similar to that reported by Seubert et al.

B. Synthesis of Zwitterionic Nanocomposite Hydrogels

Zwitterionic hydrogels were prepared by creating solutions of sulfobetaine acrylamide and 2-hydroxyethyl methacrylate monomers in deionized water. The concentration of

* Corresponding author.

I. Lackovic (ed.), *1st Global Conference on Biomedical Engineering & 9th Asian-Pacific Conference on Medical and Biological Engineering*,
IFMBE Proceedings 47, DOI: 10.1007/978-3-319-12262-5_11

monomer was 50% by weight. To these solutions, the clay (Laponite, XLS, Rockwood) was added at a weight ratio of 5 % and silver nitrate was 0.01M. For the crosslinker addition, the crosslinker Poly(ethylene glycol) methyl ether methacrylate was added at a cross-linker ratio of 1 % mole ratio to monomer. After sonication in an ice bath to prevent premature polymerization, the initiator, potassium persulfate,was added at 1M to the solutions and the catalyst,TEMED, 1ml homogenized by stirring at ice water temperature. Then, using UV 362 nm to reduce silver nanoparticle on clays surface within the hydrogel networks for 2 hours. Finally, free-radical polymerization was then allowed to proceed for 20 h at room temperature. The gels were then removed from the slides and immersed in phosphate-buffered saline (PBS) to hydrate. This hydration water was changed daily for 5 days to remove unreacted chemicals and excess salt.

C. Characterization of Silver Nanoparticle Formation of Hydrogels

The Ag nanoparticles in the hydrogels were characterized by UV-vis absorption using a JASCO V-630 spectrophotometer. The UV absorption was measured at the concentration of 0.1 g crushed sample in 3.0 ml of distilled water. The range of scanning was set from 300 nm to 800 nm.

D. Swelling Ratio of Hydrogels in Difference Solution

The nanocomposite hydrogels are placed in the presence of the solutions of difference salt concentration for determining the water absorbing properties of materials. The dried hydrogels is immersed in deionized water (ddH2O), phosphate buffered saline (PBS) and aqueous solution containing 1M NaCl for 48 hours at room temperature on a roller mixer. After swelling, the hydrogels are dried in oven 60°C for 1 day and under vacuum 60 °C 1 day. The swelling is calculated as follows:

$$Swelling(\varphi)=(W_s-W_d)/W_s*100\% \qquad (1)$$

Where W_s and W_d represent weights of swollen and dried hydrogels, respectively

E. Measurement of Mechanical Property of Hydrogels

Compressive properties of each hydrogel were determined using an Instron 4467 mechanical tester with a 10N load cell. Cylindrical samples with a size of 1 cm in diameter and ~1 cm height are compressed to failure at a rate of 1 mm/min. The modulus was calculated from the linear portion of the stress-strain curves.

F. Anti-protein Fouling Properties of Hydrogels

The adsorption of bovine serum albumin (BSA) on the hydrogel disks was evaluated using the enzyme-linked immunosorbent assay (ELISA) method. The ELISA measurement was repeated using six independent disks (n = 3 in total)for each hydrogel substrate and the average result was reported.

G. Anti-bacterial Fouling Property of Hydrogels

Staphylococcus epidermidis was used to investigate bacterial adhesion behavior on the surface of hydrogels. *S. epidermidis* was cultured in a Luria–Bertani solution over night. These cultures were incubated at 37 °C and were shaken at 100 rpm.Then,centrifugation of bacterial solution,4000 rpm,10mins,to transfer bacterial suspension into PBS buffer.Dilution of bacterial suspension concentration with UV-vis absorption 670 nm to 0.1. The hydrogel disks were incubated with 75 wt % ethanol for 1 h at 25 °C and washed by PBS 3 times in a 24-well plate. A total of 2 mL of bacteria suspension was added to sample. The bacteria were then incubated with the samples for 3 hours in incubator, 37 °C, CO_2 . The bacterial solution was removed after 3 hours and each sample was then washed with PBS 3 times to remove the attached bacteria. Bacteria adhering to the sample surfaces were stained with 20 μL of Live/Dead BacLight for 10 min. After washing with PBS three times, samples with stained bacteria were observed with a CCD camera mounted on CCD-Cool SNAP camera (Roper scientific, Inc., USA) and epifluorescent illumination through a FITC filter.

H. Anti-bacterial Property of Hydrogels

The anti-bacterial effect of hydrogels involving honey was examined on agar plates inoculated with *Staphylococcus epidermidis(S.epidermidis)* and *Pseudomonas aeruginosa(P. aeruginosa)* by using the inhibition of zone tests. The anti-bacterial experiment were prepared by smearing with 2 mL freshly grown bacterial inoculums and put on several the hydrogels(1 x 1 cm^2) on plate, then incubated at 37 °C in incubator1 for 12 h.

III. RESULTS AND DISCUSSION

A. Silver Nanoparticle Formation in Hydrogels

In Fig. 1, samples of SBAA hydrogel and hydrogel containing Ag nanoparticles were examined using a UV-vis spectrophotometer to confirm the existence of Ag. As shown, the clear absorption at λ=398 nm is observed for the sample of SBAA+Ag, which reflects the reduction of Ag^0 from Ag^+ during the polymerization of SB materials.

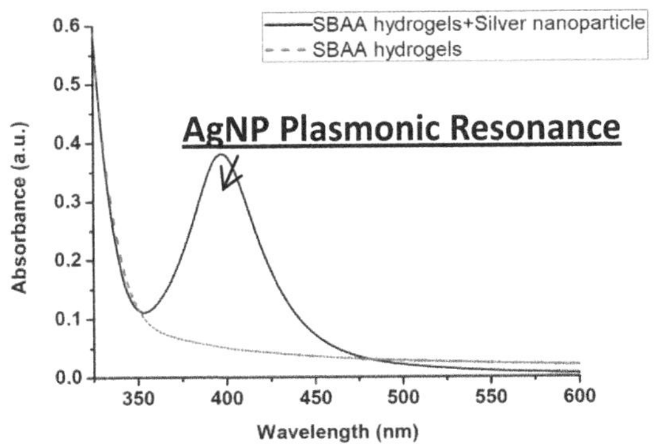

Fig. 1 The UV-vis spectroscopic spectrum for SBAA and SBAA+Ag nanocomposite hydrogels.

B. Swelling Ratio of Hydrogels in Difference Solution

We prepared nanocomposite hydrogels from SBAA, SBAA with silver nanoparticles in comparison with HEMA. The samples were immersed in deionized water, PBS and 1M NaCl solutions for 48 h, followed by weighting for swelling ratios. The different hydrogels swelling ratios in difference solutions were shown in Fig. 2. The swelling ratios for SBAA in DI, PBS and 1N NaCl are $\varphi = 77\pm0.4$ %, 84 ± 0.3 % and 84 ± 0.3 %. The swelling ratios for SBAA with silver nanoparticles in DI, PBS and 1N NaCl are $\varphi = 75\pm0.2$ %,85 ± 1.3 % and 84 ± 1.4 %. The swelling ratios for HEMA in DI, PBS and 1N NaCl are $\varphi =$ and 72 ± 1.5 %, 61 ± 0.1 % and 56 ± 0.9 %.

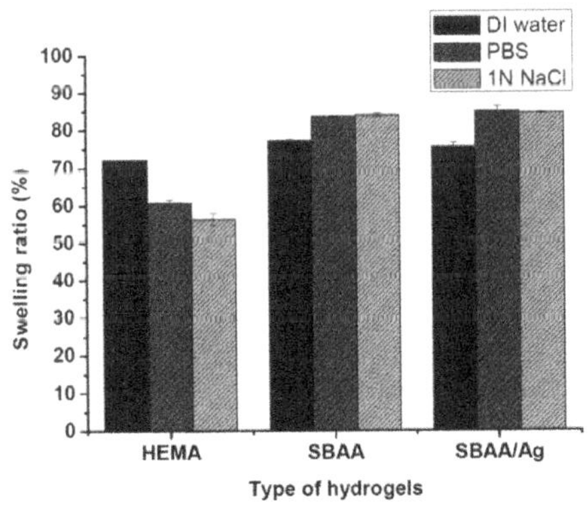

Fig. 2 Hydrogel swelling ratios in difference solutions.

Obviously, the swelling ratios change with composition of gels and environments. The SBAA-based materials exhibited higher water contents in all conditions than HEMA-based materials. Presence of silver nanoparticles does not influence the hydration of nanocomposites significantly. Meanwhile, the finding indicates that the nanocomposite hydrogels absorbed water molecules in high ionic strength environments, such as PBS, particular for the SBAA-based hydrogels. This proves the unique properties of zwitterionic materials, i.e. the "anti-polyelectrolyte effect"[1] the ion-induced hydration enables us to manipulate the architecture and conformation of zwitterionic materials to be responsive smart polymeric devices for future applications.

C. Measurement of Compression Modulus of Hydrogels

The zwitterionic hydrogels studied so far have shown low mechanical strength, which limits their potential biological uses[2]. So,we added clay into zwitterionic hydrogels to improve stiffness of materials.In Fig. 3, we added difference weight percentage of clay in hydrogels and measure the compressive modulus.

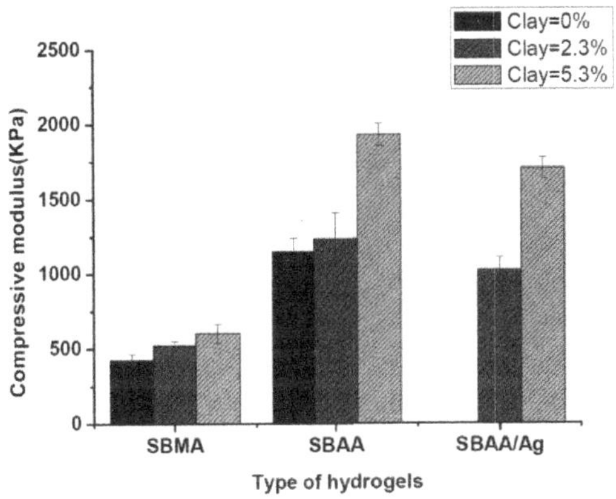

Fig. 3 The compressive modulus histogram of difference weight percentage clay in hydrogels.

In Fig. 3,we can find the positive correlation of compressive modulus when clay percentage increases in all hydrogels. But the compressive modulus of SBAA-based hydrogels exhibited higher compressive modulus than SBMA-based hydrogels. In the Zhao et al. study, they proved the acrylamide structure have more hydrogen bond between water molecules than acrylate structure. So, we suggested acrylamide exhibits inter/intra molecular interaction via hydrogen boding.

D. Anti-protein Fouling Properties of Hydrogels

In the present work, we investigated the non-specific protein adsorption of bovin serum albumin(BSA) on the hydrogel. The adsorption of BSA on the hydrogel was evaluated using the enzyme-linked immunosorbent assay (ELISA) method. The result in the Fig. 4.

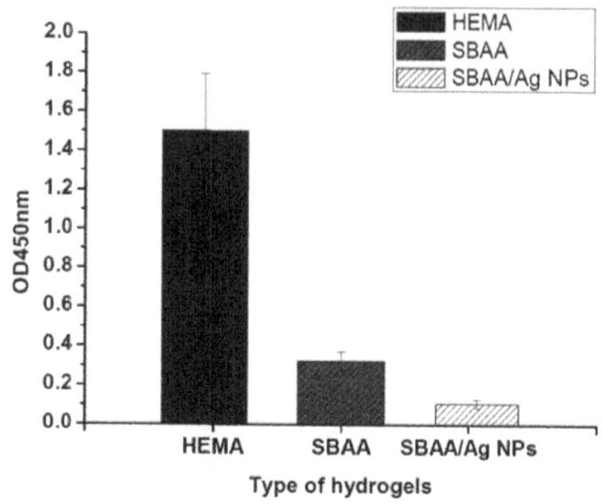

Fig. 4 The relative comparison of protein adsorption on hydrogels surface was evaluate by ELISA,detected absorption on 450nm.

From Fig. 4, the hydrogels of SBAA and SBAA/Ag NPs have lower degree of protein adsorption than HEMA hydrogel. So,we suggested that the hydrogels of SBAA and SBAA/Ag NPs can reduce protein fouling when frequency change wound dressings.

E. Anti-bacterial Fouling Property of Hydrogels

In Fig. 9, *S. epidermidis* was in contact with SBAA (left)and HEMA(right) hydrogel for 3 h, and observed under fluorescence microscope after staining. The amount of adherent bacteria on HEMA hydrogel was significantly higher than that on SBAA hydrogel. We nearly cannot see the existence of bacteria on SBAA hydrogel, which proves the excellent antifouling properties of pSBAA hydrogels.

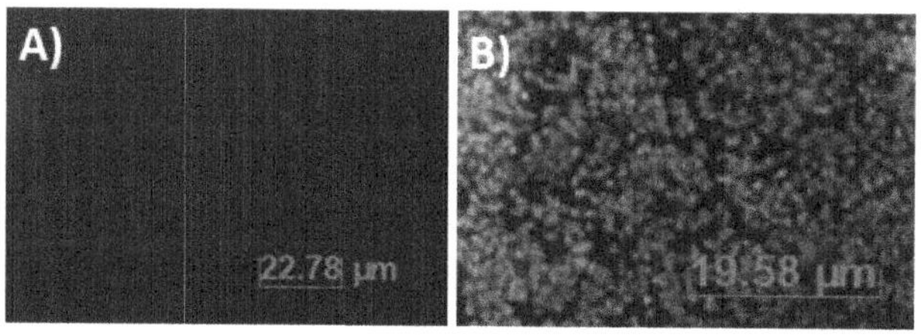

Fig. 5 The *S. epidermidis* was in contact with SBAA hydrogel (a) and HEMA hydrogel (b) for 3 hours, and observed under fluorescence microscope after staining.

F. Anti-bacterial Property of Hydrogels

In Fig. 6 shows the effectiveness of nanocomposite hydrogels to kill bacteria on agar plates. The parallel comparison experiment was performed with SBAA/MA hydrogel without reduction of Ag nanoparticles and SBAA/MA nanocomposite with Ag nanoparticles . The white hazy areas indicate bacterial growth, whilst the more transparent areas surrounding the Ag nanocomposite hydrogel indicate bacteria free region or zones of inhibition. This result provides strong evidence of anti-microbial properties of nanocomposite hydrogels arising due to the presence of the Ag nanoparticles.

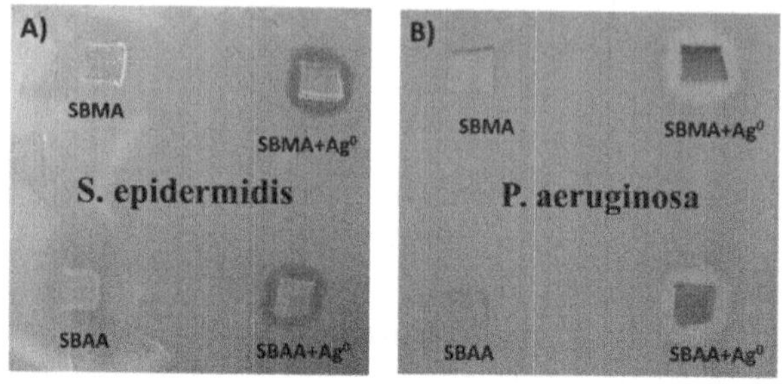

Fig. 6 The *S. epidermidis*(A) *and P. aeruginosa*(B) was in contact with SBAA/MA and SBAA/MA+Ag hydrogel.

IV. Conclusion

In this work, we successfully synthesized novel nonfouling zwitterionic nanocomposite hydrogels and present the functions of materials as wound dressing. The zwitterionic nanocomposite hydrogels have higher water absorption than nonionic hydrophilic hydrogel in physiological environment (i.e. PBS). In the bio-fouling tests, the zwitterionic nanocomposite hydrogels can reduce bovine serum protein and *S. epidermidis* to adsorption on surface. We confirmed the presence of Ag nanoparticles in the network of hydrogel by using UV-vis spectroscope. This nanocomposite hydrogel exhibits excellent capability to repress the growth of bacteria.Finally, the mechanical property of hydrogel was enhanced by adding clay to increase durability in operation. This novel zwitterionic nanocomposite hydrogel has potential to become a new generation of chronic wounds dressing.

Acknowledgment

This work was supported by the National Science Council (NSC101-2911-I-008-001).

References

1. Lowe,A.B.,N.C. Billingham, and S.P. Armes et al. (1999) *Synthesis and properties of Low-Polydispersity Poly(sulfopropylbetaine)s and Their Block Copolymer*. Macromolecules, 32(7):2141-2148
2. Zhang, Z.,T. Chao,and S. Jiang et al. (2008) *Physical, Chemical, and Chemical-Physical Double Network of Zwitterionic Hydrogels*. The Journal of PhysicalChemistryB,112(17):5327-5332

The Transfectability and Cell Motility on Materials with Different Physico-chemical Properties

Nien-Chi Huang[1] and Shan-Hui Hsu[1,2,*]

[1] Institute of Polymer Science and Engineering, National Taiwan University, Taipei, Taiwan
[2] Research Center for Developmental Biology and Regenerative Medicine, National Taiwan University, Taipei, Taiwan

Abstract— **Gene delivery by non-viral vectors is limited by cytotoxicity. In this study, we transferred plasmid DNA into stem cells by seeding cells on substrates with different physico-chemical properties. Gene entry was facilitated by the activation of integrins and cell motility on different material surface. The finding could be used to screen materials that promote cell migration and endocytosis.**

Keywords— **substrates, gene delivery, cell motility, integrin.**

I. INTRODUCTION

Cells are very sensitive to the cell culture surface. Substrate topography can modulate stem cell function and endocytosis [1]. The culture substrates can enhance mesenchymal stem cells forming three-dimensional spheroids and facilitate the transfection efficiency [2]. The topography may also activate the integrins. The distribution and turnover of integrin receptors influence cell behavior and endocytosis [3,4]. Knockdown of integrin β1 by siRNA inhibits the cell migration and endocytosis [5].

Since substrates can modulate integrin receptor [3] and endocytosis [2] while integrin receptor is associated with endocytosis and migration [5], we assume that substrates that promote cell motility may mediate endocytosis (Fig 1a). In this study, the migration and gene transfer of human umbilical cord mesenchymal stem cells (UCMSCs) were investigated on substrates with different physico chemical features. This could be used to design materials for promoting gene delivery.

II. WRITING THE PAPER

A. Preparation of Hyaluronan-Modified Chitosan (CS-HA) Membranes

The Chitosan powder molecular weight was ~ 510 kDa and the degree of deacetylation was ~77%. Hyaluronan molecular weight was about 2,500 kDa. To prepare CS-HA membranes, chitosan was dissolved in 1% acetic acid, and coated on coverslip glass (~300 µl). After dry, the HA solution (3mg/ml, ~300 µl) was dropped onto the glass. The CS-HA coated coverslip glass was crosslinking by ethyl(dimethylaminopropyl) carbodiimide/N-hydroxysuccinimide for 48 h and then washed with PBS before the cell study.

B. Preparation of Polyurethane (PU) Films and Grooves

To prepare PU films (Flat), 300 µl of PU dispersion was directly coated on coverslip glass. To prepare PU grooves (Groove), templates were first made of micropatterned silicon wafer (microgrooves with 3 µm depth and the aligned ridges and grooves with spacing size of 20 µm). Poly(dimethylsiloxane) (PDMS) was used to produce the submaster templates. The PDMS templates were covered by 2.5 ml of PU dispersion and the coverslip glass was placed on the template to print the pattern. After dried, the coverslip glass with PU grooves was removed from the templates.

C. Electrospinning of PU Random Fibers and Aligned Fibers

Thin PU films were first cast on coverslip glass from 100 µl of PU dispersion at 5000 rpm for 20 s. On the thin PU films, random and aligned PU fibers were deposited by electrospinning. Dried PU was dissolved in a co-sovlent comprising 2,2,2-Trifluoroethanol (TFE) and N,N-Dimethylacetamide (DMAc) (TFE:DMAc= 54.5:35.5 weight ratio) to achieve a concentration of 10 wt% PU. The flow rate was fixed at 10 µl/min and the high-voltage power supply was set at 20 kV. For random fibers (ES), the coated glass was placed on an aluminum plate at a distance of 32 cm for collection. For aligned fibers (Aligned-ES), the coated glass was taped on a rotating disk at a distance of 5 cm with a rotation speed of 900 rpm. The collection time was 20 min for both fibers.

D. Stem Cell Culture and Transfection of Plasmid DNA

Human UCMSCs (BIONET Corp) were used passages 6 to 8 for the study. UCMSCs were seeded (5×10^4 cells) onto different substrates and cultured with 1 ml of serum-free medium that contained 1 µg naked GATA4 plasmid (encoded GFP fluorescence is shown in Fig. 1b) for 12 h and then the medium was changed to 10% serum-containing medium without plasmids. At 60 h after cell seeding, cells were collected for gene expression experiment. Real-time RT-PCR was used to analyze the gene expression. The

* Corresponding author.

I. Lackovic (ed.), *1st Global Conference on Biomedical Engineering & 9th Asian-Pacific Conference on Medical and Biological Engineering*,
IFMBE Proceedings 47, DOI: 10.1007/978-3-319-12262-5_12

expression of ITGα5, and ITGβ1 were determined at 12 h, and for the expression of GATA4 were determined at 60 h. All expression levels were normalized to GAPDH.

E. Analysis of Cell Migration

For time-lapse examination of UCMSCs motility, the data were recorded by a real-time Cultured Cell Monitoring System for 48 h at 10 min intervals. Cell migration distance was determined by the ImageJ software. The cell migration rate was calculated as the travelling distance divided by the total recording time (60 h).

III. RESULTS

The morphology of UCMSCs cultured with the naked GATA4 plasmid on TCPS, CS-HA, Flat, ES, Aligned-ES, and Groove for 24 h are shown in Fig. 2a. UCMSCs on CS-HA formed spheroids and those on TCPS and ES were attached with fully spread morphology. In contrast, a part of cells formed spheroids and the other part of cells were attached with spread morphology on Flat, aligned-ES, and Groove.

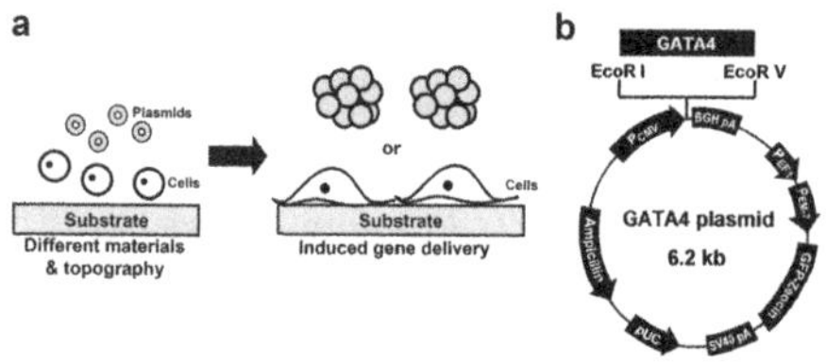

Fig. 1 (a) Schematics of the different materials and topography inducing naked gene delivery. (b) The structure map of the GATA4 plasmid DNA.

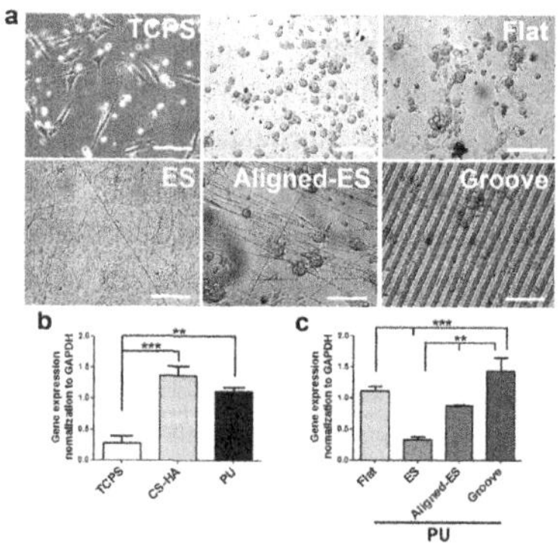

Fig. 2 (a) The morphology of UCMSCs cultured on TCPS, CS-HA, PU Flat, ES, Aaligned-ES, and Groove. (b,c) Transfectability of UCMSCs expressed as the level of GATA4 gene expression on different materials. The statistical significance difference was evaluated by one-way analysis of variance (ANOVA). **, p< 0.01; ***, p< 0.001.

The GATA4 expression levels of UCMSCs after transfection of the naked GATA4 plasmid on various materials are shown in Fig. 2b-c. In particular, cells transfected on CS-HA, Flat, Aligned-ES and Groove showed more GATA4 expression than those on TCPS and ES.

The ITGβ1 and ITGα5 gene expressions of UCMSCs for 12 h on various materials are shown in Fig. 3a-d. The gene expression of ITGα5 had the same tendency as that of ITGβ1 on different materials. The highest expression levels of these two genes were observed on Groove. The migration rate of UCMSCs cultured on various materials for 60 h is shown in Fig. 3e-f. The cell migration rates on CS-HA and on Groove were similar (~150 μm/h). Cells on TCPS and ES migrated slower (~80 μm/h) than those on the other materials.

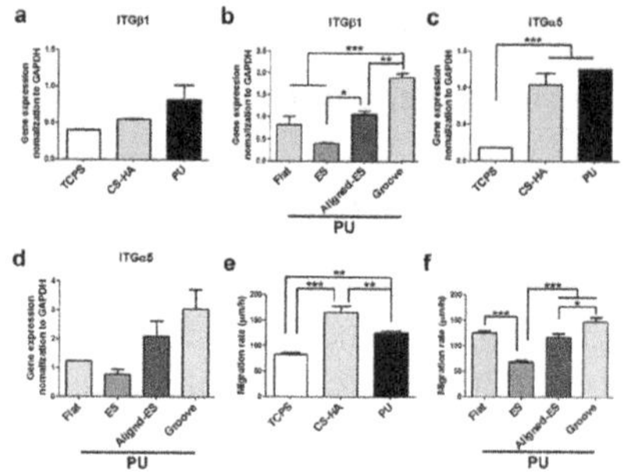

Fig. 3 The expression of integrin at 12 h post cell seeding, including that of (a,b) ITGβ1, and (c,d) ITGα5 on different materials. (e,f) The cell migration rate on different materials. *, p<0.05; **, p<0.01; ***, p<0.001.

IV. DISCUSSION

Previous literature has explored the surface designs of material to affect cell function [6] and improve gene delivery [7]. The surface structures may also play a key role in gene delivery and cell morphology. The activation of integrins can affect the cell motility and endocytosis [5].

We hypothesized that the surface properties of a culture substrate may change the cell morphology and then affect the endocytosis. Cells that formed spheroids may move faster and enhance the transfection efficiency. We also suggested that different integrins may be activated by the substrate materials, changing cell motility and endocytosis.

V. CONCLUSIONS

Substrate materials may be designed to increase the transfection of GATA4 plasmid into UCMSCs. The materials with unique physico-chemical properties can activate the integrins and affect the cell motility, thereby enhancing the transfectability.

CONFLICT OF INTEREST

The authors declare that they have no conflict of interest.

REFERENCES

1. Kong HJ, Hsiong S, and Mooney DJ (2007) Nano Lett 7:161-166.
2. Hsu Sh, Ho TT, and Tseng TC (2012) Biomaterials 33:3639-3650.
3. Webb DJ, Parsons JT, and Horwitz AF (2002) Nat Cell Biol 4: E97-E100.
4. Caswell P, and Norman J (2008) Trend Cell Biol 18:257-263.
5. Chao WT, and Kunz J (2009) FEBS Lett 583:1337-1343.
6. Kim DH, Han K, Gupta K et al. (2009) Biomaterials 30:5433-5444. 7. Teo BKK, Goh SH, Kustandi TS et al. (2011) Biomaterials 32:9866-9875.
7. Teo BKK, Goh SH, Kustandi TS et al. (2011) Biomaterials 32:9866-9875.

Author: Nien-Chi Huang
Institute: Institute of Polymer Science and Engineering,
Street: No. 1, Sec. 4, Roosevelt Road
City: Taipei
Country: Taiwan
Email: yuemoon27@hotmail.com

In Situ Circular Compression and Doppler Optical Coherence Tomography Studies on Effects of Diabetic Mellitus on Vesa Nervonum of Sciatic Nerve

Eric Chia[1], Chou-Chin Lin[2], Chung-Yi Sue[1], and Ming-Shaung Ju[1,*]

[1] Department of Mechanical Engineering, National Cheng Kung University, Tainan, Taiwan
[2] Department of Neurology, National Cheng Kung University Hospital, Tainan, Taiwan

Abstract— **Diabetes mellitus is one of the most common diseases in the world and can causemany types of neuropathies, and even mortality. It is therefore important to understand how diabetes mellitus alters the mechanical properties of nerve tissues and their blood vessels. In this study, in situ compression-and-hold circular compression tests were applied to the sciatic nerves of both diabetic rats and normal rats. Doppler optical coherence tomography (Doppler OCT) was then utilized to monitor the configuration of the arterioles in two groups of rats. The force data acquired in the compression tests were fitted by using Fung's quasi-linear viscoelastic model (QLV) to determine the viscoelasticity of the nerves. The results show that the nerves in the diabetic group had a longer relaxation time than those in the normal group. Consequently, the Doppler OCT observations reveal that in contrast to the normal arterioles, the diabetic arterioles did not dilate in the relaxation phase. The results of the force data integrated with the corresponding arteriole dilatation images may explain why the diabetic patients are more prone to carpal tunnel syndrome. The results may facilitate developing new approaches for treating diabetic neuropathy and for nerve repair and regeneration.**

Keywords— **diabetic mellitus, nerve tissue, arterioles, quasi-linear viscoelasticity, Doppler optical coherence tomography.**

I. INTRODUCTION

Diabetes mellitus is one of the most common diseases in the world and can cause many types of neuropathies, and even mortality. Diabetes induces abnormalities in the blood vessels within nerve tissues and causes nerve ischemia, which leads to a degeneration of the nerve fiber. In developing new treatments for diabetes, it is therefore important to understand how diabetes mellitus alters the mechanical properties of nerves and their blood vessels.

Sunderland and Walsh [1] investigated the axial stress-strain properties of human nerves removed from autopsy specimens within 12 hours. The results showed that the peripheral nerve trunks elongated elastically with an increasing load to a certain point and then showed a semi-plastic deformation behavior thereafter. Rydevik and Lundborg [2, 3] used a specially designed compression chamber to examine the variation of the nerve conduction speed due to external pressure. It was shown that under a pressure of 200-400 mmHg, the nerve was injured even when the pressure was applied for only a few minutes. Kwan and Hanno [4] examined the viscoelastic property of living nerves, but did not consider how the material constants of the nerves could be determined using a viscoelastic model. In general, the above studies investigated the mechanical properties of nerves and try to explain how traumas result in nerve tissue injury. However, chronic diseases, e.g., diabetes mellitus, are another important category of etiologies in causing neuropathies.

In our past studies [5], *in situ* compression-and-hold circular compression was used to analyzed the material properties of diabetic nerves using Fung's QLV model [6]. The results revealed that in contrast to normal nerves, diabetic nerves took a longer time to reach equilibrium during the relaxation phase. However, the study did not consider the effect of compression on arterioles (vesa nervonum).

Accordingly, in this study, the compression-and-hold testing device is integrated with the Doppler optical coherence tomography (**OCT**) to acquire the force responses and corresponding images of arterioles of nerves in both diabetic rats as well as normal rats. The main goal of this study is to investigate the differences of responses to compression in diabetic and normal arterioles within their sciatic nerves.

II. MATERIALS AND METHODS

A. Samples Preparation

The present experiments were performed using a normal and a diabetic neuropathic Wistar rats with weights ranging from 550-700 g. Diabetes mellitus was induced in the six rats by means of a single injection of streptozotocin (STZ) three months prior to the experiments. All of the rats were anesthetized by injecting 0.05 ml/100 g of Zoletil- 50, and a cut with a length of around 5-7 cm was made at the lateral thigh in order to reveal the sciatic nerve. The nerve was encircled by a polypropylene (PP) sheet and the rat was then transferred to the experimental system shown in Fig. 1 in order to perform the compression tests.

* Corresponding author.

I. Lackovic (ed.), *1st Global Conference on Biomedical Engineering & 9th Asian-Pacific Conference on Medical and Biological Engineering*,
IFMBE Proceedings 47, DOI: 10.1007/978-3-319-12262-5_13

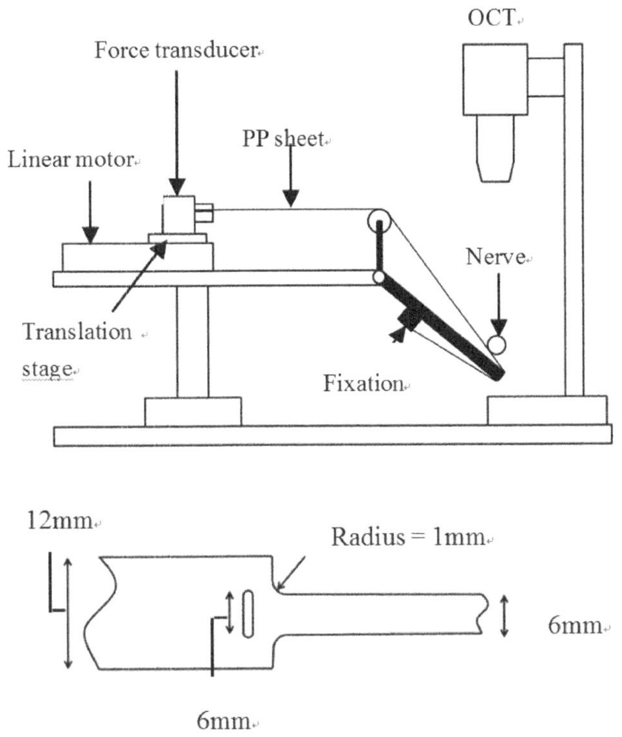

Fig 1. Circular compression apparatus and OCT setup and the geometry of polypropylene (PP) sheet

B. Experimental Setup

Prior to each compression test, the nerve was preconditioned by repeated (6 times) cyclic compression to a strain of 0.1 at the strain rate 0.01 s^{-1} in order to stabilize the internal structure of the nerve[6]. Compression-and-hold tests were performed to obtain the stress and strain histories of the sciatic nerves in both the normal and the diabetic rats. The nerve was compressed to a final strain of 0.1 under strain rate of 0.01 s^{-1}. After that the nerve was held at the final strain of 0.1 for 240 s and then the compression force was removed.

For each sample, the force data collected during the three compression tests were converted to the radial compressive stress ($\bar{\sigma}_r$) and strain (ε_r) according to our previous study [5] as:

$$\overline{\sigma}_r = \frac{1}{2\pi r w \mu}\left(T_1 - \frac{T_1}{e^{2\pi\mu}}\right) \quad (1)$$

$$\varepsilon_r = \frac{r_0 - r}{r_0} \quad (2)$$

where T_1 is the tension of the PP sheet, w is the width of the PP sheet, μ is the kinetic friction coefficient between the PP sheet and the nerve, and r and r_0 are the radius of the nerve under tension T_1 and the initial radius of the nerve, respectively.

C. Image and Data Analysis

The cross-sectional images of the sciatic nerves were captured by THORLABS SS-Doppler OCT software and were rendered to image sequence format to better examine the dilatation of the arterioles. The image was then integrated with the stress data in order to establish the relationship between the recorded stress values and the arteriole dilation. Finally, the viscoelasticity of the nerve were fitted by using the QLV model[6], which was described in details in the previous study [5].

III. RESULTS AND DISCUSSIONS

Figure 2 shows the typical stress-strain curve of a normal rat nerve tissue and its corresponding images captured by Doppler OCT. The typical curve fitting result is shown in the lower plot of Figure 2(a). The stress responses are fitted by QLV model with the relaxation time constant $\tau_\varepsilon = 112.9$. From Figure 2(b), the dilatation of the arteriole can be clearly seen in the normal rats. At the beginning, the arteriole collapses due to the compression (Fig. 2(b) i & ii). After 110 seconds (Fig. 2(b) iii), the arteriole dilates gradually and finally returns to its original size after 190 seconds (Fig. 2(b) iv).

Figure 3 shows the typical stress-strain curve of a diabetic rat nerve and its corresponding images captured by Doppler OCT. In contract to the normal rat nerve, in diabetic rat nerve τ_ε value is greater ($\tau_\varepsilon = 1000$), which means the diabetic nerve takes longer time to relax to steady stress state. From Figure 3(b), the arteriole does not dilate even to the end of the recording in the relaxation phase (Fig. 3(b) ii, iii, iv).

The results show that the relaxation time of a nerve will influence the dilatation of arteriole. The arteriole inside a normal nerve dilates at the relaxation phase but that in the diabetic nerve tissue does not. In physiological environment, a nerve is usually compressed by muscle around it. If the material properties of the nerve change, the arterioles will collapse when the muscles contract, just as similar to the condition observed in the experiment. In addition, the dilatability of diabetic blood vessel is smaller than normal blood vessel[7]. This will cause ischemia of the nerve and result in nerve degeneration [2, 3].

The methodology developed in this study may offer an objective and relatively non-invasive way to evaluate the mechanical properties of vessels inside a nerve and the results may help to explain the pathophysiology of diabetic polyneuropathy. Further analyses on the loads on the buckling of arterioles are on-going.

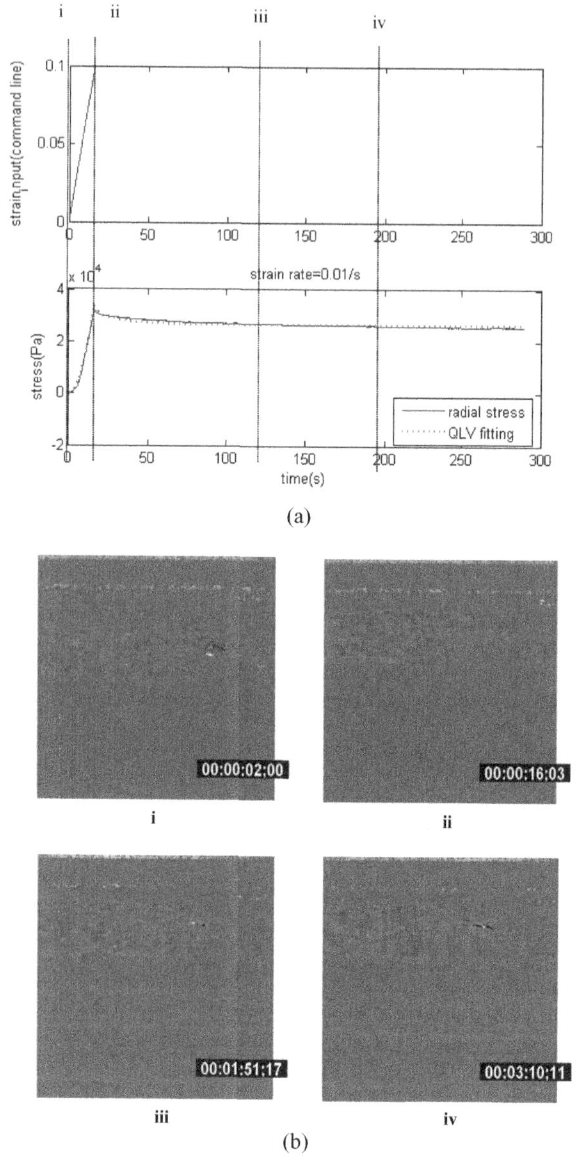

Fig 2. (a) Stress-strain curve of normal nerve tissue measured (blue solid line) and analyzed by QLV model curve fitting (red dotted line). (b) Corresponding tissue images captured by Doppler OCT

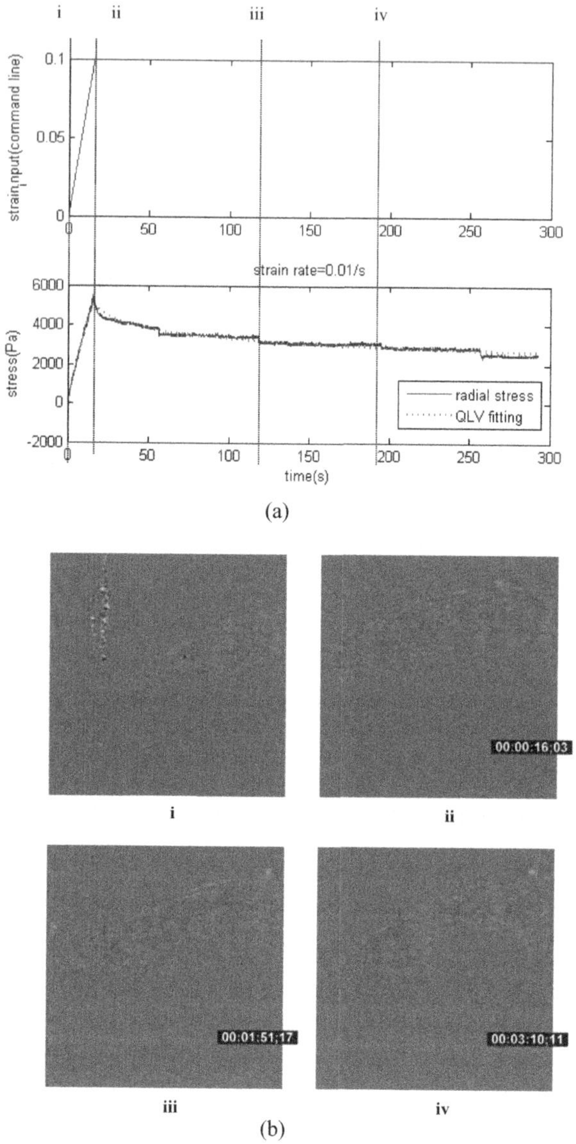

Fig 3. (a) Stress-strain curve of diabetic nerve tissue measured (blue solid line) and analyzed by QLV model curve fitting (red dotted line). (b) Corresponding diabetic tissue images captured by Doppler OCT

IV. CONCLUSIONS

This study has successfully acquired *in situ* force responses of the nerve and corresponding images of arteriole dilatation. The nerve of diabetic rats has a longer relaxation time than that of normal rats and thus the arterioles do not dilate under compression. The nerve tissue in diabetic rats may be prone to ischemia and a lack of nutrient, which may lead to a degeneration of the nerve fiber. This finding may explain why diabetic patients are more prone to compartment syndromes.

ACKNOWLEDGMENT

The support from NSC 102-2221-E-006-025-MY3 of Taiwan is gratefully acknowledged.

CONFLICT OF INTEREST

The authors declare that they have no conflict of interest.

STATEMENT OF ANIMAL RIGHTS

The research protocol was approved by animal ethics committee of National Cheng Kung University.

REFERENCES

1. Sunderland, S (1968) Nerves and nerve injuries. New York: CHURCHILL LIVINGSTONE.
2. Rydevik, B. and G. Lundborg (1977) Permeability of intraneural microvessels and perineurium following acute, graded experimental nerve compression. Scandinavian journal of plastic and reconstructive surgery. 11(3): p. 179-187.
3. Rydevik B Fau and C. Nordborg (1980) Changes in nerve function and nerve fibre structure induced by acute, graded compression. Journan of Neurology Neurosurgery and Psychiatry, (0022-3050 (Print)).
4. Kwan, M.K., et al. (1992) Strain, stress and stretch of peripheral nerve. Rabbit experiments in vitro and in vivo. Acta orthopaedica Scandinavica. 63(3): p. 267-272.
5. Chen, R.J., C.C. Lin et al. (2010) In situ biomechanical properties of normal and diabetic nerves: an efficient quasi-linear viscoelastic approach. J Biomech. 43(6): p. 1118-24.
6. Y.C.Fung (1993) Biomechanics: Mechanical Properties of Living Tissues. 2nd edition ed. New York: Springer-Verlag.
7. Zahnd, G., et al. Intramural shear strain can highlight the presence of atherosclerosis: A clinical in vivo study. in Ultrasonics Symposium (IUS), 2011 IEEE International. 2011.

* Corresponding Author.

Author:	Prof. Ming-Shaung Ju
Institute:	National Cheng Kung University
Street:	No.1, University Road
City:	Tainan
Country:	Taiwan (R.O.C)
Email:	msju@mail.ncku.edu.tw

Characterisation of the Stability and Bio-functionality of Tethered Proteins on Bioengineered Scaffolds: Implications for Stem Cell Biology and Tissue Repair

Ting-Yi Wang[1], Kiara A.F. Bruggeman[2], Rebecca K. Sheean[1], David R. Nisbet[2,*], and Clare L. Parish[1,*]

[1] Florey Institute of Neuroscience & Mental Health, The University of Melbourne, Parkville, Australia, 3010
[2] Research School of Engineering, The Australian National University, Canberra, Australia, 0200

Abstract— **In the context of biological applications, the timely delivery of molecules can be critical for cellular and organ function. As such, previous studies have demonstrated the superior long-term protein delivery, by way of protein tethering onto bioengineered scaffolds, compared to conventional delivery of soluble protein *in vitro* and *in vivo*. Despite such benefits little knowledge exists regarding the stability, release kinetics, longevity, activation of intracellular pathway and functionality of these proteins over time. By way of example, here we examined the stability, degradation and functionality of a protein, glial derived neurotrophic factor (GDNF), which is known to influence neuronal survival, differentiation and neurite morphogenesis. Enzyme-linked immuno-sorbent assays revealed that GDNF, covalently tethered onto polycaprolactone electrospun nanofibrous scaffolds, remained present on the scaffold surface for 120 days, with no evidence of protein leaching or degradation. The tethered GDNF protein remained functional and capable of activating downstream signalling cascades, as revealed by its capacity to phosphorylate intracellular Erk in a neural cell line. Furthermore, immobilisation of GDNF protein promoted cell survival and differentiation in culture at both 3 and 7 days. This study provides important evidence of the stability and functionality kinetics of tethered molecules.**

Keywords— **protein tethering, scaffolds, stability, neurons.**

I. INTRODUCTION

Soluble proteins in their natural physiological environment execute their function and are then degraded by enzymes, oxidation, hydrolysis and other reactions over relatively short periods of time, thereby losing their original bio-functionality. As such, repeated synthesis and delivery from the local environment is required for ongoing activity [1]. Consequently there is increasing interest to develop improved methodologies to enable the stable delivery of molecules and proteins, and to ensure these factors can be administered in temporally and spatially appropriate manners. Work by us has already demonstrated demonstrated that when tethered onto electrospun nanofibrous scaffolds both brain derived neurotrophic factor (BDNF) and glial-cell derived neurotrophic factor (GDNF) were capable of promoting neural stem cell proliferation and influencing differentiation in vitro to a greater extent than culturing cells in the presence of soluble protein [2, 3]. Furthermore, tethered GDNF maintained long-term biofunctionality *in vivo*, supporting the survival, differentiation, and integration of transplanted neural stem cells for up to 28 days [3].

Despite evidence for the benefit of immobilised proteins, little attention has been paid to the amount of protein tethered to biomaterial surfaces, stability and longevity of tethered proteins, activation of intracellular signalling pathway. Here we investigated the stability of a tethered protein, GDNF, its activation of intracellular signalling pathway, and its functionality. GDNF represents an example whereby prolonged protein delivery could have a significant impact on stem cell populations in vitro, disease progression and disease treatment.

II. EXPERIMENTAL PROCEDURES

A. Synthesis of Electrospun Scaffolds and Protein Tethering

Electrospun fibres were produced from polycaprolactone (PCL, Mn 70-90k), dissolved in a 3:1 (v/v) solution of chloroform and methanol respectively. Spinning was performed at room temperature using a 20 kV voltage, a 21G needle, a 2 mL/hr flow rate, and a 13 cm working distance. The scaffolds were then aminolysed by immersion in 0.05 M ethylene diamine (ED), diluted in 2-propanol (Merck Pty) for 15 minutes. For immobilisation of GDNF onto PCL scaffolds, 4-(N-maleimidomethyl) cyclohexane-1-carboxylic acid 3-sulfo-N- hydroxy-succinimide ester sodium salt (sulfo-SMCC) was used as a cross-linker. The PCL scaffolds were immersed in the sulfo-SMCC solution (2.5 mg/mL in PBS) for 2 hours at room temperature, then transferred to a GDNF solution (4 mg/ml) overnight at 4 °C.

B. Enzyme-linked immunoabsorbent assay (ELISA)

Scaffolds were incubated in 1 mg/mL of goat anti-GDNF antibody (R & D Systems) containing 5% donkey serum in PBST (PBS containing 0.05% Tween-20) for 2 hours. The scaffolds were washed three times in PBST before being immersed in anti-goat horseradish peroxidase (HRP, 1:2000 in PBST solution containing 2% donkey serum) for 1 hour. Scaffolds were assessed by colour development using TMB

* Corresponding authors.

I. Lackovic (ed.), *1st Global Conference on Biomedical Engineering & 9th Asian-Pacific Conference on Medical and Biological Engineering*,
IFMBE Proceedings 47, DOI: 10.1007/978-3-319-12262-5_14

microwell peroxidase system (R & D). 30 μl of 1M HCl was added to stop the reaction, and the absorbance (at 450 nm) was measured with a plate reader (SpectraMax).

C. BET Surface Area Analysis of PCL Scaffolds

Brunauer-Emmett-Teller (BET) surface area analysis was performed using a micromeritics TriStar II surface area and porosity instrument to determine the surface area of the scaffolds [4], and subsequently the amount of GDNF tethered onto the PCL surface.

D. Immunoblotting

The dopaminergic neural stem cell line, SN4741, was cultured in DMEM, 10% FBS, L-glutamine (2 mM), penicillin/streptomycin (50 U/ml), and glucose (0.6%). For analysis of intracellular GDNF signalling, 100,000 cells were seeded; and at 70% confluency the cells were changed into serum-free media with or without GDNF (soluble, 30ng/ml or immobilised) prior to being lysed in ice-cold buffer (containing 20 mM Tris-Cl, pH 7.5, 150 mM NaCl, 1% Triton X-100, 1% protease inhibitor cocktail, 50 mM NaF, and 0.2 mM Na_3VO_4) for 20 minutes on ice. Lysates were centrifuged at 14,000 rpm for 20 minute at 4 °C to collect supernatants. Protein was quantified using the bicinchoninic acid assay kit. Protein (50 μg) was electrophoresed through 12.5% SDS polyacrylamide gels and transferred to Immobilon PVDF-FL membarne (Millipore). Membranes were blocked with 5% skim milk in Tris-buffered saline with Tween-20 (TBST), and incubated with mouse pErk1,2 (1:2,000) and rabbit total Erk1,2 (1:1,000) antibodies in 3% BSA in TBST overnight at 4 °C. Blots were washed and incubated with IRDYe 680 and 800CW conjugated secondary antibodies (1:10,000) and detected using the Odyssey Classic system.

E. Microdissection and Culturing of Cortical Neural Stem Cells/Progenitors

All procedures were conducted in accordance with the Australian National Health and Medical Research Council's published Code of Practice for the Use of Animals in Research, and experiments were approved by the Florey Neuroscience Institute animal ethics committee. The collected embryos (embryonic day 11.5) were immersed in chilled L15 medium (invitrogen), the brains removed and ventral midbrain microdissected. Subsequently the tissue was incubated in 0.1% DNase and 0.05% trypsin (in HBSS) for 15 minutes. Finally, the tissue was dissociated in N2 media consisting of a 1:1 mixture of F12 and MEM supplemented with 15 mM HEPES buffer, 1 mM glutamine, 6 mg/ml glucose, 1.5 mg/ml bovine serum albumin, and 1% N2 supplement. Cells were seeded at a density of 175,000 cells/cm^2 and incubated at 37 °C in 5% CO_2.

F. Immunocytochemistry

Fixed cultures were incubated overnight in the following primary antibodies: mouse anti-β tubulin (TUJ1, 1:1500) and rabbit anti-tyrosine hydroxylase (TH, 1:400). Cultures were then washed in PBS before secondary antibodies were added for an hour. Secondary antibodies (1:300): DyLight 488 donkey anti-rabbit, DyLight 549 donkey anti-mouse.

III. RESULTS AND DISCUSSION

A. Confirmation of Protein Immobilisation and Maintained Presentation without Degradation

The electrospun PCL scaffolds were treated with ethylenediamine (ED) to produce amine groups on the fibre surface for protein (GDNF) attachment via a crosslinker, SMCC [2]. The amount of fluorescamine on the scaffolds after aminolysation was measured to be 1.2×10^{-11} mol/g. Subsequent GDNF attachment onto the scaffolds (24 cm^2), via SMCC crosslinking, was confirmed by ELISA. Results showed significant levels of GDNF on the scaffold (PCL_iGDNF; 975 ± 115 pg), compared to PCL scaffolds alone (75 + 45 pg) or in the absence of the SMCC crosslinker (PCL_sGDNF, 180 + 30 pg; reflective of physically absorbed GDNF into the scaffold), Figure 1A. In light of BET analysis, demonstrating a total surface area of 24cm^2 for the 0.6cm diameter PCL scaffold, and a total of 975 + 115 pg GDNF on the scaffold, we were able to estimate a total of 41 pg of tethered GDNF per cm^2 of PCL scaffolds.

To confirm that the majority of the protein was tethered, and not absorbed onto the scaffolds, we vortexed the scaffolds that had been immobilised with GDNF to 'shake off' any protein embedded but not tethered to the PCL fibres. Under these conditions, no significant difference was seen in GDNF levels on PCL_iGDNF and PCL_iGDNF with vortexing (PCL_iGDNF: 975 ± 115 pg, and PCL_iGDNF(v): 650 ± 60 pg, respectively, Figure 1A), indicating that the majority of the protein was covalently attached.

Importantly, we confirmed that freezing of scaffolds had no effect on the stability of the protein, with no significant difference observed in the amount of tethered protein at day 0 from fresh versus frozen PCL_iGDNF samples (Figure 1A-B). Examination of PCL_iGDNF scaffolds, with or without vortexing, showed no significant difference in GDNF concentration over time, demonstrating that the protein remained tethered on the scaffold without degradation for at least 120 days (Figure 1B) and thereby highlighting the potential application of these scaffolds for long-term protein presentation. Results from the supernatant revealed that any absorbed protein leached from the scaffold within 24 hours (225 + 75 pg, Figure 1C). Interestingly,

GDNF was only marginally detectable in the supernatant at 3, 7, and 14 days, indicating that the protein measured in the supernatant after 24hrs had likely degraded, and thereby further highlighting the benefit of protein tethering for biological applications.

Here we demonstrate the ability to covalently tether GDNF onto the surface of electrospun PCL scaffolds using the sulfo-SMCC protein crosslinking reaction. This linking is dependent on the protein of interest possessing sulfhydryls (thiols, -SH), which readily react with the maleimide group within the sulfo-SMCC at pH 6.5-7.5. However, it is still possible for maleimides to react with amines, such as those found on the N-terminus of a protein or peptide [5]. At pH > 7.5 the reactivity of maleimides to amines begins to increase and as our reactions were conducted in PBS (pH 7.4); the same chemistry can be used to tether a protein that does not posses a free sulfhydryl group, although the reaction will be slower.

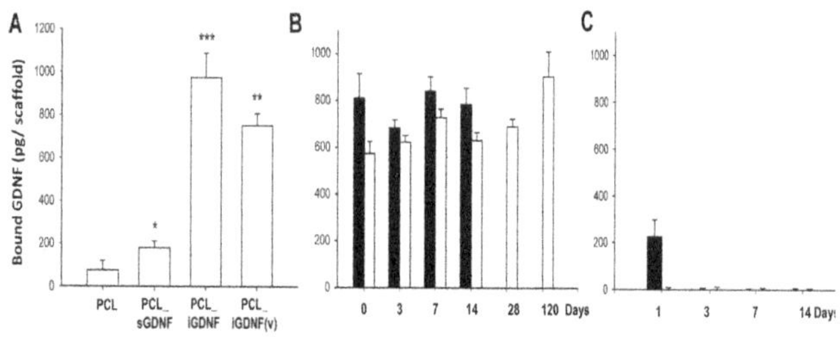

Fig. 1 Confirmation of protein tethering and stability on electrospun nanofibers.

(A) Immobilisation of GDNF on PCL scaffolds (iGDNF) significantly increases the presentation of protein in culture.. (B) Amount of GDNF presents on scaffolds after attachment without vortexing (black bars) and after attachment with vortexing (white bars). (C) A small amount of GDNF was absorbed onto the scaffolds at the time of tethering, which leached from the biomaterial within the first day. Data represents Mean ± SEM. *P < 0.05, **P < 0.01, ***P < 0.001, One-way ANOVA with Tukey post-hoc test.

B. The Biofunctionality of Tethered GDNF in Vitro

Next we investigated the bio-functionality of tethered GDNF on a neural stem cell line. Using the dopaminergic cell line (SN4741), known to express the GDNF receptors, c-ret and GFRa1, we examined the ability of tethered GDNF to induce intracellular phosphorylation of ErK1 and ErK2, key components of the GDNF-ErK signalling pathway. Comparable levels of total ErK1 and 2 could be detected in cells cultured on both PCL and PCL_iGDNF. However, the presence of GDNF significantly increased the phosphorylation of ErK (Figure 2A), indicating that tethered GDNF was capable of mediating intracellular GDNF signalling. Quantification of band density revealed a significant (4.4-fold) increase in the ratio of phospho-ErK to total ErK following culturing on tethered GDNF, Figure 2B. Next we examined the duration of functionality of tethered GDNF. While soluble GDNF (30 ng/ml) significantly increased pErK levels after 1 hour of stimulation, by 3 days in culture pErK levels were not significantly different to untreated cultures, reflective of degradation of the GDNF protein. By comparison, tethered GDNF resulted in a significant increase in pErK levels at 1 day and was maintained for 3 days in culture (Figure 2C-D). Here we demonstrate tethered protein is capable of activating intracellular Erk and maintain sustainable signalling (i.e. phospho-Erk levels), and may therefore present a superior method to prolong functional protein delivery for *in vitro* and *in vivo* applications.

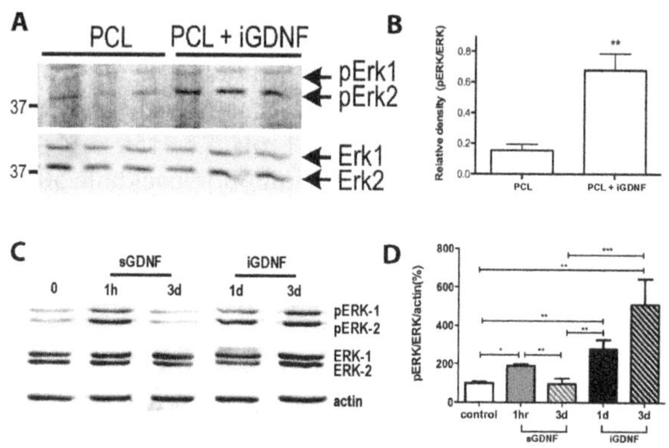

Fig. 2 Phosphorylation of intracellular ERK confirms functionality and longevity of tethered GDNF.

(A) Culturing of SN4741 neural cells on PCL and PCL+iGDNF (B) Ratio of phospho-ERK/total ERK level. (C-D) Phospho-ERK levels were significantly elevated after 1 hour of stimulation of SN4741 cells with soluble GDNF, but returned to basal levels within 3 days. By contrast culturing cells on iGDNF resulted in maintained elevated pERK levels (at 1 and 3 days in culture). Data represents Mean ± SEM. *P < 0.05, **P < 0.01, ***P < 0.001, Students t-test and One-way ANOVA.

Finally we examined the ability of tethered GDNF to not only induce an intracellular response, but also provide a prolonged effect on neural progenitors in culture. Here we demonstrate that soluble GDNF increased cell survival at 3 days, however viability significantly diminished thereafter to levels not different from untreated controls, presumably reflecting insignificant GDNF levels in the media beyond this time. By contrast, tethering GDNF onto the scaffold surface significantly increased and maintained cell survival. After 3 days in culture, we demonstrated that tethered GDNF significantly improved the viability of VM cells in culture compared to cells cultured in control (56.37% ± 0.96 and 44.04% ± 1.78, respectively), or PCL scaffolds alone (46.74% ± 2.86), Figure 3A,C-F. Similarly immobilised

GDNF enhanced the number of dopaminergic cells (TH+) in culture, Figure 3B,K-N. After 7 days, cells cultured in the presence of immobilised GDNF showed no decrease in cell viability or the proportion of dopaminergic neurons compared to 3 days in culture, demonstrating maintained activity of GDNF (Figure 3).

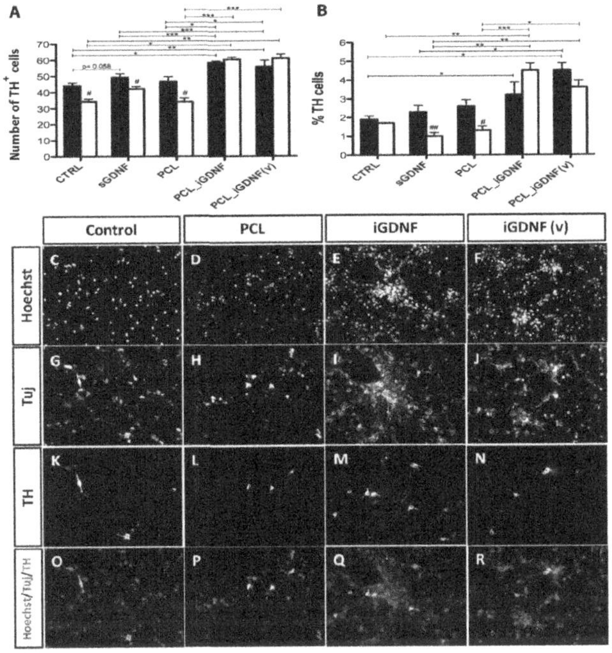

Fig.3 GDNF immobilisation enhances cell viability and differentiation.

(A)Protein tethering with or without vortexing, significantly increased the viability and (B) proportion of tyrorine Hydroxylase-immunoreactive (TH+) cells in ventral midbrain cultures. Black bars: 3 days *in vitro* (DIV), White bars: 7 DIV. (C-F) Hoechst labelled nuclei, (G-J) TUJ+ neurons, (K-N) TH+ dopaminergic neurons, and (O-R) merged images of VM cells. Data represents Mean + SEJM. *P< 0.05, **P< 0.001.

IV. CONCLUSION

Protein immobilisation on the surface of tissue engineering scaffolds has been investigated for their potential to influence cellular responses *in vitro* and *in vivo*. While the benefits of tethered proteins have been recognised for some years now, there has been a notable lack of research concentrating on their stability and bio-functionality kinetics. Here we demonstrate, by way of GDNF as an example, that tethered proteins on electrospun scaffolds are stable for prolonged periods of time (with no evidence of degradation), activate intracellular signalling cascades, and maintain cellular effects (GDNF influencing cell viability and differentiation). These findings hold significant potential for the use of biomaterials in presenting and maintaining the activity of proteins *in vitro* and *in vivo*.

Abbreviations— iGDNF, immobilised GDNF; iGDNF(v), immobilised GDNF scaffolds that have been exposed to vortexing; sGDNF, soluble GDNF.

REFERENCE

1. Tessmar, J. K., and Gopferich, A. M. (2007) Matrices and scaffolds for protein delivery in tissue engineering. *Advanced drug delivery reviews* **59**, 274-291
2. Horne, M. K., Nisbet, D. R., Forsythe, J. S., and Parish, C. L. (2010) Three-dimensional nanofibrous scaffolds incorporating immobilized BDNF promote proliferation and differentiation of cortical neural stem cells. *Stem cells and development* **19**, 843-852
3. Wang, T. Y., Forsythe, J. S., Nisbet, D. R., and Parish, C. L. (2012) Promoting engraftment of transplanted neural stem cells/progenitors using biofunctionalised electrospun scaffolds. *Biomaterials* **33**, 9188-9197
4. Nisbet, D. R., Rodda, A. E., Finkelstein, D. I., Horne, M. K., Forsythe, J. S., and Shen, W. (2009) Surface and bulk characterisation of electrospun membranes: problems and improvements. *Colloids and surfaces. B, Biointerfaces* **71**, 1-12
5. Sharpless, N. E., and Flavin, M. (1966) The reactions of amines and amino acids with maleimides. Structure of the reaction products deduced from infrared and nuclear magnetic resonance spectroscopy. *Biochemistry* **5**, 2963-2971

Author: Ting Yi Wang
Institute: Florey Institute, the University of Melbourne
Street: 30 royal parade
City: Parkville
Country: Australia
Email: ting.wang@florey.edu.au

Growth and Albumin Secretion of AML-12 Hepatocytes with Low Frequency-Low Intensity Ultrasound Stimulation

Kuan-Ting Kuo, Ching-Wen Huang, Ioannis Manousakas, Benjamin Teong, and Shyh-Ming Kuo

Department of Biomedical Engineering, I-Shou University, Kaohsiung, Taiwan

Abstract— **Clinically, physical, electrical or ultrasound stimulation is used to promote cell and tissue self-repairing. Though research on ultrasound stimulation mostly uses high frequency ultrasound stimulation, in our project, we use low frequency ultrasound stimulation of different intensities to treat AML-12 hepatocytes. The cells growth condition and albumin secretion was tested. The results show no difference related to ultrasound intensity for the growth condition and albumin secretion of AML-12, but ultrasound did not cause apoptosis.**

Keywords— **Ultrasound stimulation, AML-12, Hepatocytes, Albumin.**

I. INTRODUCTION

The largest organ in our body is the liver which has the ability of metabolism, detoxification, protein synthesis, secretion, and excretion. The liver is the only organ which can regenerate itself, but with limited functionality. In our study, in order to enhance the ability of regeneration, we consider the use of one of the physical stimulations, low intensity ultrasound. Experimental conditions in this study involved ultrasound stimulation of low frequency and with different intensities. AML-12 hepatocytes were cultured and exposed to ultrasound. These cell cultures were then tested for proliferation and albumin secretion [1], [2].

II. MATERIALS AND METHODS

A. Cell Cultures

AML-12 liver cells were cultured in 75-Tflasks, and placed in an incubator at 37 °C, 5% carbon dioxide for 7 days. While testing the growth condition, on days 0, 1, 3 and 7, the culture medium was changed on days 2, 4 and 6. For albumin secretion testing, the cells were cultured for 7 days but with no medium changes.

B. Ultrasound Stimulation

In order to use the ultrasound transducer on the bench, a silicon case was fit around the transducer. The transducer was then connected to a custom-made matching circuit and then to an RF amplifier. A diagram showing the experimental configuration is presented in Fig.1. A photograph of the experimental configuration for the ultrasound stimulation is shown in Fig.2. The 75T-flask containing the AML-12 hepatocytes was put on the ultrasound transducer on which ultrasound transmission gel was applied. A function generator generated a continuous sine wave signal of 32.8 kHz frequency. The signal passed through the RF amplifier and through the matching circuit to the ultrasound transducer. The output powers used were at 30mW and 100 mW. Zero output power was used for a control group. The exposure to ultrasound stimulation was 20 minutes per day. Albumin secretion tests were performed on the days 0, 1, 3 and 7. Albumin secretion tests and cell growth condition tests were performed on the days 0, 1, 3 and 7. The experimental protocol is presented in Fig.3.

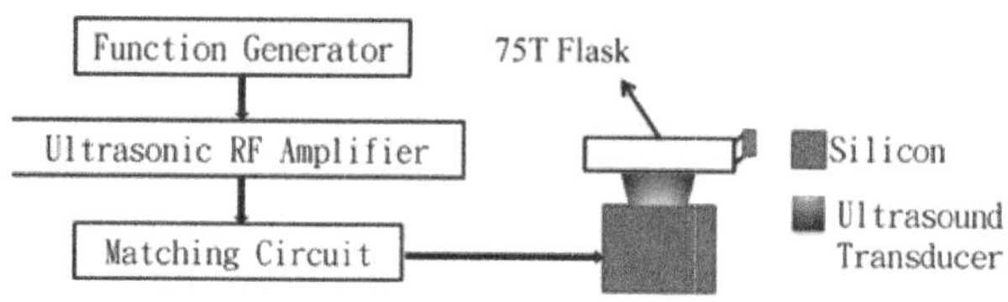

Fig. 1 Ultrasound stimulation system.

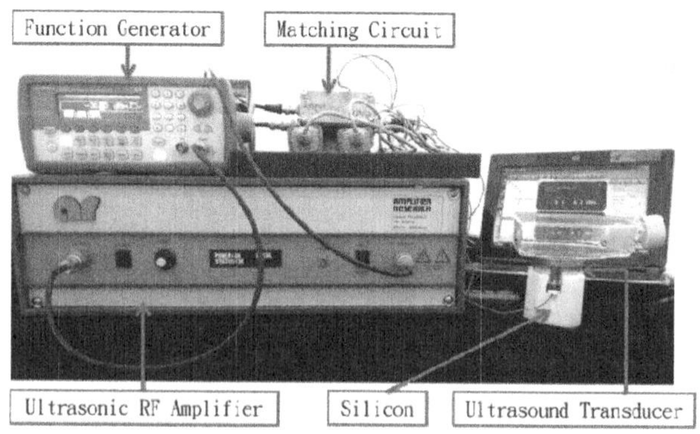

Fig. 2 Ultrasound stimulation system.

I. Lackovic (ed.), *1st Global Conference on Biomedical Engineering & 9th Asian-Pacific Conference on Medical and Biological Engineering*, IFMBE Proceedings 47, DOI: 10.1007/978-3-319-12262-5_15

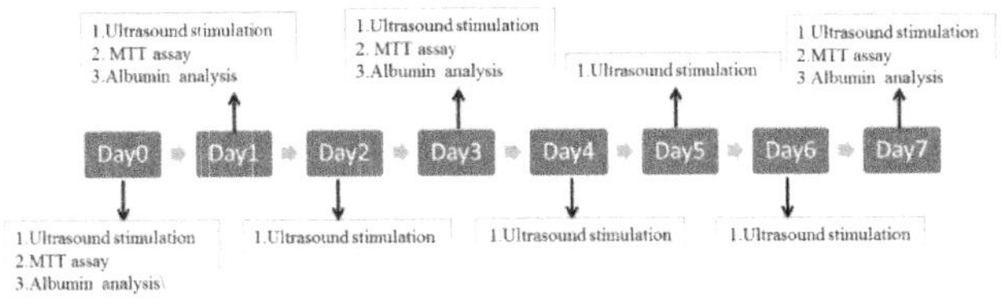

Fig. 3 Experimental protocol.

C. Cell Growth Condition Test

MTT reagent was added into the 75T-flasks, and react in the incubator for 3 hours. Then the liquid was withdrawn and centrifuged.

The supernatant was removed and DMSO was added to dissolve. An OD value was obtained by an ELISA Reader.

D. Albumin Secretion

The medium collected from the 75T-flasks and concentrated using concentrating tubes, the upper liquid was withdrawn, and coloring agents were added. Finally, OD values were obtained by an ELISA reader.

III. Results

In Fig. 4, pictures of the cell cultures are shown from day0 to day7 and for all the ultrasound power conditions. Fig. 5 shows the result of the MTT tests and Fig. 6 shows the albumin secretion results. Observed with an optical microscope, at the group of 30mW, the number of cells and their activity has increased along with the days, but its albumin secretion, does not have any significant change within 7 days. In addition, as the number of cells and cell activity also increased with 100mW stimulation, the albumin secretion was not significantly changed.

Although in this study changes cannot be seen in the AML-12 hepatocytes proliferation due to the ultrasound stimulation, it seems that ultrasound does not affect negatively the cells or cause apoptosis.

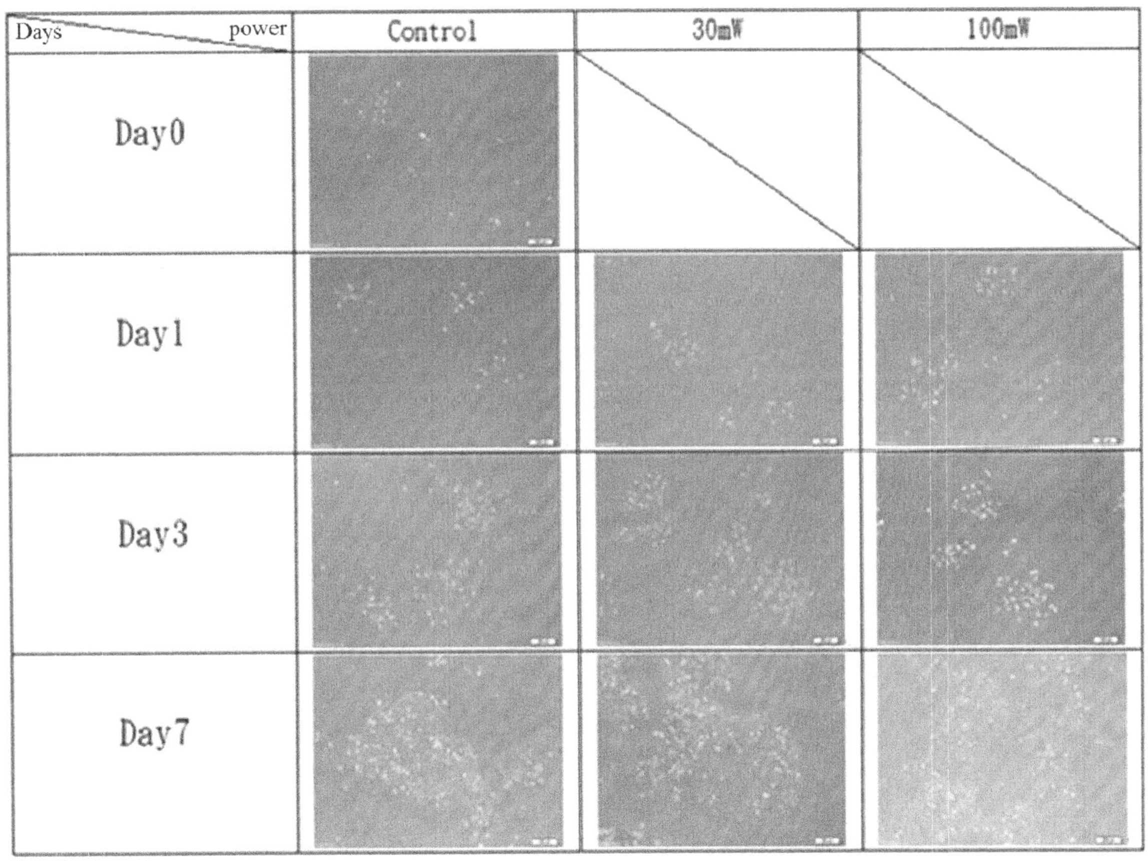

Fig. 4 AML-12 Hepatocytes with Low Frequency-Low Intensity Ultrasound Stimulation.

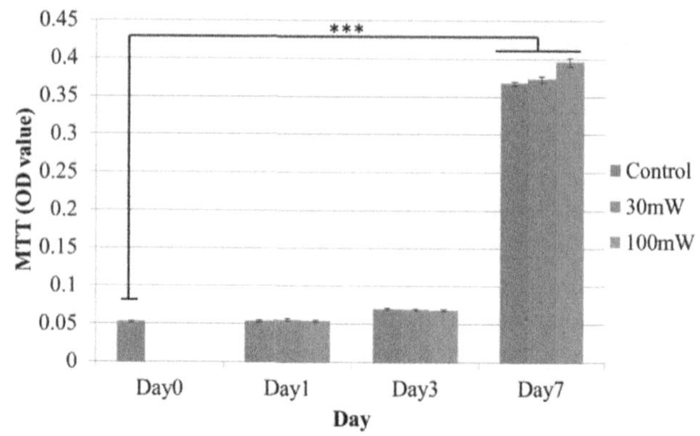

Fig. 5 Cell growth condition test.

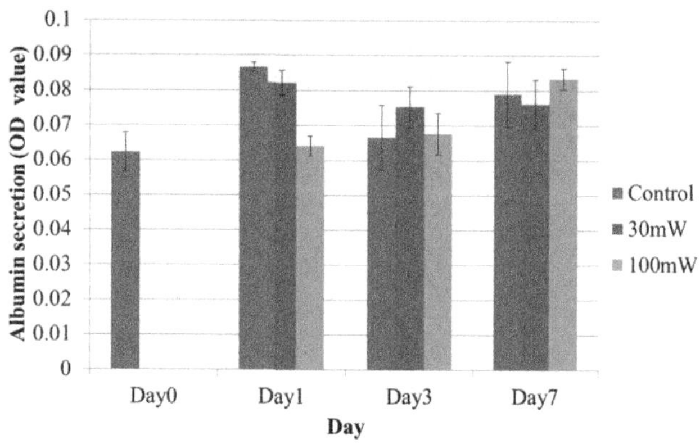

Fig. 6 Albumin secretion.

IV. Conclusions

From this study it can be concluded that low frequency low intensity ultrasound stimulation does not cause apoptosis for AML-12 hepatocytes. It shows that the powers of 30mW and 100mW may be too low to cause a significant change. In the future, we will try higher intensities and exposure times, and further study the cell growth condition and albumin secretion.

Conflict of Interest

The authors declare that they have no conflict of interest.

References

1. Nelson L J, Treskes P, Howie A F et al. (2013) Profiling the Impact of Medium Formulation on Morphology and Functionality of Primary Hepatocytes in vitro. Sci Rep 3:2735 DOI 10.1038/srep02735
2. Toyama Y, Sasaki K, Tachibana K et al. (2012) Ultrasound stimulation restores impaired neovascularization-related capacities of human circulating angiogenic cells. Cardiovasc Res 95(4):448-59 DOI: 10.1093/cvr/cvs173

Author: Ioannis Manousakas
Institute: Department of Biomedical Engineering, I-Shou University
Street: Jiaosu Village Yanchao District
City: Kaohsiung
Country: Taiwan
Email: i.manousakas@ieee.org

Overlapping Bare-Metal Stents Strategy in Treatment of Thoracic Aortic Aneurysm: A Numerical Study

P. Zhang, A.Q. Sun*, F. Zhan, and X.Y. Deng*

Key Laboratory for Biomechanics and Mechanobiology of Ministry of Education, School of Biological Science and Medical Engineering, Beihang University, Beijing, China, 100191

Abstract— **To investigate the hemodynamic performance of overlapping bare-metal stents treatment of thoracic aortic aneurysms (TAA), three simplified geometric models, named, no stent, with one single stent and two overlapped stents were studied and compared in terms of velocity profiles and wall shear stress (WSS) distributions by means of computational fluid dynamics (CFD). The results showed that overlapping bare-metal stents intervention significantly decreased the WSS and the blood flow velocity in the aneurysm sac, meanwhile the vortex in the sac became weaker and weaker. The results indicated that overlapping stents intervention may effectively isolate the thoracic aortic aneurysm, protecting it from rupture. In conclusion, overlapping bare-metal stents may serve a similar purpose to that of the multilayer flow modulator (MFM) manufactured by Cardiatis SA (Isnes, Belgium).**

Keywords— **thoracic aortic aneurysm, overlapping bare-metal stents, hemodynamics, numerical simulation.**

I. INTRODUCTION

Since the debut of endovascular repair of abdominal aortic aneurysm in the 1990s, it was introduced as a less invasive method than traditional open repair [1]. However, if an aneurysm is adjacent to or involving major arterial branches, stent-grafts would occlude the branches as well [2].

To solve this, a new type of multilayer flow modulator (MFM) technology manufactured by Cardiatis SA (Isnes, Belgium) has been developed that may offer an endovascular alternative to surgery in such cases [2, 3]. Clinically, it has shown positive superiority in reducing blood flow velocity and inducing the formation of organized thrombus in the aneurysm sac, hence provides protection for the aneurysm wall [2, 4-6]. The MFM, however, is now in high cost and still in clinical trials [7].

Some researchers proposed that several overlapping bare-metal stents can serve a similar purpose to the multilayer stent. Several clinical trials using overlapping bare-metal Wallstents (Boston Scientific, Natick, Mass) have been carried out to repair aortic aneurysms in the Peking University Third Hospital, China (unpublished data, personal communication). Rare studies, regretfully, have been reported to the aortic aneurysm treatment by using overlapping bare-metal stents and its hemodynamic performance is still unclear. Therefore, it is very necessary to investigate the hemodynamic features of overlapping bare-metal stents by means of numerical simulations.

The aim of the present work is to evaluate the hemodynamic performance of this treatment using CFD method. To do so, simplified TAA models in three cases, namely, without stent, with a single stent and with double stents overlapped, were constructed and compared numerically in terms of velocity profiles and WSS distributions.

II. METHODS

A. Fluid Dynamic Models

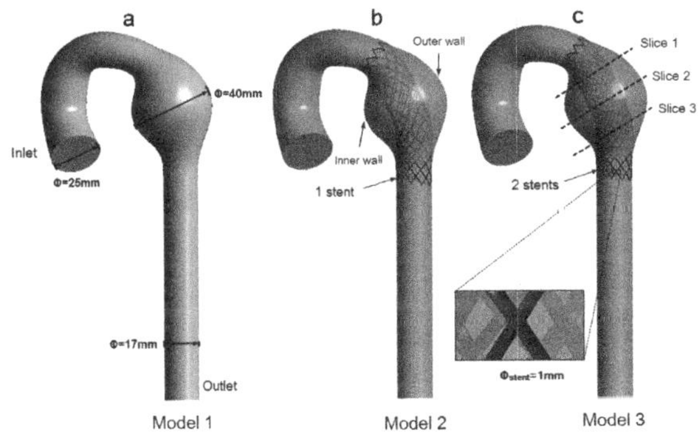

Fig. 1 The schematic of 3 aneurysm models. (a) Model 1 is the aneurysm geometry without stent intervention,(b) Model 2 is the aneurysm geometry with a single stent intervention; (c) Model 3 is the aneurysm geometry with double stents overlapping.

Three simplified geometrical models of thoracic aortic aneurysm were created using commercial software Solid Works (Solid Works Corp, Concord, MA), named Model 1, Model 2 and Model 3 (Fig. 1). The geometry of the artery was created according to Liu's aorta model [8], in which the diameters of inlet and outlet sections were 25mm and 17mm [8]. A typical aneurysm was created at the descending aorta with the maximum diameter of 40mm (Model 1). One single stent and double stents overlapped were set in Model 2 and 3 respectively. The stents have a total length l=70 mm

* Corresponding authors.

I. Lackovic (ed.), *1st Global Conference on Biomedical Engineering & 9th Asian-Pacific Conference on Medical and Biological Engineering*, IFMBE Proceedings 47, DOI: 10.1007/978-3-319-12262-5_16

and 20 wires with 1mm circular cross-section, which are fixed to the proximal and distal necks of the aneurysm. Specifically, the stent was assumed to have half of its thickness embedded into the arterial wall and the two stents were stagger completely spatially (Fig.2B).

B. Numerical Grids

The meshing software ANSYS ICEM CFD (ANSYS Inc., Canonsburg, PA, USA) was used in all the models. A hybrid discretization method which used both tetrahedral and hexahedral elements was applied to the stented models (Fig.2A). After an appropriate mesh independence study, the final volume grids were 191,268 cells for Model 1, whereas 2,957,879 cells and 4,157,954 cells, respectively, for Model 2 and Model 3.

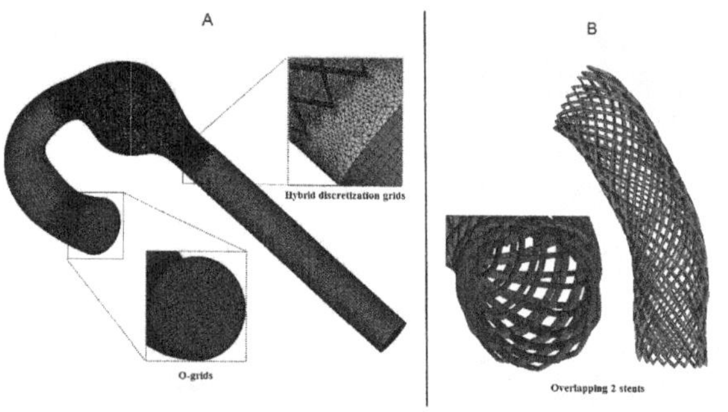

Fig. 2 The schematic of grids in the stented model (A) and the spatial structure of overlapping double stents (B).

C. Numerical Approaches

1. Assumptions

Flow simulation under steady-state condition was performed in the present work. The artery walls and the stent surfaces were defined as rigid and no-slip [9]. Blood was assumed as incompressible, laminar, non-Newtonian fluid [10]. The Carreau model was used to calculate the blood viscosity:

$$\eta(\dot{\gamma}) = \eta_\infty + (\eta_0 - \eta_\infty)\left[1 + (\lambda\dot{\gamma})^2\right]^{\frac{n-1}{2}} \quad (1)$$

where $\eta_\infty = 3.45\times10^{-3}$ kg/(m.s), $\eta_0 = 5.6\times10^{-2}$ kg/(m s), n = 0.3568, $\lambda = 3.313$s[11].

2. Governing Equations

The flow simulation is based on the three-dimensional incompressible Navier-Stokes and continuity equations:

$$\rho\left(\frac{\partial u}{\partial t} + u\cdot\nabla u\right) = -\nabla p + \nabla\cdot\tau \quad (2)$$

$$\nabla\cdot u = 0 \quad (3)$$

where u and p represent, respectively, the fluid velocity vector and the pressure. $\rho = 1050$ kg/m^3[10].

3. Boundary Conditions

At the inlet, a flat spatial velocity profile was imposed, assuming the time-average Re= 790 based the MRI measurements [12]. At the outlet section, the outflow boundary condition was set, that is, the flow at the outlet was set as a fully developed flow.

4. Computation

The numerical calculations were carried out using a validated finite volume-based algorithm ANSYS FLUENT CFD (ANSYS Inc., Canonsburg, PA). The discrete form of the differential governing equations of blood flow follows the second-order upwind scheme. Pressure was solved through the pressure-velocity coupling method known as the SIMPLE algorithm. The convergence criterion was set to 10-5 for continuity and velocity residuals.

III. RESULTS

A. Velocity Profiles

To facilitate the presentation of the velocity profiles in the aneurysm sac, three representative slices were selected along the longitudinal direction of the centerlines shown in Fig.1 (Model 3). Slice 1 is located at the proximal neck of the aneurysm sac, Slice 2 at the middle part of the sac, Slice 3 at the distal neck of the sac. The view of the velocity profiles for all the slices is shown in Fig.3.

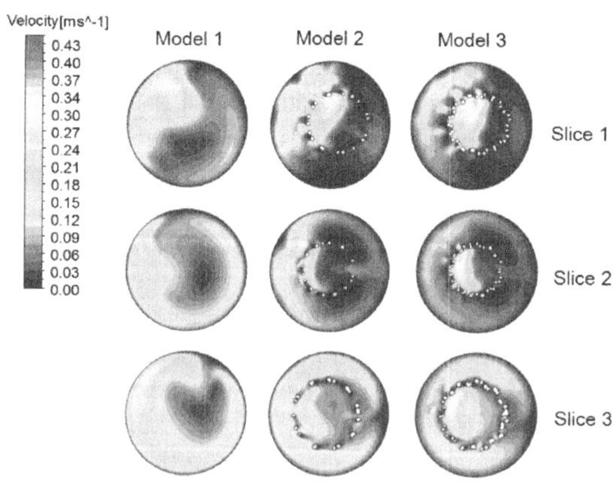

Fig. 3 Contours of velocity at different locations of the aneurysm indicated by the slice letters. Slice 1 is the cross-section in the proximal neck of the aneurysm. Slice 2 is the middle cross-section of the aneurysm. Slice 3 is the cross-section in the distal neck of the aneurysm.

In Model 1, the velocity of blood flow near the outer surface of the aneurysm is higher than that near the inner surface. In particular, the flow velocity in central area of the sac is high relative to the surrounding area. In Model 2, this kind of velocity distribution is changed, and the flow velocity near the outer surface of the sac decreases. This trend is more obvious in Model 3, presenting more uniform distribution of velocity. In addition, the flow velocity near the central area of the stents has been enhanced in Model 3 when compared with that of Model 1 and 2.

Streamlines in these 3 models are shown in Fig. 4, colored by velocity magnitude. The flow field is characterized by evident vortex in Model 1, presenting recirculation and stagnation emerged in the aneurysm sac. While in Model 2 and 3, the vortex in the sac becomes weaker and weaker due to the stent(s) introduced.

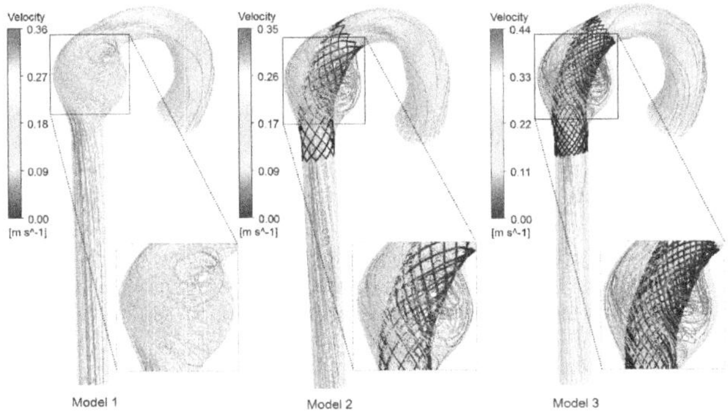

Fig. 4 Velocity streamlines in the three models.

B. WSS Distribution

Contours of WSS on the surface of the aneurysm are shown in Fig. 4. On the whole, the WSS on the aneurysm wall is reduced after stent implantation and in Model 3 WSS is reduced to no more than 0.4-0.6 Pa in most of the aneurysm area. Specially in Model 1, the WSS distribution is uneven, presenting a relative high WSS area at the outer surface close to the distal neck of the aneurysm, which is worthy of notice. By stent(s) implantation, high WSS in this area has been reduced in Model 2 and 3.

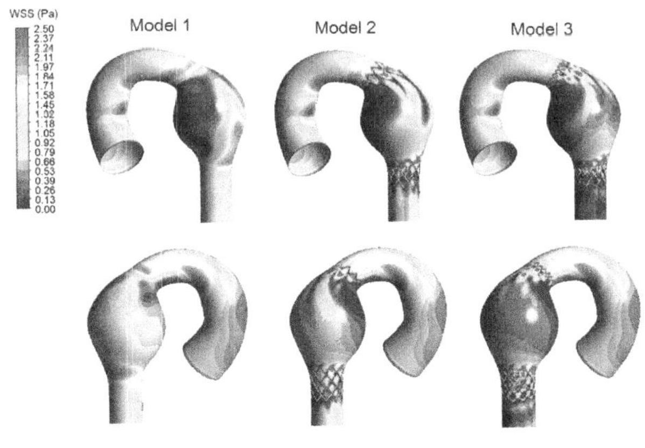

Fig. 5 WSS distributions on the aneurysm wall of the three models.

IV. DISCUSSION

The clinical trials at the Peking University Third Hospital in China indicate that overlapped bare-metal stents might serve a similar purpose to that of the MFM in treatment of aortic aneurysms (unpublished data, personal communication). In the present article we numerically analyzed the hemodynamic features of this overlapping stents intervention treatment by using a simplified TAA model with two overlapped stents deployed in the aneurysm sac. We compared the double overlapping treatment model with aneurysm models without stent or with only one single stent deployed in terms of velocity profiles and wall shear stress distributions.

The numerical results confirmed that overlapping stents intervention led to an evident decrease in blood flow velocity near the aneurysm wall and significantly reduced WSS. The resulted hemodynamic features by the overlapping stents may certainly provide favorable conditions for the formation of thrombus in the aneurismal sac, which may effectively isolate the aneurysm and serves a similar result to this of the multilayer stent.

The recent clinical trials of the multilayer stent indicate that it instigates a process of aortic remodeling involving initial thrombus deposition [6] and significantly reduces blood flow velocity and WSS, while inducing laminar flow in the aneurismal sac[4, 6, 13, 14]. This can facilitate the formation of organized thrombus in forms of stable layers, which gives protection against rupture of the aneurysm [5, 15, 16]. The present numerical study showed that the double overlapping stents could also induce a similar flow field of slow velocity and low shear stress in the aneurysm sac (Figs. 3 and 5), hence provide protection for the aneurysm.

In this pilot study, as a main limitation, smoothed wall and simplified aorta model without the existence of arch branches was used in the present study, which may have a non-negligible influence on flow patterns in the TAA.

V. CONCLUSION

In conclusion, overlapping bare-metal stents can create a favorable blood flow environment promoting thrombus formation in the aneurismal sac, hence effectively isolate the thoracic aortic aneurysm. It can be considered as an alternative option for the treatment of TAAs, serving a similar purpose to that of the MFM.

Acknowledgment

This work is supported by Grants-in-Aid from the National Natural Science Research Foundation of China (No. 11332003, 11228205, 11202016, 11102014) and the National Key Technology R&D Program (2012BAI18B02, 2012BAI14B04).

Conflict of Interest

There is no conflict of interest involved.

References

1. De Bruin, J.L., et al. (2010) Long-term outcome of open or endovascular repair of abdominal aortic aneurysm. New England Journal of Medicine, 362(20): p. 1881-1889.
2. Henry, M., et al. (2008) Treatment of renal artery aneurysm with the multilayer stent. Journal of Endovascular Therapy, 15(2): p. 231-236.
3. Carrafiello, G., et al. (2011) Endovascular repair of a celiac trunk aneurysm with a new multilayer stent. Journal of Vascular Surgery, 54(4): p. 1148-1150.
4. Vaislic, C.D., et al. (2014) One-year outcomes following repair of thoracoabdominal aneurysms with the Multilayer Flow Modula-tor: report from the STRATO trial. Journal of Endovascular Therapy, 21(1): p. 85-95.
5. Benjelloun, A., et al. (2012) Endovascular treatment of a tuberculous thoracoabdominal aneurysm with the Multilayer stent. Journal of Endovascular Therapy, 19(1): p. 115-120.
6. Sultan, S., M. Sultan, and N. Hynes. (2014) Early mid-term results of the first 103 cases of multilayer flow modulator stent done un-der indication for use in the management of thoracoabdominal aortic pathology from the independent global MFM registry. The Journal of cardiovascular surgery, 55(1): p. 21-32.
7. Kahn, S.L., et al. (2014) In vivo construction of a multilayer bare-metal stent for the treatment of an aortic mycotic pseudoaneu-rysm. Journal of vascular surgery.
8. Liu, X., et al. (2009) A numerical study on the flow of blood and the transport of LDL in the human aorta: the physiological signifi-cance of the helical flow in the aortic arch. American Journal of Physiology-Heart and Circulatory Physiology, 297(1): p. H163-H170.
9. Chiastra, C., et al. (2013) Computational fluid dynamic simulations of image-based stented coronary bifurcation models. J R Soc Inter-face, 10(84): p. 20130193.
10. Liu, X., et al. (2011) Effect of non-Newtonian and pulsatile blood flow on mass transport in the human aorta. Journal of Biomechanics, 44(6): p. 1123-1131.
11. Cho, Y. and K. Kensey. (1990) Effects of the non-Newtonian viscosity of blood on flows in a diseased arterial vessel. Part 1: Steady flows. Biorheology, 28(3-4): p. 241-262.
12. Hope, T.A., et al. (2007) Comparison of flow patterns in ascending aortic aneurysms and volunteers using four-dimensional mag-netic resonance velocity mapping. J Magn Reson Imaging, 26(6): p. 1471-9.
13. Henry, M., et al. (2013) The multilayer flow modulator stent for the treatment of arterial aneurysms. The Journal of cardiovascular surgery, 54(6): p. 763-783.
14. Tolva, V.S., et al. (2012) Multiple multilayer stents for thoracoabdominal aortic aneurysm: a possible new tool for aortic endo-vascular surgery. Int J Gen Med, 5: p. 629-32.
15. Chen, C.Y., et al. (2014) Effects of Intraluminal Thrombus on Patient-Specific Abdominal Aortic Aneurysm Hemodynamics via Stereoscopic Particle Image Velocity and Computational Fluid Dynamics Modeling. Journal of Biomechanical Engineering-Transactions of the Asme, 136(3).
16. Balderi, A., et al. (2013) Treatment of visceral aneurysm using multilayer stent: two-year follow-up results in five consecutive patients. Cardiovascular and interventional radiology, 36(5): p. 1256-1261.

Author: Deng X.Y. & Sun A.Q.
Institute: Key Lab for Biomechanics and Mechanobiology of Minis-try of Education, School of Biological Science&Medical Engineering , Beihang University
Street: XueYuan Road No.37,HaiDian District
City: Beijing
Country: China
Email: dengxy1953@buaa.edu.cn; saq@buaa.edu.cn

Simulation and Wave Intensity Analysis of Intra-aortic Counterpulsation

Bo-Wen Lin[1,2] and Pong-Jeu Lu[1,2]

[1] Department of Aeronautics and Astronautics, National Cheng Kung University, Tainan 701, Taiwan
[2] Heart Science and Medical Devices Research Center, National Cheng Kung University, Tainan 701, Taiwan

Abstract— **This work aims at developing a system dynamic model that can simulate various hemodynamic and wave characteristics associated with the counter-pulsation circulation support. A novel hybrid circulation model consisting of a one-dimensional (1-D) flow model and a lumped parameter Windkessel model was constructed. High-resolution Roe-splitting was developed for wave capturing and Runge-Kutta method was used for time-stepping this coupled hybrid circulation system. Wave propagation phenomenon in the arteries was successfully simulated. By adjusting the time-varying elastance of the ventricles, the healthy and failed heart conditions can be simulated. Failing heart supported by intra-aortic balloon pump (IABP) was simulated. These simulation results indicate that for 40 ml IABP support, cardiac output was elevated 4.1%. During systolic unloading, IABP deflation generated a backward decompression wave, with a "sucking" effect toward the aortic root, resulting in a reduced left ventricular afterload. During diastolic augmentation, IABP inflation generated a backward compression wave, with a "pushing" effect toward the aortic root to help coronary diastolic perfusion. Wave patterns of counterpulsation can be investigated using wave intensity analysis, which is able to quantitatively assess diastolic augmentation and systolic unloading of IABP counterpulsation based on a strict energy transport theory of wavelet.**

Keywords— **Intra-aortic balloon pump, Lumped parameter method, Hybrid circulation model, Heart failure, Ventricular assist device.**

I. INTRODUCTION

The development of left ventricular assist devices (LVADs) has been advanced substantially for treating heart failure in recent years. The intra-aortic balloon pump (IABP) is the most widely used acute LVAD to date, with beneficial hemodynamic outcomes reported clinically [1]. IABP operates on the principle of counterpulsation, which has two key effects: 1) reduction of aortic pressure during systole to decrease ventricular ejection afterload, namely systolic unloading and 2) augmentation of diastolic pressure to enhance coronary perfusion during diastole, namely diastolic augmentation [2].

Counterpulsation effectiveness has been assessed using peak and trough values of aortic and left ventricular pressure waveforms, and the pressure-derived indexes such as tension time index and endomyocardial viability ratio [3]. Strictly speaking, these traditional measures have been made with assumptions and hence are sometimes inaccurate, or even misleading in the evaluation of counterpulsatile support efficacy [4]. Moreover, none of these traditional indexes connect to the wave phenomena of pulsatile blood ejection and the IABP-generated counterpulsation. This work proposes a new assessment method using system dynamic model for simulating the characteristic hemodynamic features of intra-aortic counterpulsation. Wave intensity analysis (WIA) was employed to analyze and assess IABP counterpulsation, providing an alternative perspective stressing pulse wave mechanics in the circulatory blood flow.

II. METHODOLOGY

A. Governing Equations for Intra-aortic Balloon Pump

Pulse waves propagating along vascular segments have been modeled using one dimensional (1-D) flow conservation laws of mass and momentum augmented by a structural state equation representing vessel wall mechanics. The newly derived 1-D equations with IABP being inserted in the aorta (see Fig. 1) can be expressed as [5]:

$$\begin{aligned} &\frac{\partial \tilde{A}}{\partial t}+\frac{\partial q}{\partial x}=0 \\ &\frac{\partial q}{\partial t}+\frac{\partial}{\partial x}\left(\frac{q^2}{\tilde{A}}\right)+\frac{\tilde{A}}{\rho}\frac{\partial p}{\partial x}=-\frac{2\pi\nu q(R+R')}{\delta\tilde{A}} \end{aligned} \tag{1}$$

where $\tilde{A}=A-A'$ is the effective lumen area of the tubular conduit with A and A' representing aortic lumen and IABP outer cross-sectional area, respectively; q is the flow rate, ρ is the blood density, ν is the kinematic viscosity (assumed to be constant), δ is the boundary layer thickness (assumed to be constant), R is lumen cross-sectional radius, and p is the static pressure. The independent variables x and t represent, respectively, the spatial and time coordinates of the postulated 1-D equations.

To close up the above flow equations with three state variables (A, q, and p), a third equation is necessary, namely the state equation of the tube structure, which is presently modeled as a two-dimensional thin-walled elastic structure described by the tube law [6]:

I. Lackovic (ed.), *1st Global Conference on Biomedical Engineering & 9th Asian-Pacific Conference on Medical and Biological Engineering*,
IFMBE Proceedings 47, DOI: 10.1007/978-3-319-12262-5_17

$$p(x,t)-p_0=\frac{4}{3}\frac{Eh}{r_0(x)}\left[1-\sqrt{\frac{A_0(x)}{A(x,t)}}\right] \tag{2}$$

where p_0 is the ambient or tissue pressure, A_0 is the cross-sectional area with radius r_0 at zero transmural pressure (i.e., at $p=p_0$), and E and h are the Young's modulus and thickness of the vascular wall, respectively.

B. System Dynamic Modeling

Wave propagation phenomenon in aorta with IABP embedded is presently simulated using 1-D flow model. This 1-D flow model is coupled with other segments of the cardiovascular system, represented by lumped parameter models (Windkessels), forming a closed-loop hybrid circulation model that simulates the IABP-assisted circulation (see Fig. 1). The system dynamic model, after semi-discretized in space, can be expressed in a state-space form as:

$$\begin{bmatrix} \frac{dV_1}{dt} \\ \frac{dV_2}{dt} \\ \frac{dV_3}{dt} \\ \frac{dV_4}{dt} \\ \frac{\partial \tilde{A}_{5,i}}{\partial t} \\ \frac{\partial q_{5,i}}{\partial t} \\ \frac{dV_6}{dt} \\ \frac{dV_7}{dt} \end{bmatrix} = \begin{bmatrix} \frac{V_7}{C_7R_7}-\frac{V_1}{C_1}\left(\frac{1}{R_7}+\frac{1}{R_1}\right)+\frac{V_2}{C_2R_1} \\ \frac{V_1}{C_1R_1}-\frac{V_2}{C_2}\left(\frac{1}{R_1}+\frac{1}{R_2}\right)+\frac{V_3}{C_3R_2} \\ \frac{V_2}{C_2R_2}-\frac{V_3}{C_3}\left(\frac{1}{R_2}+\frac{1}{R_3}\right)+\frac{V_4}{C_4R_3} \\ \frac{V_3}{C_3R_3}-\frac{V_4}{C_4R_3}-Q_{4,5} \\ -\frac{\partial q_{5,i}}{\partial x} \\ -\frac{\partial}{\partial x}\left(\frac{\tilde{q}_{5,i}^2}{\tilde{A}_{5,i}}+\tilde{B}_{5,i}\right)+S_{5,i} \\ Q_{5,6}-\frac{V_6}{C_6R_6}+\frac{V_7}{C_7R_6} \\ \frac{V_6}{C_6R_6}-\frac{V_6}{C_6}\left(\frac{1}{R_6}+\frac{1}{R_7}\right)+\frac{V_1}{C_1R_7} \end{bmatrix} \tag{3}$$

where the state variable V is the volume, C is the compliance, and R is the resistance. The subscript i indicates the i-th cell of the 1-D flow model whereas the digital numbers 1 to 7 denote the seven lumped blocks depicted in Fig. 1. Left and right hearts are modeled using the pressure-volume relationship suggested by Suga et al. [7], in which the ventricular contractility is controlled by the amplitude of a time-varying elastance. The inserted IABP balloon is modeled using a predetermined volume time series. The detailed derivation of this hybrid circulation model can be found in [5].

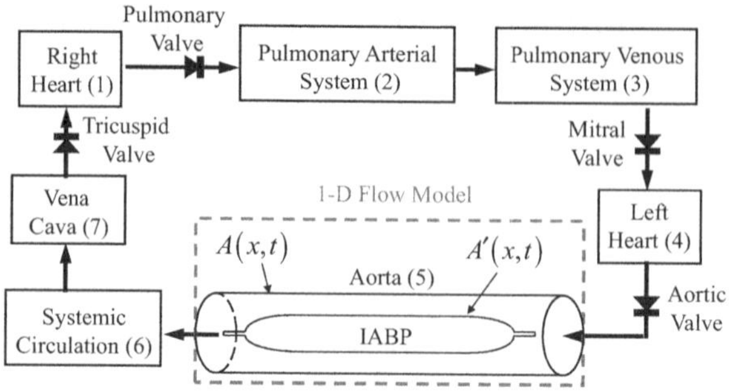

Fig. 1 Hybrid circulation model

C. Numerical Methods

A high-resolution finite-volume Roe-splitting flux-difference method in conjunction with a time-accurate Runge-Kutta marching method was developed to solve the hybrid circulation model, Eq. 3 [5,8]. As heart contraction and IABP pumping are put into action, pulsatile blood flow can be generated with various kinds of waves propagating and reflecting in the closed-loop circulation circuits.

D. Wave Intensity Analysis (WIA)

The wave splitting introduced by Parker and Jones [9] for calculating wave intensity (WI) was used in this work. The net WI, or the energy of a wavelet sampled over an infinitesimal time period is defined by:

$$dI = dPdU \tag{4}$$

where dP and dU are the pressure and velocity differences between two consecutive instances of time, respectively. WI can be decomposed into contributions associated with the forward (+) and backward (−) propagating wave components:

$$dI_{\pm}=\pm\frac{1}{4\rho c}\left(dP\pm\rho c dU\right)^2 \tag{5}$$

where c is the wave speed. Note that forward propagating waves have $dI_+>0$ always, while backward propagating waves having $dI_-<0$ always.

E. Inflation/deflation Timing Definition

Inflation/deflation (or augmentation/unloading) timing plays a critical role in determining counterpulsation efficacy [4,10,11]. The temporal zero-point references for inflation and deflation timings are defined to be at the dicrotic notch (aortic valve closure) and at the onset of blood ejection, respectively. The notation of 1 count (50 milliseconds) was used to denote the unit inflation or deflation time interval after the reference zero-point.

F. Simulation Scenarios

Numerical simulations including healthy, heart failure, and IABP-assisted cases are present. Peak values of the isovolumetric time-varying elastance of left heart are set 2.6 and 0.78 mmHg/ml for the healthy and heart failure subjects, respectively. In the device assisted case, IABP with 40 ml stroke volume and with inflection/deflection timing of 1/-1 (count) are used to treat heart failure. All simulations are conducted using the heart rate (HR) of 60 beats/min.

III. RESULTS

A. Baseline in healthy and heart failure subjects

The simulated hemodynamic characteristics are shown in Table 1 and Fig. 2. In the healthy subject, the systolic/diastolic aortic pressure (AOP), stroke volume (SV), and cardiac output (CO) are 129.8/75.0 mmHg, 81.0 ml, and 4.8 L/min, respectively. These hemodynamic characteristics and features are clinically similar to what generally observed. In the heart failure case, however, CO reduces 23.8% by reducing the elastances of the right and left hearts.

Table 1 Simulated hemodynamic characteristics

Parameter	Healthy	Failure	IABP
Aortic pressure (mmHg)	129.8/75.0	92.6/57.5	75.1/39.6
Left heart pressure (mmHg)	140.0/0.5	98.6/10.4	75.0/7.5
Left heart volume (ml)	151.6/70.6	215.0/153.4	181.2/116.5
Stroke volume (ml)	81.0	61.6	64.7
Cardiac output (L/min)	4.8	3.66	3.81
Stroke work (mmHg*ml)	9235.07	4652.5	3288.32

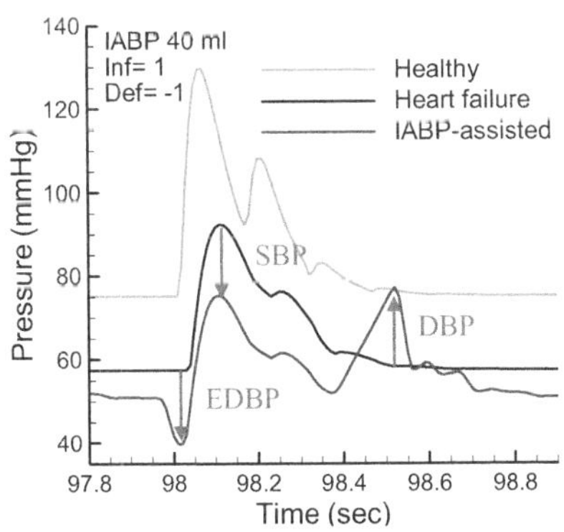

Fig. 2 Pressure waveforms for healthy, heart failure and IABP-assisted heart failure cases. SBP: systolic blood pressure, EDBP: end-diastolic blood pressure, DBP: diastolic pressure. Balloon inflation (Inf) and deflation (Def) are timed using count units (1 count=50 milliseconds).

B. Counterpulsation Features

For the IABP-assisted failing heart, CO is elevated 4.1%. The efficacy of counterpulsatile support is evident by comparing the pressure characteristics between the heart failure and the IABP-assisted cases. Systolic unloading decreases both end-diastolic blood pressure (EDBP) and systolic blood pressure (SBP), whereas diastolic augmentation increases diastolic blood pressure (DBP), as shown in Fig. 2.

C. Deflation Timing Control

The effect of deflation timing is evaluated under IABP counterpulsatile support with deflation timings ranging from 1 to 3 counts before blood ejection while keeping inflation timing fixed at 1 count after dicrotic notch. The aortic pressure and the deduced wave intensity characteristics are depicted in Fig. 3. There are 3 intensity peaks (marked with Eu1, Cu2, and Ca3) that are essential to the counterpulsation performance. Upper case letters "C" and "E" denote the compression (pushing) or expansion (pulling or sucking) nature of the wave, respectively, and the numeric value represents the sequence in which the waves arise. Lower case letters "a" and "u" refer to IABP-generated augmentation and unloading waves. It is seen that backward propagating Eu1 and Ca3 waves are IABP generated as a result of balloon deflation and inflation, respectively, whereas Cu2 corresponds to the accelerated systolic ejection caused by the balloon-induced contraction unloading.

IV. DISCUSSION

The main wave corresponding to systolic unloading in the aorta was characterized by the Eu1 backward decompression wave (Fig. 3) that was generated by IABP deflation. Cu2 wave was the subsequent forward compression wave generated by left ventricular ejection. The main wave corresponding to diastolic augmentation in the aorta was characterized by the Ca3 backward compression wave that was generated by IABP inflation. These wave patterns are consistent with those previously found with the in-vivo IABP support [4].

IABP-generated backward-traveling waves have been shown predominantly in driving aortic and coronary blood flow to achieve counterpulsatile support [4,10]. During systolic unloading, IABP deflation generated the Eu1 wave, with a ''sucking'' effect toward the aortic root that translates to reduced left ventricular afterload, resulting in the reduction of the subsequent systolic Cu2 wave. During diastolic augmentation, IABP inflation generates the Ca3 wave, with a ''pushing'' effect toward the aortic root that helps coronary diastolic perfusion.

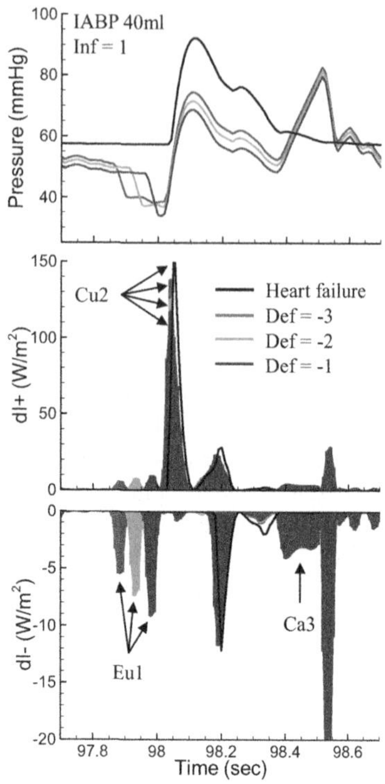

Fig. 3 Deflation timing influence on the aortic hemodynamic and wave intensity characteristics. See text for definitions of Eu1, Cu2, and Ca3. Deflation timings are set at 1, 2, and 3 counts before the onset of ejection.

The aortic wave intensities were found sensitive to the timing of the balloon deflation. When the deflation timing was set preceding to ejection onset by -1 to -3 counts, the wave intensities Eu1 corresponding to systolic unloading were progressively weakened and the following ejection-induced compression waves Cu2 became less depleted due to decreased compression-decompression wave merging and cancellation, as shown in Fig. 3.

Via WIA, complex wave interaction can be decomposed into wave motion events disclosing the onset, strength and direction of the forward- or backward-going wave components. This analysis is very instrumental in quantifying the energy carried by these constituent wavelets in the explanation of the pulsatile blood flow characteristics.

V. CONCLUSION

A system dynamic model that can simulate the hemodynamic features of the intra-aortic balloon counterpulsation was developed. With the aid of wave intensity analysis, counterpulsation effectiveness can be better quantified with propagating wave features revealed. During systolic unloading, balloon deflation generates a backward decompression wave, with a ''sucking'' effect toward the aortic root that translates to reduced left ventricular afterload. During diastolic augmentation, balloon inflation generates a backward compression wave, with a ''pushing'' effect toward the aortic root that helps coronary diastolic perfusion. These waves are sensitive to inflation/deflation control timings. Premature balloon deflation leads to much weaker backward decompression wave sent toward aortic root and results in lesser afterload reduction. Wave intensity analysis is shown to be effective in revealing wave characteristics and is able to quantify balloon- and heart-generated waves when interacted together.

CONFLICT OF INTEREST

The authors declare that they have no conflict of interest.

REFERENCES

1. Bolooki H (1998) Clinical application of intra-aortic balloon pump. 3rd edn. Futura Publishing Company, NY.
2. Papaioannou TG, Stefanadis C (2005) Basic principles of the intraaortic balloon pump and mechanisms affecting its performance. ASAIO J 51 (3):296-300.
3. Sarnoff SJ, Braunwald E, Welch GH, Case RB, Stainsby WN, Macruz R (1958) Hemodynamic determinants of oxygen consumption of the heart with special reference to the tension-time index. Am J Physiol 192 (1):148-156.
4. Lu PJ, Yang CFJ, Wu MY, Hung CH, Chan MY, Hsu TC (2011) Wave energy patterns of counterpulsation: A novel approach with wave intensity analysis. J Thorac Cardiovasc Surg 142 (5):1205-1213.
5. Lin BW (2007) Wave intensity analysis of counter-pulsation circulation support. Master Thesis, National Cheng Kung University, Tainan, Taiwan.
6. Olufsen MS (1999) Structured tree outflow condition for blood flow in larger systemic arteries. Am J Physiol-Heart C 276 (1):H257-268.
7. Sagawa K, Maughan L, Suga H, Sunagawa K (1988) Cardiac contraction and the pressure-volume relationship, vol 480. Oxford University Press New York.
8. Lin BW, Lu PJ (2014) High-resolution Roes scheme and characteristic boundary conditions for solving complex wave reflection phenomena in a tree-like arterial structure. J Comput Phys 260:143-162.
9. Parker KH, Jones CJH (1990) Forward and backward running waves in the arteries: Analysis using the method of characteristics. J Biomech Eng 112 (3):322-326.
10. Lu PJ, Yang CFJ, Wu MY, Hung CH, Chan MY, Hsu TC (2012) Wave intensity analysis of para-aortic counterpulsation. Am J Physiol-Heart C 302 (7):H1481-H1491.
11. Lu PJ, Lin PY, Yang CF, Hung CH, Chan MY, Hsu TC (2011) Hemodynamic and metabolic effects of para- versus intraaortic counterpulsatile circulation supports. ASAIO J 57 (1):19-25.

Author: Bo-Wen Lin
Institute: National Cheng Kung University
Street: No.1, University Road
City: Tainan
Country: Taiwan (R.O.C.)
Email: baldwincafa@gmail.com

Enhanced Accumulation of LDLs within the Venous Graft Wall May Account for Its Accelerated Atherogenesis

Z.Z. Wang, X. Liu, H.Y. Kang, A.Q. Sun, and X.Y. Deng*

Key Laboratory for Biomechanics and Mechanobiology of Ministry of Education,
School of Biological Science and Medical Engineering,
Beihang University, Beijing, China

Abstract— **To test the hypothesis that the venous graft when implanted in an arterial bypass might endure a fast infiltra-tion/accumulation of low-density lipoproteins (LDLs) within the vessel and hence the accelerated atherogenesis. we meas-ured measured DiI-LDLs uptake by both arteries and veins under arterial condition. The experimental results showed that that the amount of DiI-LDLs uptake by the venous wall was much higher compared with arterial wall, which was con-sistent with our hypothesis.**

Keywords— **venous graft, Low-density lipoprotein, acceler-ated atherosclerosis.**

I. INTRODUCTION

Arterial grafts made by synthetic polymers have achieved a great success in vascular bypass surgery and arterial re-construction for more than 50 years[1], but when the coro-nary arteries and the low extremity peripheral arteries char-acterized by small caliber and low flow are bypassed, autologous veins (for example the greater saphenous vein) are the prior option. Nevertheless, once a vein implanted into the arterial system as graft, it will develop atheromatous lesions at an accelerated rate, which is the major cause of venous graft late failure[2 , 3].

It has been demonstrated that the hydraulic conductivity (filtration flow) and endothelial permeability of blood ves-sel walls are key factors affecting lipids transport and de-velopment of atherosclerotic lesions[4, 5]. Because the venous wall is much thinner than the arterial wall, under arterial pressure the venous graft might have a much higher filtration rate than the artery[6, 7]. Moreover, the excessive distension of the venous graft under arterial pressure will certainly disrupt its wall structure, in turn augmenting its permeability[8]. Based on this reasoning, we hypothesize that the pathologically enhanced filtration rate and permea-bility of the venous graft might lead to fast infiltra-tion/accumulation of lipids within the graft wall. This may account for the accelerated genesis and development of atherosclerosis in the venous graft.

* Corresponding author.

To verify this hypothesis, in the present study, we meas-ured the DiI-LDLs uptake by both artery and vein under arterial condition.

II. METHOD

A. Preparation of Vessel Segments

Swine femoral artery and lateral saphenous vein were harvested from farm pigs weighing 120–140 kg at a local abattoir. Our experiment was approved by the university ethics review board. Immediately after the swine was sacrificed, the leg was excised and transported to our labora-tory in low temperature. In a laboratory biological safety cabinet, the vessel was exposed and the surrounding tissue was carefully removed. A 6 to 7 cm-long segment of blood vessel was cannulated on both sides using thin-walled stain-less steel pipes. Then the two cannulas were fixed rigidly onto a specially designed metal supporting frame to hold the vessel at its in vivo length and minimize endothelial damage. The vessel was flushed internally with Krebs solution (con-centrations in mmol/L: NaCl, 118; KCl, 4.7; NaHCO3, 25; KH2PO4, 1.2; MgSO4, 1.2; CaCl2, 2.5; glucose, 11) to wash away all remaining blood. In order to check its integri-ty, the blood vessel was pressurized with a head tank filled with Krebs solution. Any points on the vessel that leaked were sealed by coagulating with an electrical fulgurator and all branches were ligated. The cannulated vessel was then dissected from the body and transferred to a stainless steel chamber (Fig. 1A).

B. Perfusion Solution

Krebs solution containing DiI-LDL (5μg/mL) was fresh-ly prepared as the perfusion solution, in which the pH value was adjusted to 7.4. Before the experiment, DiI-LDL (Bio-medical Technologies Inc, Stoughton, MA, USA) were diluted in RIPA Lysis Buffer (biomiga) with a concentration range of 0-0.5 μg/mL. Fluorescence measurements were performed using a spectrofluorometer (Cary Eclipse, Varian, UT, USA) with excitation and emission wavelengths set at 549 and 564 nm, respectively. Then, the standard curve could be obtained (Fig. 2).

I. Lackovic (ed.), *1st Global Conference on Biomedical Engineering & 9th Asian-Pacific Conference on Medical and Biological Engineering*,
IFMBE Proceedings 47, DOI: 10.1007/978-3-319-12262-5_18

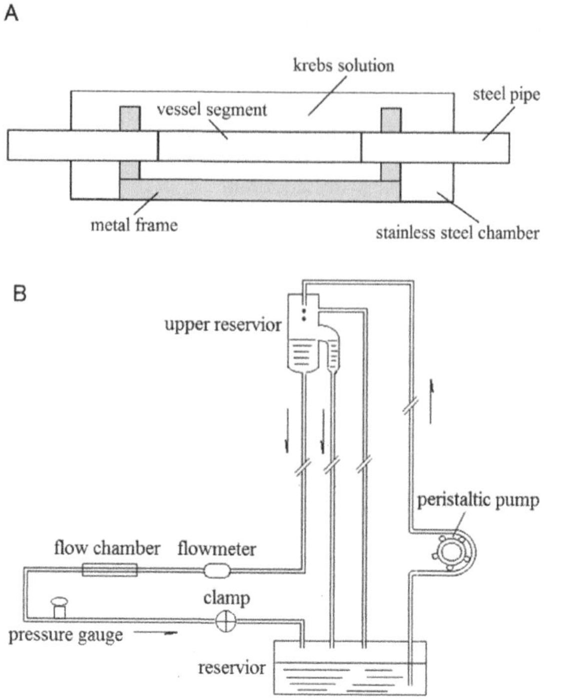

Fig. 1 (A) Schematic drawing of the stainless steel chamber encasing the test blood vessel. (B) Schematic drawing of the experimental perfusion system. The over flow head-tank provides a steady flow to the test vessel segment. The pressure gauge and the flowmeter are for monitoring the pressure and flow rate in the test vessel.

C. *Experimental Procedure*

Firstly, the harvested vessel segment was connected into the perfusion system (Fig. 1B) and the stainless steel cham-ber was filled with the Krebs solution. Then, the test vessel segment was perfused under arterial condition at a tempera-ture of 23°±0.5°C.

(i) Analysis of DiI-LDLs distribution: After 3-h perfu-sion with saline solution plus 5μg/ml DiI-LDL, the vessel was embedded in Tissue-Tek optimum cutting temperature (OCT, Sakura Finetek USA, Torrance, CA) medium and frozen quickly on dry ice mixed with methanol bath. Then the frozen vessel was sliced into 6 μm sections by using a Leica CM1950 cut machine. After mounting with Anti-fade Fluorescence Mounting Medium with DAPI (HelixGen, Guangzhou, China), the sections were imaged under a Leica TCS SPE confocal microscope (Leica Microsystems, Wetzlar, Germany) by using a 40× oil objective lens.

(ii) Measurement of the amount uptaken by vessel wall: during the experiment, the outer diameter and length of the test vessel were measured with a caliper, which was later used to determine the volume of the vessels. After three-hour perfusion, the vessel segment was flushed with Krebs solution to wash off the dissociative DiI-LDLs, and then the vessel segment was dissected from the cannulas and given a brief rinse in Krebs solution. Then, the vessel segment was digested in RIPA Lysis Buffer (biomiga) and complete lysis of the tissues was achieved by gentle pipetting of the lysate, followed by removal of cell debris by centrifugation(1000 rpm, 15 min). The fluorescence of the vessel tissue was measured with a spectrofluorometer (Cary Eclipse) with excitation and emission wavelengths set at 549 and 564 nm, respectively. The fluorescence intensity was then converted to the concentration of lipoproteins with the standard curve of DiI-LDL. The uptake by the vessel wall was expressed as the weight of DiI-LDL taken up per volume (μg/mm_3).

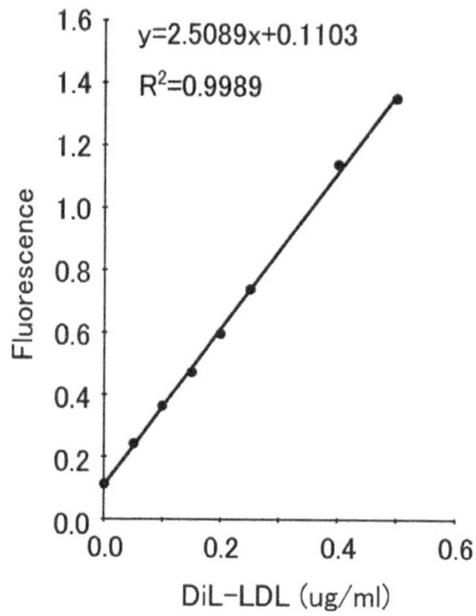

Fig. 2 Standard calibration curve of DiI-LDLs used in the experiment.

D. *Statistical Analysis*

SPSS19.0 (SPSS Inc.) software was used for statistical analysis. All experimental results are expressed as means ± the standard deviation (SD). One-way ANOVA was used to compare mean values of the measured data of the vein and artery. Differences were considered significant at $P<0.05$.

III. RESULT

The distribution of DiI-labeled LDLs (DiI-LDLs) across the test vessel wall is depicted in Fig. 3. It shows the fluorescence intensity of venous wall is higher compared with arterial wall. The concentration of DiI-LDLs within the vessel walls is presented in Fig. 4. As evident, the amount of DiI-LDLs uptaken by venous wall (48.26±6.56×10_{-3} μg/mm3) is significantly higher than that by the arterial wall (1.30±0.24×10_{-3} μg/mm3) (n=4, $P<0.05$).

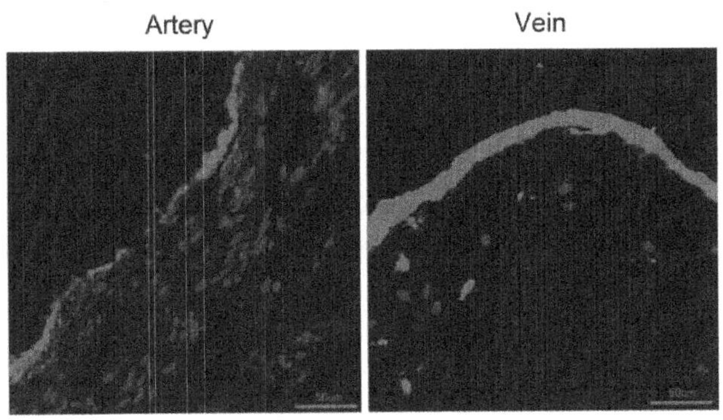

Fig. 3 Micro-images of the DiI-LDLs distribution across the venous and arterial wall under the arterial hemodynamic condition. Scale: 50μm. The fluorescence intensity of venous wall was higher than that of arterial wall.

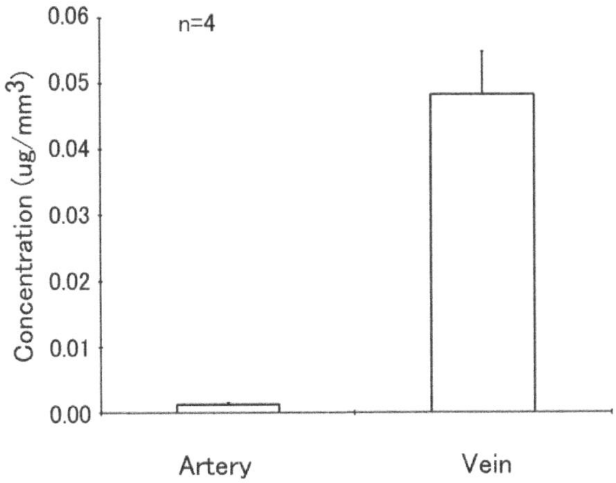

Fig. 4 Experimental result of the DiI-LDLs concentration within the ve-nous and arterial wall under the arterial hemodynamic condition. The vertical bars indicate the standard deviations. The amount of the DiI-LDLs uptake by the venous wall was significantly higher when compared the arterial wall (n=4, $P<0.05$).

IV. DISCCUSION

When implanted into the arterial system as grafts, veins will develop atheromatous lesions at an accelerated rate, which is the major cause of venous graft late failure. The process of atherogenesis in venous grafts is very similar to the one in the arterial system, in which the deposi-tion/ accumulation of lipids such as low density lipoproteins (LDLs) within the arterial wall is the initial event[9], and the high LDLs concentration within vessel wall could accel-erate the atherogenesis[10, 11].

When subjected to the arterial pressure, the filtration rate and endothelial permeability of the venous wall would be elevated sharply, we therefore believe that the LDL would be fast accumulated within the wall of venous graft and hence the accelerated atherogenesis.

To verify this hypothesis, we carried out an experiment in which the harvested artery and vein was perfused with DiI-LDL solution under arterial condition, and then the DiI-LDLs concentration within vessel wall were compared. Our measurement showed that the amount of DiI-LDLs uptaken by the venous wall was much higher than that by the arterial wall.

We suppose that two reasons might account for the fast accumulation of LDL within the graft wall. First of all, the higher filtration rate of venous graft can not only cause enhanced concentration polarization of LDLs at the luminal surface of the graft, in turn enhancing the transport of LDLs into the venous graft wall by the mechanism of concentra-tion gradient, but also can directly lead to high influx of LDLs to the vessel wall. Secondly, the higher endothelial permeability of venous graft also could increase the LDL infiltration and accumulation within the vessel wall[5].

Nevertheless, in this preliminary study, we failed to measure the endothelial permeability and hydraulic conduc-tivity (filtration flow) of the venous wall. Therefore, it is difficult to quantify the relative importance of them in LDL uptakes by the venous graft.

V. COMPLIANCE WITH ETHICAL REQUIREMENTS

A. Conflict of Interest

There is no conflict of interest involved in the article.

B. Statement of Human and Animal Rights

Our animal experiment was approved by the university ethics review board.

VI. CONCLUSIONS

When implanted into the arterial system, the venous graft will endure a fast infiltration/accumulation of atherogenic lipids (LDLs) within the vessel wall. This may contribute to the accelerated genesis and development of atherosclerosis in the venous graft.

ACKNOWLEDGMENT

This work was supported by Grants-in-Aid from the Na-tional Natural Science Research Foundation of China [31170904, 11332003, 11228205]; the Specialized Research Fund for the Doctoral Program of Higher Education [20121102110031]; Special Fund for Excellent Doctor

Degree Dissertation of Beijing [20131000601]; and the Innovation Foundation of BUAA for PhD Graduates.

Conflict of Interest

There is no conflict of interest involved in the article.

References

1. Kent KC, Whittemore AD, Mannick JA. (1989) Short-term and midterm results of an all-autogenous tissue policy for infrainguinal reconstruction. J Vasc Surg 9: 107-114.
2. Motwani JG, Topol EJ. (1998) Aortocoronary saphenous vein graft disease: pathogenesis, predisposition, and prevention. Cir-culation 97: 916-931Otsuka F, Yahagi K, Sakakura K, et al. (2013) Why is the mammary artery so special and what protects it from atherosclerosis? Ann Cardiothorac Surg 2: 519-526.
3. Campeau L, Enjalbert M, Lesperance J, et al. (1984) The rela-tion of risk factors to the development of atherosclerosis in sa-phenous-vein bypass grafts and the progression of disease in the native circulation. A study 10 years after aortocoronary bypass surgery. N Engl J Med 311: 1329-1332.
4. Baldwin AL, Wilson LM, Simon BR. (1992) Effect of pressure on aortic hydraulic conductance. Arterioscler Thromb 12: 163-171.
5. Stangeby DK, Ethier CR. (2002) Coupled computational analy-sis of arterial LDL transport -- effects of hypertension. Comput Methods Biomech Biomed Engin 5: 233-241.
6. Deng X, Marois Y, Guidoin R, et al. (1996) Efficiency of an ex-ternal support to reduce lipid infiltration into venous grafts: in vitro evaluation. Artif Organs 20: 1208-1214.
7. Wilens SL, McCluskey RT. (1952) The comparative filtration properties of excised arteries and veins. Am J Med Sci 224: 540-547.
8. Dabagh M, Jalali P, Tarbell JM. (2009) The transport of LDL across the deformable arterial wall: the effect of endothelial cell turnover and intimal deformation under hypertension. Am J Physiol Heart Circ Physiol 297: H983-996.
9. Stary HC. (1989) Evolution and progression of atherosclerotic lesions in coronary arteries of children and young adults. Arte-riosclerosis 9: I19-32.
10. Schwenke DC, Carew TE. (1989) Initiation of atherosclerotic le-sions in cholesterol-fed rabbits. II. Selective retention of LDL vs. selective increases in LDL permeability in susceptible sites of arteries. Arteriosclerosis 9: 908-918.
11. Schwenke DC, Carew TE. (1989) Initiation of atherosclerotic le-sions in cholesterol-fed rabbits. I. Focal increases in arterial LDL concentration precede development of fatty streak lesions. Arteriosclerosis 9: 895-907.
12. Prosi M, Zunino P, Perktold K, et al. (2005) Mathematical and numerical models for transfer of low-density lipoproteins through the arterial walls: a new methodology for the model set up with applications to the study of disturbed lumenal flow. J Biomech 38: 903-917.

Author: X.Y. Deng
Institute: Key Laboratory for Biomechanics and Mechanobiology of Ministry of Education, School of Biological Science and Medical Engineering.
Street: XueYuan Road No.37, HaiDian District
City: Beijing
Country: China
Email: dengxy1953@buaa.edu.cn

Osteogenic Differentiation of Human Mesenchymal Stromal Cells Promoted by Acoustic Vibration

X. Chen, D.Y. Zhong, F. He, and Z.P. Luo

Orthopedic Institute, Soochow University, Suzhou, China

Abstract— **In order to verify whether differentiation of human stem cells toward bone tissue is promoted by higher acoustic vibration (≥90 Hz), human mesenchymal stromal cells (hMSCs) were mechanically stimulated with vibration (400 and 800 Hz, 0.3 g acceleration) for 30 min every 24 h for 7 or 14 days in vitro. Cells were seeded in osteogenic medium, which enhanced differentiation towards bone tissue. The osteogenic differentiation of hMSCs under the vibrated and non-vibrated conditions was assessed by examining mRNA expression of various osteoblast-associated markers (ALP, Runx2, osterix (Osx), collagen type I (Col I) and osteopontin (OPN)), and matrix mineralization. Our results indicated that acoustic vibration at frequency 800 Hz was more favorable for hMSCs osteogenic differentiation: the gene expression involved in osteogenic differentiation was significantly increased after 7 and 14 days, and deposition of calcium was almost 1.5-fold. Further studies are necessary to verify the long-term viability and commitment to osteogenic differentiation of hMSCs in vitro and in vivo, and select the optimum sensitive acoustic frequency, with the purpose of determining whether acoustic vibration could become a novel means to treat osteoporosis.**

Keywords— **Acoustic vibration, Human mesenchymal stromal cells, Osteogenic differentiation, Osteoporosis.**

I. INTRODUCTION

Osteoporosis is a disease characterized by progressive deterioration of bone tissue due to an imbalance in the breakdown and rebuilding of bone, giving rise to increased bone fragility and susceptibility to fracture. Current methods for the prevention and treatment of osteoporosis are primarily drug-based, which delay disease progression but do not fully restore the balance in bone resorption and formation[1, 2].

As bone is a dynamic and self-regulating organ capable of adapting its mass and morphology according to its mechanical environment, some researchers have turned to a biomechanical approach to treating osteoporosis[3].

In fact, in recent years application of mechanical vibration in clinical trials has greatly increased for osteoporosis. And there is abundant in vivo evidence of osteogenic activity both in whole body and in local repair[4].

Recent studies suggest that low acoustic vibration (20-90 Hz) has the ability to direct the lineage commitment of bone marrow mesenchymal stromal cells (BMSCs), the progenitors of osteocytes and osteoblasts, by biasing cell fate in favor of osteogenesis over adipogenesis[5, 6]. If there existed the optimum acoustic vibration — that enhances BMSCs toward bone formation, which could be a cue for recovering bone loss arising from osteoporotic conditions. More specially, vibration frequency in these studies mostly focused on the range of low acoustic frequency[7, 8]. However, the effect of higher acoustic frequency (90-20000 Hz) vibration applied on BMSCs has not been studied.

Therefore, in this study, we aimed to delineate whether acoustic vibration(≥90 Hz) signals could influence human mesenchymal stromal cells (hMSCs) toward bone formation in vitro. hMSCs were exposed to repeated bouts of the stimulus at an acceleration of 0.3 g and different frequencies of 0, 400 and 800 Hz. hMSCs markers of osteoblastic differentiation, and their functional capacity to form mineralized bone nodules were examined.

II. MATERIALS AND METHODS

A. Culture of hMSCs

Primary hMSCs were isolated from human umbilical cord blood of a healthy donor (aged 4 yrs). The cells were cultured up to 80% confluence in 175 cm^2 cell culture flasks using α-MEM medium supplemented with 10% fetal bovine serum (10% FBS), 100 U/ml penicillin, and 100 mg/ml streptomycin in humidified atmosphere of 5% CO_2 at 37°C. Cells were then harvested using 0.25% trypsin and seeded in 12-well plate, then incubated in osteogenic medium: DMEM containing 10% FBS, 100 U/ml penicillin, 100 mg/ml streptomycin, 10 nM β-glycerophosphate disodium salt hydrate, 0.1 μM dexamethasone and 50 mg/L lascorbic acid and subjected to mechanical strain detailed described as follows. The medium was changed every 3 days.

B. Acoustic Frequency Mechanical Loading Platform

A vibration loading of cell cultures was developed to stimulate hMSCs with different vibrations. 12-well plates cultured with hMSCs were mounted onto the platform of

I. Lackovic (ed.), *1st Global Conference on Biomedical Engineering & 9th Asian-Pacific Conference on Medical and Biological Engineering*, IFMBE Proceedings 47, DOI: 10.1007/978-3-319-12262-5_19

a vibration shaker which was excited by one channel of functional generator providing the amplitude, waveform, and frequency of the vibration. When the platform was placed in the cell culture incubator, hMSCs cultures received perpendicular mechanical stimuli (magnitude of 0.2 g, frequencies of 400 and 800 Hz) for 30 min every 24 h for various time periods as indicated in each experiment. Cells that were not stimulated with mechanical stimuli served as the negative control. The effects of acoustic vibration on hMSCs proliferation, osteogenic differentiation and mineralization were evaluated.

C. RNA Extraction and RT-PCR Analysis

After the acoustic vibration of 7 and 14 days, total RNA was isolated from cells using TRIzol reagent according to the manufacturer's protocol. For the detection of the mRNA level of osteogenic genes, the total-RNA was reverse-transcribed with a 5 × PrimeScript RT Master Mix and the transcription level of GAPDH was validated as the normalizer. Real-time quantitative PCR was performed with SYBR Green PCR Master Mix on Chromo4 Real-Time PCR Detection System. ΔCt was calculated by subtracting the Ct of GAPDH mRNA from the Ct of the mRNA of interest genes. The relative mRNA level was calculated according to the equation $2^{-\Delta\Delta Ct}$. All reactions were done in triplicate. The sequences of primers for RT-PCR are listed in Table 1.

D. Alizarin Red Stain

Following the experiment, cells were washed twice with ice-cold PBS and fixed in 4% polyoxymethylene for 30 min at 14 days. Cultures were stained for 30 min with a 1% alizarin red solution for calcium detection. Following the stain, cultures were rinsed with ddH_2O. Graphs express mineralization as a percent of the experimental control. The calcium deposition was then dissolved with perchloric acid and quantified by measuring the absorbance at 420 nm.

E. Statistics

Values were calculated as means ± standard deviation (SD). The expression of osteogenic genes and quantity of calcium deposition in cells between different groups were compared by t test. $P < 0.05$ was considered statistically significance. All tests were two-sided and were conducted using SPSS 16.0 software.

Table 1 Primers used for Real-time RT-PCR

Gene	Primer sequence(5'- 3')	GeneBank accession
GAPDH	F: AGAAAAACCTGCCAAATATGATGAC	NM_002046
	R: TGGGTGTCGCTGTTGAAGTC	
Col I	F: CAGCCGCTTCACCTACAGC	NM_000088
	R: TTTTGTATTCAATCACTGTCTTGCC	
ALP	F: AGCACTCCCACTTCATCTGGAA	NM_000478.3
	R: GAGACCCAATAGGTAGTCCACATTG	
OPN	F: GCGAGGAGTTGAATGGTG	NM_013227.2
	R: CTTGTGGCTGTGGGTTTC	
Runx2	F:AGAAGGCACAGACAGAAGCTTGA	NM_001015051.3
	R:AGGAATGCGCCCTAAATCACT	
Osx	F: CACTCACACCCGGGAGAAGA	NM_152860.1
	R:GGTGGTCGCTTCGGGTAAA	

III. RESULTS

A. Changes in mRNA Expression of Osteogenic Genes

Real-time RT-PCR revealed that the expression of osteogenic differentiation related genes, ALP, Col I, OPN, Runx2, and Osx were all up-regulated in vibrated cells at 7 days. The highest response of these related genes was due to the 800 Hz regime. It enhanced ALP, Col I and Osx mRNA expression most significantly, which exhibited 5.3-, 2.4 and 4.6-fold increases, respectively, compared with the non-vibrated cells, and significantly larger than the response to 400 Hz (Fig.1).

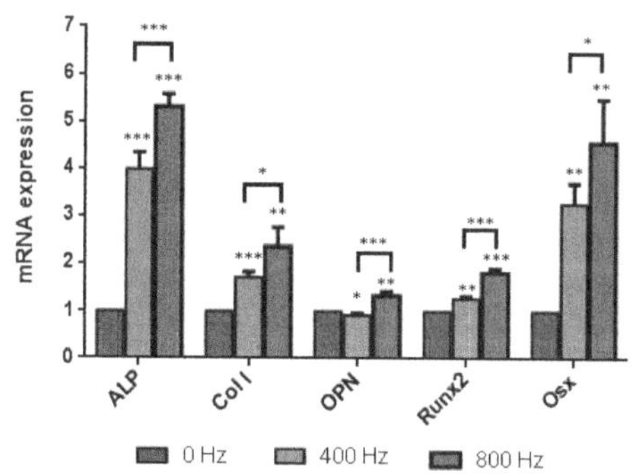

Fig. 1 Real-time RT-PCR of osteoblastic differentiation markers, ALP, Col I, OPN, Runx2 and Osx was performed after 7 days of vibration(0, 400 and 800 Hz). Statistically significant values are indicated as *, $P< 0.05$; **, $P< 0.01$; ***, $P< 0.001$.

However, after 14 days of acoustic vibration, RNA level of ALP, Col I , OPN, Runx2, and Osx were inhibited in the

400 Hz group. In particular, hMSCs vibrated at 800 Hz displayed significantly higher osteogenic-related gene expression, with increases of 2.3- fold at ALP, 1.2- fold at Col I, 1.8-fold at OPN and 1.8-fold at Osx, respectively, with respect to controls (Fig.2).

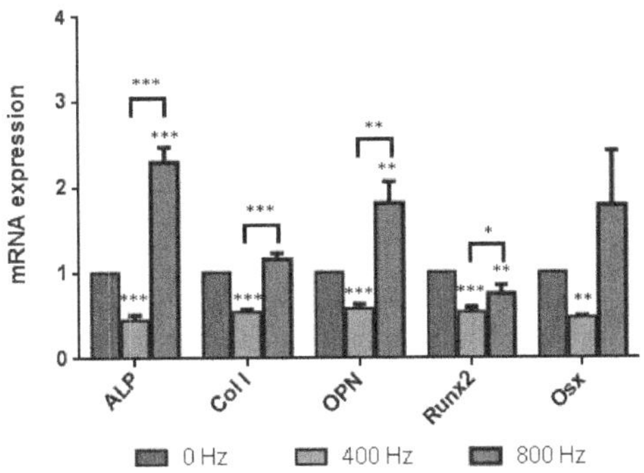

Fig. 2 Real-time RT-PCR of osteoblastic differentiation markers, ALP, Col I, OPN, Runx2 and Osxwas performed after 14 days of vibration (0, 400 and 800 Hz). Statistically significant values are indicated as *, $P< 0.05$; **, $P< 0.01$; ***, $P< 0.001$.

Calcium deposition was determined by assessment of the destained amount of alizarin red S after the stained images were captured (Fig.3). 800 Hz vibration for 14 days significantly accelerated matrix mineralization, as shown by an approximately 1.5-fold increase in the amount of stained alizarin red S compared with the staining observed for the non-vibrated cells (Fig.4). But 400 Hz vibration failed to increase calcium deposition, which was consistent with the PCR results.

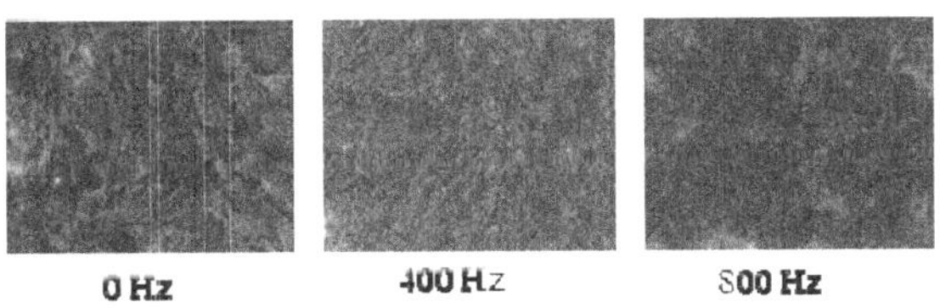

Fig. 3 Calcium deposition of hMSCs was visualized by alizarin red S staining after 14 days of vibration (0, 400 and 800 Hz).

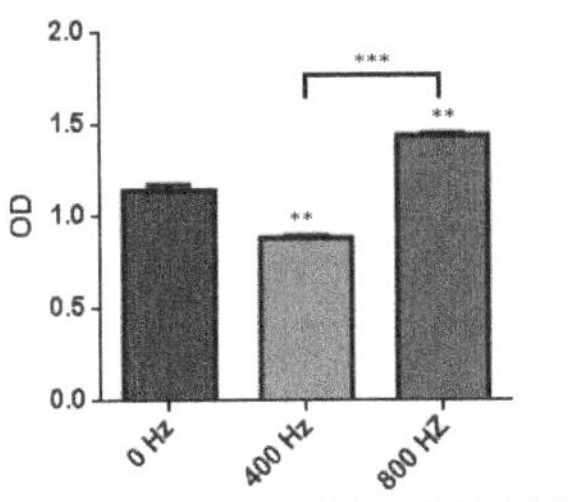

Fig. 4 Calcium deposition of hMSCs after 14 days of vibration (0, 400 and 800 Hz) was quantified by measurement of the amount of alizarin red S staining, as detailed in the Methods section. Statistically significant values are indicated as *, $P< 0.05$; **, $P< 0.01$; ***, $P< 0.001$.

IV. DISCUSSION

Vibration is a mechanical treatment widely utilized in clinical and rehabilitation centres. Of recent interest is a mechanical vibration signal—that has been shown to increase bone formation in animal models, including young mice[9], ovariectomized rats[10], and rats subjected to hind limb disuse by tail-suspension[11].

Despite the obvious promotion of vibration on bone metabolism in vivo, the molecular and cellular basis for this effect remains relatively unclear. hMSCs was chosen in this study because it is a good source of osteoblast precursor cells, which can differentiate into bone with the appropriate conditions. In addition, some studies have elucidated that low acoustic vibration has the ability to direct the lineage commitment of BMSCs toward osteogenesis over adipogenesis in vivo [5, 6]. Therefore, if there existed the optimum acoustic vibrations — that enhanced BMSCs toward bone formation, which would be a new method for recovering bone loss arising from osteoporotic conditions.

More specially, vibration frequency in above studies mostly focused on the range of 20-90 Hz frequency, except that Dumas et al. reported extracellular matrix produced by osteoblasts under 400 Hz vibration was favorable to BMSC osteodifferentiation[12]. Consistent with this report, our current study hypothesized acoustic vibration (≥90 Hz) signals would induce hMSCs toward osteogenic differentiation. With the utilization of amplitude detection device on the mechanical loading platform, 400 and 800 Hz could generate the similar acceleration of 0.3 g, which was widely considered as the suitable vibration amplitude by most previous studies[7]. Therefore, 400 and 800 Hz were chosen for this study.

The effect of different acoustic vibration on hMSCs osteogenesis was evaluated by measuring mRNA levels of early to late osteoblast associated markers. Based on the results of the RT-PCR analysis, vibration at 400Hz in the earlier 7 days significantly enhanced mRNA level of ALP, Col I, Runx2 and Osx. However, 400Hz significantly decreased expression of these osteogenetic genes after later 7 days vibration, when compared to the non-vibrated controls. Consistent with these changes, the amount of matrix mineralization decreased upon acoustic vibration at 400 Hz after 14 days of vibration. Taken together, these findings demonstrate that 400 Hz could promote hMSCs osteogenesis in earlier stage to some extent, but inhibited osteogenesis in later stage.

Notably, when hMSCs were stimulated at 800 Hz acoustic vibration after 7 and 14 days, we all observed a large vibration-induced increase in the expression of most osteogenic genes compared with the non-vibrated group or 400 Hz group. As Osx considered as a more specific marker of osteoblasts and crucial for osteoblast formation, the increase in Osx expression might have contributed to the acceleration of matrix mineralization observed in the 800 Hz vibrated cultures.

In this study, we might consider that hMSCs responded to acoustic vibration (800 Hz) toward osteogenic differentiation. These differential sensitivities reflect gene-specific preferences for specific frequencies. This finding is quite interesting, and it is possible that vibration at 800 Hz might activate the signaling pathways involved in osteogenesis. We speculate some specular acoustic frequency vibration might have affected the phosphorylation pattern of proteins that regulate the cell cycle. Thus, further investigations are necessary to test these hypotheses and to better understand the molecular mechanisms underlying the cellular responses to acoustic frequency.

As we known, acoustic frequencies cover a wide range of 20 ~ 20000 Hz. The frequency we employed in our study was a small part of acoustic frequency. It is necessary to systematically investigate the response of hMSc to acoustic frequencies and find a series of the specific sensitive frequencies. These studies will pave the way for the development of an acoustic based therapeutic system for osteoporosis in the elderly.

V. CONCLUSION

Our study provided a glimpse at how hMSCs respond to acoustic vibration at the level of gene transcription and matrix mineralization. At 400 Hz vibration, we observed markers of osteogenesis increased after 7 days, then decreased significantly after 14 days. Our results indicate that acoustic vibration at frequency 800 Hz, with a 0.3 g acceleration was more favourable for hMSCs osteogenic differentiation. Further studies are necessary to verify the long-term viability and commitment to osteogenic differentiation of hMSCs in vitro and in vivo, with the purpose of determining whether acoustic vibration could become a novel means to treating osteoporosis.

ACKNOWLEDGMENT

This work was supported by the National Natural Science Foundation of China under Grant no. 31270995.

CONFLICT OF INTEREST

The authors declare that they have no conflict of interest.

REFERENCES

1. Lau E, Lee W D, Li J et al. (2011) Effect of low - magnitude, high - frequency vibration on osteogenic differentiation of rat mesenchymal stromal cells. J Orthop Res 29(7):1075-1080
2. Si L, Winzenberg T, Palmer A et al. (2014) A systematic review of models used in cost-effectiveness analyses of preventing osteoporotic fractures. Osteoporosis Int 25(1):51-60
3. Rubin C, Turner A S, Bain S et al. (2001) Anabolism: Low mechanical signals strengthen long bones. Nature 412(6847): 603-604
4. Zhao L, Dodge T, Nemani A et al. (2014) Resonance in the mouse tibia as a predictor of frequencies and locations of loading-induced bone formation. Biomech Model Mechan 13(1): 141-151
5. Luu Y K, Capilla E, Rosen C J et al. (2009) Mechanical stimulation of mesenchymal atem cell proliferation and differentiation promotes osteogenesis while preventing dietary - induced obesity. J Bone Min Res 24(1): 50-61
6. Rubin C, Capilla E, Luu Y et al. (2007) Adipogenesis is inhibited by brief, daily exposure to high-frequency, extremely low-magnitude mechanical signals. Proc Natl Acad Sci USA 104 (45):17879-17884
7. Kim I, Song Y, Lee B et al. (2012) Human mesenchymal stromal cells are Mechanosensitive to Vibration stimuli. J Dent Res 91(12): 1135-1140.
8. Judex S, Rubin C. (2010) Is bone formation induced by high-frequency mechanical signals modulated by muscle activity? J Musculoskelet Neuronal Interact 10(1): 3
9. Xie L, Jacobson J M , Choi E S et al. (2006) Low-level mechanical vibrations can influence bone resorption and bone formation in the growing skeleton. Bone 39(5): 1059-1066
10. Oxlund B, Ørtoft G, Andreassen T T et al. (2003) Low-intensity, high-frequency vibration appears to prevent the decrease in strength of the femur and tibia associated with ovariectomy of adult rats. Bone 32(1): 69-77
11. Garman R, Gaudette G, Donahue L R et al. (2007) Low - level accelerations applied in the absence of weight bearing can enhance trabecular bone formation. J Orthop Res 25(6): 732-740
12. Dumas V, Ducharne B, Perrier A et al. (2010) Extracellular matrix produced by osteoblasts cultured under low-magnitude, high-frequency stimulation is favourable to osteogenic differentiation of mesenchymal stem cells. Calcified Tissue Int 87 (4): 351-364

Author: Xi Chen, Dong-Yan Zhong, Fan He, Zong-Ping Luo
Institute: Soochow University Orthopedic Institute
Street: 708 Renmin Rd, Rm 304, Bldg 1, Orthopedic Institute, Soochow University (South Campus), Suzhou
City: Suzhou
Country: China
Email:cxtracy1126@163.com

Discuss the Epithelial to Mesenchymal Transition by the View of Mechanics

Ho-Kai Huang[1] and Ming-Long Yeh[2]

[1] Department of Biomedical Engineering, National Cheng-Kung University, Tainan, Taiwan
[2] Department of Biomedical Engineering, National Cheng-Kung University, Tainan, Taiwan

Abstract— **The epithelial to mesenchymal transition (EMT) involves several physiological and pathological phenomena and endows cells with invasive and migratory properties. We use the microplate measurement system (MMS) to measure cells stiffness. The EMT cells will have higher stiffness. However, treating inhibitor Cyto-D and ML-7 will lower cells' stiffness. Based on this, we can use mechanical properties, to be a principle of the EMT process.**

Keywords— **EMT, microplate measurement system, cell stiffness.**

I. INTRODUCTION

The epithelial to mesenchymal transition (EMT), which converts polarized epithelial cells into motile mesenchymal cells and promotes invasive and migration properties plays a key role in the early stages of metastasis. Cancer metastasis remains the leading cause of death worldwide. Thus, identifying and prohibiting cells undergoing EMT has important clinical relevance, especially in cancer diagnosis and therapy.

Recently, stiffness has been recognized as a quick and quantitative measure to differentiate the types of cells[1], such as compressive stiffness of cells might possibly be used to predict the onset of leukostasis [2] and tensile stiffness of cells could be used to grade the metastatic potential of tumor cells [3]. The importance of cell mechanical properties (CMs) to cancer is appreciated, yet the contributions of specific cytoskeleton to cells undergoing EMT and their physiological significance are needed further elucidation.

II. MATERIALS AND METHODS

MMS was modified version of previous set-up [4] to axially compress-relax-retract individual cells captured between a rigid plate and an AFM tip which were oriented horizontally in order to simultaneously observe cells and measure their stiffness. In addition, the commercial product as AFM cantilever overcame the inconvenience of glass microplate reproduction [5]. Though prior research has investigated the TGF-β1 effects on the cell in resisting compression, those studies only examined forces applied locally onto the cell [6, 7]. However, cells typically experience mechanical forces applied along them entirety [8]. A schematic representation of the experimental geometry and optical phase contrast images are shown in Fig. 1(a), (b) and (c).

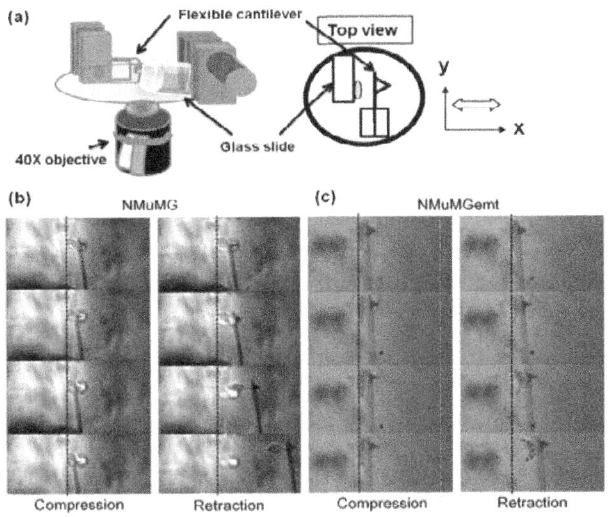

Fig. 1 (a) Schematic drawings of the MMS setup A cell is placed between two plates symmetrically mounted on each side of the microscope stage. The Cartesian coordinate axes of the images are defined by the indicated plot, and the flexible cantilever is driven along the X-axis by a stepper motor. (b) Representative phase contrast images of NMuMG cells undergoing mechanical measurements. The dotted line represents the edge of the glass slide, where the measured cell adhered. (c) Representative phase contrast images of NMuMGemt cells. The dotted curve in red indicates the speculated end-reinforced adhesion of NMuMGemt during retraction.

A. Experimental Setup of Force Measurements Using MMS

Glass microscope slides were sterilized in 70% ethanol overnight and exposed to UV irradiation for 15 minutes. To coat an extracellular substrate layer, the slides were incubated in 10 μg/cm^2 type I collagen from rat tails (BD Bioscience, California, USA) overnight followed by washing in PBS twice. Suspended NMuMG or NMuMGemt cells (2×105 cells/ml) were allowed to adhere to the collagen-coated slides in a 6 cm dish. Meanwhile, the NMuMGemt cells were additionally treated with TGF-β1 for EMT induction. What's more, we treat Cyto-D and ML-7 to inhibit NMuMGemt cells. After a 48 h incubation, the cell seeding glass slides were perpendicularly placed in a 10 cm

I. Lackovic (ed.), *1st Global Conference on Biomedical Engineering & 9th Asian-Pacific Conference on Medical and Biological Engineering*,
IFMBE Proceedings 47, DOI: 10.1007/978-3-319-12262-5_20

dish. Culture medium containing 30 mM HEPES was added to the dish to prevent pH changes over the course of the experiment. The dish was placed on an inverted microscope (AE31, Motic, China) that was positioned on an anti-vibration table, and all experiments were performed in an incubation chamber at constant temperature with controlled CO2 levels. Selected cells were observed using a 40× objective for all experiments. To obtain a calibration scale, a standard grid image was taken using the same objective with a CCD camera (TCA-10, Tucsen, China). These images were subsequently examined to obtain a 4.8 pixels/μm calibration constant.

B. Cantilever Calibration

For calibration, a PDMS substrate of Young's modulus E=5kPa was estimated in advance using a material testing system (LRX5K, Lloyd Instrument, England). According to a previous study [9] for simulating this substrate as a spring, in this case, the spring constant of PDMS, kp ,was equal to the relationship between the pulling force, and the elongated deformation was given by Eq1:

$$k_p = \frac{EL}{(1-v^2)} \qquad (1);$$

Where L (≒10μm) is the length of the cantilever-PDMS contact area and ν (≒0.25) is the Poisson's ratio of the substrate and Young's modulus E (≒5 kPa). We can get k_p was 0.09 μN/μm. The mechanical equivalence between the cantilever and PDMS then implied that

$$k_p\delta_p = k_c\delta_c \qquad (2);$$

The tensile force generated by the drag force from cantilever deflection induced tension force onto the PDMS substrate. During a cantilever-PDMS separation experiment, we could measure the elongated deformation of PDMS, where (δ_p) was 3μm and the deflection of cantilever (δ_c) was 30μm. Therefore, the estimated k_c was 0.009μN/μm according to equation (2), and this was then applied as a spring constant for the standard cantilever. Each flexible cantilever used in our experiments was calibrated with respect to the standard cantilever. The resolution of MMS was calculated from the deflection and spring constant of cantilever by using minimum unit (1 pixel=0.21μm) multiplied by the calibrated spring constant (0.009μN/μm) of the cantilever. Therefore, the estimated resolution was 2nN.

C. Image Analysis and Mechanical Properties Estimation

Each cell was recognized as either a spheroid or hemi-spheroid with rotational symmetry around the x-axis. The x- and y-dimensions were defined as the cell height and diameter, respectively. Axial strain (ε) was calculated as a change in cell height (measured immediately) divided by the initial cell height (measured prior to compression). In addition, the contact area (Ac) between cells and the cantilever was assumed to be circular because of the symmetry between the cell shape, and its value was estimated from the measured cell diameter, which changed progressively during measurement. The deflection of the calibrated cantilever was measured by synchronizing images. The measured force (F) was calculated by using Hooke's law from the deflection of cantilever multiplied by the calibrated spring constant of the cantilever. An image analysis program was encoded using the MATLAB software. Stress (σ) was calculated using Eq3: $\sigma = \frac{F}{Ac}$ (3) ;

Stiffness (E) was estimated by the Eq4: $E = \frac{\sigma}{\varepsilon}$ (4) ;

III. Results and Discussions

First, we use the MMS to measure cells mechanical properties. We compared control and EMT cells and

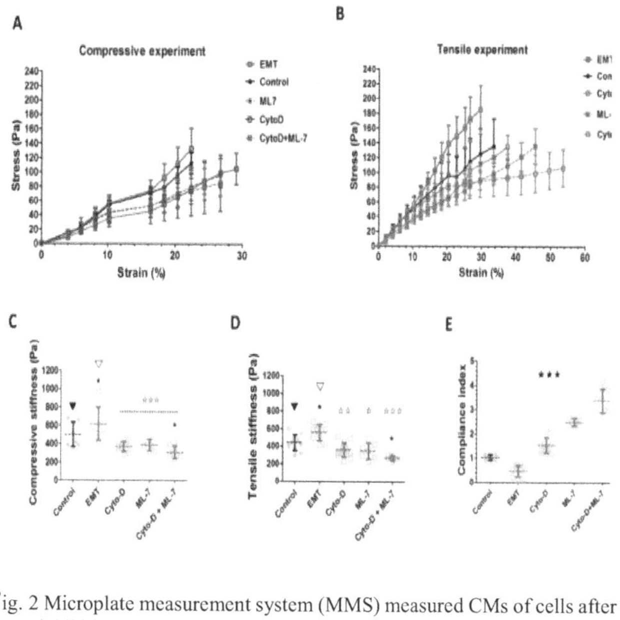

Fig. 2 Microplate measurement system (MMS) measured CMs of cells after drugs inhibition and its additive effects with TGF-β1. The stress verse strain curves of both (A) compressive and (B) tensile experiment were shown. The untreated EMT cells (red line with square-markers) had the stiffest slope. And each marker with the upper and lower bars indicated the mean and SD from a group of applied stress at specific strain value. (C and D) When compare to control cells (indicated by ▼), the cells after EMT (indicated by ▽) had significantly higher stiffness. When compare with untreated-EMT cells (indicated by ▽), the drug-inhibited EMT cells had significantly lower stiffness. (E) The compliance index (CI) of each condition showed that, the cells with lower stiffness were more compliant to the constant external force. Between each group, there are significant differences in CI. ☆: $p<0.05$, ☆☆: $p<0.01$, ☆☆☆: $p<0.001$

treating inhibitor cells (Fig. 2). In compressive experiment, all groups presented an increment of stress, when the acquired strain was above 16%, meanwhile, the nucleus was compressed (Fig. 2A). We estimated the compressive stiffness (CS) of cells from the slope of curve wholly. From the whole-cell-mechanics aspect, we prefer to consider the stiffness as the combined contribution from membrane, nucleus and cytoskeleton. After drug inhibition, alone or combined, the slope of curves seemed flatten in the same way, which depicted that the CS was responsive to drugs but was not distinguishable. We compressed cell with the constant pre-setting working distance, the acquired strain of drug-inhibited cells was as high as 30%, indicated that had higher compliance.

The stress-strain curves of tensile experiments (Fig. 2B) revealed the tensile stiffness (TS) divergence between groups, and demonstrated that TS had an extraordinary distinguishable character. Additionally, the compliance of cells under tension was intricately responding to the TGF-β1 and addictive effects of drug-inhibition specifically.

To compare with control cells, the compressive and tensile stiffness were increased after EMT by 23.2% and 10.2%, respectively (Fig. 2C and D). This increment in CMs might contribute to the early process of cancer cell metastasis[10], permit cancer cells access to dissemination sites such as the lymphatic and blood vasculature through EMT[11].

The effectiveness of Cyto-D and ML-7 was confirmed in EMT cells, whereas, the EMT cells was not varied from the control cells in stiffness, after inhibited by Cyto-D or ML-7. More than 30% decrease in stiffness after Cyto-D or ML-7 inhibition indicated that there was an antagonist relationship with TGF-β1. Furthermore, combined Cyto-D and ML-7 had addictive effect on EMT cells, decreased by 48% and 49% in compressive and tensile stiffness, respectively (Fig. 2C and D), indicating the different inhibiting mechanism of Cyto-D and ML-7.

After Cyto-D or ML-7 inhibition, the dynamic cell morphology adaptation disappeared due to the inhibition of F-actin assembly and depression of the self-contractile forces at the adhesion sites via connections with the myosin II[12].

Remarkably, the cell strain progressively increased with applied tensile force, represented as compliance index (CI). Subsequently, the CI of EMT cell was only a half of control cells (Fig. 2E) Consistently, the CI of EMT cells was increased by 2, 4 and 5.8 folded after Cyto-D, ML-7 and Cyto-D+ML-7 inhibition (Fig. 2E) ($p<0.001$).

The main advantage of MMS was that we can observe the cell deformation and measure the mechanical properties at the same time. The inspection of cell strain was indicated as CI in this study, which demonstrated a high responsiveness to cell stiffness in a reverse relationship.

IV. Conclusion

The stiffness is an important signal to discuss the EMT process. Through the modified MMS system, we can test the cells stiffness. The results showed that normal cells through EMT will change its properties. The EMT cells have larger stiffness than normal cells. But if we add inhibitors, we can find that the stiffness of the cells significantly decreased. Based on this, we can easily distinguish the normal cells and cancer-induced cells. Therefore, this property can be used to detect cancer cells more quickly in the future.

V. References

[1] White cell mechanics: basic science and clinical aspects. Proceedings of a symposium held at the Kroc Foundation, Santa Ynez Valley, California, May 2-6, 1983. Kroc Foundation series. 1984;16:1-318.

[2] Lam WA, Rosenbluth MJ, Fletcher DA. Increased leukaemia cell stiffness is associated with symptoms of leucostasis in paediatric acute lymphoblastic leukaemia. British journal of haematology. 2008;142:497-501.

[3] Swaminathan V, Mythreye K, O'Brien ET, Berchuck A, Blobe GC, Superfine R. Mechanical stiffness grades metastatic potential in patient tumor cells and in cancer cell lines. Cancer Res. 2011;71:5075-80.

[4] Nagayama K, Yanagihara S, Matsumoto T. A novel micro tensile tester with feed-back control for viscoelastic analysis of single isolated smooth muscle cells. Med Eng Phys. 2007;29:620-8.

[5] Mitrossilis D, Fouchard J, Pereira D, Postic F, Richert A, Saint-Jean M, et al. Real-time single-cell response to stiffness. Proc Natl Acad Sci U S A.107:16518-23.

[6] Canetta E, Duperray A, Leyrat A, Verdier C. Measuring cell viscoelastic properties using a force spectrometer: influence of protein-cytoplasm interactions. Biorheology. 2005;42:321-33.

[7] Thoelking G, Reiss B, Wegener J, Oberleithner H, Pavenstaedt H, Riethmuller C. Nanotopography follows force in TGF-beta1 stimulated epithelium. Nanotechnology. 2010;21:265102.

[8] Guilak F, Mow VC. The mechanical environment of the chondrocyte: a biphasic finite element model of cell-matrix interactions in articular cartilage. Journal of biomechanics. 2000;33:1663-73.

[9] Mitrossilis D, Fouchard J, Guiroy A, Desprat N, Rodriguez N, Fabry B, et al. Single-cell response to stiffness exhibits muscle-like behavior. Proc Natl Acad Sci U S A. 2009;106:18243-8.

[10] Labelle M, Begum S, Hynes RO. Direct signaling between platelets and cancer cells induces an epithelial-mesenchymal-like transition and promotes metastasis. Cancer cell. 2011;20:576-90.

[11] Birchmeier W. Cell adhesion and signal transduction in cancer. Conference on cadherins, catenins and cancer. EMBO reports. 2005;6:413-7.

[12] Stewart MP, Helenius J, Toyoda Y, Ramanathan SP, Muller DJ, Hyman AA. Hydrostatic pressure and the actomyosin cortex drive mitotic cell rounding. Nature. 2011;469:226-30.

The Relationship of Coloboma of Cortical Plate attaching Sigmoid Sinus and Vascular Pulsatile Tinnitus: A Numerical Study

Shan Tian[1], Rui Mao[1], Zhaohui Liu[2], Lizhen Wang[1], and Yubo Fan[1,*]

[1] Key Laboratory for Biomechanics and Mechanobiology of Ministry of Education, School of Biological Science and Medical Engineering, Beihang University, Beijing, 100191, China

[2] Department of Radiology, Beijing Tongren Hospital, Capital Medical University, Beijing, 100730, China

Abstract— **Vascular pulsatile tinnitus is a common and serious symptom, but no clear biomechanism. According to clinical radiographic reports, coloboma of cortical plate attaching sigmoid sinus occurs widely among patients, and most of them can be cured through cortical plate reconstruction surgery. Therefore cortical plate coloboma is a high-possibility etiology causing vascular pulsatile tinnitus. To study the mechanical relationship between cortical plate coloboma and vascular pulsatile tinnitus, finite element models of sigmoid sinus flow field and cortical plate were developed based on CT images. The generation and propagation of tinnitus noise were simulated separately. The model with and without cortical plate were analyzed to make comparison. The evaluation result provided a mechanical conclusion that coloboma of cortical plate attaching sigmoid sinus would remarkably amplify the noise generated in sigmoid sinus, therefore directly leading to audible perception. The conclusion also positively supported the cortical plate reconstruction surgery to cure vascular pulsatile tinnitus.**

Keywords— **vascular pulsatile, tinnitus, sigmoid sinus, simulation, vibration, noise.**

I. INTRODUCTION

Vascular pulsatile tinnitus (PT) is a common symptom in otology and neurology. There are about 9 million patients in China at present. Prolonged vascular PT would seriously harm the quality of daily life of patients, and may even lead to mental disorders [1]. The mechanism of vascular PT remains unclear. Several etiology hypotheses have been suggested in previous researches, including abnormal or high velocity blood flow in sigmoid sinus (SS) [2,3], coloboma of cortical plate (CP) attaching SS[4] and change of air cell density in temporal bone [5] are all thought to be possible responsibilities to vascular PT. Among them, coloboma of CP attaching SS was reported as a common character of vascular PT patient [6]. According to anatomy structure, CP is an important part in the propagation route of noise vibration generated by blood flow in SS to the air cells in temporal bone (Fig. 1). Coloboma of CP would lead to exposure of SS vessel wall to air cells in temporal bone, which are connected to tympanic cavity directly by air. Fixing CP by surgery has been applied to be an effective method against vascular PT, 80% patients were reported to be cured by this surgery [7,8]. However, there is still no quantitative study about the mechanism of how coloboma of CP might cause vascular PT, and why CP fixing surgery is effective curing vascular PT.

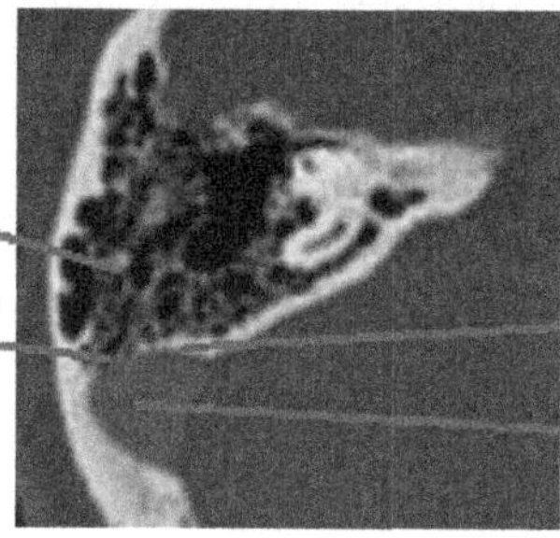

Fig. 1 Horizon CT image of vascular PT patient

In order to study the mechanism of CP coloboma hypothesis, numerical simulations were performed by the author to reveal the relationship between PT sound intensity and CP coloboma. The flow field and noise generation in SS were simulated by Fluent, and the propagation of sound vibration was simulated in Abaqus CAE using explicit dynamic simulation. One finite element model with intact CP and another without CP were established based on computed tomographic (CT) scanned images of a typical vascular PT patient. The simulation result was validated with subjective PT sound intensity report by typical patient. This study would draw a conclusion that the coloboma of CP would remarkably increase the noise vibration received in tympanic cavity, and that CP fixing surgery would effectively reduce the tinnitus intensity.

II. METHOD

The 3D model of flow field in SS, 2D model of SS vessel wall and CP were all developed based on CT scanned images of a typical vascular PT patient. 2 cases were established, one with intact CP, while the other without CP due to coloboma. The generation of sound in SS flow field and the propagation of sound in SS vessel wall and CP were evaluated separately using different simulation methods.

* Corresponding author.

I. Lackovic (ed.), *1st Global Conference on Biomedical Engineering & 9th Asian-Pacific Conference on Medical and Biological Engineering*, IFMBE Proceedings 47, DOI: 10.1007/978-3-319-12262-5_21

A. Evaluation of Sound Generation

The 3D geometric model of SS was meshed with tetrahedral elements. The static flow field in SS with peak velocity in a pulse was achieved by FLUENT 14.0 to be the sound source of vascular PT. The flow field was simulated with static laminar model. The value of mass-flow-inlet of SS was set to be 0.0075kg/s according to the average MRI measurement result of 14 vascular PT patients. Pressure-outlet was applied in this case.

After the static peak flow field in a pulse was achieved, the case was converted to be a transient one, and Fflowcs-Williams & Hawkings model was applied to evaluate the sound spectrum at a certain point in the flow field. The receiver was set at the CP coloboma point on the inner wall of SS. The sound spectrum result at the receiver was then dealt with fast Fourier transform, translating to be an equivalent sound pressure load on the model of SS vessel wall and CP.

B. Evaluation of Sound Propagation in SS Vessel Wall and Cortical Plate

The sound propagation in SS vessel wall and CP was then simulated by evaluating the vibration of vessel wall and CP under the equivalent sound pressure loading using explicit dynamic analysis in Abaqus CAE 6.11. The 2D model size in 2 cases was shown in table 1. As the average intact CP thickness among 200 people is reported as 1mm, the CP thickness in case 2 was set to be 1mm. The SS vessel thickness was set to be 0.5mm according to measurement on SS specimen. The 2D geometry model of SS vessel wall and CP were meshed into quadrangle elements in Hypermesh (Fig. 2). The material property of SS vessel wall and CP was illustrated in table 2. Shell edge load was set on edge A (the inner wall of SS) according to the equivalent sound pressure——0.028N, 250Hz. Edge B and D were fixed in all degrees of freedom. The time period of simulation process was set to be 1s to observe the steady vibration response. The normal velocity of point at edge C was monitored in the whole simulation process. The vibration velocity amplitude of edge C would directly determine the noise intensity in air cells. The steady vibration result in 2 cases was recorded and analyzed in the result section, and also be used in validation as the velocity boundary sound source.

Table 1 CP thickness in 2 cases

Case number	CP thickness (mm)	SS wall thickness (mm)
1	0	0.5
2	1	0.5

Table 2 Material property of SS vessel wall and CP[8,9]

	Elastic module (MPa)	Poisson's ratio	Density (kg/m^3)
Vessel wall	0.5	0.45	1150
Cortical plate	12000	0.25	1900

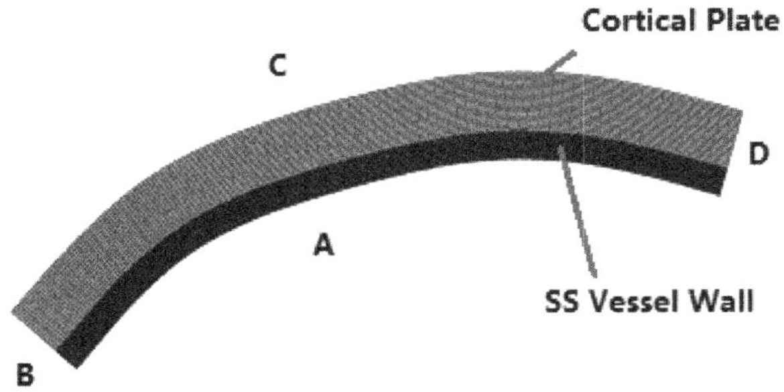

Fig. 2 Meshed model of SS vessel wall and cortical plate

C. Validation

The subjective PT intensity report by a typical vascular PT patient with CP coloboma was used to validate the result of this article. The 2D model of air cells in temporal bone was developed based on CT images. The sound source was set according to the steady vibration velocity result in 2 cases. The sound field in air cells was simulated using Virtual Lab REV 11, and the sound intensity in air cells was recorded and compared with the subjective intensity feeling of PT.

III. RESULT

The inner surface sound intensity distribution in SS (Fig. 3) was firstly achieved in FLUENT, and the sound intensity spectrum at CP coloboma point (Fig. 4) was obtained by Fflowcs-Williams & Hawkings model. After the Acoustic superposition process, the sound intensity spectrum was displaced with an equivalent simple harmonic sound pressure in a single frequency——0.0028Pa, 250Hz.

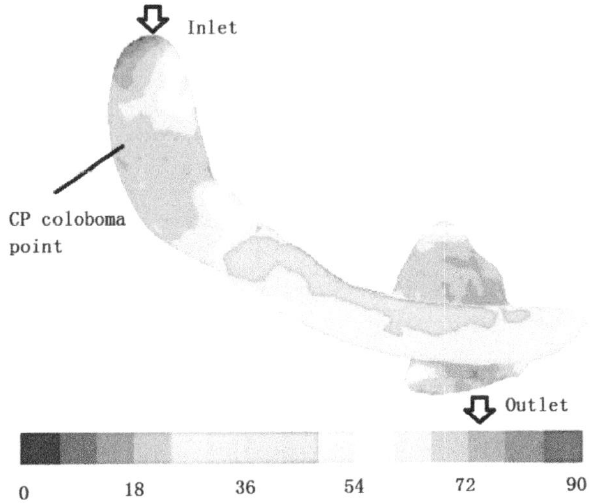

Fig. 3 Inner surface sound intensity distribution in SS (Unit: dB, preference pressure 2×10^{-5}Pa.)

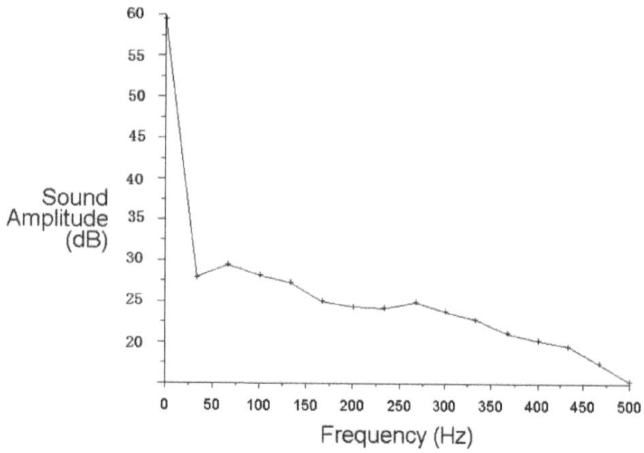

Fig. 4 Sound intensity spectrum at CP coloboma point, reference pressure 2×10^{-5}Pa.

Then this simple harmonic sound pressure load was applied on the 2D model of SS vessel wall and CP besides SS. The vibration velocity history output of edge C in case 1 was shown in Fig. 5. The steady vibration velocity amplitude and the sound intensity received in air cells were illustrated in table 3. It indicates that with an intact CP beside SS, the noise generated in SS flow field cannot propagate into air cells in temporal bone. But once CP is moved away from the model, the vibration of SS vessel wall would be considerable enough to cause PT.

Validation was based on the subjective PT sound intensity report by a typical vascular PT patient with CP coloboma, who had provided the CT images to the author. The PT intensity was described around 45dB. Compared to the sound intensity simulation result in air cells (30dB with CP coloboma), the author successfully evaluated the sound intensity in generation and propagation process, and obtained a convincing relationship between CP thickness and PT noise vibration propagation.

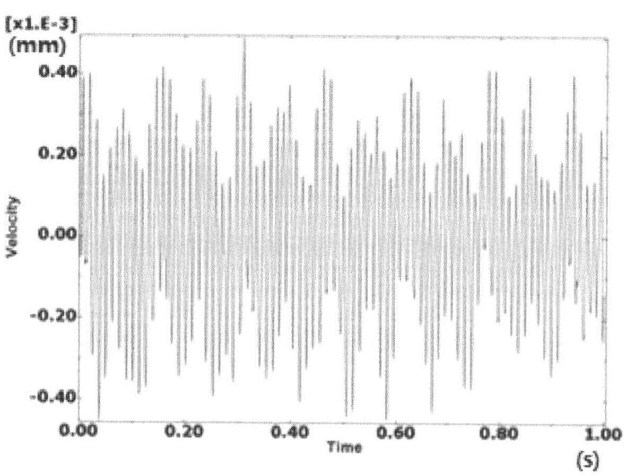

Fig. 5 Velocity history output of edge C in case 1.

Table 3 Velocity output average result and sound intensity validation

Case number	Average velocity (nm /s)	Sound intensity in air cells (dB)
1	5000	30
2	10	-14

IV. DISCUSSION

To find out the mechanism of how CP coloboma might be an important pathogeny leading to vascular PT, the author used numerical method to evaluate the generation and propagation of PT noise. The generation of PT noise was obtained by computing the peak flow field in 3D SS model, and the sound propagation process in SS vessel wall and CP was simulated by explicit dynamic method in 2D model. Finally the vibration result in 2 cases was validated with the subjective PT intensity report by a typical patient.

Numerical study is generally thought to be not accurate enough to achieve precise result data, so this study used simulation method to make comparison between the result of 2 cases. As experimental study on vascular PT is much harder than simulation to implement at present, this numerical study provided a feasible way for the mechanism research of vascular PT.

The validation positively supported the accuracy of this numerical study, indicating that the error range in the whole simulation process is acceptable, and that the comparing conclusion obtained from 2 cases is convincing. As the simulation of vascular PT model is still in primary stage, the accuracy of this study is limited in many aspects, and some of them can be improved in further research. Firstly, the simulation of blood flow field in SS was done statically at the peak velocity moment in this study. If possible, the varying velocity of blood in one pulse should be simulated in the flow field, as the sound source may be related to the velocity variation in flow field. Secondly, the sound pressure was simplified to one simple harmonic load in this study. However, octave frequency band should be applied in this simplification to enumerate several simple harmonic pressure loads without interference with each other. Thirdly, in the simulation of sound vibration propagation in SS vessel wall and CP, the 2D geometric models with different CP thickness is not equivalent to coloboma of one piece of CP shown in the CT images. 3D model should be established for better result accuracy in future study.

The result of this study validated the CP fixing surgery——using material with high elastic module to fill coloboma of CP could remarkably reduce the PT sound vibration propagated into air cells in temporal bone.

Although this surgery is a main clinical method for vascular PT at present, it is still with high risk, so further study should focus on vascular PT mechanism, making attempts on discovering new safer therapeutic methods to cure vascular PT. There is a promising prospect of this study in the future.

V. Conclusion

Through this numerical mechanism study, we can draw a conclusion that coloboma of cortical plate attaching sigmoid sinus would amplify the sound amplitude generated in sigmoid sinus flow field for nearly 3 orders of magnitude, which would be a direct pathogeny leading to vascular pulsatile tinnitus. The feasibility of cortical plate fixing surgery applied to cure vascular pulsatile tinnitus is validated in this study.

Acknowledgment

I would like to show my deepest gratitude to my supervisor, Professor Yubo Fan, who has provided me with valuable guidance in every stage of study. I would extend my thanks to Dr. Lizhen Wang and Dr. Zhaohui Liu for their patient guidance and specialized suggestion. I shall also say thanks to my schoolmates who have helped me with specific simulation operations.

This work was supported by Grant 81371545 and 81171311 from the National Natural Science Foundation of China, and Grant 13JL03 from capital medical university.

Conflict of Interest

The authors declare that they have no conflict of interest.

References

1. Okazaki H, Doi T, Izumikawa M, et al (2011) Pulsatile tinnitus as a first symptom of essential thrombocythemia. Am J Otolaryngol 32(3): 263-264.
2. Cowley PO, Jones R, Tuch P, et al (2009) Pulsatile tinnitus from reversal of flow in an aberrant occipital artery: resolved after carotid artery stenting. AJNR Am J Neuroradiol 30(5): 995-997.
3. Topal O, Erbek SS, Erbek S, et al (2008) Subjective pulsatile tinnitus associated with extensive pneumatization of temporal bone. Eur Arch Otorhinolaryngol 265(1): 123-125.
4. Xue J, Li T, Sun X, et al (2012) Focal defect of mastoid bone shell in the region of the transverse-sigmoid junction: a new cause of pulsatile tinnitus. J Laryngol Otol 126(4): 409-413.
5. Tüz M, Doğru H, Yeşildağ A (2003) Subjective pulsatile tinnitus associated with extensive pneumatization of temporal bone. Auris Nasus Larynx 30(2) : 183-185.
6. Eisenman DJ (2011) Sinus wall reconstruction for sigmoid sinus diverticulum and dehiscence: a standardized surgical procedure for a range of radiographic findings. Otol Neurotol 32(7): 1116-1119.
7. Liang X, Chen G, Gong S, et al (2011) CT and DSA of vascular pulsatile tinnitus patients. Radial Practice 26(3): 256-259.
8. Guo J, Wang Z, Xian J, et al (2011) CT arteriography and venography diagnosis in pulsatile tinnitus caused by sigmoid sinus diverticulum CHIN ARCH OTOLARYNGOL HEAD NECK SURG 18(4): 178-180.
9. Zhao S, Gu L, Stacey R. Froemming (2012) Finite element analysis of the implantation of a self-expanding stent: impact of lesion calcification. Journal of Medical Devices 6: 021001-1-021001-6.
10. F. Gaynor Evans (1975) Mechanical properties and histology of cortical bone from younger and older men. ANAT. REC 185: 1-12.

Author: Yubo Fan
Institute: School of Biological Science and Medical Engineering, Beihang University
Street: 37# Xueyuan Road, Haidian District
City: Beijing
Country: China
Email: yubofan@buaa.edu.cn

Numerical Simulation of the Dynamic Response of Thoracolumbar Spine in Impact of Ejection

Cheng-Fei Du[1], Li-Zhen Wang[1], Song-Yang Liu[2], and Yu-Bo Fan[1,*]

[1] School of Biological Science and Medical Engineering Beihang University, Beijing, China
[2] Institute of Aviation Medicine, Air force, Beijing, China
yubofan@buaa.edu.cn

Abstract— **Pilots have been often sustained ejection-induced spine trauma and investigation of dynamic response of spine benefit for the insight of injury mechanism and design of protective device under ejection condition. This study developed a nonlinear finite element (FE) model of the thoracolumbar spine and a multi-body dynamic model of dummy respectively. The kinetic data of multi-body model and stress information of FE model have been analyzed. It can be found that ejection impact induces obvious axial compression and anterior flexion of the spine, which may contribute to the incidence of spinal injury. The high stress was located in T1 and L1 which has more risk of injury during impact loading. The combination of FE method and multi-body dynamic approach provides a convenient tool for studying occupants restrained by seat belts, such as drives, aviators, etc.**

Keywords— **finite element, multi-body, dynamic response, biomechanics, ejection.**

I. INTRODUCTION

Military aircrew maybe more prone to develop musculoskeletal disabilities involving the spine due to the characteristic of anatomy of spine and complex accelerative environment. According to the investigation of Lewis [1], the overall percentages of ejection survivals who sustained spinal fractures was 29.4% and the majority of fractures was located on the thoracolumbar region.

The method of numerical simulation has been widely used to investigate the structural response of the spine to impact loading, while these investigations have not concerned ejection-induced injury. Therefore, the aim of this study was to investigate the dynamic response of multi-segment thoracolumbar spine in ejection scenario, which may provide the insight of mechanism into spine trauma and benefit for design of protective device under ejection condition. To realize it, two kinds of model have been developed. One was the Multi-body dynamics model of dummy to provide overall kinematic data of segmental body, the other was the finite element model of thoracolumbar spine from which internal stress and strain information could be obtained.

* Corresponding author.

II. MATERIALS AND METHODS

A. FE Model of Thoracolumbar Spine

A serial CT images of a healthy male (age: 35, height: 174cm, weight: 75kg) from T9 to S1 were obtained. A medical image processing software((Mimics 10.0, Belgium) was used to separate the geometrical information of the bone and a CAE pre-processoring software (Hypermesh 11.0; USA) was used to mesh. The intervertebral disk involved a nucleus pulposus and fiber-reinforced annulus ground substance proportioned according to histological findings (44% nucleus, 56% annulus) [2]. The crisscross fibers were divided into 8 layers in the radial direction and were oriented at an average angle of ±30°to the endplates. Seven major ligaments (All, Pll, Itl, Fl, Ssl, Isl and Cl) were created according to the anatomical observations and measurement [3]. All the fibers and ligaments were taken as 3D cable elements which only sustained tension.

The pelvis and the seat were meshed using 4-node tetrahedral solid elements and 4-node shell elements respectively. All the material properties and element types of components of FE model of the thoracolumbar spine in Table 1. Abaqus 6.11 and Ls-dyna 971 were used to conduct static and dynamic simulation respectively. The interaction between facet joints was assumed as frictionless surface to surface contact. During dynamic analysis, an hourglass coefficient of 0.01 was used to avoid the emergence of an hourglass scenario.

B. Validation of FE Model

Validation was undertaken by comparing the predicted data by the current model with the results from other literature. In vitro experimental results from the investigation of Renner was chose to validated the model in quasi-static condition [4].

The T12-L1 segment was chosen to conduct dynamic validation and the material parameters of the annulus ground substance and nucleus pulposus were increased to get the dynamic stiffness. The simulated results were compared with experimental data [5].

I. Lackovic (ed.), *1st Global Conference on Biomedical Engineering & 9th Asian-Pacific Conference on Medical and Biological Engineering*,
IFMBE Proceedings 47, DOI: 10.1007/978-3-319-12262-5_22

C. Multi-body Dynamic Model

A facet dummy model of the pilot was developed, having the same weight and height as the subject which provide the scan data to the previous FE model. This model consisted of 16 interconnected rigid segments as follows: head, neck, upper torso, lower torso, thighs, legs, feet, upper arms, forearms, hands. These segments were connected with joints and the properties of each joint, such as range of motion, stiffness, friction, and damping, were included.

The rigid seat model was built and the retractor and pretensioner were included. A PCU/15P harness restraint was modeled directly in Hypermesh 11.0. The geometric information and material properties of the harness restraint were derived from the related specifications or experimental measurement. The dummy was adjusted to the position before ejection and the restraint systems were pretensioned beforehand.

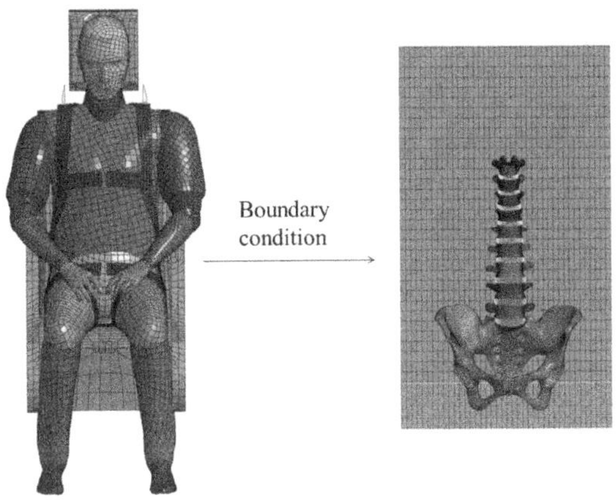

Fig. 1 Multi-body dynamics model of pilot (left) and FE model of thoracolumbar spine

To use the kinematic data of dynamics model in the FE model, the hip joints points and a point corresponding to the center of the superior endplate of T9 were chosen as reference points. The translation and rotation of these reference points relative to the seat were recorded and taken as the boundary condition to use in the finite element analysis.

D. Simulation of Ejection

To consider the inertia force of body during impact, two nodal points were created in the mid-sagittal plane: one was connected with the upper endplate of T9; the other was positioned 10mm anterior to the L2L3 disk and 200mm superior to the upper endplate of T9 to represent the weight of the rest of the upper body. These two points were connected by a rigid beam. Mass points were created in the center of mass of each segment [6]. For each vertebra, a rigid beam was constructed to connect the middle region of cortical bone with the mass point of each segment.

The accelerative load with peak value of 15G, duration of 0.2s, and onset rate of 150G/s, was exerted on the seat pan at an angle of 5° to the seat back. During simulation, all components in the finite element model were constrained to move only in the sagittal plane of the pilot, and the pelvis and T9 were allowed to rotate only around the reference axis of the seat.

III. RESULTS

A. Validation Results

As shown in Figures 2 & 3, the results predicted by the present model were in close agreement with published experimental data and FE models. Accordingly, this model can be further used for study the dynamic response of the thoracolumbar spine under various impacts.

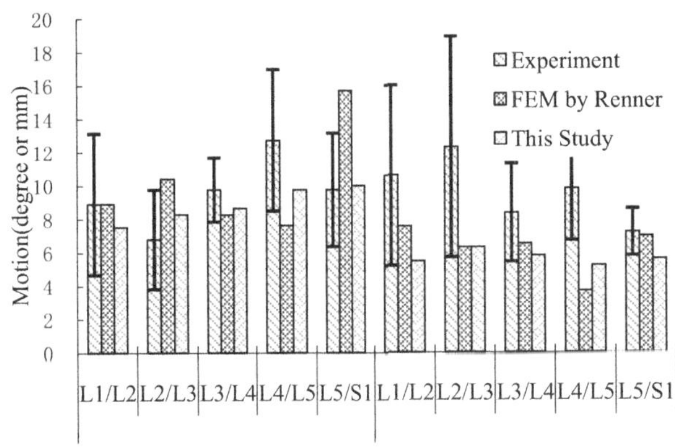

Fig. 2 Comparison of predicted results by the current FE model against investigation by Renner [4]

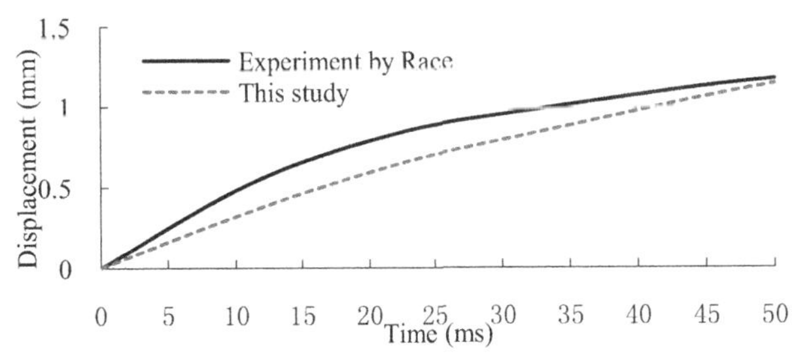

Fig. 3 Comparison of the FE model with dynamic experimental data

B. Dynamic response predicted by dynamic multi-body model

The motion (rotation and translation) of the thorax (near T9) and hip is shown in Figure 4. The site of thorax and hip have the similar rotational displacement. While the translational displacement in thorax was far more than it in hip joint. This was partly due to the anterior flexion of upper trunk before the retractor was activated to be locked.

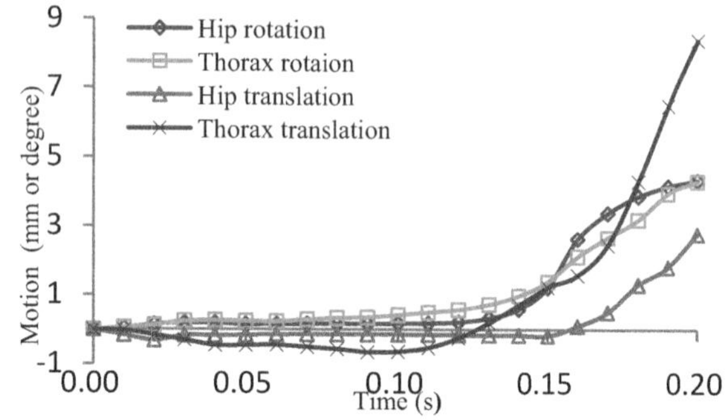

Fig. 4 Motion of different sites of trunk during ejection

C. Dynamic Response Predicted by FE model

During the first stage of ejection, a typical pattern of stress distribution on the thoracolumbar spine is shown in Figure.5. The high stress (vonMises) regions were located in anterior parts of the cortical bone of T12 and L1 and gradually shifted to the pedicle bases in the lower lumbar vertebrae.

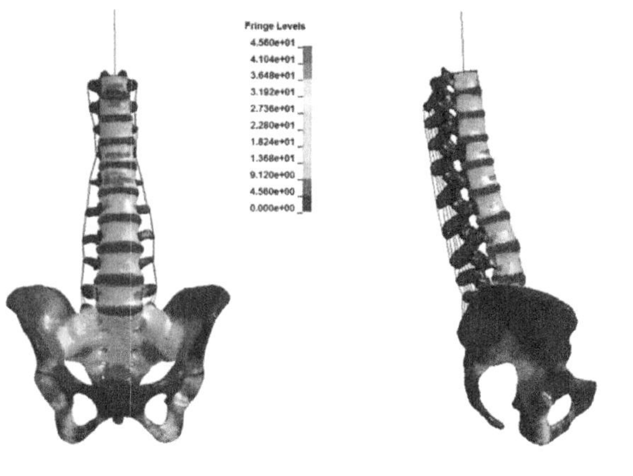

Fig. 5 Stress distribution on thoracolumbar spine during ejection (t=0.12s)

Variations of maximal stress in the cortical bone and endplate during impact loading are shown in Figure.6. During the acceleration onset stage (0-0.1s), the tremendous thrust force exerted on the buttocks resulted in a continuous increase in maximal stress of cortical bone and endplate. After 0.1s, the imposed acceleration remained constant and the maximum stress alternated up and down in a little range.

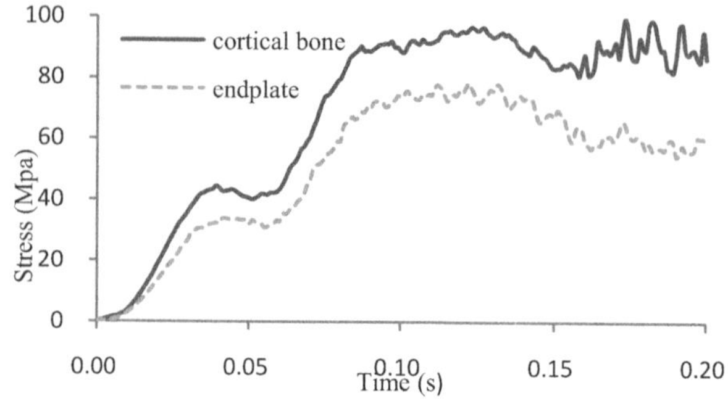

Fig. 6 History of maximum stress in the cortical bones and endplates during ejection impact

IV. DISCUSSION

Compared to experiment, numerical simulations provide more detailed information at lower costs and offer better repeatability. The dynamic response index (DRI) and multi-body dynamic are two methods of numerical simulation which have been widely used in the biodynamic investigation of ejection scenario [7,8].However it is hard for these two methods to provide the detailed and accurate mechanics information of internal tissue such as bone and ligament. The FE method allow the calculation of local deformations and stress in body during impact loading, but it require excessive computing power and time in constructing model, choice of materials and mesh of medium.

This study combined FE and multi-body models to investigate the dynamic response of pilot trunk especially the location of spine in the event of ejection. Based on the predicted results from multi-body dynamics, the upper trunk flexed anteriorly and the buttocks titled backward and moved forward along with the seat pan due to the center of gravity anterior to the spine and the direction of ejection being angled away from the seat back. The rotation and translation of the buttocks were all significantly less when compared to similar thoracic measurements. Also, compression of intervertebral discs caused slackening of the shoulder harness during ejection, which contributed to the flexion of the upper torso. The results of finite element model indicated that high stresses were mainly concentrated on the anterior parts of T12, L1 and the region close to pedicle bases of the lower lumbar spine. Similar stress distribution was reported by Qiu [10] and ejection induced spinal injuries have been occurred in these locations. In this model, the maximum stress on the cortical bone reached 97.1MPa, which is close to the yield stress of cortical bone (110MPa).

Many studies have shown that impact loading causes fracture of the endplate or vertebral body, although there is a lack of consensus on which region fails first. In this study, the maximum stress in structure of endplate was less than it

Table 1 Element Information and Material Properties used in the Finite Element Model

Components Name	Young's Modulus (MPa)	Poisson's Ratio	Density (kg/mm^2)	Cross- sectional Area(mm^2)	Type of Element	Number of Elements
Cortical bone	14000	0.30	1.83E-06		Hexahedral	4744
Cancellous bone	100	0.2	0.17E-06		Hexahedral	68186
Posterior elements	3500	0.25	1.83E-06		Hexahedral	40234
Endplate	10000	0.25	1.06E-06		Hexahedral	11916
Pelvis	5000	0.2	1.83E-06		Tetrahedral	40327
Disc						
Annulus	Mooney–Rivlin c1 = 0.12, c2 = 0.045		1.0E-06		Hexahedral	17010
Nucleus pulpous	Mooney–Rivlin c1 = 0.12, c2 = 0.03		1.2E-06		Hexahedral	12780
Collagenous fiber	Calibrated stress-strain curves				Cable	38880
Ligament						
ALL			1.0E-06	63.7	Cable	72
PLL			1.0E-06	20	Cable	64
FL			1.0E-06	40	Cable	63
ITL	Calibrated deflection-force curves		1.0E-06	3.6	Cable	36
ISL			1.0E-06	40	Cable	45
SSL			1.0E-06	30	Cable	9
CL			1.0E-06	60	Cable	180

ALL, anterior longitudinal ligament; PLL, posterior longitudinal ligament; FL, ligamentum flavum; ITL, intertransverse ligament; ISL, interspinous ligament; SSL, supraspinous ligament; CL, capsular ligament.

in cortical bone throughout the duration of ejection impact. It is hard to determine that initial failure occurs in the vertebral body or endplate during ejection because the failure strengths of these regions are still not very clear.

It should be noted that there are some limitations to this study. In the multi-body dynamic model, the effect of clothing, soft tissues (skin, muscles, etc.) on the dynamic response of the pilot under ejection impact were not considered. The ligaments were all modeled as 1-dimensional nonlinear springs for the convenience of computation. More accurate geometrical and material properties should be considered in future work.

V. CONCLUSIONS

The combination of multi-body and FE models provided a suitable tool to study the biodynamic response of restrained pilot under ejection scenario. Ejection impact could induce obvious axial compression and anterior flexion of the spine, which may contribute to the incidence of spinal injury. The high stress was located in T1 and L1 which has more risk of injury.

REFERENCES

1. Lewis M E (2006). Survivability and injuries from use of rocket-assisted ejection seats: analysis of 232 cases. Aviation, space, and environmental medicine 77(9): 936-943.
2. Schmidt H, Heuer F, Drumm J (2007). Application of a calibration method provides more realistic results for a finite element model of a lumbar spinal segment. Clin Biomech 22(4):377-84
3. Agur A Mr, Dalley A F (1999). Grant's Atlas of Anatomy, 10th ed., Williams and Wilkins, Baltimore, MD.
4. Renner S M, Natarajan R N, Patwardhan A G (2007). Novel model to analyze the effect of a large compressive follower pre load on range of motions in a lumbar spine. Journal of Biomechanics 40(6):1326-1332
5. Race A, Broom N D, Robertson P (2000). Effect of loading rate and hydration on the mechanical properties of the disc. Spine 25(6): 662-669.
6. Pearsall D J, Reid J G, Livingston LA (1996). Segmental inertial parameters of the human trunk as determined from computed tomography. Annals of biomedical engineering 24(2): 198-210.
7. Payne, P R (1961). The dynamics of human restraint systems, impact acceleration stress. National Academy of Sciences, National Research Council, Washington, DC.1961.
8. Belytschko T L. Schwer, and Privitzer E (1987). Theory and application of a three-dimensional model of the human spine. Aviation, Space, and Environmental Medicine 49(1 Pt. 2):158.
9. Qiu T X, Tan K W, Lee V S, et al (2006). Investigation of thoracolumbar T12–L1 burst fracture mechanism using finite element method. Medical engineering & physics 28(7): 656-664.

Carpal Tunnel Biomechanics – Displacement and Associated Intra-Carpal Tunnel Pressure Studies during Finger Flexion

K. Liong[1], S.J. Lee[2], A. Lahiri[3], and H.P. Lee[1]

[1] National University of Singapore/Department of Mechanical Engineering, Singapore
[2] National University of Singapore/Department of Surgery, Singapore
[3] National University Hospital/Department of Hand & Reconstructive Microsurgery, Singapore

Abstract— **Idiopathic carpal tunnel syndrome (CTS) affects a significant portion of the population, although its exact etiology remains unknown. Based on dynamic ultrasonographic examination of the carpal tunnel inlet, in thumb and index finger (IF) flexion, we observed that the tendon(s) moves in the volar-ulnar direction, displacing the median nerve in the same direction. In middle finger (MF) flexion, however, the tendon moves dorsa-radially, leading to the volar-ulnar movement of the nerve. Median nerve and tendon displacements increased from thumb, IF and MF flexion. These general motion patterns were applied to a patient-specific computer-generated model of the carpal tunnel to determine the associated pressures. Motions in which the tendons move volarly, as in IF and thumb flexion, elicit greater nerve contact and von Mises stresses than those in which the tendons move in a dorsal-ulnar direction, as in MF flexion. Nerve displacement was also not directly correlated with nerve stress. The utilization of finite element modeling allows direct quantification of stresses within the tunnel without any invasive procedures, and may provide insight into the changing intra-carpal mechanics as CTS develops, which may lead to more effective CTS treatment.**

Keywords— **Carpal tunnel syndrome, median nerve, displacement, intra-carpal tunnel pressure.**

I. INTRODUCTION

Idiopathic carpal tunnel syndrome (CTS) affects a significant portion of the population. Although thickening of the subsynovial connective tissue[1], and repetitive hand motions[2] have been associated with CTS development, its exact etiology remains unknown[3]. The pathological changes do not explain the cause of dynamic symptoms that are aggravated during finger motion. This highlights the need for a greater understanding of carpal tunnel dynamics that could lead to the development of more effective CTS preventive therapies and treatment.

Thus far, previous ultrasonographic studies on median nerve displacement have reported differing results. Van Doesburg, et al.[4] studied thumb, index finger (IF) and middle finger (MF) flexion, and reported a volar-ulnar movement of the median nerve and the associated tendons in the latter two cases. Yoshii, et al.[5], however, described a dorso-radial movement of the tendon and a volar-ulnar movement of the median nerve during MF flexion. In addition, transverse ultrasonographic studies were conducted by Ugbolue, et al.[6] on cadaveric specimens during IF and MF flexion, and found the transverse displacements to be small and irregular. This lack in consistency demonstrates the need for a more detailed study into intra-carpal tunnel dynamics[2,6].

While nerve displacement is useful in understanding nerve-tendon interaction, it offers limited insight into the stress that the nerve experiences. Previous studies[7,8] conducted in-vivo pressure measurements via a catheter connected to a pressure transducer. The use of catheters, unfortunately, implies that pressure may only be quantified at a single point, and that only fluid pressure may be obtained. Contact pressure may only be measured in cadaveric wrists, while the stress actually experienced by the median nerve cannot be determined at all. These difficulties highlight the necessity for the use of a different modality to observe intra-carpal tunnel pressure.

In the first part of this study, based on dynamic ultrasonographic examination at the carpal tunnel inlet, movement of the median nerve and the associated tendon in thumb, IF and MF flexion in normal candidates, was quantified. These structures are found to exhibit a general movement in each motion. In the second part of the study, these motion patterns were applied to a finite element model of the carpal tunnel. The associated pressures were then determined. In this way, the motion that elicits the greatest pressure in the median nerve may be quantitatively determined.

II. METHODS

This study was approved by our institutional review board and all participants gave informed consent.

A. Ultrasound Studies

A cohort of normal volunteers (11 males and 4 females, within the age-group of 30 to 45 years) was studied. We utilized the routine 3D ultrasound machine General Electric RSP6-16-D 3D/4D linear transducer probe (General Electric Voluson E8 expert system, Milwaukee, WI, USA). The subjects were seated with the hand in a neutral supine

I. Lackovic (ed.), *1st Global Conference on Biomedical Engineering & 9th Asian-Pacific Conference on Medical and Biological Engineering*,
IFMBE Proceedings 47, DOI: 10.1007/978-3-319-12262-5_23

position. The probe was placed at 90-degrees, at the proximal inlet of the carpal tunnel. Candidates were instructed to gradually flex the thumb, IF or MF separately, until the fingertip touched the hand palm, and then to extend the finger again. The real-time videos were recorded and evaluated using digital image morphometry.

The ultrasonographic video images were digitized with VirtualDub (v1.9.11, GNC General Public License), and the images were input into ImageJ (v1.44, Public Domain License) and scaled according to the 1cm grid. The median nerve was observed in all motions. The flexor pollicis longus (FPL) tendon was outlined in the case of thumb flexion, flexor digitorum superficialis (FDS) 2 and FDP 2 in IF flexion, and FDS 3 in MF flexion. The hyper-echogenic rim of the median nerve and tendon was then outlined in each image and their centroids calculated. These centroids were then plot in Microsoft Excel (Microsoft Office 2008, Redmond, WA) to determine the structural displacement.

B. *Finite Element Analysis of the Carpal Tunnel*

MRI scans from a single healthy candidate in the neutral supine position were utilized to create a 3D model of the carpal tunnel. Images were superimposed in MIMICS (v14.1, Materialise, Leuven, Belgium) to create a 3D model, which encompassed the transverse carpal ligament (TCL), surrounding bone boundary, flexor tendons, the median nerve and the interstitial matter. The bone boundary was created in the place of the dorsal carpal bones to simplify analysis (Fig. 1). 3D tetrahedral meshes were created in HYPERMESH (v11.0, Altair Hyperworks, Huntsville, AL), then exported into ABAQUS (v 6.12, Dassault Systemes Technologies, Providence, RI) for modeling and simulation.

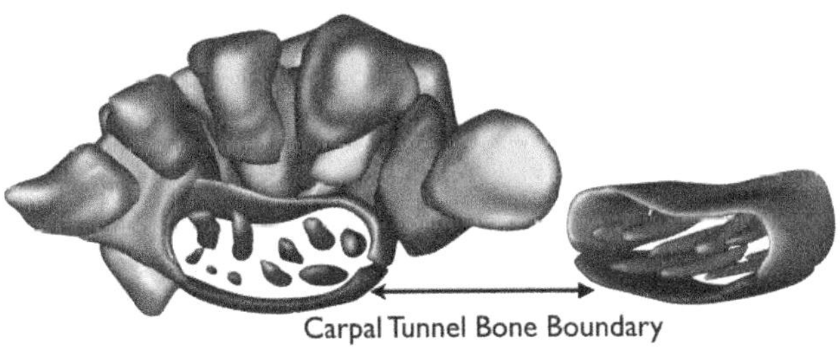

Fig. 1 Creation of carpal tunnel bone boundary from carpal bones

In this study, coupled Eulerian-Lagrangian (CEL) analysis was employed to simulate the movement of the tendons through the interstitial fluid. The median nerve, flexor tendons, bone boundary and TCL were assigned with solid Lagrangian elements. The initial position of the interstitial fluid between the nerve and tendons was defined in the Eulerian boundary.

Material Properties: The median nerve, flexor tendons and TCL were prescribed an Ogden hyperelastic model definition (Eq. (1)), as reported by Main et al.[9,10]. W, defines strain energy as a function of deviatoric principal stretches, λ_i. The values for μ and α, of each individual structure are detailed in Table 1. FDS 5 was not tested due to its small size, and will be assigned FDS 4 properties. An estimated density of 1100 kg/m^3 was prescribed to flexor tendons, and a minimally higher density of 1250 kg/m^3 was prescribed to the nerve.

$$W(\lambda_1, \lambda_2, \lambda_3) = \frac{2\mu}{\alpha^2}(\lambda_1^\alpha + \lambda_2^\alpha + \lambda_3^\alpha - 3) \quad (1)$$

Table 1 Ogden hyperelastic coefficients of median nerve & tendons

Structure	μ (kPa)	α
Nerve	6.45	6.50
FPL	12.45	10.90
FDS 2	19.85	7.70
FDS 3	16.30	7.8
FDS 4	16.85	10.00
FDP 2	21.65	11.80
FDP 3	23.50	7.70
FDP 4	13.85	8.00
FDP 5	19.75	9.20
TCL	38.75	16.82

Elastic properties were assigned to the carpal bones boundary, and the interstitial matter was modeled as a fluid to replicate its tissue continuity[11] nature (Table 2).

Table 2 Elastic Properties of Carpal Bones & Interstitial Fluid Properties

Carpal Bones Material Properties	Young's Modulus, E (MPa)	10 000
	Poisson's Ratio, ν	0.3
	Density (kg/m^3)	1200
Interstitial Fluid Properties	Viscosity, η (Ns/m^2)	0.3
	Bulk Modulus, K (GPa)	0.5
	Density, ρ_f (kg/m^3)	1063

Boundary Conditions & Constraints: The carpal bone boundary was prescribed a fixed condition. A perfectly bonded interface was defined between the TCL and bone boundary. Free inflow and outflow boundary conditions were prescribed in ABAQUS.

Prescribed Displacements & Velocities: Transverse tendon displacements associated with individual finger flexion were obtained from the ultrasound study. To simulate the average physical time for a single finger flexion cycle would take an extensively long time. Therefore, since the hyperelastic properties of the median nerve and flexor tendons were strain-rate independent, a physical simulation time of 0.01s was utilized instead. The displacement was maintained, and the resultant velocity calculated (Table 3).

III. RESULTS

A. Ultrasound Study

A predominant pattern of motion between the nerve and associated tendon was observed in each motion. In thumb flexion, we observed that the FPL moves in the volar-ulnar direction, displacing the nerve in the same direction. A similar displacement pattern is also observed in the case of IF flexion, where FDS 2 and FDP 2 tendons push against the nerve. In MF flexion, however, the FDS 3 tendon moves dorsa-radially, and pushes up against the dorsal side of the median nerve, leading to its volar-ulnar movement (

Fig 2). Median nerve displacements increased from thumb, IF and MF flexion, although this difference is only significant between thumb and MF flexion (p=0.0280). Tendon displacements increase from thumb to MF flexion, although this increase was not statistically significant (Table 3).

B. Finite Element Analysis of the Carpal Tunnel

Fluid pressure in the whole model, middle and distal end of the carpal tunnel, and median nerve contact pressure and von Mises stress were measured. The greatest median nerve contact pressure and von Mises stress was encountered in IF followed by thumb and MF flexion (Fig 3). This is in spite of the fact that the greatest displacement and fluid pressure is associated with MF flexion, followed by IF flexion and thumb flexion. Motions in which the tendons move volarly (IF and thumb flexion) appear to elicit greater median nerve contact pressure and von Mises stresses than those in which the tendons move in a dorsal-ulnar direction (MF flexion).

IV. DISCUSSION

In this study, we have established that a predominant general motion exists for finger flexion. In each individual finger flexion action, regardless of CTS symptomology, a general nerve-tendon pattern of movement was observed.

Table 3 Experimental and simulated distance and physical times in thumb, index finger (IF) and middle finger (MF) flexion actions. The resultant velocities simulated were also included.

Finger Flexion		Thumb	IF		MF
Structure		FPL	FDS 2	FDP 2	FDS 3
Experimental Data	Distance (mm)	1.439 (0.4219)	1.508 (0.9566)	1.513 (1.028)	1.671 (1.110)
	Physical Time (s)	0.8624 (0.4118)	1.013 (0.2353)		0.8097 (0.3737)
Simulated Scenario	Distance (mm)	1.910	2.336	2.034	3.616
	Physical Time (s)	0.01			
Resultant Velocity (mm/s)	V_x	-56.33	203.9	-130.1	166.4
	V_y	180.3	34.29	140.7	-309.3
	V_z	-28.69	108.6	-68.19	86.37

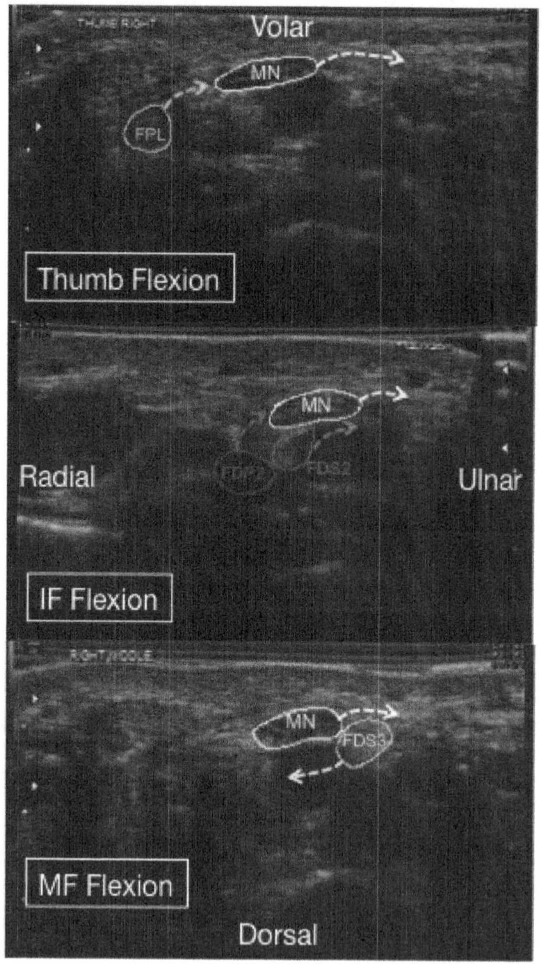

Fig. 2 Predominant motions patterns of the median nerve and associated tendon(s) in different finger flexion actions.

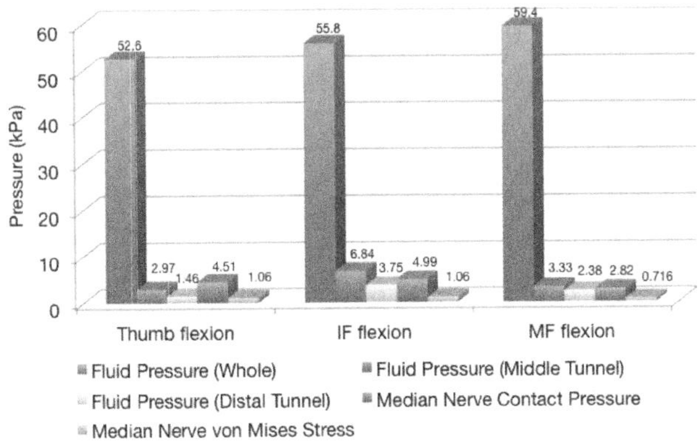

Fig. 3 Maximum pressures recorded for thumb, IF and MF flexion.

MF flexion displayed the greatest nerve and tendon displacement, followed by IF and thumb flexion.

It was also determined that IF flexion elicits the greatest nerve stress, followed by thumb and MF flexion (Fig 3). This suggests that the resultant nerve stress is dependent upon the path of the associated tendon. Volarly-moving tendons, as in a thumb of IF flexion, elicit greater nerve stress than dorsally-moving tendons, as in MF flexion. Our finding also suggests that a greater median nerve displacement does not necessarily imply a greater nerve stress, as MF flexion, although exhibiting the greatest displacement, presented with a lower von Mises stress. This further highlights the importance of determining the movement directions of tendons in various hand or finger actions to estimate the amount of stress the nerve may be experiencing.

The present findings suggest that high pressures are indeed elicited on the median nerve during finger flexion actions, especially in IF flexion. The maximum stress the median nerve experiences, albeit for a short duration, is significantly elevated. This could explain the dynamically provoked symptoms that are often encountered in mild idiopathic CTS candidates[12]. As they perform repetitive hand movements, the median nerve experiences heightened stress. Consequently, the subject experiences numbness, tingling[13] and sensory disturbance along the median nerve distribution[14]. These findings further elucidate intra-carpal tunnel mechanics, which may lead to more effective CTS prevention and treatment.

V. CONCLUSION

In conclusion, we have demonstrated that the stress the nerve experiences is dependent upon the path of the associated tendon. In addition, median nerve displacement is not directly correlated with nerve stress. The utilization of computational modeling in the study of patient-specific carpal tunnel mechanics allows direct quantification of stresses without any invasive procedures. This may provide valuable insight into the changing intra-carpal mechanics as CTS develops, leading to more effective CTS treatment.

ACKNOWLEDGEMENTS

The authors would like to acknowledge the help of Ms Dawn Chia from National University Hopsital, in the ultrasonographic examination of candidates.

CONFLICT OF INTEREST

The authors declare that they have no conflict of interest.

REFERENCES

1. Oh S, Belohlavek M, Zhao C et al. (2007) Detection of differential gliding characteristics of the flexor digitorum superficialis tendon and subsynovial connective tissue using color doppler sonographic imaging. J Ultras Med 26: 149-155
2. Thomsen JF, Gerr F, Atroshi I. (2008) Carpal tunnel syndrome and the use of computer mouse and keyboard: A systematic review. BMC Musculoskelet Disord 9: 1-12
3. Uchiyama S, Itsubo T, Nakamura K et al. (2010) Current concepts of carpal tunnel syndrome: pathophysiology, treatment, and evaluation. J Orthop Sci 15: 1-13
4. Van Doesburg MHM, Henderson J, van der Molen ABM et al. (2012) Transverse plane tendon and median nerve motion in the carpal tunnel: ultrasound comparison of carpal tunnel syndrome patients and healthy volunteers. PLoS One 7: 1-5
5. Yoshii Y, Villarraga HR, Henderson J et al. (2009) Ultrasound assessment of the displacement and deformation of the median nerve in the human carpal tunnel with active finger motion. J Bone Joint Surg Am 91: 2922-2930
6. Ugbolue UC, Hsu WH, Goitz RJ et al. (2005) Tendon and nerve displacement at the wrist during finger movements. Clin Biomech 20: 50-56
7. Seradge H, Jia Y-C, Owens W. (1995) In vivo measurement of carpal tunnel pressure in the functioning hand. J Hand Surg - Am 20: 855-859
8. Keir PJ, Wells RP, Ranney DA et al. (1997) The Effects of Tendon Load and Posture on Carpal Tunnel Pressure. J Hand Surg - Am 22: 628-634
9. Main EK, Goetz JE, Baer TE et al. (2012) Volar/dorsal compressive mechanical behavior of the transverse carpal ligament. J Biomech 45: 1180-1185
10. Main EK, Goetz JE, James Rudert M et al. (2011) Apparent transverse compressive material properties of the digital flexor tendons and the median nerve in the carpal tunnel. J Biomech 44: 863-868
11. Guimberteau JC, Delage JP, Wong J. (2010) The role and mechanical behavior of the connective tissue in tendon sliding. Chirurgie De La Main 29: 155-166
12. Ibrahim I, Khan WS, Goddard N et al. (2012) Carpal Tunnel Syndrome: A Review of the Recent Literature. Open Orthop J 6: 69-76
13. Carpal Tunnel Syndrome at http://www.faculty.kw.edu/vlhview.asp
14. Seffinger MA, Hruby RJ. (2007) Carpal Tunnel Syndrome. W.B. Saunders, Philadelphia

Numerical Modeling to Calculate Thermal Lesion Formation Using Internally-Cooled Electrodes during Radiofrequency Ablation of Liver Tumors

Huang-Wen Huang

Department of Innovative Information and Technology, Langyang Campus, Tamkang University, Ilan 26247, Taiwan

Abstract— **Radio-frequency ablation (RFA) heat treatment is a popular "minimally invasive" treatment method for both primary and metastatic liver tumors, and the heat treatment is studied by numerical calculation. Most of numerical modeling in radio-frequency ablation use commercial finite element methods package. The present paper describes the model used finite difference methods to simulate RFA with internally-cooled electrode, and large blood vessels cooling simultaneously. A finite difference model is used to solve all partial differential equations (PDEs) for a simple three dimensional (3-D) cubic geometry model. Maximum tissue temperature is used as a critical index for reaching thermal lesion during RFA. Cylindrical RF cool-tip electrode is internally cooled at constant water temperature. The use of series and parallel thermal resistances of composite materials are presented in the model. Results show consistency with experimental results.**

Keywords— **Radio-frequency ablation (RFA), thermal lesion formation, finite difference method, liver tumors.**

I. INTRODUCTION

Radio-frequency ablation (RFA) has been an important tumor removal treating modality around the globe, particularly for liver tumors. In recent years, RFA technology has been improved continually and it is applied in treating other tumors in kidney, lung and other solid organs[1-4]. The ablation is less expensive than other treatment options and it provides excellent alternative means of treatment which is hard to perform by surgical resection.

Typical setting of RFA includes a RF generator and two electrodes: one needle electrode directly inserted into the tumor and one dissipative electrode (ground pad)[5]. During RFA procedure, the needle electrode is inserted under image guidance and an alternating current (about 500 kHz) is then applied across the inserted electrode and the ground pad for around minutes. When electric current travels through tissue, Joule heat is generated due to the movement of ions in cellular fluids against friction, resulting in temperature elevation. As tissue temperature is raised beyond 50 °C, irreversible cellular damage occurs, and then an area of coagulation necrosis is formed around the electrode [5-6]. The cool-tip RFA system platform makes the straight-needle maximum energy delivery possible to create larger ablation zones.

The incomplete RF tumor ablation leads to local recurrence rate of around 40% [7,8]. Thus many research groups around the world have conducted both experiments and computer analysis to obtain better understanding to perform precise tumor treatments. However conducting experiments cost time and money in comparison with computer simulation. However, few computer simulation works published to date addressed this problem[9-13]. Some addressed temperature distribution during RFA using computer models but without considering heat-sink impact of large blood vessel,[14-16]as most computer models of RFA used finite element method in calculation.

Some[17]considered a blood vessel with constant 37 °C which was a worst case scenario during RFA. This paper used RF heating power source, and revealed thermal lesion deflection caused by thermally significant convective blood vessels (with various mean blood temperatures along vessel's path according to the law of energy conservation): particularly orthogonal vessel cooling impact on RFA lesion. The combination of these studies has not been reported. Shih *et al.*[18]used ideal external power source, and heating domain was assigned in parallel to single blood vessel which are significant differences as compared to this study. The presented paper implement finite difference model of internally-cooled electrode during RFA. The use of series and parallel thermal resistances of composite materials are presented in the model. Results show consistency with experimental results[19].

II. METHODS

A. *Pennes Bio-heat Transfer Equation*

After obtaining the power p_e, the Pennes bio-heat transfer equation is used to calculate tissue temperatures. That is,

$$\nabla \bullet (k \nabla T(x,y,z)) - \dot{w}_b c_b (T(x,y,z) - T_a) + p_e = 0 \qquad (1)$$

where k, c_b, w_b, and p_e are thermal conductivity of soft tissue, specific heat of blood, blood perfusion rate and absorbed thermal power density, respectively. The metabolism effect is neglected in the bio-heat equation due to its limited effect on temperature distribution during heat treatment.

I. Lackovic (ed.), *1st Global Conference on Biomedical Engineering & 9th Asian-Pacific Conference on Medical and Biological Engineering*, IFMBE Proceedings 47, DOI: 10.1007/978-3-319-12262-5_24

B. Thermal Conductivity near Electrode

We modeled the thermal conductivity near the wall of electrode according to modeling of ferromagnetic implement hyperthermia[20].In Fig.1(a), the thermal conductivity *k* between node *i* and adjacent *i-1* for the one-dimensional case in x-y plane,

$$k_{i-\frac{1}{2}} = \frac{k_t k_c h'_{i-\frac{1}{2}}}{k_c(h'_{i-\frac{1}{2}} - (r_c - r_s)) + k_t(r_c - r_s)} \tag{2}$$

$$h'_{i-\frac{1}{2}} = h_{i-\frac{1}{2}} - r_s \tag{3}$$

where subscript s represents seed, c represents catheter, and t represents tissue. This formulation is equivalent to the use of series of thermal resistances of composite materials. The distance between the edge of the seed and the adjacent node is modified grid size (normal grid size minus the radius of seed) as shown in Equation (3). The correctness of this expression has also been confirmed by comparing numerical results with an analytical solution. The conduction term in the z-direction, the thermal conductivity k can be,

$$k_{k+\frac{1}{2}} = [\pi r_s^2 k_s + (\Delta x \Delta y - \pi r_s^2) k_c] / \Delta x \Delta y \tag{4}$$

which is equivalent to the use of parallel thermal resistances of composite materials.

C. Considering Internally-Cooled Electrode

The circulating water temperature is assumed constant due to convective energy dominance. Therefore, we may utilize the Equation (2). Catheter is replaced by electrode and seed is replaced by flowing water. Equation (2) of thermal conductivity in x-y plane is modified to the following,

$$k_{i-\frac{1}{2}} = \frac{k_t k_e h'_{i-\frac{1}{2}}}{k_e(h'_{i-\frac{1}{2}} - (r_e - r_w)) + k_t(r_e - r_w)} \tag{5}$$

where subscript w represents water, e represents electrode, and t represents tissue. This formulation is then reduced approximately to,

$$k_{i-\frac{1}{2}} \cong k_t \tag{6}$$

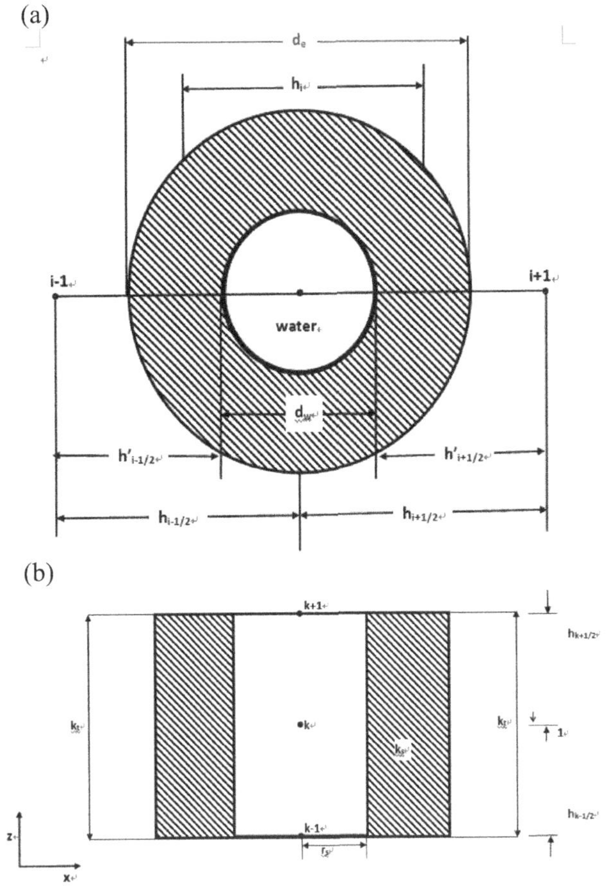

Fig. 1 (a) Illustration of simulating the internally-cooled electrode in lateral cross-sectional view. Here *h* s are normal grid size, and *h*'s are modified grid size around seed used to account for its finite size. (b) in longitudinal view.

when $(r_e - r_w)/h'_{i-\frac{1}{2}}$ is small and k_e / k_t is large. The electrode's thermal conductivity varies ranging from 71 to 401 W/(m.K) in different materials and the ratio of k_e / k_t approximates to 142 to 802 [21]. As it is indicated that only minor increases in thermal lesion dimensions with electrode materials of higher thermal conductivity [21]. These observed differences likely do not provide a significant advantage during clinical procedures. Thus, the Equation (6) make the thermal conductivity in-between electrode node and adjacent node reasonable.

The conduction term in the z-direction, the thermal conductivity k of Equation (4) is modified to be,

$$k_{k+\frac{1}{2}} = [\pi r_w^2 k_w + (\Delta x \Delta y - \pi r_w^2) k_e] / \Delta x \Delta y \tag{7}$$

With considering conduction contribution from tissue, Equation (7) is modified to

$$k_{k+\frac{1}{2}} = [\pi r_w^2 k_w + (\pi r_e^2 - \pi r_w^2)k_e + (\Delta x \Delta y - \pi r_e^2)k_t] / \Delta x \Delta y \quad (8)$$

Since circulating constant water temperature within electrode, the constant water temperature is assumed. This implies high thermal transport in water which is mainly due to convective energy and it can be treated as the same as thermal conductivity of electrode. Then the Equation (8) is modified to

$$k_{k+\frac{1}{2}} = [\pi r_e^2 k_e + (\Delta x \Delta y - \pi r_e^2)k_t] / \Delta x \Delta y \quad (9)$$

Equation (9) describes thermal conductivity along electrode nodes in z-direction, except for end nodes at both top and bottom which are direct contact with tissue; the thermal conductivity is approximated as

$$k_{k+\frac{1}{2}} \cong k_t \quad \text{at the top} \quad (10)$$

$$k_{k-\frac{1}{2}} \cong k_t \quad \text{at the bottom} \quad (11)$$

Table 1 Material properties used in computational model for electrical conductivity of liver tissue and RF cool-tip electrode

Element	Material	ρ (kg/m^3)	c (J/kg K)	k (W/m K)	σ (S/m) (at 25 ℃)
Active RF probe tip	Stainless steel	21500	132	71	$4 \cdot 10^6$
Tissue	Liver	1000	4000	0.5	0.333
Blood vessel	Blood	1000	4000	0.5	0.333

III. RESULTS

A. Simulating Two-Electrode with Different Electrode Spacing

Fig. 1 shows (a)The geometry of numerical configuration is a cube. (b) The central x-z plane reveals an artery blood vessel running in positive Z direction which is parallel to the RF probe located at the center of the cube and the vein is running in opposite direction (red dash line). For an orthogonal blood vessel, it is running in positive Y direction at the center of x-y planes.

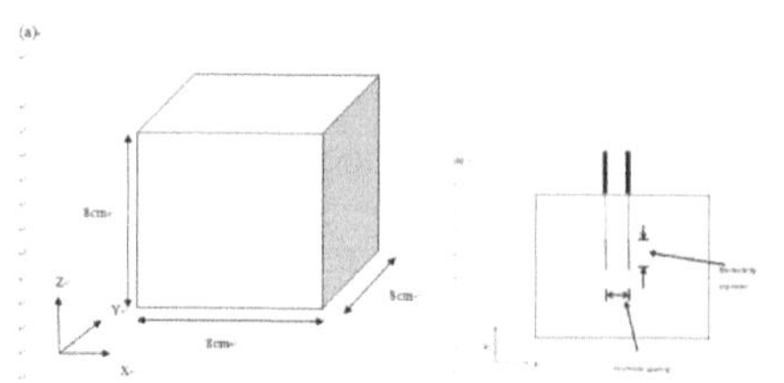

Fig. 1

Figure 2. (a), (b), (c) and (d) Temperature distributions for two-electrode radiofrequency ablation with the electrode tip exposure length of 2-cm at different electrode spacing. Figure 2(a) of X-Z and Figure 2(b) of X-Y planes are at the central planes with the electrode spacing of 2-cm. The internally-water cooled electrodes are placed along z-dir. Figure 2(c) of X-Z and Figure 2(d) of X-Y planes are at the central planes with the electrode spacing of 1-cm. The internally-water cooled electrodes are placed along z-dir. (e) RF Ablation-induced coagulation zone volume generated by two parallel internally cooled electrodes which are apart at various distances in liver. The vertical axis value represents a ratio of coagulation zone volume by two electrdoes to that by single electrode. (i.e. 1.0 mean the thermal lesion size is identical to the lesion size generated by single internally cooled electrode only.) Two coagulation necrosis threshold temperatures are used here: 55°C and 60°C.

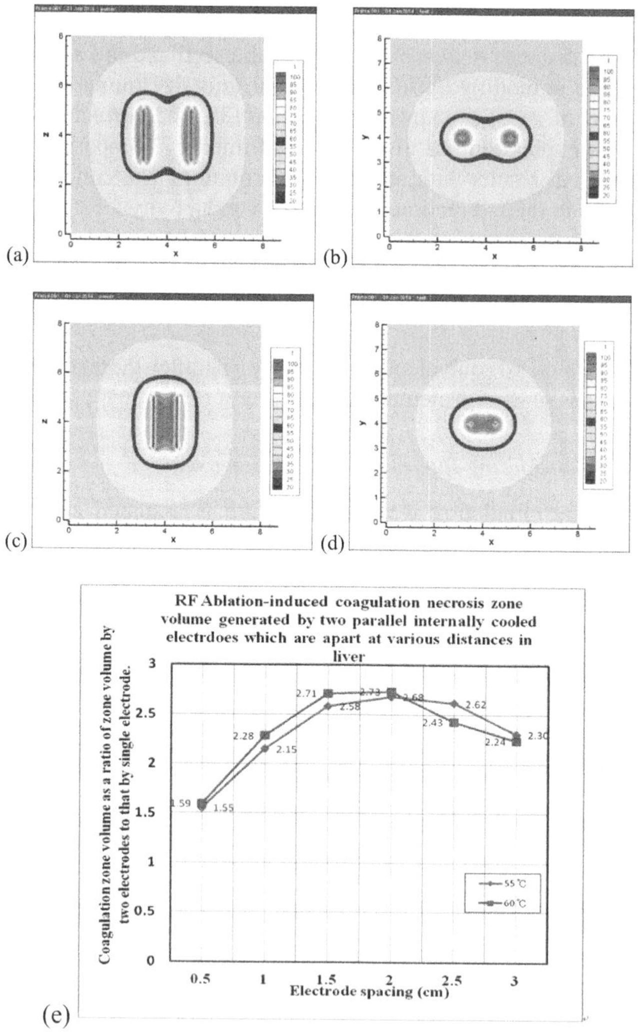

Fig. 2

Figure 2(e) demonstrated that when threshold temperature is 55 ^oC, and the thermal lesion size could reach maximum value of 2.68, as the electrode spacing gradually increases from 0.5-cm to 2.0-cm. The value of 2.68 indicated 2.68 times the thermal lesion size generated by single internally cooled electrode during RFA. It signified that overlapping effect of heat contributions from each electrode was intensifying until reaching the maximum at the distance of 2-cm. The situation is the same when threshold temperature is 60 ^oC.

IV. CONCLUSIONS

A numerical model using finite difference method to calculate temperature distributions via RF heating has established. The model is used to study the influence of blood perfusion rate, high thermal gradients within lesion, and large vessels around the thermal lesion formation. A fast numerical model is capable of predicting thermal lesion formation by multiple parallel internally-cooled electrodes. Results demonstrated that larger coagulation necrosis zone volume is generated with the multiple-electrode technique in minimum invasive localized RF ablation of liver tumor treatment. Overlapping thermal effect from each electrode and clover-shaped thermal lesion formation of three-electrode RFA system are highlighted in the numerical simulations which are consistent with the experimental results.

ACKNOWLEDGMENT

The author would like to thank the National Science Council of Taiwan for partially supporting this research under no. NSC 102-2221-E-032-006-.

CONFLICT OF INTEREST

The author declare that they have no conflict of interest.

REFERENCES

1. D A Gervais, F J McGovern, R S Arellano, W S McDougal, P R Mueller, "Renal cell carcinoma: clinical experience and technical success with radio-frequency ablation of 42 tumors," Radiology **226,** 417-24 (2003).
2. M Ahmed, C L Brace, F T Jr Lee, S N Goldberg, "Principles of and advances in percutaneous ablation," Radiology **258,** 351-69 (2011).
3. D E Dupuy, T DiPetrillo, S Gandhi, N Ready, T Ng, W Donat, W W Mayo-Smith, "Radiofrequency ablation followed by conventional radiotherapy for medically inoperable stge I non-small cell lung cancer," Chest **129,** 738-45 (2006).
4. T Livraghi, L Solbiati, M F Meloni, G S Gazelle, E F Halpern, S N Goldberg, "Treatment of focal liver tumors with percutaneous radio-frequency ablation: complications encountered in a multicenter study," Radiology **226,** 441-51(2003).
5. S N Goldberg, "Radiofrequency tumor ablation: principles and techniques," Eur. J. Ultrasound **13,** 129-47 (2001).
6. D Haemmerich, "Biophysics of radiofrequency ablation," Crit. Rev. Biomed. Eng. **38,** 53-63 (2010).
7. L. Solbiati, T. Livraghi, S. N. Goldberg, T. Ierace, F. Meloni, M. Dellanoce, L. Cova, E.F. Halpern, and G. Scott Gazelle, "Percutaneous Radio-frequency Ablation of Hepatic Metastases from Colorectal Cancer: Long-term Results in 117 Patients", *Radiology*, vol. 221,pp. 159–166 (2001).
8. R. Gillams and W. R. Lees, "The Importance of Large Vessel Proximity in Thermal Ablation of Liver Tumours", *RSNA 1999*, Chicago, IL, (1999).
9. M Ahmed, Z Liu, S Humphries, S N Goldberg, "Computer modeling of the combined effects of perfusion, electrical conductivity, and thermal conductivity on tissue heating patterns in radiofrequency ablation," Int. J. Hyperth. **24,** 577-88 (2008).
10. S N Goldberg, P F Hahn, K K Tanabe, P R Mueller, W Schima, C A Athanasoulis, C C Compton, L Solbiati, G S Gazelle," Percutaneous radiofrequency tissue ablation: does perfusion-mediated tissue cooling limit coagulation necrosis?" J. Vasc. Interv. Radiol. **9,** 101-11 (1998).
11. S N Goldberg, P F Hahn, E Halpern, R Fogle, G S Gazelle, "Radiofrequency tissue ablation: effect of pharmacologic modulation of blood flow on coagulation diameter," Radiology **209,** 791-9 (1998).
12. Z Liu, M Ahmed, A Sabir, S Humphries, S N Goldberg, "Computer modeling of the effect of perfusion on heating patterns in radiofrequency ablation," Int. J. Hyperth. **23,** 49-58(2007).
13. W Schramm, D Yang, B J Wood, D Haemmerich, "Contribution of direct heating, thermal conduction and perfusion during radiofrequency and microwave ablation," Open Biomed. Eng. J. **1,** 47-52 (2007).
14. D. Haemmerich, D. M. Mahvi, F. T. Lee Jr., J. G. Webster, *RF Ablation at Audio Frequencies Preferentially Targets Tumor – A Finite Element Study*, Proceedings of the scond Joint EMBS/BMES conference, Houston, TX, USA oct. 23-26 (2002).
15. S. M Lobo, K S. Afzal, M Ahmed, J B. Kruskal, R. E. Lenkinski and S. N. Goldberg, "Radiofrequency ablation: modeling the enhanced temperature response to adjuvant NaCl pretreatment," Radiology 230:175–182 (2004).
16. G. Suárez, F. Hornero and E. J. Berjano ,"Mathematical modeling of epicardial RF ablation of atrial tissue with overlying epicardial fat," Open Biomed. Eng. J. **4,** 47-55 (2010).
17. Dieter G. Haemmerich, *Finite Element Modeling Of Hepatic Radio Frequency Ablation,* Ph.D. dissertation, University Of Wisconsin – Madison, USA (2001).
18. T.-C. Shih, H.-S. Kou and W.-L. Lin, "Effect of effective tissue conductivity on thermal dose distributions of living tissue with directional blood flow during thermal therapy." International Communications in Heat and Mass Transfer 29(1). 115-126, (2002).
19. Huang-Wen Huang, *Influence of blood vessel on the thermal lesion formation during radiofrequency ablation for liver tumors*, Med. Phys. 40 (7), July 2013.
20. Z-P Chen, R. B. Roemer and T. C. Cetas, "Three-dimensional simulations of ferromagnetic implant hyperthermia" Med. Phys. **19** (4) 989-997 (1992).
21. David Schutt Enrique J. Berjano and Dieter Haemmerich, Effect of electrode thermal conductivity in cardiac radiofrequency catheter ablation: A computational modeling study, International Journal of Hyperthermia, 2009, Vol. 25, No. 2 : Pages 99-107.

Author: Huang-Wen Huang
Institute: Tamkang University
Street: No.180, Linwei Rd., Jiaoxi Township
City: Yilan County 26247
Country: Taiwan, ROC
Email: hhw402@mail.tku.edu.tw

Image Based Simulation for Liver Tumor Ablation by Focused Ultrasound

M.A. Solovchuk[1], T.W.H. Sheu[1,2], and M. Thiriet[3]

[1] Center for Advanced Study in Theoretical Sciences (CASTS), National Taiwan University, Taipei, Taiwan
[2] Department of Engineering Science and Ocean Engineering, National Taiwan University, Taipei, Taiwan
[3] Sorbonne Universities, UPMC Univ Paris 06, UMR 7598, Laboratoire Jacques-Louis Lions, F-75005, Paris, France

Abstract— **The present computational model is aimed at predicting the temperature field in a region of the hepatic parenchyma with a cancer resulting from applied high-intensity focused ultrasounds (HIFU) for thermal ablation of the tumor in a patient-specific geometry. The three-dimensional (3D) acoustic–thermal–hydrodynamic coupling model computes the pressure, temperature, and blood velocity fields expressed by the nonlinear Westervelt equation with relaxation effects and bioheat equations in both the hepatic parenchyma and blood vessels (sink). The classical nonlinear Navier–Stokes equations related to mass and momentum conservation in large hepatic blood vessels are employed both for convective cooling and acoustic streaming. This 3D three-field coupling demonstrates that both convective cooling and acoustic streaming change the temperature considerably near large blood vessels. In addition, acoustic streaming cannot be neglected due to resulting velocity magnitude and blood redistribution between different branches. The results presented in the current work can be further used to construct a surgical planning platform.**

Keywords— **HIFU, liver tumor, 3D reconstruction, blood flow.**

I. INTRODUCTION

Liver cancer is the second leading cause of cancer death in men and the sixth leading cause among women in the world [1, 2]. At an early stage liver cancer can be successfully treated with surgery or liver transplantation. For a patient diagnosed at an advanced stage of disease fewer surgical options exist. Unfortunately, no more than 20 percent of patients can be treated with the surgery. In addition to the open and minimally invasive surgery, cryotherapy, radio-frequency (RF) ablation, microwave coagulation therapy, laser-induced thermotherapy, and catheter-based infusion chemotherapy followed by transarterial chemoembolization chemotherapy (TACE), high-intensity focused ultrasound (HIFU)-based treatment is noninvasive, nonionizing technique. High intensity focused ultrasound (HIFU) is a promising method for the tumor ablation and it can be used when other methods cannot be applied. Thermal ablation relies on the observation that a temperature above 56°C applied during one second by energy source (pressure or electromagnetic waves) causes irreversible tissue damage.

The target tissue temperature should rises to lethal levels without affecting healthy surrounding tissue, especially blood vessels to avoid vascular damage, although some organs such as the liver has a strong self-renewal, which enables fast regeneration. On the other hand, blood flow cooling reduces the necrosed volume [3, 4].

Creating a medico surgical platform requires proper HIFU equipment and a simulation device that incorporates multiple GPU processors for fast and efficient computations. Image processing tools are mandatory for optimized procedures. Simulations carried out on patient-specific geometries are aimed at training, predicting, and planning the treatment. Numerical investigation also enables to relatively easily test the effects of nonlinear wave propagation, blood flow cooling, and acoustic streaming on HIFU tumor ablation.

The three-dimensional (3D) acoustic–thermal–hydrodynamic coupling model computes the pressure, temperature, and blood velocity fields expressed by the nonlinear Westervelt equation with relaxation effects and bioheat equations in both the hepatic parenchyma and blood vessels. The classical nonlinear Navier–Stokes equations related to mass and momentum conservation in large hepatic blood vessels are employed both for convective cooling and acoustic streaming. The 3D problem is solved using the finite-volume method [3-4].

II. METHODS

A. Mathematical Model

The three-dimensional (3D) acoustic-thermal-hydrodynamic coupling model is proposed to compute the pressure, temperature, and blood flow velocity.

The mathematical model [3-5] relies on a coupling of: (1) nonlinear Westervelt equation with relaxation effects being taken into account; (2) heat equations in biological tissues; and (3) acoustic streaming hydrodynamic equations. The computational domain is meshed from a patient-specific 3D reconstruction that includes the hepatic and portal veins (Fig. 1). The total number of tetrahedral elements is 910,000. In the focal region, the grid is refined, thereby generating a cell length of 0.2mm.

Acoustic field generated by a HIFU source was modeled using the nonlinear Westervelt equation

I. Lackovic (ed.), *1st Global Conference on Biomedical Engineering & 9th Asian-Pacific Conference on Medical and Biological Engineering*,
IFMBE Proceedings 47, DOI: 10.1007/978-3-319-12262-5_25

$$\nabla^2 p - \frac{1}{c_0^2}\frac{\partial^2 p}{\partial t^2} + \frac{\delta}{c_0^4}\frac{\partial^3 p}{\partial t^3} + \frac{\beta}{\rho_0 c_0^4}\frac{\partial^2 p^2}{\partial t^2} + \sum_{i=1}^{2} \mathbf{P}_i = 0$$
$$(1+\tau_i \frac{\partial}{\partial t})\mathbf{P}_i = \frac{2}{c_0^3} c_i \tau_i \frac{\partial^3 p}{\partial t^3} \quad (1)$$

In the above, p is the sound pressure, β is the coefficient of nonlinearity, and δ is the diffusivity of sound resulting from viscosity and heat conduction, τ_n is the relaxation time and c_n is the small signal sound speed increment for the n-th relaxation process. Two relaxation processes are considered in the present work. The first two terms describe the linear lossless wave propagating at a small-signal sound speed. The third term denotes the loss due to thermal conduction and fluid viscosity. The fourth term accounts for acoustic nonlinearity which may considerably affect thermal and mechanical changes within the tissue. The last term accounts for the relaxation processes.

For the linear Westervelt equation the intensity is equal to $I_L = p^2 / 2\rho c_0$, where c_0 is speed of sound. In the nonlinear case, the total intensity is

$$I = \sum_{n=1}^{\infty} I_n, \quad (2)$$

where I_n are the corresponding intensities for the respective harmonics nf_0. The ultrasonic power deposition per unit volume is calculated as follows

$$q = \sum_n 2\alpha(nf) I_n, \quad (3)$$

where acoustic absorption α linearly depends on frequency.

Tissue heating by ultrasound involves an energy balance in which source terms associated with metabolic heating and ultrasound power deposition are balanced by sink terms associated with convective cooling (large blood vessels), perfusion cooling (microvasculature), heat conduction, and energy storage. In order to calculate the temperature we have separated the domain of our interest into two regions: region free or large blood vessels (Eq. 4.1) and region inside large blood vessel (Eq. 4.2) with diameter d>0.5 mm. Tissue heating by ultrasound can be well described by two bioheat equations

$$\rho_t c_t \frac{\partial T}{\partial t} = k_t \nabla^2 T - w_b c_b (T - T_\infty) + \mathbf{q} \quad (4.1)$$

$$\rho_b c_b \frac{\partial T}{\partial t} = k_b \nabla^2 T - \rho_b c_b \mathbf{\bar{u}} \cdot \nabla T + \mathbf{q} \quad (4.2)$$

where T is the temperature, and ρ, c, and k are the density, specific heat, and thermal conductivity, respectively, which the subscripts t or b referring to the tissue and blood domains.

Focused ultrasound can induce an additional mass flow. This effect is known as acoustic streaming and is taken into account in the present HIFU simulation study. It can enhance blood flow cooling, representing an additional heat sink [2, 3]. The vector equation for modeling the blood flow motion, subject to the divergence free equation, in the presence of acoustic stresses is as follows:

$$\frac{\partial \vec{u}}{\partial t} + (\vec{u} \cdot \nabla)\vec{u} = \frac{\mu}{\rho}\nabla^2 \vec{u} - \frac{1}{\rho}\nabla P + \frac{\mathbf{1}}{\boldsymbol{\rho}}\vec{\mathbf{F}}, \quad (5)$$

In Eq. (5), the force vector **F** acting on the blood fluid due to ultrasound is assumed to act along the acoustic axis n. The resulting nonzero component in **F** takes the following form

$$\vec{\mathbf{F}} \cdot \vec{n} = \frac{q}{c_0}. \quad (6)$$

First the acoustic pressure was calculated. Westervelt equation is solved using the sixth-order accurate finite difference scheme [3]. The acoustic pressure was calculated only once for a given set of transducer parameters. Afterward ultrasound power deposition in Eq. (3) and acoustic streaming force in Eq. (6) were determined and stored. Blood flow velocity was computed from Eq. (5) at every time step with the acoustic streaming effect being taken into account and then substituted to the bioheat equations (4). With the known blood flow velocities and power deposition terms, temperatures in blood flow domain and in liver were calculated. The three-dimensional problem is analyzed using finite-volume method. A detailed description of the solution procedures can be found in our previous articles [2-4]. The present 3D computational model was validated by comparing our simulated results for the temperature field, with and without flow, with the experimental results [5]. Temperature elevation by HIFU in ex-vivo porcine muscle was also studied experimentally by MRI and numerically [6]. We demonstrated that for peak temperatures below 85-90 ^{0}C numerical simulation results are in excellent agreement with the experimental data in three dimensions. Both temperature rise and lesion size can be well predicted.

III. RESULTS

In the present section we are going to present numerical results for a patient specific liver model. First we are going to investigate the effect of acoustic streaming. Acoustic streaming is considered as a second order physical effect in the HIFU therapy and it is usually neglected. To investigate the importance of acoustic streaming effect during a thermal therapy, we have plotted in Figs. 2, 3 the velocity profiles at different cutting planes in portal venous network with and without acoustic streaming effect. Maximum velocity magnitudes in the portal vein for the cases considered with and without acoustic streaming are 37 and 7 cm/s, respectively. Acoustic streaming increases the velocity magnitude by more than four times. This will increase the blood flow cooling and decrease the temperature rise [3, 4].

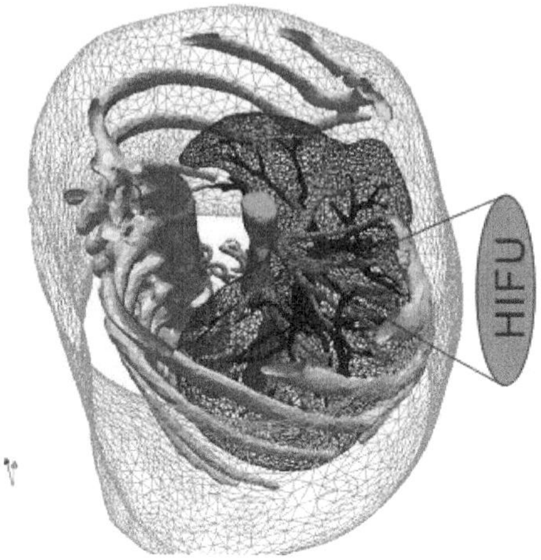

Fig. 1. Patient specific 3D geometry reconstructed from CT images.

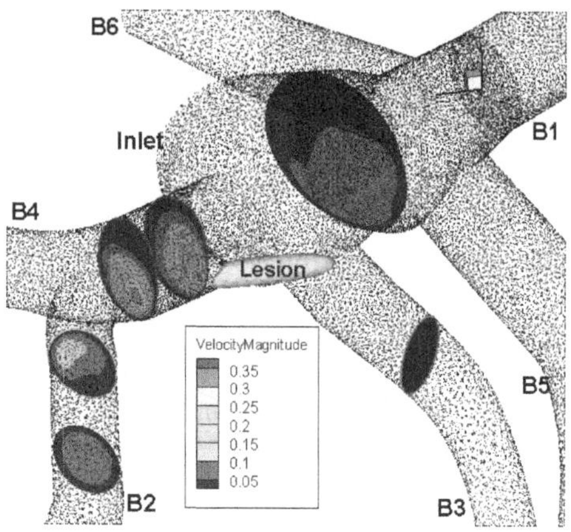

Fig. 2. The predicted velocity profiles at different cutting planes in portal venous network when acoustic streaming effect is taken into account; lesion (necrosed volume) is drawn with light blue.

In Table 1 the predicted mass fluxes at different branches of the portal vein, schematic in Fig. 2, are presented with and without acoustic streaming. The mass fluxes at branches 2 and 4 are increased more than twice; the mass flux at branch 3 is decreased by seven times. Hence, acoustic streaming can lead to sufficient mass flux redistribution among different branches. This effect can be used to control drug delivery.

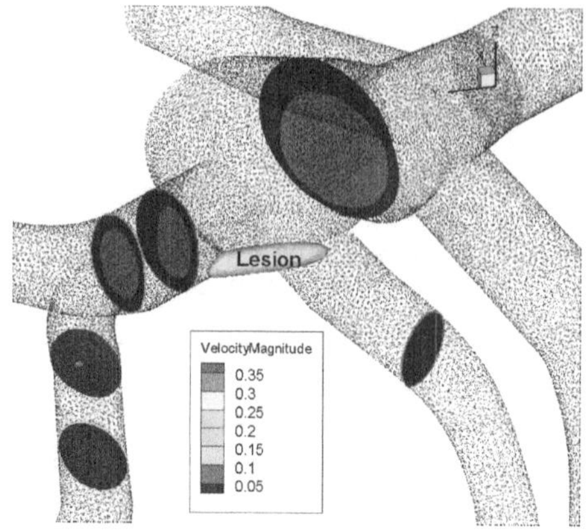

Fig. 3. The predicted velocity profiles at different cutting planes in portal venous network when acoustic streaming effect is **not** taken into account; lesion (necrosed volume) is drawn with light blue.

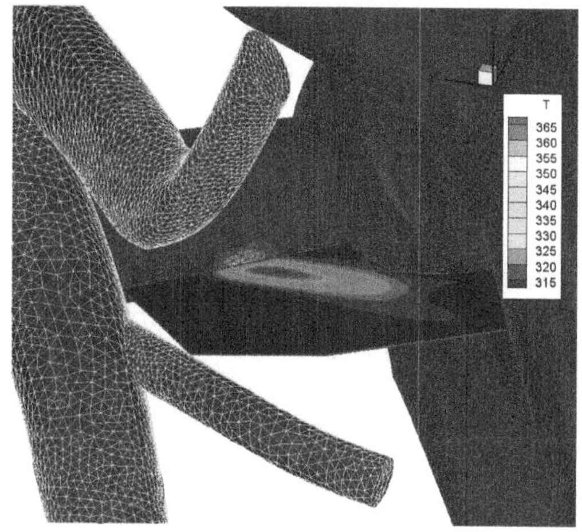

Fig. 4. The predicted temperature contours in tumor and in portal vein at the selected cutting plane z=0.16 m for the case with sonication time 0.4 s.

Table 1 Acoustic streaming effect on blood mass flow (10^{-3} kg/s) distribution among different branches (B) of the portal vein marked in Fig.2

	B1	B2	B3	B4	B5	B6	Inlet
Without AS	3.3	0.58	0.53	1.5	1.28	1.13	8.32
With AS	2.2	1.27	0.07	3.3	0.69	0.76	8.32
Difference (%)	-32	+120	-87	+121	-46	-33	

The simulated temperature contours in tumor and in the portal vein at the cutting plane $z=0.16$ are presented in Fig. 4 at time $t=0.4$ s (end of sonication). The temperature 56 ^{0}C can be achieved on the blood vessel wall; therefore tumor close to blood vessel can be ablated. The temperature inside the blood vessel remains almost unchanged except in the boundary layer close to the focal point. Therefore focused ultrasound can be a safe therapy to ablate tumors close to blood vessel wall. However, more experimental studies in vitro and in vivo are necessary. Previously it was shown [2, 4] that in the moderate-intensity regime thin layer of tissue close to blood vessel wall remained viable and could not be ablated. High focal intensities and small exposure time, used in the current study, are two factors that help to ablate tumors proximal to large blood vessels. Nonlinear propagation effects also help to ablate tumor in this case. Simulation results can help to optimize an appropriate set of sonication time, ultrasound power and focal point location.

IV. CONCLUSIONS

The proposed three-dimensional computational model of HIFU therapy is carried out on a mesh derived from 3D reconstruction of the liver and its major vessels. A priori, the lower the flow velocity, the smaller the ablation zone volume should be due to the presence of a large blood vessel with respect to a target parenchyma free of large blood vessels. However, the treatment efficiency is markedly influenced not only by blood flow cooling, but also acoustic streaming. At high intensities, cooling by acoustic streaming can prevail over the simple cooling by the blood flow through large intrahepatic blood vessel. Acoustic streaming may thus enhances therapy safety. These results can be further used to construct a surgical planning platform for the non-invasive HIFU tumor ablating therapy in real liver geometry from MRI image and can lead in the future to a substantial improvement of the focused ultrasound ablation of liver tumor. The presented model can be used in planning tools for the thermal ablation of tumor in other organs and is also applicable to acoustic hemostasis treatment [7].

ACKNOWLEDGMENT

The authors would like to acknowledge the financial support from the Center for Advanced Study in Theoretical Sciences (CASTS) and from the National Science Council of Republic of China under Contract No. NSC102-2811-M-002-125.

CONFLICT OF INTEREST

The authors declare that they have no conflict of interest.

REFERENCES

1. Sheu TWH, Solovchuk MA, Chen AWJ, Thiriet M (2011) On an acoustics–thermal–fluid coupling model for the prediction of temperature elevation in liver tumor. International Journal of Heat and Mass Transfer 54:4117–4126
2. Solovchuk MA, Sheu TWH, Lin WL, Kuo I, Thiriet M (2012) Simulation study on acoustic streaming and convective cooling in blood vessels during a high-intensity focused ultrasound thermal ablation. International Journal of Heat and Mass Transfer 55:1261–1270
3. Solovchuk MA, Sheu TWH, Thiriet M (2013) Simulation of nonlinear Westervelt equation for the investigation of acoustic streaming and nonlinear propagation effects. J. Acoust. Soc. Am. 134:3931–3942
4. Solovchuk MA, Sheu TWH, Thiriet M, Lin WL (2013) On a computational study for investigating acoustic streaming and heating during focused ultrasound ablation of liver tumor. Applied Thermal Engineering 56:62-76
5. Huang J, Holt RG, Cleveland RO, Roy RA (2004) Experimental validation of a tractable numerical model for focused ultrasound heating in flow-through tissue phantoms. J. Acoust. Soc. Am. 116:2451–2458
6. Solovchuk MA, Hwang SC, Chang H, Thiriet M, Sheu TWH (2014) Temperature elevation by HIFU in ex vivo porcine muscle: MRI measurement and simulation study. Medical physics 41(5), 052903.
7. Solovchuk MA, Sheu TWH. (2013) Computational model for investigating acoustic hemostasis, Proc. "Int. Workshop on Computational Science and Engineering" PoS(IWCSE 2013)019, 11 pp.

Author: Maxim Solovchuk
Institute: National Taiwan University
Street: Roosevelt Road
City: Taipei
Country: Taiwan
Email: solovchuk@gmail.com

Development of a Novel Micro-motion Dental Implant System

Y.Y. Chen[1], W.P. Chen[1,*], H.H. Chang[2], S.H. Huang[2], and C.P. Lin[2]

[1] Department of Mechanical Engineering, National Taipei University of Technology, Taipei, Taiwan
[2] Graduate Institute of Clinical Dentistry, School of Dentistry, National Taiwan University, Taipei, Taiwan

Abstract— **Dental implantation has brought about not only the occlusive capability restoration for edentulous patients, but also provided a better choice for the tooth reconstruction. With the advancements of science and technology, a satisfactory success rate of the dental implantation was reported. However, the mechanical behavior of the dental implant is still not similar to a natural tooth with the periodontal ligament. The micro-motion mechanism is the main difference between the natural tooth and the dental implant. Therefore, the aim of this study was to develop a novel dental implant abutment with a micro-motion mechanism that imitates the biomechanical behavior of the periodontal ligament, with the goal of not only maintaining the primal success rate but also increasing the long-term survival rate of dental implants. Firstly, computer-aided design software was used to design a novel dental implant abutment with an internal resilient component with a micro-motion capability. The feasibility of the novel system was investigated via finite element analysis. Then, a prototype of the novel dental implant abutment was fabricated, and the mechanical behavior was evaluated. The compression test of the novel dental implant was performed to prove micro-motion function. Moreover, the fatigue test of the novel dental implant was executed on the basis of the ISO 14801 standard. The results of the finite element analysis and the compression test confirmed that the novel dental implant abutment possessed the anticipated micro-motion capability. The nonlinear force-displacement behavior apparent in this micro-motion mechanism imitated the movement of a human tooth. Furthermore, the novel dental implant accomplished the fatigue test successfully at 5,000,000 cycles with frequencies of 5 Hz. The maximum endured load of the fatigue resistance of the novel dental implant is 160 N according to the ISO 14801 standard.**

Keywords— **Dental implant, micro-motion, finite element analysis, fatigue test, ISO 14801, natural tooth.**

I. INTRODUCTION

Dental implant systems are important for edentulous patients. Although dental implantation now has a high success rate greater than 90% [1]. However, an ideal dental implant should provide the stability as well as the micro-motion of a natural tooth. None of the current commercial dental implant systems provides the micro-motion capability to imitate a natural tooth. The inconsistent movements between the dental implant and the natural tooth limit the design and success of an implant system [2]. Therefore, the aim of this study is to develop a novel dental implant abutment with a pericementum-like mechanism that can imitate the biomechanical behavior of a natural tooth. Such a novel dental implant abutment would not only maintain the primal success rate but also increase the long-term survival rate of the implant.

II. MATERIALS AND METHODS

It was comprised of four main stages: design, finite element analysis (FEA), compression test and fatigue test for the development of the novel dental implant system with a micro-motion capability in this study. First, the novel dental implant abutment was designed. The internal structure of a commercially available abutment was ameliorated to provide a micro-motion mechanism. Moreover, an elastic ring was assembled inside the abutment to provide a resilience function (Fig. 1). Second, the FEA of this novel dental abutment was executed to evaluate its feasibility. A three-dimensional model of the dental abutment was meshed to establish an FE model. The material properties, contact, boundary and loading conditions were reasonably defined in the FEA [3, 4]. The displacement and the stress were obtained to estimate the mechanical response of the novel dental abutment. The prototype of the novel dental abutment was fabricated before the mechanical experiments. Finally, two mechanical experiments of the novel dental abutment were orderly performed. One was a compression test to ensure the credibility of the FEA (Fig. 2). The other was a cyclic fatigue test to evaluate the life of the novel dental abutment according to the ISO 14801 standard [5] (Fig. 3).

The novel dental abutment was designed for the Straumann dental fixture (Fig. 1g) of the other commercially available dental implant. The connection of the Straumann dental implant belongs to the type of an internal hexagon. The outer contour of the Straumann dental abutment was adopted to design the novel dental abutment. The novel dental abutment included the coping component (Fig. 1d), the resilient ring component (Fig. 1e), and the abutment component (Fig. 1f). The novel dental implant and the relevant apparatuses were fabricated, as shown in Fig. 1.

* Corresponding author.

I. Lackovic (ed.), *1st Global Conference on Biomedical Engineering & 9th Asian-Pacific Conference on Medical and Biological Engineering*,
IFMBE Proceedings 47, DOI: 10.1007/978-3-319-12262-5_26

The function and the life of the second prototype of the novel dental implant were respectively evaluated by way of the compression experiment and the fatigue test in this study. The specimen of the novel dental implant was prepared for both mechanical experiments (Fig. 1b). First, the compression test of the novel dental implant was executed using the MTS universal testing machine (Model: 858 Mini Bionix, MTS Corporation, Eden Prairie, MN, USA) and the laser displacement sensor (Model: LB-1103, Keyence, Elmwood Park, NJ, US). An axial load of 150 N was applied upon the coping component, as shown in Fig. 2. The novel dental implant was tested repeatedly nine times in the compression test. The force-displacement curves were acquired to evaluate the mechanical behavior of the novel dental implant.

The fatigue test of the novel dental implant was performed via the MTS and the angular jaw. The metal holder was used to fix the novel dental implant (Fig. 3). A 30 ° oblique load of 200 N with a 5 Hz in frequency was applied upon the novel dental implant through a hemispherical head. The load varied sinusoidally between a nominal peak value (200 N) and 10 % of this value (200 N × 10% = 20 N). The intention of the hemispherical loading member is to ensure a single force on the test specimen. The number of load cycles was recorded until five million cycles or failure in the fatigue test of the novel dental implant. Besides, the data for the cycle number were obtained by testing specimens at a series of loads until a lower limit is reached according to the ISO 14801 standard. Therefore, the cyclic load could be decreased when the testing specimen was failed.

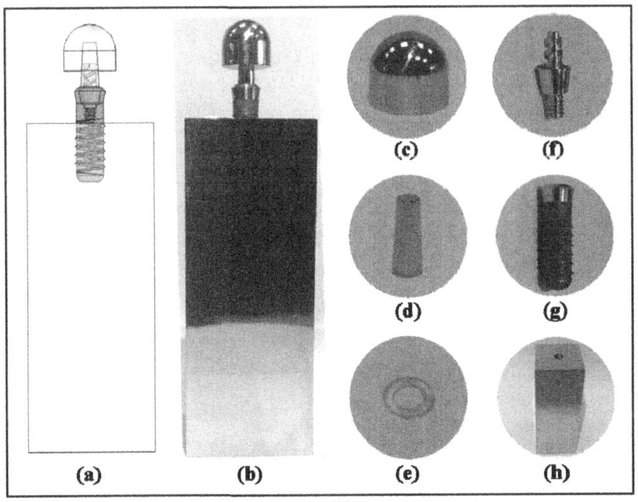

Fig. 1 Three-dimensional model (a) and prototypes (b) of the novel dental implant system. (c) hemispherical head. (d) coping. (e) resilient ring. (f) abutment. (g) fixture. (h) specimen holder.

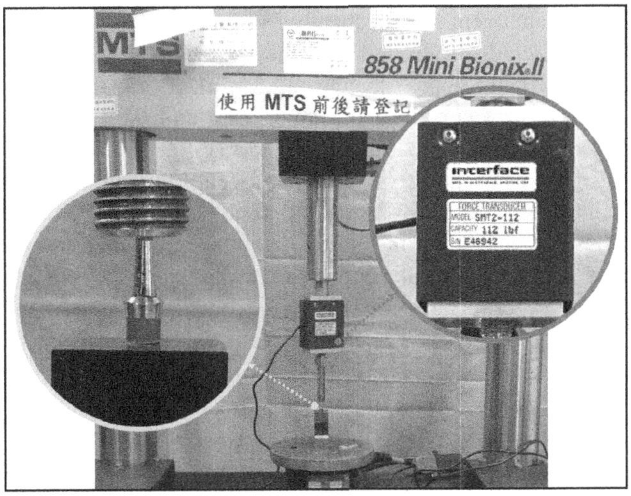

Fig. 2 Experimental setup of the novel dental implant on a universal testing machine in the compression test

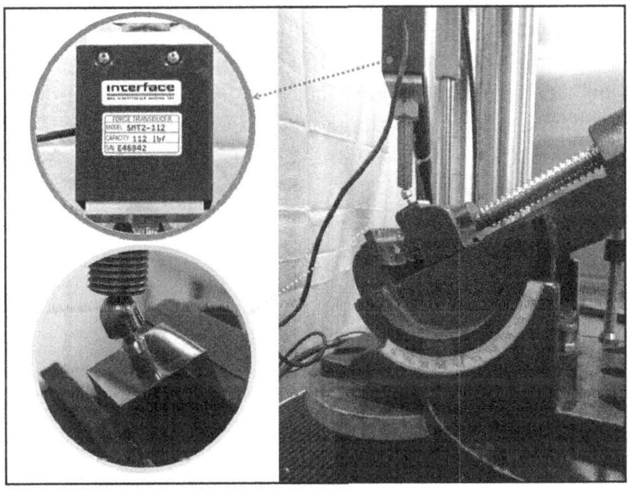

Fig. 3 Experimental setup of the novel dental implant on a universal testing machine in the fatigue test

III. RESULTS AND DISCUSSIONS

The von Mises stress distribution of the novel abutment was mainly concentrated at the annular fillister of the abutment and the bottom of the coping. The maximum von Mises stress of the coping was 516.5 MPa, the maximum von Mises stress of the abutment was 321.35 MPa, the maximum von Mises stress of the ring was 85.15 MPa, and the maximum von Mises stress of the fixture was 73.25 MPa under the 150-N loading condition (Fig. 4). When the force was increased from 0 N to 0.75 N, the displacement was increased to approximately 0.02 mm in the FEA of the novel abutment. Subsequently, when the force was increased gradually from 0.75 N to 5 N, the displacement was increased to approximately 37.5 μm. Both the force-displacement curves of the experiment and the FEA exhibited similar mechanical behavior (Fig. 5). The force-displacement curves of the novel dental implant were obtained under the 150-N loading condition in the compression test, as shown in Fig. 5. A total of nine experimental data had an excellent repeatability in this study. The quality of the experimental procedure is satisfactory. The nonlinear behavior of the novel dental implant was presented in the compression test. The reaction displacement of the novel dental implant was 0.1 mm by the loading force of approximately 17.6 N. When the load reached 150 N, the reaction displacement of the novel dental implant was 0.19 mm. It proves that a design of the novel dental implant with the micro-motion mechanism is practicable through the FEA and the experiments in this study. It is to be regretted that the novel dental implant is failed in the fatigue test again according to the ISO 14801 standard. Finally, the novel dental implant has accomplished the fatigue test successfully under the cyclic load of 160 N until 5,000,000 cycles in this study. The maximum endured load of the novel dental implant is 160 N according to the ISO 14801 standard.

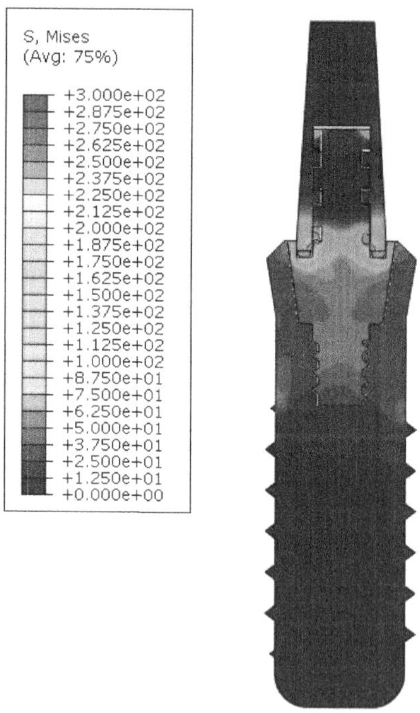

Fig. 4 The sectional view of the von Mises stress distribution of the novel implant under the 150-N load in the finite element analysis

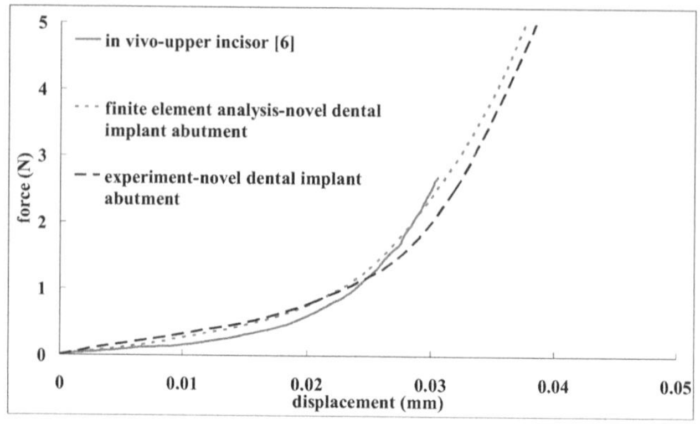

Fig. 5 Force-displacement curves of the novel abutment (the FEA and the mechanical experiment) and a natural tooth [6]

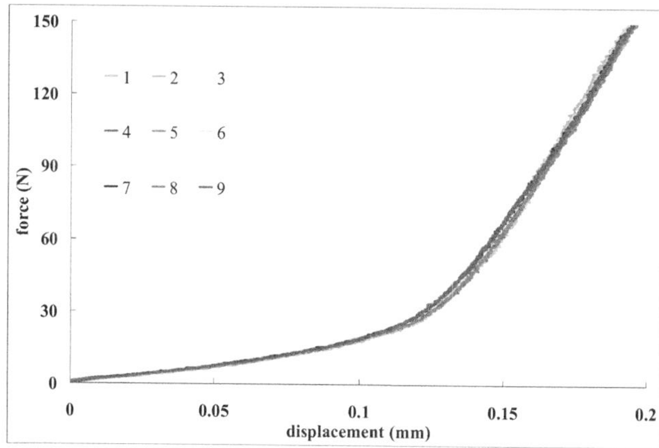

Fig. 6 Force-displacement curves of the novel micro-motion dental implant in the compression experiment

IV. Conclusions

Within the limitations of the present study, the ability of a novel dental implant to provide a micro-motion mechanism was validated by FEA and experiments. The mechanical behavior of the novel dental implant was similar to that of a natural tooth during mastication.

Conflict of Interest

The authors declare that they have no conflict of interest.

References

1. Mangano C, Mangano F, Shibli JA, Tettamanti L, Figliuzzi M, d'Avila S, Sammons RL, Piattelli A. (2011) Prospective Evaluation of 2,549 Morse Taper Connection Implants: 1- to 6-Year Data. J Periodont 82:52–61.

2. Lekholm U, Gröndahl K, Jemt T. (2006) Outcome of oral implant treatment in partially edentulous jaws followed 20 years in clinical function. Clin Implant Dent Relat Res 8:178–186.
3. Toms SR, Lemons JE, Bartolucci AA, Eberhardt AW. (2002) Nonlinear stress-strain behaviour of periodontal ligament under orthodontic loading. Am J Orthod Dentofac Orthop 122:174–179.
4. Toms SR, Dakin GJ, Lemons JE, Eberhardt AW. (2002) Quasi-linear viscoelastic behavior of the human periodontal ligament. J Biomech 35:1411–1415.
5. ISO/FDIS 14801:2007, Dynamic fatigue test for endosseous dental implant.
6. Parfitt GJ. (1960) Measurement of the physiological mobility of individual teeth in an axial direction. J Dent Res 39:608–618.

Author: Yen-Yin Chen
Institute: Department of Mechanical Engineering, National Taipei University of Technology
Street: No.1, Sec. 3 Chung-Hsiao E. Rd., Da-an District, Taipei City 106, Taiwan R.O.C.
City: Taipei
Country: Taiwan
Email: yychenbrian@yahoo.com.tw

Corresponding Author: Weng-Pin Chen
Institute: Department of Mechanical Engineering, National Taipei University of Technology
Street: No.1, Sec. 3 Chung-Hsiao E. Rd., Da-an District, Taipei City 106, Taiwan R.O.C.
City: Taipei
Country: Taiwan
Email: wpchen@ntut.edu.tw

Author: Hao-Hueng Chang
Institute: Department of Dentistry, School of Dentistry, National Taiwan University and National Taiwan University Hospital
Street: No.1, Changde St., Jhongjheng District, Taipei City 100, Taiwan R.O.C.
City: Taipei
Country: Taiwan
Email: changhh@ntu.edu.tw

Author: Shih-Hao Huang
Institute: Graduate Institute of Clinical Dentistry, School of Dentistry, National Taiwan University
Street: No.1, Changde St., Jhongjheng District, Taipei City 100, Taiwan R.O.C.
City: Taipei
Country: Taiwan
Email: d97422003@ntu.edu.tw

Corresponding Author: Chun-Pin Lin
Institute: Department of Dentistry, School of Dentistry, National Taiwan University and National Taiwan University Hospital
Street: No.1, Changde St., Jhongjheng District, Taipei City 100, Taiwan R.O.C.
City: Taipei
Country: Taiwan
Email: pinlin@ntu.edu.tw

Experimental Investigation of Aerodynamic Dust Resuspension Due to Foot Step

Y. Kubota[1] and O. Mochizuki[2]

[1] Faculty of Science and Engineering, Toyo University, Saitama, Japan
[2] Department of Biomedical Engineering, Toyo University, Saitama, Japan

Abstract— **The particulate matter on the floor is at first detached and resuspended from the floor and then redistributed by human activities (i.e. walking). The objective of this paper is to investigate experimentally particle resuspension and redistribution due to human foot motion. The flow visualization with actual foot tapping was also carried out to demonstrate the particle resuspension. The experiments were carried out by flow visualization and Particle Image Velocimetry (PIV) measurements. To define the measurements better, the foot was modeled either as a disk, an elongated plate or a slipper-wearing foot model, that moved normal to the ground. The results indicate that particles can be resuspended with the walking process by aerodynamic mechanism. The particles resuspension is caused by wall jet between the foot and floor, and the particles redistribution takes place by the vortex dynamics.**

Keywords— **Dust Particle Resuspension, Idealized foot, Wall jet, Vortex, PIV measurement.**

I. INTRODUCTION

An indoor air quality is affected by an amount of particulate matter (PM) suspended in air. The particulate matter is first detached from the floor (resuspended), and then entrained into the human thermal plume, where it can ultimately be inhaled. Resuspension of particles is caused by human activities such as walking. Ferro et al. examined that once resuspended the particulate matter can affect the human health[1]. Question at issue is how the human motion causes the resuspension of particles.

The particles are strongly attracted to the floor via various forces (adhesion, electrostatic, Van Der Waals forces and can be detached via either ballistic or aerodynamic mechanism, or combination of both[2, 3]. The ballistic mechanism occurs when colliding particles break the cohesive bond, which exists between particles. Whereas the aerodynamic mechanism occurs when the particles are resuspended by purely flow disturbances generated by the body. The dust resuspension due to a sphere impacting the wall was investigated by Eames et al., and the associated vortex dynamics around a sphere impacting the wall was studied by Leweke et al. [4]. The present paper examines the aerodynamic mechanism of particle resuspension excluding floor vibration, etc.; to focus on the wall jet and the vortex dynamics caused by the idealized foot motion. Also, this article addresses the subsequent redistribution of the particles by the aerodynamics mechanism.

Modeling the human walking motion and the associated foot kinetics is complex with both a vertical and a rotational component [5]. In the present laboratory experiment, the stepping motion is modeled as normal motion to the floor and both the downward portion of the walking cycle as well as the foot stomping are examined for the first approximation. In these experiments, the motion is stopped just before touching the floor, ensuring no floor vibration to focus on the aerodynamic resuspension mechanism. Here, the idealized foot is modeled as one of the followings: a disk, an elongated plate and a slipper. The disk and elongated plate have the equivalent area to a US 8 size human shoe. Khalifa et al. studied analytically and numerically the aerodynamic resuspension mechanism of particle "attached" to the wall beneath a falling disk [6]. The present study is focused on the global flow field and associated particle resuspension around the immediate the neighborhood the idealized foot.

II. EXPERIMENTAL SETUP AND CONDITIONS

Particle flow visualization with the human foot tapping was first conducted. Actual tapping motion consists of foot pivoting around the heel touching the floor. The subject wore a slipper. The angular velocity during in the portion of downward motion was 4.3rad/sec as measured with a Photron high-speed camera.

A sketch of the setup for an idealized foot is shown in Fig. 1 a). Three different geometries were used as the idealized foot model. The models were (1) a 152.4mm diameter disk, (2) an elongated plate and (3) an indoor slipper. All had smooth bottom surface. The geometry of the elongated plate was a rectangle with two half circles at the both ends, and the overall dimensions are 71.7mm in width and 269.8mm in length. The idealized foot motions were driven vertically by a computer-controlled linear servomotor. The motor could be controlled by programming the maximum velocity, acceleration, deceleration and stroke. Both flow visualization and flow-field velocity measurement were conducted in a 1.2m x 1.2m sealed acrylic case to ensure that no cross flow drafts were present.

I. Lackovic (ed.), *1st Global Conference on Biomedical Engineering & 9th Asian-Pacific Conference on Medical and Biological Engineering*,
IFMBE Proceedings 47, DOI: 10.1007/978-3-319-12262-5_27

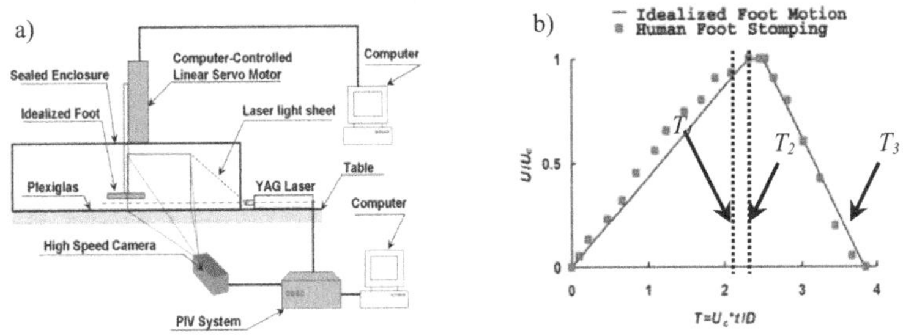

Fi g. 1 Experimental configurations. a) Sketch of the setup, b) Velocity time histories of both human foot stomping and idealized foot motion.

III. RESULTS

A. *Resuspension of Particle by a Human Foot Tapping*

The sequence of particle flow visualization with an actual foot tapping motion is shown in Fig. 2. The toe is facing the reader in the sequence of figures. The time increment is 0.1sec. At *t*=0sec., the foot stopped from downward motion, and the following two show the results during upward potion of the motion. The particles were initially seeded just underneath the foot. The particles were expelled from beneath the floor, and entrained in the vortex at *t*=0sec. Later, the resuspended particles were redistributed at *t*=0.1sec. It can be seen that once resuspended, particles are easily levitated into the air (see figure at *t*=0.2sec.) affecting the indoor air quality. In upward motion, the particles were resuspended behind the upward-moving foot at *t*=0.2sec. Thus, both downward and upward motions are shown to be equally important for the resuspension and redistribution of particles. To understand the process of particles resuspension and redistribution in more detail, the experiments were carried out using an idealized foot in prescribed motion.

B. *Idealized Foot Experiment: Effect of Initial Seeding Pattern with a Disk during Downward Motion*

The particle visualization and the velocity field measurements with a disk model have been reported earlier by Kubota, et al.[7]. In the present follow-up study with a disk, the particles flow visualizations were conducted with different types of seeding patterns. The streak patterns in Fig. 3 indicate the final particle distribution after the disk stops immediately above the wall. Four types of initial seeding patterns were examined: (a) the particles spread over the same diameter as the disk, (b) spread over half diameter of disk, (c) in annular distribution beneath the disk between half diameter from the center to the edge of the disk and (d) annular pattern immediately outside the disk seeded in 2.54cm width from the edge of the foot. The result in Figure 3a) shows that the axisymmetric particle distribution on the wall. The vortex ring forming behind a disk in rapid acceleration and deceleration both was studied experimentally and numerically by Higuchi et al.[8]. Comparison among various seeding patterns reveals that the initial position of particles affects to the particle redistribution. For example, the particles are expelled from near the edge of the foot, whereas the particles remain under the foot in Fig. 3b). This is in good qualitative agreement with analysis of projected particle trajectory by Khalifa et al.[6]. Radial streaks of particle paths are seen in Fig. 3 a), c) and d). They are believed to be due to the azimuthal vortex instability. Eames et al. and Leweke et al. and showed similar instability waves under an impacting sphere[3, 4]. The latter examined the azimuthal instability due to the sphere impact in detail experimentally and by direct numerical simulation (DNS). The present streak pattern under the disk appears to have much higher wave number than expected (see e.g., Balligand), and further study is needed including possible particle-particle interactions [9].

Table 1 Parameters used for stomping experiment

U_c [m/s]	Z_i [mm]	Z_f [mm]	Acc [m/s^2]	Dec [m/s^2]	T_1	T_2	T_3	Re_{Uc}
1.9	300	0.1	10.6	-16.0	2.18	2.34	3.78	18,500

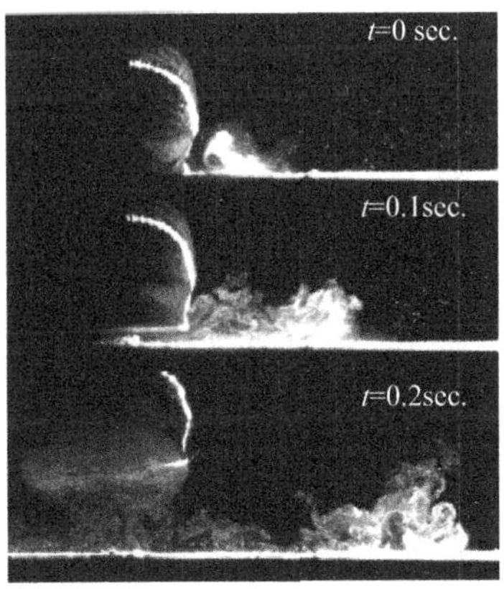

Fig. 2 Sequence of particle flow visualization with actual foot tapping.

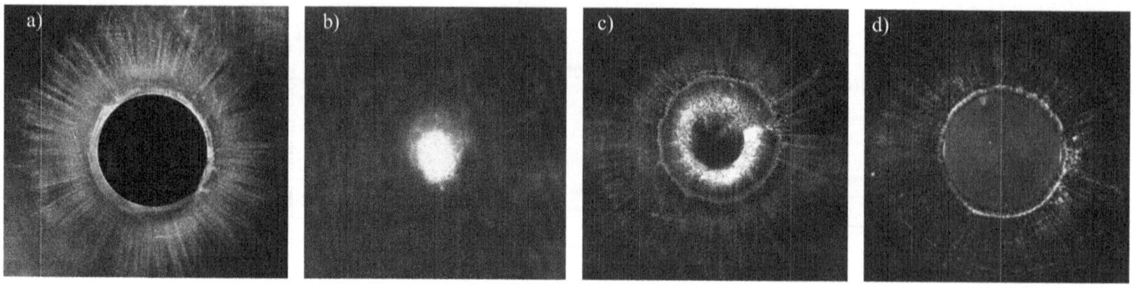

Fig. 3 Bottom views of particles trajectories due to downward disk motion with the different seeding patterns at T=T_{final}. a) Same diameter as the disk, b) A half diameter of the disk beneath the foot, c) Annular pattern beneath the foot, d) Annular pattern immediately outside the disk.

C. Particle Resuspension with an Elongated Plate

The particle streaks under an elongated plate are shown in Fig. 4, where the idealized motion simulates the downward stomping motion shown in Fig. 1b). The particles were initially seeded beneath the foot in the same pattern as the elongated plate. The particles were ejected from the wall by aerodynamic effect. The strong ejection of particles can be seen at the mid-section of the foot. Fig. 5 show the results of the particles flow visualization in downward stomping motion in side view cross-sections and compare the particle dynamics in the longitudinal and the lateral directions. As in the case of the disk we may conclude that the particle resuspension is caused by the wall jet beneath the foot and the particles redistribution is associated with the vortex dynamics[7]. The scale of vortex is clearly larger in the lateral direction than in the longitudinal direction. The strong trajectories in mid-section in Fig. 4 are considered to be associated with this larger scale vortex as well as difference in wall jet. Though not shown, a simple numerical simulation of the 3-dimensional vortex method (see, e.g., Higuchi et al) indicated an evolution of vortex geometry to enhance in the lateral direction[8]. In short, the elongated plate caused a strong three-dimensional flow and the particle redistributions.

The velocity field measurements with the elongated plate during downward stomping motion are shown in Figures 6. The foot is masked in black. The large-scale vortex is also seen in the lateral cross section (Fig. 6b)). The high velocity region in the lateral direction can be seen within the present vortex, whereas the magnitude of resulting velocity in the longitudinal cross section (Fig. 6a) is relatively small.

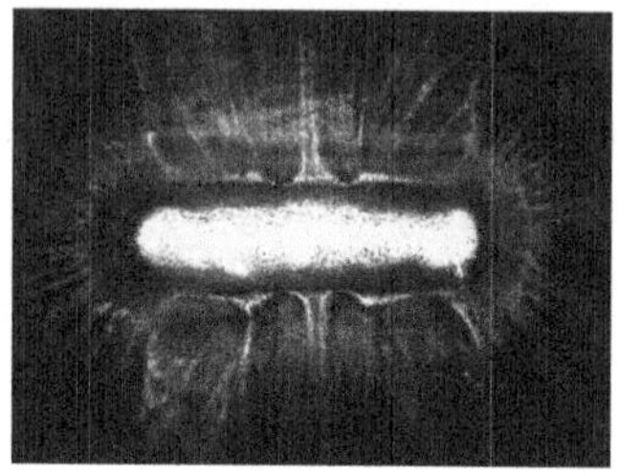

Fig. 4 Particles trajectories caused by an elongated plate in downward stomping motion at T=T_{final}, Z=Z_f (bottom view).

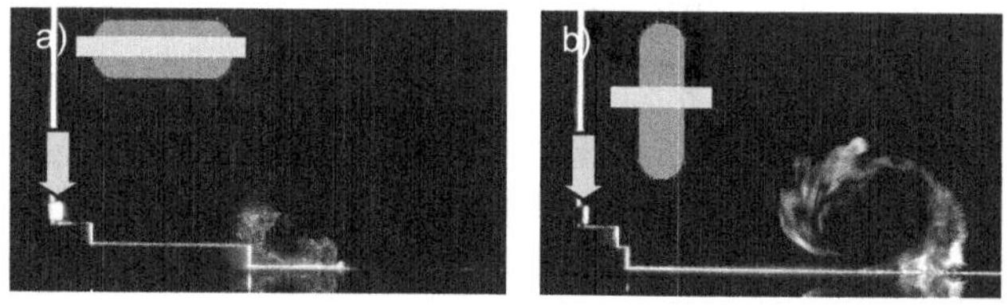

Fig. 5 Particles flow visualization in downward stomping motion with an elongated plate, a) T=4.92, Z=Z_f in longitudinal direction, b) T=4.92, Z=Z_f in lateral direction.

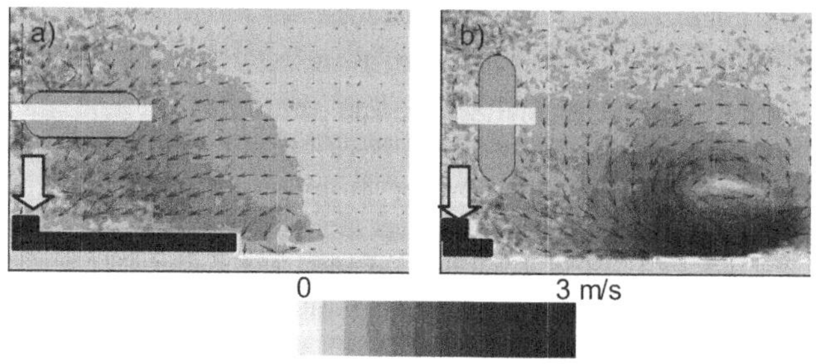

Fig. 6 Velocity measurement around an elongated plate in downward stomping motion , a) T=4.92, Z =Z_f in longitudinal direction, b) T=4.92, Z=Z_f in lateral direction.

D. Particle Resuspension with an Indoor Slipper

The particle trajectories underneath a slipper during downward stomping motion are shown in Fig. 7. A commercially available indoor slipper was used. The particles were initially seeded just underneath the slipper. By T=3.71, the particles were expelled from underneath the slipper, and most resuspended particles were ejected from near the mid-section of the slipper. Later in T= T_{final}, trajectories of particles are in the diagonal direction in the mid-section of the slipper as shown in Fig. 7b).

Side view of resuspended particles in downward stomping motion of the slipper is shown in Fig. 8 These results correspond to the typical trajectories in Fig. 7. The result near the heel of the slipper is shown in Fig. 8 a), clearly shows a vortex emanating from the heel. In the cross-sectional views at mid-section at a diagonal angle (Fig. 8 b)) and across the ankle (Fig. 8 c)), both trajectories show larger amount of resuspension of particles. The three-dimensional aerodynamic effect on particle resuspension from a simplified elongated plate as well as an actual slipper has been demonstrated. With more realistic shoe geometries, resuspension and redistribution of particles are expected to be even more three-dimensional and the sole roughness and indentation would play a major role.

IV. DISUCUSSION AND CONCLUSION

Particle flow visualizations and velocity measurements were carried out with the actual foot tapping and the idealized foot. Both downward and upward portion of the actual foot tapping caused the resuspension and redistribution of particles, so the both downward and upward motions are equally affected to the particles resuspension.

Flow visualization with the idealized foot motion shows that the particles beneath the foot were expelled and resuspended due to a wall jet between the foot and floor in general accord with the mechanism for particle resuspension proposed by Khalifa et al., though with high density particle deposited prior to the experiment, most particles were not attached via Van Der Waals forces[6]. Khalifa et al. predicted that much higher speed jet within 0.5mm from the wall is needed to detach the particles from the wall[6]. Khalifa et al. also examined the initial particle position and particle trajectories relative to the free falling disk[6]. The particles near the center were not ejected from beneath the disk. This analytical result is in agreement with the present results from particles flow visualization. The importance of large-scale structure in flow-field was shown in present results.

Both the elongated plate and the indoor slipper have caused the strong three-dimensional aerodynamics effects during the foot motion. The resuspension and redistribution of particles from mid-section of foot were more significant. This three-dimensional vortex dynamics affected the strength of resuspension of and particularly redistribution of particles. Since the large-scale flow structures play such an important role in particle redistribution, and the present results are likely sensitive to the details of the walking kinematics, an investigation with more accurate foot kinetics and foot geometries is needed.

CONFLICT OF INTEREST

The authors declare that they have no conflict of interest.

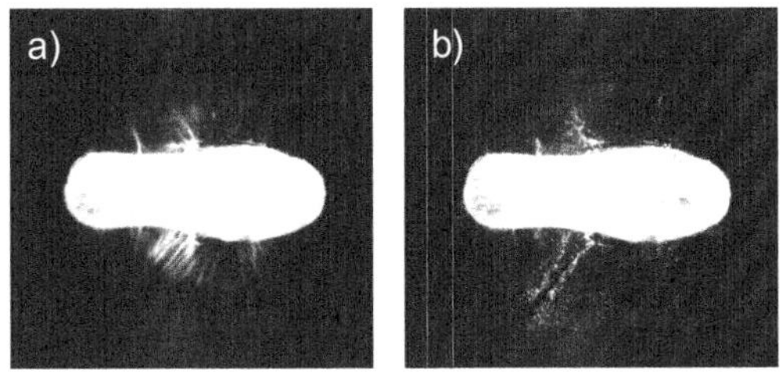

Fig. 7 Particles trajectories with a slipper in downward stomping motion from bottom view, a) T=3.71, Z/D=0.001, b) $T=T_{final}$, $Z=Z_f$=0.1mm.

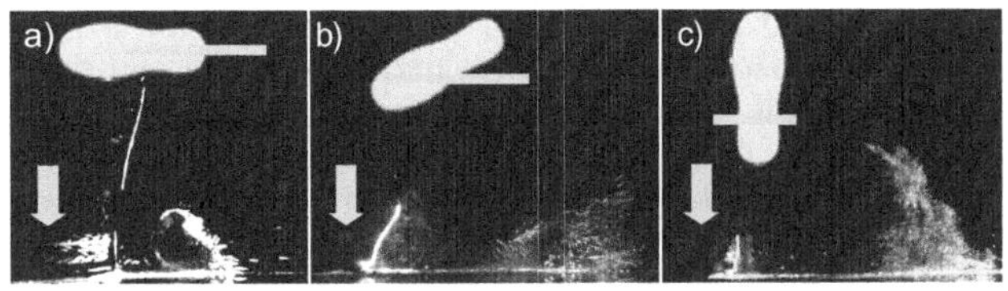

Fig. 8 Particles flow visualization from side view with a slipper in downward stomping motion ($Z=Z_f$=0.1mm), a) Near the heel at T=4.27, b) Near the mid-section at T=4.76, c) Near the ankle at T=4.76.

REFERENCES

1 Ferro A R, Kopperud R J, Hildmann L M (2004) Elevated personal exposure to particulate matter from human activities in a residence. J. Exp. Anal. Environ. Epidemiol. 14:S34-S40
2 Soltani M, Ahmadi G (1994) On Particle Adhesion and Removal Mechanisms in Turbulent Flows. J. Adhes. Sci. Technol., 8:763–785.
3 Eames I, Dalziel S B (2000) Dust resuspension by the flow around an impacting sphere. J. Fluid Mech. 403:305-328
4 Leweke T, Thompson M C, Hourigan K (2004) Vortex dynamics associated with the collision of a sphere with a wall. Physics of fluids, 16:L74-L77
5 Winter D A (2005) Biomechanics and motor control of human movement, Hoboken, N.J., USA: John Wiley & Sons.
6 Khalifa H E, Elhadidi B (2007) Particle levitation due to a uniformly descending flat object. Aerosol Sci. Technol., 41:33-42
7 Kubota Y, Hall J W, Higuchi H (2007) An Experimental Investigation of the Flowfield and Dust Resuspension Due to Idealized Human Walking: Disk Model. Proc. the 5th Joint ASME/JSME Fluid Engineering Conference, San Diego, CA, USA
8 Higuchi H, Balligand H, Strickland J H (1996) Numerical and experimental investigations of the flow over a disk undergoing unsteady motion. J. Fluids Structures, 10:705-719
9 Balligand H (2000) Unsteady wake structure behind a solid disk. Ph.D. Thesis, Syracuse University, NY, USA

Author: Yoshihiro Kubota
Institute: Toyo University
Street: 2100 Kujirai, Kawagoe
City: Saitama
Country: Japan
Email: kubota548@toyo.jp

Design a Center of Pressure Measurement Device into the Insole

Z. Dong[1], H.H. Chu[1], C. Hansen[2], and J.S. Shieh[1]

[1] Department of Mechanical Engineering, Yuan Ze University, Taoyuan, Taiwan
[2] UMR CNRS 7338, Biomécanique et Bioingénierie, Université de Technologie de Compiègne (UTC), Compiègne, France

Abstract— **The Center of pressure (COP) measurement is an important tool used for quantifying the dynamic properties of human's balance and can be used to assess the risk of falling among elderly people. This paper presents a novel COP measurement device, based on three pressure sensors and double layer-designed insoles. Via a data acquisition (DAQ) device, the collected data can be remotely transmitted to wireless receiver Bluetooth. The aim of this study is to reduce hardware costs by using low-cost materials to gain the same results as the commercial portable COP measurement products. Experimental results show that the correlation coefficient of two systems is r=0.871±0.03 for the medio-lateral direction, and r=0.835±0.078 for the anterior-posterior direction. The results suggest that the design study delivers stable and reasonable results and that a low-cost pressure system is feasible.**

Keywords— **falling, plantar pressure, center of pressure, double-layer insole.**

I. INTRODUCTION

In recent years, the proportion of the elderly population is getting higher in Taiwan, which shows that Taiwan has stepped into the aging society. In this situation, the elderly medical care ratio increased gradually. Among of all, falling down is the second biggest cause of death for the elderly, and it is also the main cause of hospitalization [1]. The reason of falling is a physiological decline to maintain balance [2] during walking and standing.

The foot center of pressure (COP) is a virtual site about the foot's plantar surface, which is the average location of all pressures acting on the foot at any given time [3][4]. The location of COP is an important measurement in gait and balance control [3][5].

COP measurement systems can be divided into force plate and in-shoe measurement devices. Referring to previous studies [6], COP measured at the foot/shoe or foot/orthotics interface may be more representative of typical foot function than COP measured at the shoe/floor interface and may be better suited for evaluating footwear and footwear modifications. This raises the importance of in-shoe pressure measurement devices. Multiple systems commercial COP measurement systems (such as Parotec System) [7] are available, however, they are very costy. Hence, the object of this study is to create a low-cost and portable dynamic balanced measurement device and compare it with a commercial COP measurement system (i.e., Advanced Mechanical Technology Inc.).

This study is structured twofold: first, we present the pressure measurement insoles, which contain three pressure sensors in each insole. Secondly we present the data receiving system, which is based on a DAQ device. The details are presented in the next two sections.

II. DESIGN OF INSOLE

A. Sensor Position Selection

Spatial plantar pressure distribution is an important and useful measurement for gait analysis [7]. According to the reference picture, the sole of foot can be divided into 4 main areas, the heel, midfoot, metatarsal, and toes [7]. Heel and metatarsal areas support most of the body weight and adjust the body balance [8][9]. In order to obtain the pressure distribution of the subjects and to optimize the sensor placement, the subjects were asked to walk over a runway with pigment on the soles of the feet. Figure 1 shows the subject's footprint. The lighter areas represent the main areas of the pressure distribution and in coherence with the literature. [7]. Therefore, the positions of three sensors were selected at heel and metatarsal areas in the prototype insoles, because these areas show high pressure during normal activities (Fig 2b).

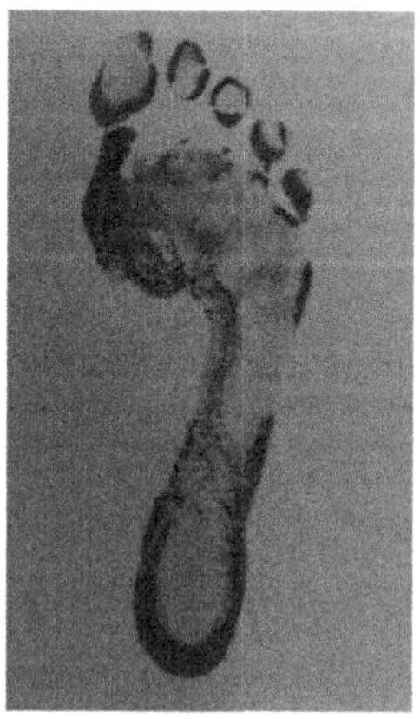

Fig. 1 The blueprint which shows the main plantar pressure distribution area

I. Lackovic (ed.), *1st Global Conference on Biomedical Engineering & 9th Asian-Pacific Conference on Medical and Biological Engineering*,
IFMBE Proceedings 47, DOI: 10.1007/978-3-319-12262-5_28

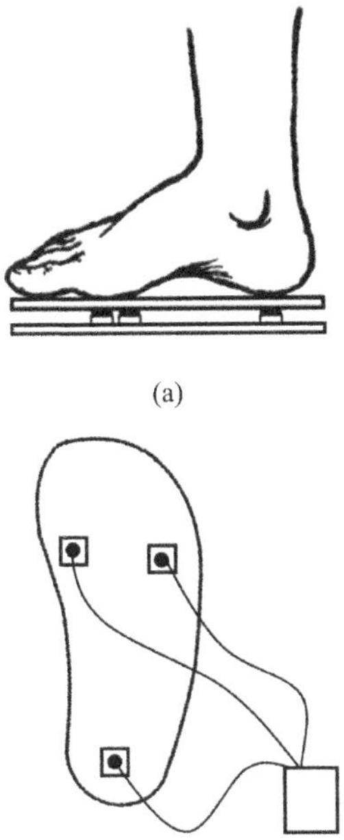

(a)

(b)

Fig. 2 Double-layer insole: (a) the side view (b) the top view

B. *Double-Layer Insole*

In preliminary tests, the sensors were directly attached to the insole. However this setup only allowed detecting 8% of the body weight, since the body weight is dispersed throughout the entire insole and will affect the accuracy of the system. To overcome this problem, the insoles were divided into one upper and one lower layer (Fig 2a). The sensors were put between two layers, and the gasket was attached to the bottom of the sensor. As a result, most of the body weight can be measured by the three sensors. The test showed a detection of 45% of body weight. The material of the layers was chosen to be hardboard to avoid deformation of the insole, because hard material can avoid the deformation of the upper layer caused by body weight.

III. DATA COLLECTION AND ANALYSIS

A. *Data Receiving System*

The pressure sensors are connected to the DAQ device, which is used to collect data. When the pressure is applying on the sensors, the voltage signals can be changed into digital signals and transferred to the remote receiver, which is laptop in our case. Bluetooth is utilized as the wireless communication technology in the present system, so that the experiment and the data acquisition process would not be limited in a short distance.

B. *Data Collection*

Five subjects voluntarily participated in the experiment after signing a statement of informed consent pertaining to the experimental procedure as required by the Helsinki declaration. The device was set on the center of the force plate, and the subjects were asked to stand on our system on one leg. Subjects should keep stable for 20 seconds at each action and tested for three times. Data was collected simultaneously from the force plate and the pressure insoles.

C. *Data Analysis*

The COP computation of the force plate was done using the general equations given by the manufacturer: And the COP computation of the pressure sensor device was done following the concept of force and torque equilibrium. The data was low-pass filtered and accuracy of our system the correlation coefficient for both COP time series was calculated. One set of COP record is shown as Figure 3, and x and y direction separated results are shown as Figure 4.

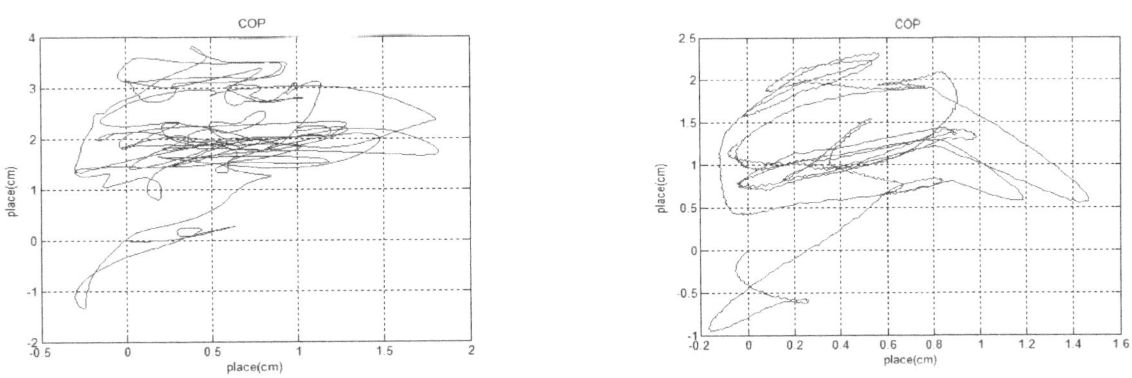

(a) (b)

Fig. 3 One set of COP record: (a) from AMTI (b) from our device

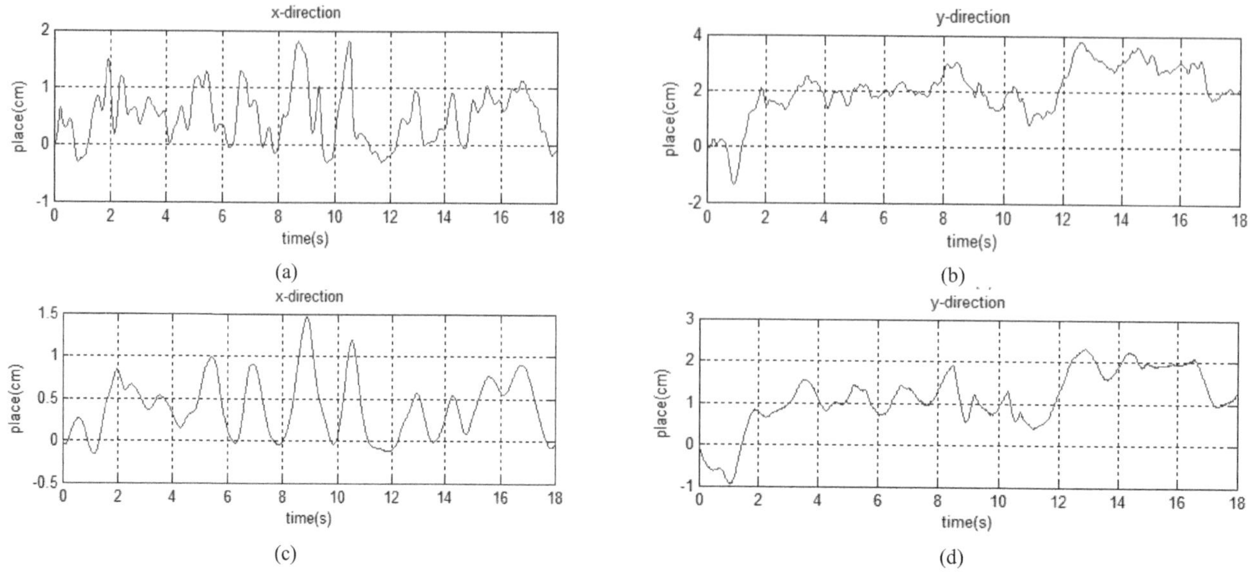

Fig. 4 X and y direction displacements of COP record: (a) x direction from AMTI (b) y direction from AMTI (c) x direction from our device (d) y direction from our device.

Table 1 correlation coefficient of AMTI and our device

Subject	1	2	3	4	5	Mean±SD
X direction	0.828±0.078	0.906±0.021	0.890±0.029	0.866±0.033	0.867±0.010	0.871±0.030
Y direction	0.913±0.078	0.722±0.139	0.800±0.076	0.839±0.107	0.899±0.046	0.835±0.078

IV. RESULT AND DISCUSSION

As shown in Table 1, the mean value of x and y direction correlation coefficient of each subject resulting in a total mean value r=0.871±0.03 for the medio-lateral direction, and a total mean value r=0.835±0.078 for the anterior-posterior direction. The results of the pressure device show similar results as the force plate. It proved that the concept of double-layer design is feasible, and our COP measurement device is also feasible in static test.

The current material of the insoles is hard board which raises the question if subjects contain their natural stance as usual. The design of the insole may need adjustments due this factor. However, the results showed good coherence between both devices. So far, only one foot static balancing tasks were tested. Future work has to implement both legs but also dynamic tests as stepping or walking.

V. CONCLUSIONS

In this paper, a COP measurement device based on three pressure sensors and double layer-designed insoles has been presented. With the design of a double layer insole, body weight can be concentrated on the area under the three sensors. The device is proved to be accurate when compared to commercially available products as a force plate while being reasonable price and affordable. The experimental result shows that the concept of double-layer insole is feasible, and it is worth to be developed.

ACKNOWLEDGMENT

This research was financially supported by Center for Dynamical Biomarkers and Translational Medicine, National Central University, Taiwan which is sponsored by the Ministry of Science and Technology (Grant Number: NSC 102-2911-I-008-001). It is also supported by Ministry of Science and Technology (Grant Number: NSC102-2221-E-155-028-MY3).

CONFLICT OF INTEREST

The authors declare that they have no conflict of interest.

REFERENCES

1. Laughton CA, Slavin M, Katdare K, Nolan L, Bean JF, Kerrigan DC, Phillips E, Lipsitz LA, Collins KJ (2003) Aging, muscle activity, and balance control: physiological changes associated with balance impairment. Gait and Posture:101-108.
2. CW Huang, PD Sue, MF Abbod, BC Jiang, JS Shieh (2013) Measuring Center of Pressure Signals to Quantify Human Balance Using Multivariate Multiscale Entropy by Designing a Force Platform. Sensors 13, 10151-10166.
3. Gill-Body KM, Popat RA, Parker SW, Krebs DE (1997) Rehabilitation of balance in two patients with cerebellar dysfunction. Physical Therapy. 77:534–52.
4. Debbia EM, Wolfa A, Goryacheva Y, Yizharb Z, Lugere E, Debid R, Haima A (2012) In-shoe center of pressure: Indirect force plate vs. direct insole measurement. The Foot 22:269-275
5. Haim A, Rozen N, Wolf A (2010) The influence of sagittal center of pressure offset on gait kinematics and kinetics. Journal of Biomechanics 43:969–77
6. Chesnin * KJ, Selby-Silverstein L, Besser MP (2000) Comparison of an in-shoe pressure measurement device to a force plate: concurrent validity of center of pressure measurements. Gait and Posture, 12: 128-133.
7. Shu L, Hua T, Wang YY, Li Q, Feng DD, Tao XM (2010) In-shoe plantar pressure measurement and analysis system based on fabric pressure sensing array. IEEE Transactions on information technology in biomedicine 14(3): 767-775
8. Kellis E (2001) Plantar pressure distribution during barefoot standing, walking and landing in preschool boys, Gait Posture 14(2): 92-97
9. M, Hessert J, Vyas M, Leach J, Hu K, L, Lipsitz A, Novak V (2005) Foot pressure distribution during walking in young and old adults, BMC Geriatr. 5:8.

Author: Prof. Jiann-Shing Shieh
Institute: Department of Mechanical Engineering
Street: 135 Yuan-Tung Road
City: Chung-Li, Taoyuan
Country: Taiwan
Email: jsshieh@saturn.yzu.edu.tw

Gait Analysis of Patients with Unilateral Piriformis Syndrome

H.P. Huang[1], C.T Wang[2], S.W. Hong[1], and T.W. Lu[1]

[1] Institute of Biomedical Engineering, National Taiwan University, Taipei, Taiwan
[2] Department of Orthopaedic Surgery, School of Medicine, National Taiwan University

Abstract— **Gait analysis has been widely used in the diagnosis of locomotors pathology and the assessment of treatment. But study of gait on Piriformis syndrome (PS) remain unclear. 3-D motion analysis was used to measure the kinematic and kinetic together with temporal-spatial parameters data of patients with PS and normal controls during walking. Patients with PS show significant increase gait speed and cadence, and peak extensor moments with increased flexion, abduction and internal rotation at the hip during the whole gait cycle. There were no significant differences in all the variables between the affected and unaffected limb in the patient group. These results may provide some advice on future work of rehabilitation and research of PS patients.**

Keywords— **Piriformis syndrome, gait analysis, sciatic nerve.**

I. INTRODUCTION

Piriformis syndrome (PS) is a condition in that the piriformis muscle spasms, and compress the surrounding structures, including the sciatic nerve and blood vessels, causing low back pain, buttock pain, and muscular weakness of the lower extremity [1], responsible for about 5-8 % of patients with low back pain and sciatica [2, 3]. Patients with PS usually have difficulty in the performance of activities of daily living due to the pain, causing patients have difficulty in hip motion. Besides, the leg paralysis by sciatica may cause patients experience difficulty in motion, such as sitting and walking for a period of time [4].

Gait analysis has been used to evaluate the pathology of locomotors and the assessment of treatment. The malfunction of the piriformis muscle leads to the increase of internal rotation or adduction of the hip joint due to the pain. On the contrary, the patient would tend to walk by a limp gait by holding the leg in a shortened and externally rotated position [5]. The other study revealed that patient would decrease hip extension during terminal stance bilaterally, and increased hip adduction, increased hip internal rotation on the affected side [6]. But the number of study base on gait analysis of PS is very small, usually case report, and lack of quantitative evidence. Research of PS base on the gait analysis can let us understand the influence of force and moment on each joint of the lower extremity.

The purpose of the current study was to identify the gait deviations, and the strategies in patients with PS by 3-dimensions kinematics and kinetics measurement during level walking.

II. MATRIAL AND METHODS

A. Subjects

Six patients with unilateral PS (age: 67.1±11.4 years; height: 158.3 ± 8.9 cm; mass: 55.9 ± 6.9 kg) and six age-matched healthy controls (age: years; height: cm; mass: kg) participated in this study, were asked to sign the letter of consent as approved by the Institutional Research Board.

The PS group was selected by the first onset piriformis syndrome patient and graded 1-3 in the Gross Motor Function Classification System (GMFCS) from the Orthopedics clinic of National Taiwan University Hospital. Besides, they should free of noticeable leg length discrepancy and without other pathology that could affect gait and cognitive function. The healthy group were selected with the criteria of free from any musculoskeletal, neurological or cardiovascular disorders. The exclusion criteria of the healthy subject were any distinct gait asymmetries, or was taking medications that might influence gait.

B. Experimental Protocol

The subjects were asked to familiar the experiment area, and a three times of practice walk on an 8-meter walkway at self-selected pace, before the recorded the trials of measuring their kinematic and kinetic data simultaneously. Each subject was stick with 39 retroreflective markers on the bony land marks for tracking the motions of the body segments, including: the pelvis (anterior superior iliac spines and posterior superior iliac spines), and each thigh (greater trochanter, mid-thigh, medial and lateral epicondyles), each shank (head of fibula, tibia tuberosity, medial and lateral malleolus) and each foot (navicular tuberosity, 5th metatarsal base and heel). By using the 8-cameras motion analysis system (Vicon T-40S, Oxford Metrics Group, UK), and measuring the ground reaction forces with 3 forceplates (AMTI, U.S.A.). Six successful trials were recorded for gait analysis.

I. Lackovic (ed.), *1st Global Conference on Biomedical Engineering & 9th Asian-Pacific Conference on Medical and Biological Engineering*, IFMBE Proceedings 47, DOI: 10.1007/978-3-319-12262-5_29

C. Data Analysis

The lower limb joints angular and internal moments were calculated using the inverse dynamics analysis from the kinematic and ground reaction force (GRF) data. We embedded an orthogonal coordinate system in each body segment, with the positive x-axis directed anteriorly, the positive y-axis superiorly and the positive z-axis to the right. A Cardanic rotation sequence (z-x-y) was used to describe the rotational movements of each joint. An optimization-based method were used to obtain the inertial properties for each body segment. The soft tissue artefacts associated with the skin markers was reduced by using a global optimization method. We normalized all the calculated joint moments to body weight (BW) and leg length (LL) defined as the length between the anterior superior iliac spine and the medial malleolus. Temporal-spatial parameters, namely walking speed, stride length normalized to leg length, stride time, cadence, and step width, were also obtained.

D. Statistical Analysis

For each of the calculated variables, independent t-tests were performed to compare each of the time-averaged values over the sub-phases between the PS and control groups All significance levels were set at α= 0.05. All the statistical analyses were performed using SPSS version 20.0 (SPSS Inc., Chicago, IL, USA).

III. RESULTS

Compared to the controls, patients with PS were found to show significantly increase gait speed and cadence ($p<0.05$), but no significant difference on stride length, stride time, and step width.

The patients with PS showed increased peak extensor moments during the mid-stance and terminal stance of the stance phase of the hip joint compared to normal controls (Fig. 1), but no significant difference in other joint, nor in other plane of the hip joint.

Compared to the control group, PS group showed significantly increased hip flexion during the whole stance phase, and hip internal rotation, and knee adduction during the whole gait cycle.

The patients with PS were found to decrease GRF in medial-lateral and vertical components (Fig. 3), especially during loading response and terminal stance phase, and smaller magnitude on the first and second peak in anterior-posterior component.

There were no significant differences in all the variables, include the joint moment, joint angle, and GRF between the affected and unaffected limb in the patient group.

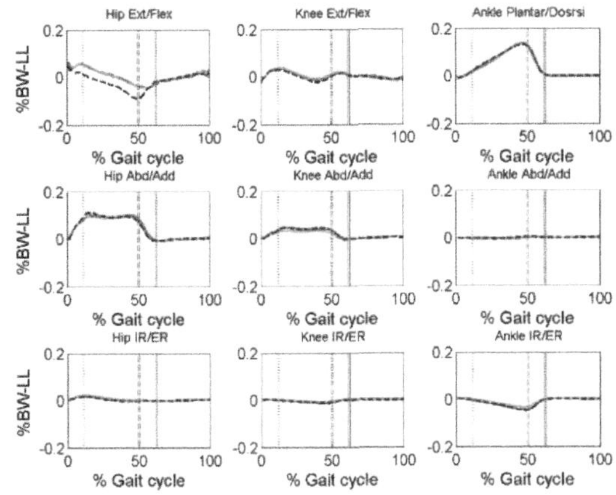

Fig. 1 Ensemble-averaged joint moments at the hip, knee and ankle in the affected limb (red lines), unaffected limb (green lines) and normal controls (dashed lines) during walking.

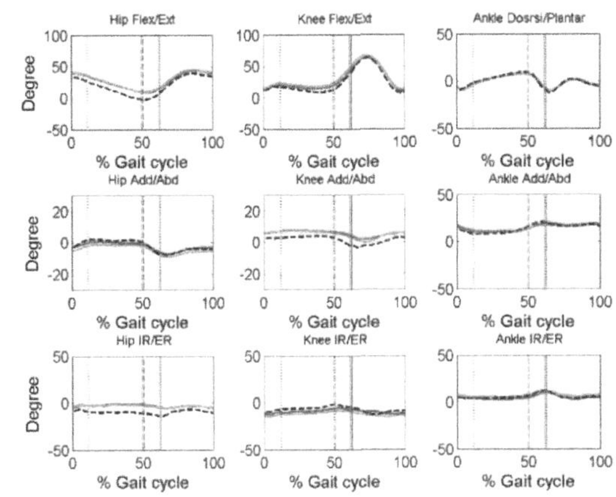

Fig. 2 Ensemble-averaged joint angles at the hip, knee and ankle in the affected limb (red lines), unaffected limb (green lines) and normal controls (dashed lines) during walking.

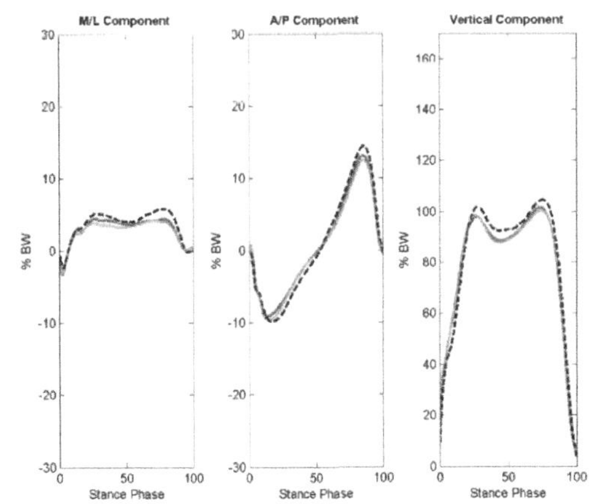

Fig. 3 Ensemble-averaged GRF in the affected limb (red lines), unaffected limb (green lines) and normal controls (dashed lines) during walking.

IV. Discussion

This study aimed to analyze the gait difference between the piriformis patient and healthy people, and discover the strategies in patients with PS by 3-dimensions kinematics and kinetics measurement during level walking.

The temporal-spatial parameters results showed that PS patients tended to walk at a faster speed together with faster step speed. But the stride length, stride time, and step width remain the same as healthy people. This may due to the pain that would increase while the hip joint extension angle increase.

The piriformis muscle origin from anterior part of the sacrum, and through the greater sciatic foramen, and insert on the greater trochanter of the femur. The anatomical location results the muscle of the lateral rotator of the hip, and the extensor and abductor the femur with hip flexion. Extension of the hip during walking may lead to overloading and pain on the injured muscle. And the joint angle data also support this deduction, with the increased hip extension and internal rotation. This movement pattern might reduce the effort of the piriformis muscle, by putting the piriformis muscle in an already shortening position during walking. GRF data showed that patients with PS tended to walk by GRF-reduced pattern. This may be the results of hip flexion and internal rotation during the stance phase. The results of this study was conflict with previous study by Rodrigue et al. (2001), but similar with the study of Tonley et al. (2010) of hip angle.

The patients with PS were found to have symmetry between the affected limb and unaffected limb. The reason of this result might due to the compensatory of the other muscle around the hip for the piriformis muscle, but this remained unclear and needed further study of Electromyography to confirm.

The observed gait changes appeared to be helpful for the reduction of pain or symptoms at the affected side. Similar changes on the unaffected side suggest that the patients adopted a symmetrical gait pattern in response to the pathology on the affected side. Symmetrical patterns helped with better weight transitions between the sides during double limb support. However, increased demands on the extensors and internal rotator at the hips may be a challenge to the patients in prolonged walking.

Limitation of this study was that the criteria of patient's inclusion did not include the value of the Visual Analogue Scale (VAS), which can provide the subjective view of pain of the patients. The level of pain of the patients may lead to different performance of the gait, and influence the results of this study. But all the patients participate in this study had the VAS score beyond 5, the results of this study might not be affected by big variation of pain.

V. Conclusions

Patients with PS were found to show specific symmetrical deviations and strategies during level walking, which appeared to be helpful for reducing the effects of the symptoms but require increased demands on the hip extensors and internal rotator. Resting and pain management are suggested to prevent long-term complications at both hips.

Acknowledgment

The authors gratefully acknowledge financial support from Nation Taiwan University Hospital, Taipei, Taiwan (103-S2465).

Conflict of Interest

The authors declare that they have no conflict of interest.

References

1. Smith J, Jones M Jr, Houghton L et al. (1999) Future of health insurance. N Engl J Med 965:325–329
2. Robinson, D.R. (1947) Piriformis syndrome in relation to sciatic pain. Am J Surg 73(3):355-358.
3. Benzon, H.T., et al. (2003) Piriformis syndrome: Anatomic considerations, a new injection technique, and a review of the literature. Anesthesiology 98(6):1442-1448.
4. Pace, J.B. and D. Nagle. (1976) Piriform syndrome. West J Med 124(6):435-439.
5. Durrani, Z. and A.P. Winnie. (1991) Piriformis muscle syndrome: An underdiagnosed cause of sciatica. J Pain Symptom Manage 6(6)374-379.
6. Rodrigue, T. and R.W. Hardy. (2001) Diagnosis and treatment of piriformis syndrome. Neurosurg Clin N Am 12(2):311-319.
7. Tonley, J.C., et al. (2010) Treatment of an Individual With Piriformis Syndrome Focusing on Hip Muscle Strengthening and Movement Reeducation: A Case Report. J Orthop Sports Phys Ther 40(2)103-111.

Author: Hsing-Po Huang
Institute: Institute of Biomedical Engineering, National Taiwan University
Street: No.1, Sec. 4, Roosevelt Rd., Da'an Dist.
City: Taipei City
Country: Taiwan
Email: hsingpohuang@gmail.com

Development of an Image-Based Algorithm for the Motility Characterizations of the Nematode *Caenorhabditis Elegans*

Wan-Jung Kuo[1] and Han-Sheng Chuang[1,2,*]

[1] Department of Biomedical Engineering, National Cheng Kung University, Tainan 701, Taiwan
[2] Medical Device Innovation Center, National Cheng Kung University, Tainan 701, Taiwan
oswaldchuang@mail.ncku.edu.tw

Abstract— **The nematode *Caenorhabditis (C.) elegans* has been widely used as a model animal for fundamental biological research. In order to investigate the effect of exercise on degenerative behaviors of *C. elegans*, such as physiological (lifespan, progeny) and biomechanical (propulsion, total power and swimming gait) properties, we developed a flow visualization technique to characterize the motility of *C. elegans*.**

Quantifying the motility of micro-organisms is always essential in understanding their biomechanical properties. Up to date, however, the direct measurement of the motility of *C. elegans* remains a big challenge due to lack of proper tools. Therefore, a simple image-based algorithm using a micro-particle image velocimetry (μPIV) for deriving the kinetic power and propulsive force of the nematode *C. elegans* was developed in this study. For the measurement, each worm was confined in a 0.5 μL droplet which was sandwiched between two glass slides separated by two tapes. The motility of the confined worm was derived from the fluid motion according to the law of conservation of energy. The experimental result showed that our measured values appear to be in good agreements with the prior data. The image-based algorithm was proven to be a simple and automated measure for characterizing the dynamic motility of micro-swimmers. The study will eventually provide valuable information for treating and preventing degenerative diseases in higher animals.

Keywords— **μPIV, *C. elegans*, propulsion, power, motility.**

I. INTRODUCTION

Evidence has shown that regularly physical exercise is effective in prevention of neurodegenerative diseases. It is also well known that exhaustive exercise causes muscle fatique or cell damage [1]. Therefore, characterizing the relationship between biomechanical properties and exercise is key to understanding the effectiveness of exercise.

Among all model animals, *C. elegans* is particularly useful in the genetic and neuronal research. Currently, however, biomechanical characterization of micro-sized organisms remains a big challenge due to lack of proper tools. It is difficult to achieve the direct measurements of nematode body because the worm's body is too small and adapt for environmental changes [2-3]. Alternatively, indirect measures are used to analyze the worms. Most commonly, the worm swimming gait was assumed to be a perfect sinusoidal waveform to obtain a theoretical model. Although the model simplified the calculation, the prediction actually deviated from the real situation [4]. After consistantly studying the neurophysiological and the behavior of worm , we found that *C. elegans* will adjust its body to adapt different environments. Therefore, some research used granular medium to determine the locomotion of *C. elegans* [5]; others used the deformation of mechanical structures, such as polydimethylsiloxane (PDMS) pillars, to sense the worm's forces [6-7]. However, these methods are too complicated to make the experiments and they have some unavoidable disadvantages.

To simplify the measurement process, we developed an image-based algorithm using a μPIV system to derive the kinetic power and propulsive force of *C. elegans*. These measurements eventually provide quantitative clues of the worm's physiological changes in response to exercise and can be potentially applied for higher animals.

II. MATERIALS AND METHODS

A. Strains of Worms and Culture Conditions

In this study, Bristol strain N2 and the mutant, KG532 *[kin-2(ce179) X]* were used. N2 is a wild-type strain representing reference behavior in this research. KG532 is a hyperactive strain carrying defective gene *kin-2*. The worm of N2 (n=4) and KG532 (n=4) are placed in the NGM buffer. The other group (n=4) is the wild-type worms in high viscosity medium which mixing dextran with the NGM buffer to achieve a 6% dextran solution. All worms were grown and maintained on nematode growth medium agar plates at 20℃ incubator and fed the *Escherichia coli (E. coli)* strain OP50 [9]. To obtain young adult worms for measurements, L4 stage worms were picked and transferred to a new agar plate spread with a lawn of *E. coli*. The isolated worms were then allowed to grow for 8 h in an incubator until turned to the stage of one-day-old adult.

* Corresponding author.

I. Lackovic (ed.), *1st Global Conference on Biomedical Engineering & 9th Asian-Pacific Conference on Medical and Biological Engineering*,
IFMBE Proceedings 47, DOI: 10.1007/978-3-319-12262-5_30

B. *Derivation of Kinetic Power and Propulsive Force*

The motility of *C. elegans* herein is derived from velocity fields based on micro particle image velocimetry (μPIV). μPIV is a flow visualization technique used for velocity measurements in microfluidics. More detailed information of PIV can be referred to the past literature [10]. The fluid is seeded with tracer particles in the flow field and is visualized by an epifluorescent microscope. A digital camera is used to capture the flow fields. Each pairs of particle images are divided into numerous interrogation windows and process with the spatial cross-correlation algorithm [11]. When the velocity and direction of the flow are determined, an acceleration field is obtained simultaneously (Fig. 1). The acceleration hence can be used for the derivation of the biomechanical properties, such as kinetic power and propulsive forces.

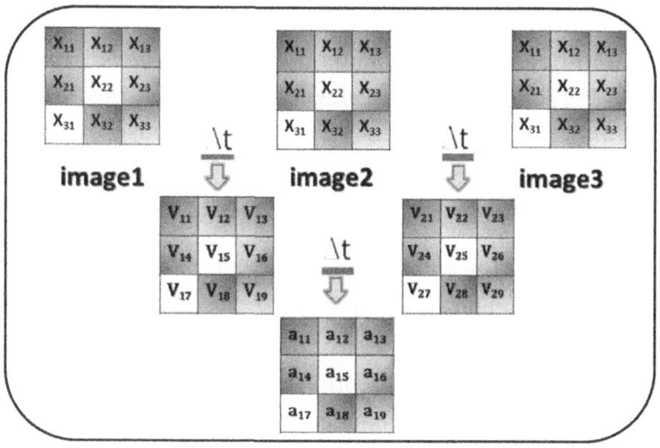

Fig. 1 Derivation of acceleration from displacements.

To implement the assessment of the motility, a worm is confined in an aqueous droplet. Base on the conservation of energy, the total force from the fluid is equivalent to the force exerted by the worm in the isolated droplet. As shown in Fig. 2, the energy of worm is obtained from the inner product of the total force and the displacement of interrogation window. In addition, the propulsive force is obtained from the inner product of the total force and the unit displacement of worm.

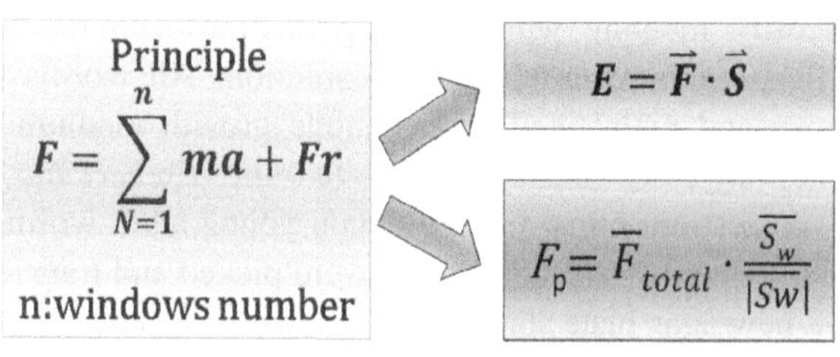

Fig. 2 Derivation of the kinetic power and propulsion.

C. *Method of Measurement*

A self-developed μPIV system was used to measure the velocity field induced by a worm in the droplet as shown in Fig. 3. An inverted epifluorescent microscope (IX71, Olympus) equipped with a 10x objective was used for visualizing the fluid motion in a droplet. In the microchip, a 0.5-μL aqueous droplet containing *C. elegans* and tracer particles (d_p =3.2 μm, Thermo Fisher Scientific) was sandwiched between two glass slides separated by a spacer of 110 μm. A high speed camera (GX3, NAC) was used to capture consecutive particle images induced by the worm's locomotion. The inset in the lower right of Fig. 3 is a contour of an instantaneous acceleration field from a swimming N2 worm.

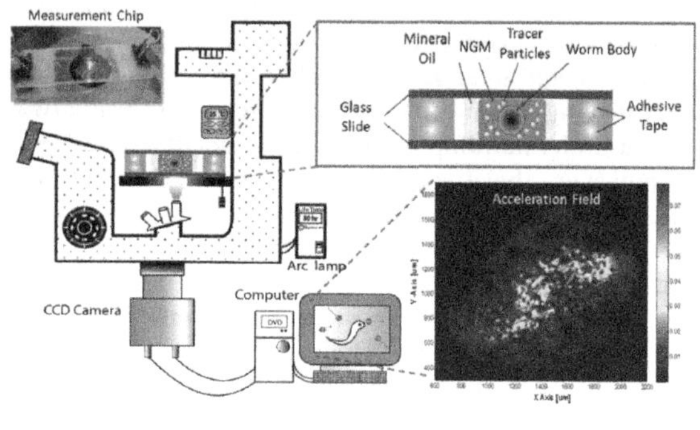

Fig. 3 Schematic of the experimental setup. The upper right corner shows measurement chip.

III. Results and Discussion

A. *Measurements of Kinetic Power and Propulsion*

The movements of N2 worms over three cycles based on the proposed algorithm were analyzed. In Fig. 4, the black solid line represents a trajectory projected by the centroid of the wild-type worm over a swimming cycle. Five postures in different time phases (i), (ii), (iii), (iv) and (v) show corresponding changes thereof.

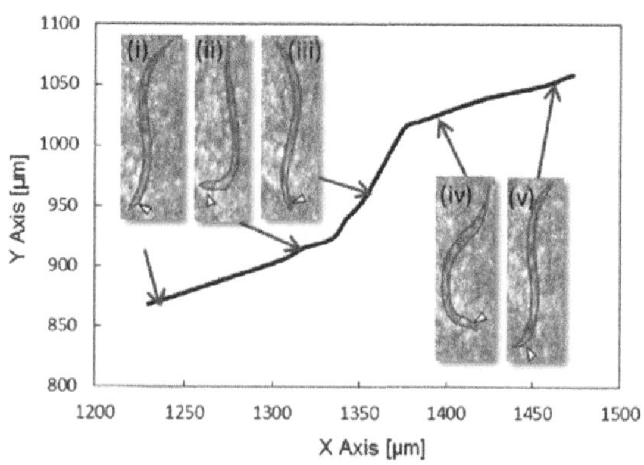

Fig. 4 Trajectory of the worm's body centroid over a swimming cycle. (i) ~ (v) show five postures in different time phases.

According to Fig. 5, the output power is high in phases (i), (iii), and (v), because the worm elongates its body; whereas the power decreases in phases (ii) and (iv) when the worm experiences a bending posture. To reflect the periodic behavior during swimming, the trend of the kinetic power (blue line) looks like a letter "W" while that of the propulsion looks like a letter "M". Noted that the opposite peaks of the power and propulsion is because the negative propulsion is designated as forward movement herein. Nevertheless, both the power and propulsive force becomes significant in the phase (i), (iii), and (v) but decreases in the phase (ii) and (iv). The results suggest that the worm body will store energy (phases ii and iv) and then releases the energy for locomotion by stretching its body (phases i, iii, v).

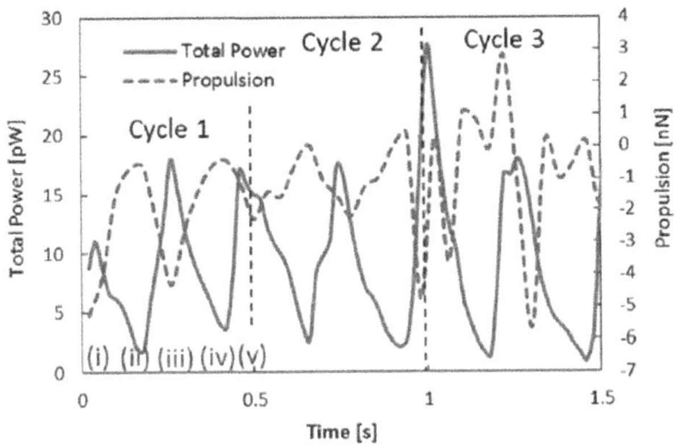

Fig. 5. Variations of power and propulsion over three cycles.

To avoid size effect, the power and propulsion were normalized with each worm's body length to form unit power and unit propulsion. For the N2 worm, the unit propulsion and power are 0.6 ± 0.5 nN/mm and 3.9 ± 2.2 pW/mm. Fig. 6 shows our measured values compared with the prior studies [12-15]. The reported power and propulsion range from 1.3 pW to 3 pW and from 1.7 to 7.6 nN, respectively. Our measured motility data appear to show good agreements and on the same order with the prior data.

However, the hardware limitation prohibited (*i.e.*, a high resolution camera for small tracer particles is required) the number of interrogation window and the measurement uncertainties between worms, there are the large standard deviations. Moreover, the number of the worm in each group (n = 4) is too small as well. The other groups have the same trend of power and propulsion. The unit propulsion and power of the KG532 worm are 1.0 ± 0.4 nN/mm and 12.3 ± 6.2 pW/mm, and the high viscosity group are 4.1 ± 3.2 nN/mm and 55.1 ± 35.4 pW/mm. These results showed the variations between the different strains of worms and the worms under different circumstances, our measurements value were with the predictions accurately.

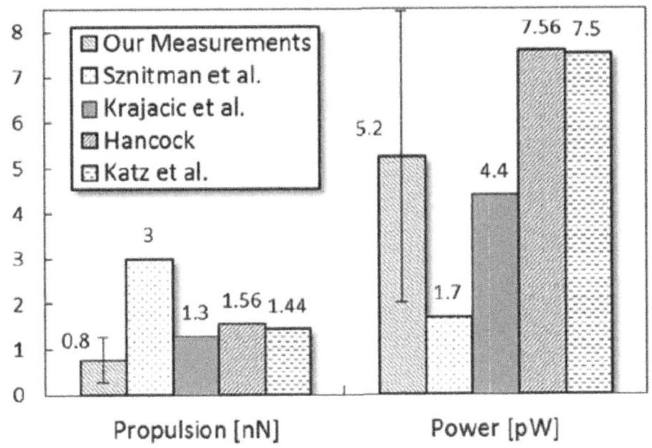

Fig. 6. Comparsions of our measurements and other studies.

B. Comparisons of Strains and Environmental Conditions

Comparisons of the motility performances between the N2 and the *kin-2* mutant are shown in Fig. 7. The *kin-2* worms have higher power and propulsion than N2 worms, and they are significant differences.

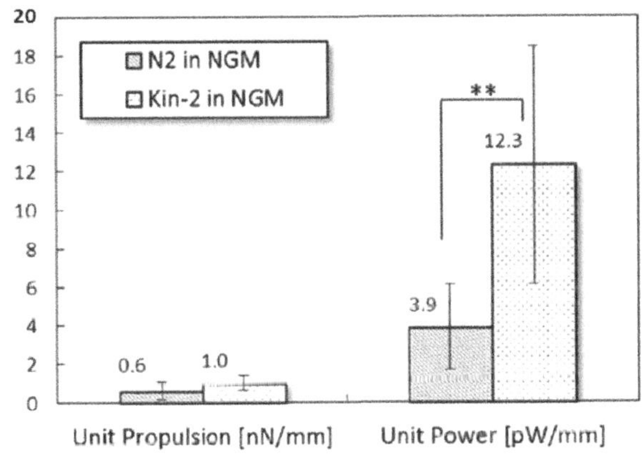

Fig. 7. Comparsions of N2 and the *kin-2* worm. ** denotes p < 0.1 based on Mann-Whitney U test.

Comparisons of the motility performances between the N2 in the NGM buffer and in the high viscosity medium are shown in Fig. 8. According to the results, the propulsion of N2 worm in the high viscosity solution is four time larger than that in the NGM. The power of N2 worm in the viscosity solution is almost fourteen times than in the NGM. In other words, the power is positively proportional to the increased viscosity because the N2 worm's power is fully contributed to its forward moving. Also, the propulsive force is stronger than the N2 in the NGM buffer.

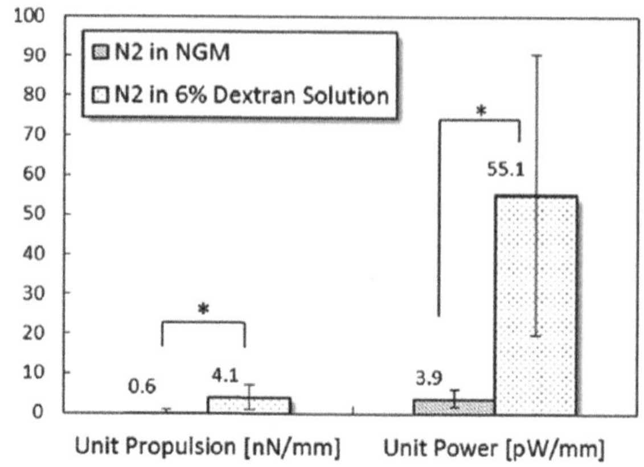

Fig. 8. Comparsions of N2 and the high viscosity group. ** denotes $p < 0.005$ based on Mann-Whitney U test.

IV. CONCLUSIONS

By incorporating the powerful tool, μPIV, into the microfluidic analysis with a self-developed image-based algorithm, the motility of *C. elegans* can be characterized in a simple way. Our study measured the different types of worms and the worms in different environments. According to the results, the N2 worms in the NGM buffer yielded a time-averaged power of 5.2 ± 3.1 pW and a time-averaged propulsive force of 1.0 ± 0.8 nN. Compared with the prior literature, our measurement results are in a reasonable range. And compared with the different groups is also in good agreements as expected. Therefore, the image-based algorithm provides a simple and automated measure for the dynamic motility of different micro-swimmers.

ACKNOWLEDGMENT

The authors are grateful to the grant 102-2221-E-006-024-MY2 funded by the Ministry of Science and Technology. The authors.also thank Dr. Chang-Shi Chen from the Institute of Biochemistry and Molecular Biology at NCKU for his generous support and technical advice in *C. elegans*.

REFERENCES

1. Mari-Carmen Gomez-Cabrera, Elena Domenech, Jose Viña. (2008) Moderate exercise is an antioxidant: Upregulation of antioxidant genes by training. Free Radical Biology & Medicine 44 (2008) 126–131
2. Fang-Yen C, Wyart M, Xie J, et al (2010) Biomechanical analysis of gait adaptation in the nematode *Caenorhabditis elegans*. PNAS 107, 20323-20328
3. Sznitman J, Shen X, Sznitman R, and P. E. (2010) Arratia. Propulsive force measurements and flow behavior of undulatory swimmers at low Reynolds number. Phys. Fluids 22, 121901.
4. Shen XN, Sznitman J, Krajacic P, et al (2012) Undulatory locomotion of *Caenorhabditis elegans* on wet surfaces. Biophys J. 102(12):2772-81
5. Jung SH. (2010) *Caenorhabditis elegans* swimming in a saturated particulate system. Phys. Fluids 22, 031903
6. Lycke R, Parashar A, PandeySmith S. (2013) Microfluidics-enabled method to identify modes of *Caenorhabditis elegans* paralysis in four anthelmintics. Biomicrofluidics 7, 064103
7. Aubry G, Lu H. (2014) A perspective on optical developments in microfluidic platforms for *Caenorhabditis elegans* research. Biomicrofluidics 8, 011301
8. Bakhtina NA, Korvink JG. (2014) Microfluidic laboratories for *C. elegans* enhance fundamental studies in biology. RSC Adv., 4691-4709
9. Brenner S. (1974) The genetics of *Caenorhabditis elegans*. Genetics. May;77(1):71-94
10. Chuang, H.S., Kumar A., Wereley S.T. (2010) CH12 Optical Flow Characterization: Micro Particle Image Velocimetry (μPIV). Methods in Bioengineering: Microfabrication and Microfluidics, Zahn, J.D. Ed., Artech House, Boston/London.
11. Keane R. D., Adrian R. J. (1992) Theory of cross-correlation analysis of PIV images. Applied Scientific Research. Volume 49,Issue3,pp191-21
12. Sznitman J. et al. (2010) Propulsive force measurements and flow behavior of undulatory swimmers at low Reynolds number. Phys. Fluids 22, 121901
13. Krajacic P. et al. (2012) Biomechanical Profiling of *Caenorhabditis elegans* Motility. Genetics 191, 1015
14. Katz D. F., Blake J. R., and Paverifontana S. L. (1975) On the movement of slender bodies near plane boundaries at low Reynolds number. J. Fluid Mech. 72, 529
15. Hancock G. J. (1953) The Self-Propulsion of Microscopic Organisms through Liquids. vol. 217 no. 1128 96-121

Influence of Mechanical Fixation on Angiogenesis during Bone Healing Process

Zhilun Zhou[1], Feng Zhao[1], Yang Yan[1], Zhen Yuan[1], Guanzhong Yang[1], Hao Yu[1], Hao Su[1], Tao Zhang[2], and Yubo Fan[1,*]

[1] Key Laboratory for Biomechanics and Mechanobiology of the Ministry of Education, School of Biological Science and Medical Engineering, Beihang University, Beijing, China

[2] Tianjin Medical University General Hospital, Tianjin, China

Abstract— **During bone fracture healing, both angiogenesis and mechanical fixation are of great significance. This study aims to obtain 3D structure of vascular network surrounding the fracture site at different healing times using vascular perfusion and micro-CT imaging technology, and to explore the influence of mechanical fixation on 3D structure of vascular network at the fracture site. To achieve the goal, transverse fracture surgery were performed on thirty six SD rats' right tibias. Half of them (SF) received stable fixation with a newly custom-designed circular external fixator and the rest (NF) didn't received any fixation devices. The imaging results indicated that compared with NF samples, SF samples contained more vascular distribution along the tibia, inferring a much more similar 3D structure to the CON samples (all of the thirty six rats' left posterior limbs were taken as control group), which tends to be beneficial to the vascular reconstruction at the fracture site.**

Keywords— **Angiogenesis, Mechanical fixation, Vascular perfusion, Micro-CT imaging, 3D structure.**

I. INTRODUCTION

Bone fracture healing is a sophisticated pathophysiological process, final results of which depend on these factors: fracture type, gap size, fixation, blood supply, neurohormonal regulation, self-condition of the patient and so forth [1]. Briefly, all of the above could be categorized into two groups: local biological and mechanical environments of the fracture site. It is possible to manipulate the regeneration of bone via control of local biological and mechanical environment.

Among all the factors of biological environment, blood supply (angiogenesis) is regarded to be of greatest importance to bone healing because of its function of transporting oxygen and nutrients and being the passage for the inflammatory cells, chondrocytes and osteoblasts to reach the fracture site [2]. Inhibiting angiogenesis could result in excessive fibrous tissues at the fracture site and cause delayed or non-union [3].

A large body of evidence indicated that bone fracture healing is rather sensitive to the local mechanical environment [4]. Degree of fixation stability determines the amount of the external callus during the process of bone repair [5]. Compressive displacement contributes more to forming new osseous tissues than distractive displacement [6].

Influence of both blood supply (angiogenesis) and mechanical environments on bone healing has been respectively studied by researchers and clinicians; however, few studies were focused on the relation or interactions between these two factors, such as how mechanical fixation has an effect on the 3D structure of neovascularization at the fracture site.

In order to explore the influence of mechanical fixation on 3D structure of vascular network at the fracture site, vascular perfusion and micro-CT imaging technology was utilized in this study.

II. MATERIAL AND METHODS

A. Custom-Designed Circular External Fixator for SD Rats

According to the current design of clinical external fixator [7], a newly custom-designed circular external fixator for SD rats was designed and manufactured. This circular fixator could provide stable fixation for a SD rat's fractured tibia diaphysis [8].

B. Experimental Animals

Thirty six healthy male SD rats with 6 weeks of average age and 200g of average weight were divided into two groups in random. One group (NF) received no fixation device after transverse fracture at right tibial diaphysis. The other group (SF) received stable fixation with the newly custom-designed fixator after surgery at right side. All of the left sides of thirty six SD rats were taken as the control group (CON). Both of the groups were again divided into three subgroups based on different sacrifice times: 2, 4 and 6 weeks postoperatively.

All of the animals were purchased from Experimental Animal Center of Beijing University. Animal treatment and care were in accordance with Regulations for the Administration of Affairs Concerning Experimental Animals promulgated by Decree No.2 of the State Science and Technology Commission of China and the Guiding Principles for the Care and Use of Animals approved by Beijing Government. All protocols were approved by the Animal Care Committee of Beihang University, China.

* Corresponding author.

I. Lackovic (ed.), *1st Global Conference on Biomedical Engineering & 9th Asian-Pacific Conference on Medical and Biological Engineering*, IFMBE Proceedings 47, DOI: 10.1007/978-3-319-12262-5_31

C. Surgical Procedure

The SD rats were placed in supine position after anesthesia. Transverse osteotomy was performed at the middle of each SD rat's tight tibial diaphysis. Stable fixation (with no inter-fragmentary gap) was given to the SF group's right posterior limbs with the new fixator and Kirschner wires. The NF group did not receive any fixation device.

D. Vascular Perfusion

At different sacrifice times, the SD rats were placed in supine position after anesthesia. And their femoral vessels at both sides were exposed after skin incision to observe the vascular perfusion effect. After opening thoracic cavity and exposing the heart, heparinized saline (100U/mL) was injected into the left ventricle until the exposed femoral vessels turned transparent and liquid flowing out of the right atrium became clear, and at the same time the right atrium was opened to substitute heparinized saline for blood in the entire circulatory system [9]. Then, in the same way, a freshly made barium sulfate suspension (30g/100mL) was injected into the circulatory system until the femoral vessels turned white and barium sulfate began to flow out of the right atrium.

After vascular perfusion, SD rats' posterior limbs of both sides were dissected off and kept in 4% paraformaldehyde solution at 4℃ overnight for fixation, and then were placed in 19% tetrasodium EDTA solution for 5 days for decalcification [9].

E. Micro-CT Imaging

In order to obtain the 3D structure of the vascular network of the fracture site, the posterior limb samples were scanned with a micro-CT scanner (Skyscan 1076, Belgium). A scan resolution of 9μm was set for all the samples and the scanning was done at 70kV and 142μA, with 1.0mm aluminum filter.

Images obtained from scanning were then reconstructed with software called Nrecon (v.1.6.4.6), with the ring artifact correction at 8, the smoothing at 0 and the beam hardening correction at 30%. Afterwards, 3D structure of the vascular network of the fracture site was gained using CTvox software (v.2.2).

III. RESULTS

Typical 3D reconstructed structures of vascular network surrounding the fracture site of different group and at different sacrifice times are shown in Fig. 1.

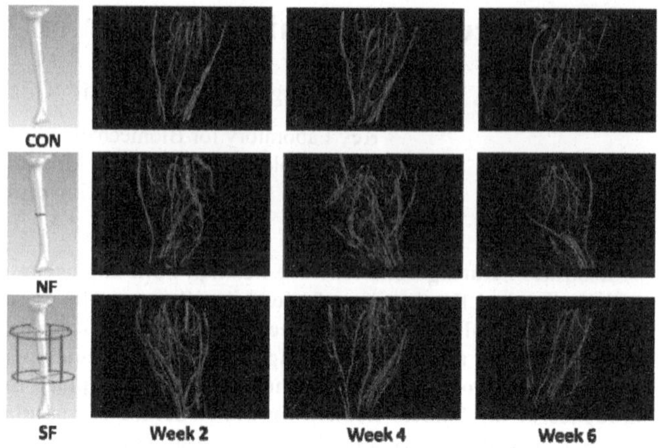

Fig. 1 Typical 3D reconstructed structures of vascular network surrounding the fracture site of different group and at different sacrifice times

The obtained images show:

(a) NF samples owned more vessels, especially micro ones than CON samples; and SF samples contained even more micro vessels than NF samples;

(b) NF samples owned more vascular distribution in the transversal direction of tibia than SF samples;

(c) SF samples owned more vascular distribution along the tibial direction than NF samples.

NF samples had more transversal vascular distribution than SF samples, which infers that there would be more shear movement and shear stress (or strain) without fixation between the fracture ends. This then induces more transversal vessels and compromises fracture healing. SF samples had more longitudinal vascular distribution than NF samples, which means that stable fixation limits the inter-fragmentary movement to mainly axial movement, and the axial stress (or strain) induces more longitudinal neovascularization formation. The stable fixation thus improves the inter-fragmentary blood fluid connectivity and enhances bone healing. The 3D structure of vascularity in SF samples was observed to be more similar to the CON samples in comparison to the NF samples, which indicates that neovascularization reconstructed in the SF samples is more optimized in comparison to the NF samples.

IV. CONCLUSIONS

In this study, vascular perfusion and micro-CT imaging technology were testified to be useful when obtaining the 3D structures of vascular network surrounding the fracture site. SF samples contained more vessels, especially micro ones than both CON and NF samples. SF samples owned more vascular distribution along the tibia, inferring a much more similar vascular distribution to natural one of CON samples, which tends to benefit the reconstruction of vascular network at the fracture site.

ACKNOWLEDGMENT

This work is kindly supported by the National Nature Science Foundation of China (11072021, 31200725 and 11120101001), National Science & Technology Pillar Program of China (2012BAI22B02, 2012BAI18B05, and 2012BAI18B07), Research Fund for the Doctoral Program of Higher Education of China (20131102130004) and SRTP of Beihang University.

CONFLICT OF INTEREST

The authors declare that they have no conflict of interest.

REFERENCES

1. Sigurdsen U, Reikeras O, Utvag SE. (2001) The influence of compression on the healing of experimental tibial fractures. INJURY 42(10): 1152-1156.
2. Hankenson KD, Dishowitz M, Gray C. (2011) Angiogenesis in bone regeneration. INJURY 42(6): 556-561
3. Hausman MR, Schaffler MB, Majeska RJ. (2001) Prevention of fracture healing in rats by an inhibitor of angiogenesis. BONE 29(6): 560-564
4. Epari DR, Duda GN, Thompson MS. (2010) Mechanobiology of bone healing and regeneration: in vivo models. P I MECH ENG H 224(12): 1543-1553.
5. Wu JJ, Shyr HS, Chao EY, et al. (1984) Comparison of osteotomy healing under external fixation devices with different stiffness characteristics. J BONE JOINT SURG AM 66(8): 1258–1264.
6. Hente R, Füchtmeier B, Schlegel U, et al. (2004) The influence of cyclic compression and distraction on the healing of experimental tibial fractures. J ORTHOP RES 22(4): 709-715.
7. Mauffrey C, Beck D, Ruhala L. (2012) Practical biomechanical considerations about external fixators. Ed. Seligson D, Mauffrey C, Roberts CS. External Fixation in Orthopedic Traumatology. London: Springer, Chap.3, pp.43-50
8. Zhao F, Zhou ZL, et al. (2013) Biomechanical evaluation of a new external fixator with axial micro-movement. In the 6th WABCE World Congress on Bioengineering, Beijing
9. Lu C, Marcucio R, Miclau T. (2006) Assessing angiogenesis during fracture healing. IOWA ORTHOP J 26: 17.

Author: Yubo Fan
Institute: Beihang University
Street: Xueyuan Road No.37, Haidian District
City: Beijing
Country: China
Email: yobofan@buaa.edu.cn

Biomechanical Behavior of a Hydrogel-Based TDR Device

C.Y. Lin[1], S.Y. Chuang[2], Y.H. Tsuang[3], and W.P. Chen[1]

[1] Department of Mechanical Engineering, National Taipei University of Technology, Taipei, Taiwan
[2] Department of Orthopaedic Surgery, Tri-Service General Hospital, National Defense Medical Center, Taipei, Taiwan
[3] Department of Orthopaedics, Shuang Ho Hospital, Taipei Medical University, Taipei, Taiwan

Abstract— **Degenerative disc disease is one of the most common diseases resulting from inflammation and instability around the affected spinal disc. Total disc replacement (TDR) is one non-fusion technique emerging as potential solutions to this condition, which can be used to restore normal motion in the spine. Although the first generation TDR devices have reasonable clinical results, similar to fusion, but several concerns in the current technologies are the inability to provide adequate shock absorption capability and time-dependent biomechanical behaviors. In order to improve this problem, second generation TDR devices incorporate more properties of a natural disc. Therefore, the objective of this study is to develop a novel biomimetic TDR device, and to demonstrate scientifically whether its biomechanical behavior is similar to that of a natural disc. Three-dimensional finite element (FE) models of a lumbar spinal motion segment (L4-5) with implants including Charité, Maverick, and the hydrogel-based TDR devices were created. With these models, the three different TDR design concepts were compared with respect to their ability to mimic the behavior of a natural disc. The analysis results indicate that the hydrogel-based TDR device could maintain the ROM well compared to that of a natural disc. However, the model with the novel TDR device predicted a marked increase of facet joint forces due to the relatively low rotational stiffness, especially in lateral bending. Although many steps are still necessary before the hydrogel-based TDR device can be used in clinical surgery to relieve back and leg pain associated with DDD. The results provide further insight into the biomechanical behavior of this novel TDR device under comparable physiologic loading conditions, and indicate that it is a feasible and promising approach.**

Keywords— **Degenerative disc disease, Total disc replacement, Finite element analysis.**

I. INTRODUCTION

Lumbar TDR devices have been used in the treatment of degenerated IVDs for over 20 years. Although the clinical success rates are reasonable, significant concerns remain over facet overloading, adjacent segment disease, and wear. Moreover, whether the long-term results of TDR implantation in DDD are as good as those of spinal fusion remains unknown. In order to improve the disadvantages of the traditional TDR devices, the second generation TDR devices have been proposed to more closely mimic the physiological behavior of a natural disc.

Under the premise of biomimetic concept, a hydrogel-based TDR device was proposed, consisting of a ball-and-socket design and a ring-shaped hydrogel in the present study. It allows for time-dependent behavior typical for a natural disc, including swelling, creep and stress relaxation. In addition, the gap design between the ball-and-socket joint provides the normal axial deformation of an IVD, and reduces the risk of hydrogel defects. The purpose of the present study was to evaluate the hydrogel-based design concepts in their ability to mimic the non-linear motion patterns of a natural disc. Finite element models of the three TDR devices (Charité, Maverick, and hydrogel-based TDR devices) were created, and their behaviors were compared to the behavior of a natural disc, within a physiological relevant loading conditions.

II. MATERIALS AND METHODS

A. Implants

In the present study, we used three different TDR designs (Fig. 1): The first design was the SB Charité III TDR device that consists of two concave endplates and a biconvex core, representing an unconstrained design. The second implant design was the Maverick TDR device that consists of a metal-on-metal, ball-and-socket articulation and incorporates a more posterior COR, representing a constrained design. The third implant design was the hydrogel-based TDR device that consists of a ball-and-socket design and a hydrogel-based, ring-shaped elastomer, also representing an unconstrained design.

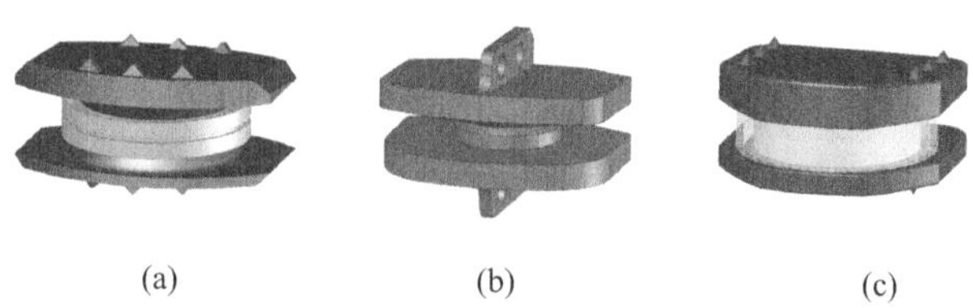

Fig. 1 The isometric view of the three different TDR devices: (a) Charité; (b) Maverick; (c) hydrogel-based TDR device.

I. Lackovic (ed.), *1st Global Conference on Biomedical Engineering & 9th Asian-Pacific Conference on Medical and Biological Engineering*, IFMBE Proceedings 47, DOI: 10.1007/978-3-319-12262-5_32

B. Finite Element (FE) Modeling

A three-dimensional FE-model of an intact L4-5 ligamentous human lumbar motion segment (Fig. 2) was created in the present study. The geometry of the lumbar vertebrae was reconstructed from computed tomography (CT) images of a 55-year-old man (The Visible Human Project, National Library of Medicine, USA). A one-millimeter scan interval for CT scanning was used from the L4 to L5 vertebrae in the transverse direction and the data files were transferred to a commercial software (Amira, TGS, San Diego, CA, USA) for image reconstruction. Each vertebral body of the model consisted of a thin cortical shell, a softer cancellous core, and a posterior bony structure. The cortical bone was modeled as a 1.0 mm thick shell surrounding the cancellous core [1], and a 1.0 mm thick endplate was inserted on the superior and inferior surfaces of the IVD [2]. Each motion segment of the FE model consists of vertebral bodies, IVD, and seven major ligaments. The IVD included the nucleus pulposus and annulus fibrosus. About 56% of the total disc cross-sectional area was defined as the disc nucleus, and the rest of the region was assumed as the disc annulus. All the ligaments were simulated by unidirectional wires with a non-linear force-displacement curve and tension-only capabilities. A FE pre-processing program, Hypermesh (AltairEngineering, Inc., Troy, MI, USA), was used to formulate the FE mesh of the intact L4-L5 vertebrae with 8-node hexahedral elements. As a result, the whole model of the L4-L5 lumbar motion segment contained 24,496 elements and 27,827 nodes. The commercial software ABAQUS v6.10 (SIMULIA, Providence, RI, USA) was utilized to perform the FE analysis. Table 1 shows the material properties used for the spinal units, and the natural IVD.

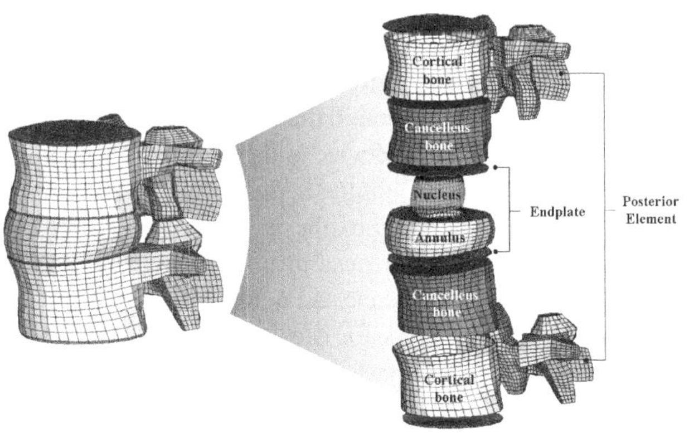

Fig. 2 FE model of the intact L4-5 lumbar motion segment.

Table 1 Element types, material types and material parameters used in the intact FE model.

Spinal Component	Element type	Material type	Material property
Cortical bone	C3D8	Linear elastic	E = 10,000 MPa $v = 0.3$
Cancellous bone	C3D8	Transverse isotropic	E = 100 MPa $v = 0.2$
Posterior elements	C3D8	Linear elastic	E = 3,500 MPa $v = 0.25$
Annulus ground matrix	C3D8	Hyperelastic-Neo-Hookean	$C_{10} = 0.3448$
Fibers of annulus fibrosus	SFM3D4	Linear elastic, tension only	E = 100 MPa $v = 0.1$
Nucleus pulposus	C3D8	Hyperelastic-Mooney-Rivlin	$C_{10} = 0.12$ $C_{01} = 0.03$
Endplates	C3D8	Hyperelastic-Neo-Hookean	$C_{10} = 0.3448$
Ligaments (ALL, PLL, ISL, SSL, ITL, LF, CL)	Wire	Nonlinear elastic, tension only	Force-displacement curve

Note: E: Modulus of elasticity; v: Poisson's ratio; ALL: Anterior longitudinal ligament; PLL: posterior longitudinal ligament; SSL: supraspinous ligament; ISL: interspinous ligament; LF: ligamentum flavum; TL: transverse ligament.

C. Implant Modeling

Both commercial implants (Charité and Maverick TDR devices) were meshed using 10-node tetrahedral elements. The hydrogel-based TDR device was meshed using 8-node hexahedral elements and 10-node tetrahedral elements. The spiked endplate surfaces of all TDR devices were simplified to a flat surface. The Charité and the Maverick TDR devices are available in different sizes. For our simulations, all TDR devices were represented with a height of 14 mm and a lordotic angle of 5°.

Both the superior and inferior components of the TDR devices were attached to the respective endplates of the vertebral bodies to simulate the absence of relative motion between the two surfaces. For all TDR devices, a standard unilateral contact was assumed at the articular surface with a friction coefficient of 0.02 [3]. The contact behavior of the facet joints, on the other hand, was simulated with the coefficient of friction set to 0.1. A CoCrMo alloy with a

Young's modulus of 300 GPa and a Poisson ratio of 0.27 was also assigned to the endplates of the three TDR devices. For the Charité TDR device, the inlays were represented by a polyethylene core (UHMWPE) with a Young's modulus of 2 GPa and a Poisson's ratio of 0.3 [3]. For the hydrogel-based TDR device, the nonlinear, compression stress-strain curves of the hydrogel and the sheath were described quantitatively with the Mooney-Rivlin model and the Ogden model, respectively.

D. *Implantation*

Disc replacement procedure for all TDR devices requires an anterior surgery for implantation. The protocol involves the stepwise removal of the anterior longitudinal ligament, the anterior portion of the annulus, and the entire nucleus pulposus. Only the posterior and lateral portion of the annulus remains in place. To mimic this surgical procedure, the elements representing these structures were removed in the FE model.

E. *Loading and Boundary Conditions*

The inferior endplate of the L5 vertebra was rigidly fixed. A follower load of 500 N was applied to simulate the combined loading of muscle forces and the upper body weight [4]. In addition to the follower load, the spinal segment was loaded with unconstrained moments of 7.5 Nm in the sagittal, lateral, and axial directions simulating flexion, extension, lateral bending, and axial rotation. The range of motion (ROM) and facet loading were compared among various designs.

III. RESULTS

A. *ROM*

In all loading conditions, the models predicted large inter-implant differences between the Charité and Maverick devices (Fig. 3), particularly in lateral bending, where the maximal percentage difference was 179%. A large difference of 72% and 125% were calculated between the Maverick and hydrogel-based TDR devices in flexion and lateral bending, respectively. The maximal percentage difference of 41% was calculated between the Charité and hydrogel-based TDR devices in axial rotation.

In flexion, only the Maverick device caused a marked decrease of 40%, while both the Charité and hydrogel-based TDR devices showed a good representation of the intact state. In extension, implantation of the Maverick and hydrogel-based TDR devices led to a slightly decreased ROM of 7% and 14% compared to the intact state, respectively. In lateral bending, the ROM predicted by the Charité and hydrogel-based TDR devices are 94% and 56% higher than that for the intact segment, respectively. In axial rotation, all three TDR designs restored almost to the intact state.

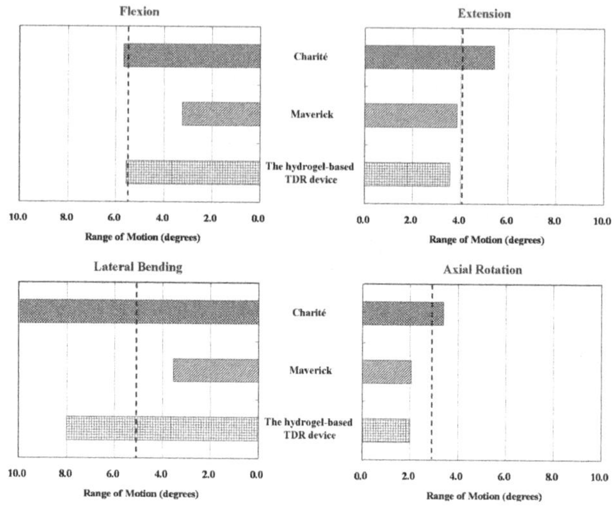

Fig. 3 Influence of implant types on the ROM in flexion, extension, lateral bending, and axial rotation. The dashed line indicates the ROM of the intact model.

B. *Facet Joint Force*

In flexion, the facet joints remained unloaded for the intact and disc prosthesis models. In extension, much larger inter-implant differences were found than was indicated under flexion (Fig. 4). The models predicted strongly increased forces for the Charité device (40%) and a marked decrease of 92% for the Maverick device compared to the intact state. In contrast, the presence of the hydrogel-based TDR device led to a better representation of the facet joint forces calculated for the intact state. In lateral bending, marked inter-implant differences were also calculated. Compared to the intact model, the facet joint force increased by 367% for the Charité device and 244% for the hydrogel-based TDR device. In contrast, the facet joints were unloaded for the Maverick prosthesis. In axial rotation, only small inter-implant differences up to 16% were calculated. The artificial disc models caused a decrease of 1.7% for the Charité device and 4.8% for the hydrogel-based TDR device compared to the intact state. In contrast, implantation of the Maverick device caused an increase of 16% compared to the intact state.

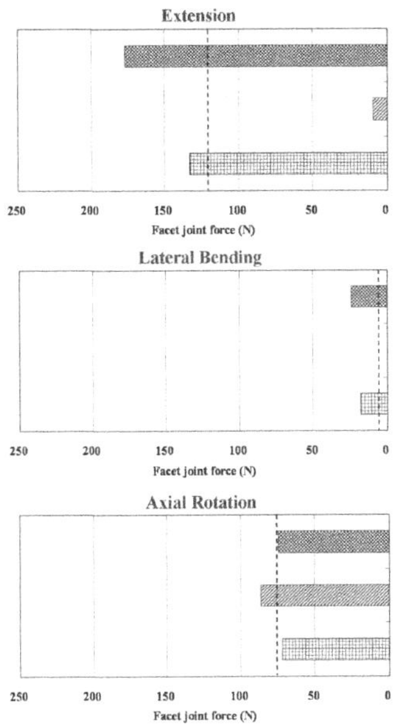

Fig. 4 Influence of implant types on acting forces in the facet joints in extension, lateral bending, and axial rotation. The dashed line indicates the facet joint forces of the intact model.

IV. DISCUSSION

The results for the Charité device in the current study are in line with the findings of Cunningham et al. [5], as they also reported about a minor increase of flexion/extension and axial rotation, but a significant increase for lateral bending after in vitro evaluation of the Charité device. Therefore, comparisons of the current numerical and previous study results showed excellent consistency, which indicated good reliability of the model to support accurate analysis and simulations. In the present study, the model with hydrogel-based TDR device mimicked the in vitro ROM of a motion segment well [6], although, similar to the Charité model, stiffness in lateral bending was relatively soft.

In the present study, the facet joint force strongly depends on the implant design. Except for axial rotation, our model predicted higher facet joint forces for the implants with an unconstrained core (Charité) and an elastomeric hydrogel compared to an implant with a constrained core (Maverick). This result can be explained by the resulting forces passing through the implant itself. An unconstrained design transfers only normal forces from the upper to the lower vertebral body. In contrast, a constrained design transfers additional shear forces through the implant and therefore, causes a higher load than the unconstrained design.

V. CONCLUSIONS

In conclusion, a model of a hydrogel-based TDR device was developed within an L4-5 motion segment. The TDR could maintain the ROM well compared to that of a natural disc. However, the model with the novel TDR device predicted a marked increase of facet joint forces due to the relatively low rotational stiffness, especially in lateral bending. Therefore, this flexibility issue needs specific attention in designing a biomimetic TDR device.

ACKNOWLEDGMENT

This study was supported by the National Science Council of Republic of China (grant No. NSC-100-2221-E-027-049-MY3).The computing facilities provided by the National Center for High-Performance Computing are greatly appreciated.

CONFLICT OF INTEREST

The authors declare that they have no conflict of interest.

REFERENCES

1. Jager M and Luttmann A. (1992) The load on the lumbar spine during asymmetrical bi-manual materials handling, Ergo 35:783-805
2. Baroud G, Nemes J, Heini P, Steffen T. (2003) Load shift of the intervertebral disc after a vertebroplasty: a finite-element study, Eur Spine J 12:421-426
3. Rohlmann A, Zander T, Schmidt H, Wilke HJ et al. (2006) Analysis of the influence of disc degeneration on the mechanical behaviour of a lumbar motion segment using the finite element method, J Biomech 39:2484-2490
4. Massey CJ, van Donkelaar CC, Vresilovic E et al. (2012) Effects of aging and degeneration on the human intervertebral disc during the diurnal cycle: a finite element study, J Orthop Res 30:122-128
5. Heuer F, Schmidt H, Klezl Z et al. (2007) Stepwise reduction of functional spinal structures increase range of motion and change lordosis angle, J Biomech 40:271-280
6. Hitchon PW, Eichholz K, Barry C et al. (2005) Biomechanical studies of an artificial disc implant in the human cadaveric spine, J Neurosurg Spine 2:339-343

Author: W.P. Chen
Institute: National Taipei University of Technology
Street: 1, Sec. 3, Zhongxiao E. Rd.
City: Taipei
Country: Taiwan
Email: wpchen@mail.ntut.edu.tw

Finite Element Simulations of Brain Responses to Soccer-Heading Impacts

P.Y. Chen[1], L.S. Chou[2], C.J. Hu[3], and H.H. Chen[1,4]

[1] Graduate Institute of Medicine Science, Taipei Medical University, Taipei, Taiwan
[2] Department of Human Physiology, University of Oregon, Eugene, OR, USA
[3] Department of Neurology, Taipei Medical University-Shuang Ho Hospital, Taipei, Taiwan
[4] Department of Physiology, College of Medicine, Taipei Medical University, Taipei, Taiwan

Abstract— **Soccer is one of the world's most popular sports, in which players must sometimes use their unprotected heads in offense or defense. In recent years, controversy surrounding the long-term effects of repeated impacts from heading has raised attention from the medical community. Previous works using numerical simulation studied the responses of the human brain during American football-related concussion. This study aims to estimate the response of the human brain to soccer-heading impacts using the finite element method. A validated full-body human model was used to analyze the impact simulation. The soccer ball flew with a translational velocity of 6 m/s or a rotational velocity of 30 rad/s. Players usually hit the ball with their foreheads or tops of heads while heading. Acceleration, Head Injury Criterion, principal strain, principal strain rate and shear stress of white matters in the brain are compared among different headings. The head motion during heading increases the acceleration of the brain during heading. The back spin of the ball increases its shear stress and strain rate during heading. When a moving player heads a ball with back spinning, the risk of mild traumatic brain injury may be high. This study shows that high strain and strain rate concentrate around the corpus callosum and shift from the impact site to the opposite direction. This observation is similar to those gathered from previous studies that simulated concussions sustained during American football.**

Keywords— **Soccer, Heading, Brain, Finite Element, Concussion.**

I. INTRODUCTION

Soccer is one of the world's most popular sports, in which players must sometimes use their unprotected heads in offense or defense. Although soccer is not traditionally identified as a sport with a high risk for head injuries, several studies have shown that concussion rates in soccer often exceed those of other contact sports [1]. In recent years, controversy surrounding the long-term effects of repeated impacts from heading has raised attention from the medical community. Previous works using numerical simulation studied the responses of the human brain during American football-related concussion. That model-predicted strain and strain rate in the corpus callosum correlate with changes in indices of concussion's white matter integrity have been confirmed preliminarily[2]. This study aims to estimate the response of the human brain to soccer-heading impacts using the finite element method. It can help us understand the risk of concussion during heading.

II. METHODS

A validated full-body human model (THUMS AM50 Model v. 4.0, JSOL Co., Osaka, Japan) was used. Finite element software LS-DYNA (Livermore Software Technology Co., Livermore, CA, USA) was used to analyze the impact simulation. Two impact sites on head, including the forehead and top of head, were simulated for two kinds of heading. The soccer ball flew with a translational velocity (6 m/s) or a rotational velocity (30 rad/s). Players usually hit the ball with their foreheads or tops of heads while heading. To simulate a powerful heading, the head can move at a velocity (3 m/s) in the opposite direction with the ball movement. There were 8 different simulations for heading, by combination of the following parameters: the impact site on the head, rotational velocity of the ball, and head motion.

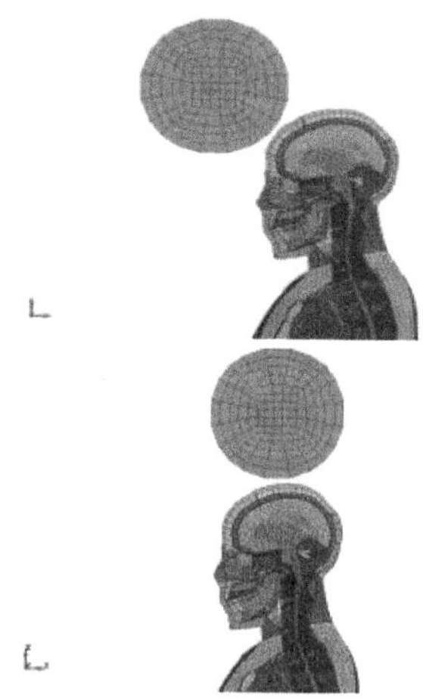

Fig. 1 Section view of the 3D model for simulation of forehead heading (upper) and top of head heading (lower)

Acceleration, Head Injury Criterion (HIC), principal strain, principal strain rate and shear stress of white matters in the brain are compared among different headings

I. Lackovic (ed.), *1st Global Conference on Biomedical Engineering & 9th Asian-Pacific Conference on Medical and Biological Engineering*,
IFMBE Proceedings 47, DOI: 10.1007/978-3-319-12262-5_33

III. RESULTS AND DISCUSSION

In cases of forehead heading, back spin of the ball and opposite motion of the head increased the resultant acceleration, max. strain, max. strain rate and max. shear stress (Table 1). The increasing trend in cases of top of head heading was the same as that in forehead heading. Heading from top of the head caused higher values than forehead heading in most of parameters except for the strain rate. Combination of back spin of the ball and head motion in both headings have a high HIC.

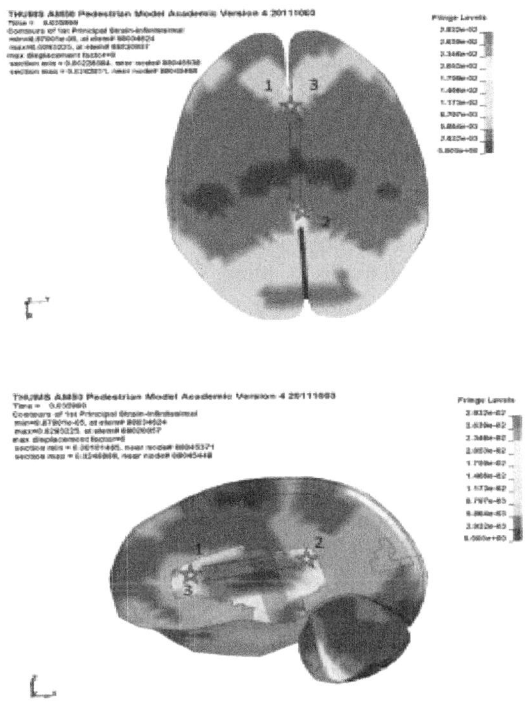

Fig. 2 Strain distribution of the brain on the sagittal plane (upper) and the coronal plane (lower) in the simulation of forehead heading; Locations of peak maximum principal strain are shown by red stars, and the time sequence is numbered.

IV. CONCLUSIONS

The head motion during heading increases the acceleration of the brain during heading. The back spin of the ball increases its shear stress and strain rate during heading. When a moving player heads a ball with back spinning, the risk of mTBI may be high. This study shows that high strain and strain rate concentrate around the corpus callosum and shift from the impact site to the opposite direction. This observation is similar to those gathered from previous studies that simulated concussions sustained during American football.

Table 1. Biomechanical parameters during the forehead heading

Parameter	Control	Ball Spin	Head Motion
Peak linear X-acceleration (G)	6.77	6.58	12.9
Peak linear Y-acceleration (G)	0.15	0.06	0.11
Peak linear Z-acceleration (G)	2.53	2.55	3.35
Peak resultant acceleration (G)	7.28	7.13	14.0
HIC	2.86	2.83	10.6
Max. Strain	0.03	0.03	0.04
Max. Strain Rate	5.21	4.44	10.3
Max Shear Stress (Pa)	0.64	1.20	3.03

Table 2. Biomechanical parameters during heading with the top of the head

Parameter	Control	Ball Spin	Head Motion
Peak linear X-acceleration (G)	1.30	0.52	1.85
Peak linear Y-acceleration (G)	0.26	0.29	0.43
Peak linear Z-acceleration (G)	4.29	4.21	7.18
Peak resultant acceleration (G)	5.33	5.38	10.1
HIC	1.30	1.23	7.02
Max. Strain	0.03	0.03	0.05
Max. Strain Rate	5.13	6.69	12.2
Max Shear Stress (Pa)	3.44	3.51	11.5

CONFLICT OF INTEREST

The authors declare that they have no conflict of interest.

REFERENCES

1. Levy ML, Kasasbeh AS, et al. (2012) Concussion in soccer: a current understand. *Word Neurosurgery* 78:535-544
2. Mcallister TW, Ford JC, et al. (2012) *Annals of Biomedical Engineering* **40**:127-140

Author: Hsiang-Ho Chen
Institute: Taipei Medical University
Street: 250 Wuxing St.
City: Taipei
Country: Taiwan, ROC
Email: hchen@tmu.edu.tw

Using Group Independent Component Analysis to Investigate Resting-State Functional Networks Underlying Motor Sequence Learning

Ho-Ching Yang[1], Chien-Ho Janice Lin[2], and Ming-Chang Chiang[1,*]

[1] Department of Biomedical Engineering, National Yang-Ming University, Taipei, Taiwan
[2] Physical Therapy and Assistive Technology, National Yang-Ming University, Taipei, Taiwan

Abstract— **Learning performance can be improved by practicing tasks with higher difficulty, a phenomenon known as the contextual interference (CI) effect. In this study, we investigated changes in the baseline functional connectivity of the brain when the participants practiced the serial reaction-time (SRT) task arranged respectively in an interleaved (higher CI) and a repetitive (lower CI) order. The resting-state functional magnetic resonance imaging (fMRI) data was analyzed using the group independent component analysis (ICA) to identify functionally homogeneous brain regions. These regions served as the nodes of the resting-state networks (RSNs) of the brain. Seven RSNs crucial for motor learning were identified, including the basal ganglia, sensorimotor, visual, auditory, visual, attentional, and the default-mode networks. We further found that the interleaved practice led to stronger functional connectivity than the repetitive practice within the default-mode network, particularly between the posterior cingulate and visual cortices, which are key regions for memory and visuospatial integration respectively. Our findings indicate that practice with higher difficulty enhances the baseline connectivity within the functional circuits of the brain, providing a neural basis for the benefits of higher CI practice on motor learning.**

Keywords— **Serial reaction time task, Contextual interference, Resting State, Independent component analysis, fMRI.**

I. INTRODUCTION

Practicing tasks with higher difficulty leads to better learning performance than practicing tasks with lower difficulty, a phenomenon known as the contextual interference (CI) effect [1]. One way to increase the contextual interference of the tasks to improve learning is to arrange the tasks in an interleaved order. Compared to the easier tasks that were arranged in a repetitive order, the more difficult interleaved tasks result in inferior practice, but better retention performance [2].Our previous work demonstrated the CI effect using functional magnetic resonance imaging (fMRI), where the interleaved practice condition invoked greater sensorimotor BOLD responses than the repetitive condition during the practice phase, but this pattern was reversed during retention [3]. Nevertheless, how various brain regions integrate to support such CI benefits on learning has remained elusive. In this paper, we investigate the functional brain network underlying the CI effects on learning based on the resting-state fMRI data [4]. The participants practiced a serial reaction-time (SRT) task arranged in either an interleaved or a repetitive order. We estimated the resting-state functional connectivity, with respect to these two practice conditions using group independent component analysis to identify functionally homogeneous brain regions as the hubs of the functional network [5]. Independent component analysis (ICA) is one of the most widely used blind source separation (BSS) techniques ,that identify the original source from noisy signals, without knowing the parameters of mixing and/or filtering processes [5, 6]. We hypothesized that, in practice phase, interleaved condition would lead to stronger resting-state functional connectivity compared with a repetitive condition. We also hypothesized that when moving on the retention phase, we would get the opposite result from resting-state functional connectivity. To our knowledge, this study is the first to apply group ICA analysis to model resting-state interregional functional connectivity with respect to motor learning of SRT tasks.

II. MATERIALS AND METHODS

A. Participants

Eighteen right-handed young adults were enrolled in the study. They were recruited from the National Yang-Ming University with the approval from the institutional review board (IRB). Participants were excluded if they had any contraindications to MRI.

B. Study Design

We adopted the design of the serial reaction time (SRT) task from our previous work [3]. The participants practiced the SRT task on two consecutive training days (Days 1 and 2). To investigate the effects of practice on learning, we tested delayed retention performance on Day 5 [7-10]. Behavioral and fMRI data were acquired concurrently on each testing day within an MRI scanner. In each day we recorded resting activity after the practice or retention sessions.

* Corresponding author.

I. Lackovic (ed.), *1st Global Conference on Biomedical Engineering & 9th Asian-Pacific Conference on Medical and Biological Engineering*,
IFMBE Proceedings 47, DOI: 10.1007/978-3-319-12262-5_34

The SRT task consisted of three different four-element sequences, presented in either a repetitive or interleaved order. The Participants positioned the four fingers of the left hand (all except the thumb) on the four light sensitive response keys of a magnet-compatible button box (Current Designs). Only one colored circle appeared at a time while the other circles were transparent [11]. The participants pressed the corresponding button as soon as possible when one of the colored circles (yellow, red, blue, and green) lighted up. The response time (RT) was recorded for each button press. We applied a within-subject crossover design, each participant started in the first week with either the repetitive practice (RP) or the interleaved practice (IP) condition; 2 weeks later, he or she performed in the other practice condition (i.e., repetitive → interleaved, or vice versa). The order of the practice conditions and the SRT task sequences was counter-balanced across participants.

C. Functional Magnetic Resonance Imaging

Images were acquired using a Siemens Trio 3.0 T MRI scanner. Functional images were acquired during and after the SRT tasks. On Days 1 and 2, each functional run lasted for 5 min and 48 s, and consisted of 153 EPI volumes (gradient-echo, TR = 2,000, TE = 30, flip angle = 90), each with 34 transverse slices, 4 mm thick, 1 mm gap, and a 64 × 64 matrix yielding an in-plane resolution of 3 × 3 mm^2. The first five volumes of each functional run were removed from analysis to allow for magnetization to approach equilibrium. On Day 5, the participants underwent three functional runs (two runs for sequence specific tests and one run for the novel sequence test). Each run lasted for 3 minutes and 48 s, and involved the acquisition of 99 EPI volumes. On each day after the SRT task we acquired resting-state data for 5 min and 48 s, where the participants were asked to think of nothing in particular, remain relaxed but awake, with their eyes closed.

D. Statistical Analysis

a) Imaging Preprocessing and First Level Analyses

Functional images were processed using the Statistical Parametric Mapping software (SPM8, Wellcome Department of Cognitive Neurology, London, UK). Image preprocessing procedures included realignment, slice-timing correction, spatial normalization that resampled the image to 3 × 3 × 3 mm^3 per voxel, and smoothing using an isotropic Gaussian filter with full width at half maximum (FWHM) = 8 mm.

b) Resting Data With Group ICA

Resting data were decomposed into functional networks by using a group-level spatial ICA as implemented in the GIFT toolbox (http://mialab.mrn. org/software/gift/). We used a relatively high-order model order (the number of components, C was set to 80) to achieve a better "functional parcellation." of the brain. To avoid otherwise prohibitive memory requirements, prior to ICA, the dimensionality of data was reduced using a two-step principal components analysis (PCA) based on the expectation-maximization (EM) algorithm, with 120 principal components (PCs) left in the first step, and then 80 PCs in the second step [12]. ICA was then performed using the Infomax algorithm [13] in the I_{CASSO} software program with 20 repetitions (http://www.cis.hut. fi/projects/ica/icasso). The group spatial maps (SMs) were estimated as the modes of the component clusters. The spatial maps and time courses (TCs, Ri) of each participant were then back-reconstruction using the GICA3 method based on PCA compression and projection [14-17]. We characterized a subset of the identified independent components (ICs) (n = 26) as our resting-state networks (RSNs), based on the assumptions that RSN should exhibit peak activations in gray matter, low spatial overlap with known vascular, ventricular, motion, and susceptibility artifacts, and have their TCs dominated by low-frequency fluctuations [2,18]. The rest of the ICs were then regarded as physiological, movement-related, or imaging artifacts (ARTs) [6].

For each participant, functional connectivity was estimated by correlating the time course of every pair of ICs, yielding an n × n correlation matrix, where n=26 is the number of ICs.

III. RESULTS

A. Resting-State Networks

Figures 1 displays seven main resting-state networks (RSNs). They were classified by their anatomical and functional properties. The basal ganglia network (BG) had functional activity focused in the thalamus. The sensorimotor network (MOT) contained the precentral and postcentral gyri. The auditory network (AUD) included Brodmann area 42 and the superior temporal gyrus. The default-mode network (DMN) was captured in five ICs. The attentional network (ATTN) included Brodmann area 7 and the parietal lobe. Finally, we identified four ICs as components of the frontal networks (FRONT), whose functional activity was stronger in Brodmann areas 6, 10, and 46, the frontal lobe, and the superior frontal gyrus.

B. Functional Network Connectivity

Figure 2 shows functional connectivity between the seven RSNs, showing that these brain regions were synchronized to function as a whole during the resting state.

Figure 3 shows that functional connectivity across seven main RSNs respectively under each practice condition and on each day. Red arrows indicate that connectivity between the two RSNs was significant. We further focused on functional connectivity patterns within the default-mode network. On day 2, the interleaved practice led to stronger functional connectivity from the posterior cingulate cortex (Brodmann area23) to the cuneus (Figure 4). This finding suggests that tasks with higher difficulty evoked more functional connections between memory-related (the posterior cingulate cortex) and cuneus in the brain.

IV. Conclusion

Our study applied the group ICA method to investigate longitudinal changes in resting brain networks that support the beneficial effects of CI on learning. We found that motor learning involved various functional specialized regions in the brain, such as sensorimotor, visual, and attentional areas. The CI effects on learning may be mediated by increased connectivity between memory and visual regions in the default-mode network, suggesting that learning changes the baseline configuration of the brain circuits.

Acknowledgement

This study was supported in part by the Ministry of Science and Technology (NSC 102-2221-E-010 -007-MY3), the National Health Research Institutes (NHRI-EX103-10219EC) and the 3T MRI Core Facility in NYMU.

Conflict of Interest

The authors declare no relationship, financial or otherwise, with individual or organizations that could influence the author's work inappropriately.

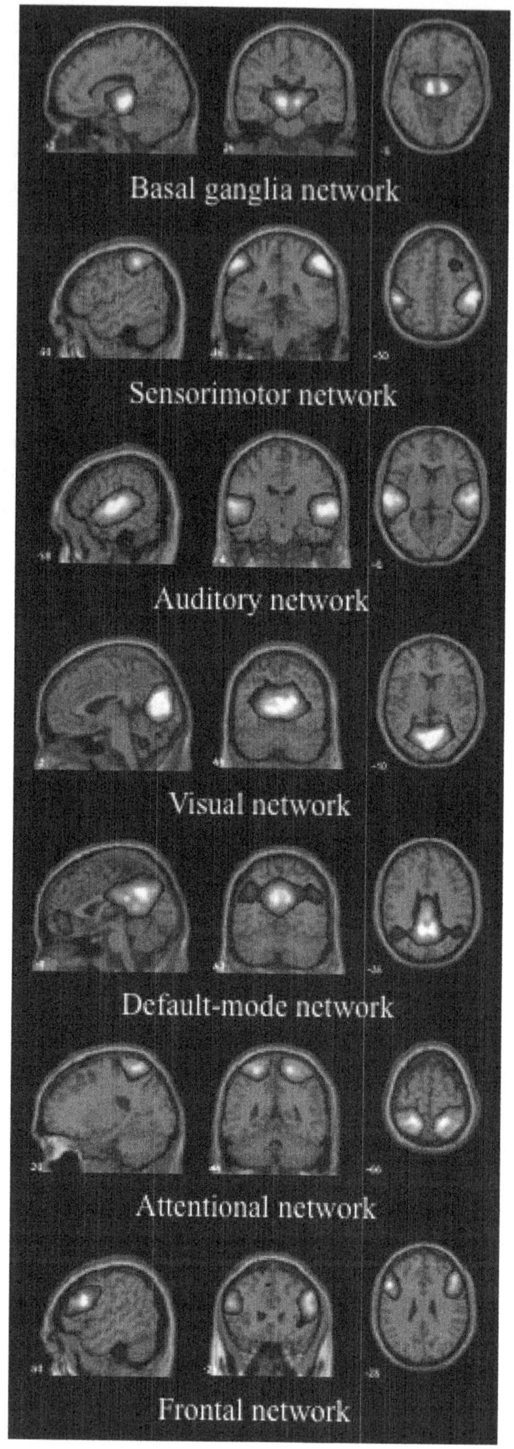

Fig. 1 Functional network connectivity within RSNs.

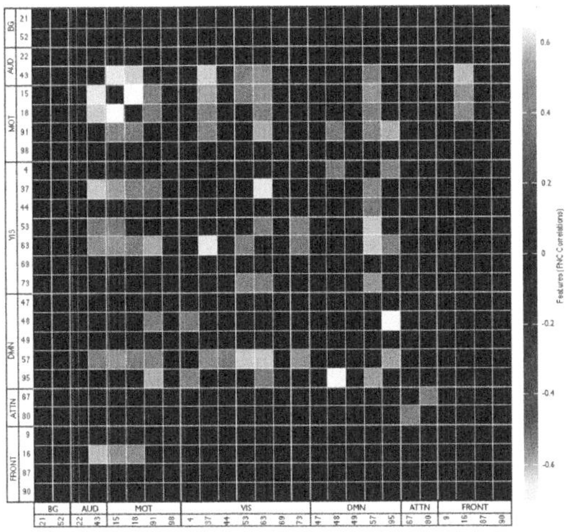

Fig. 2 Functional network connectivity between RSNs.

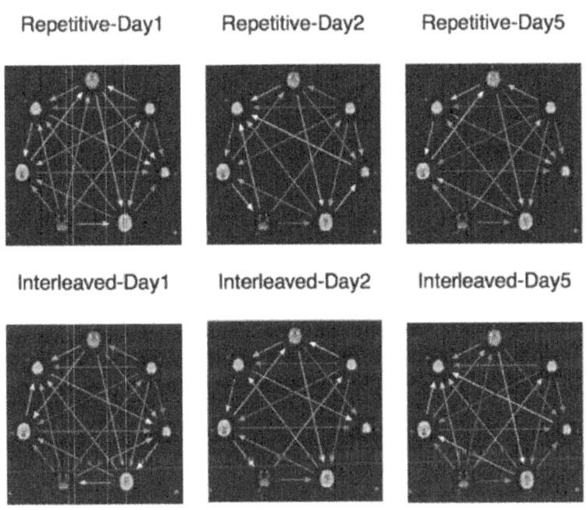

Fig. 3 Default-mode network in different practice conditions

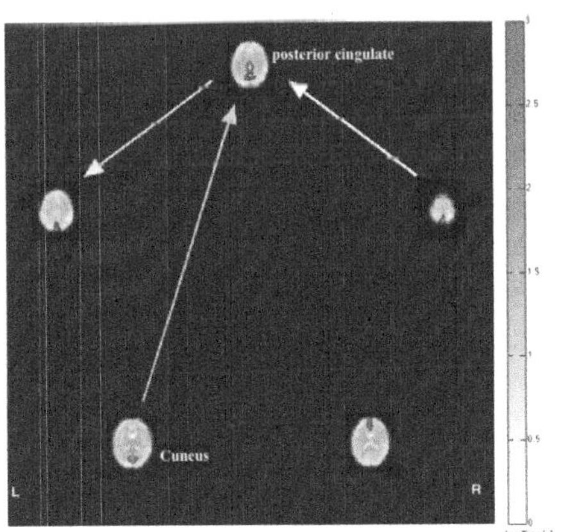

Fig. 4 Interleaved practice led to stranger functional connectivity on day 2

REFERENCES

1. Schmidt RA, Bjork RA (1992) New conceptualizations of practice: common principles in three paradigms suggest new concepts for training. Psychol. Sci. 3, 207–217.
2. Brady F, (2008) The contextual interference effect and sport skills. Percept. Mot. Skills 106, 461–472.
3. Lin CH, Knowlton BJ, Chiang MC et al. (2011) Brain–behavior correlates of optimizing learning through interleaved practice. NeuroImage. 56, 1758–1772.
4. Sami S, Miall RC (2013) Graph network analysis of immediate motor-learning induced changes in resting state BOLD. Frontiers in Human Neuroscience, Volume 7, Article 166
5. Naik GR, Kumar DK (2011) An Overview of Independent Component Analysis and Its Applications. Informatica. 35, 63-81
6. Allen EA, Erhardt EB, Damaraju E et al. (2011) A base- line for the multivariate comparison of resting-state networks. Front Syst Neurosci. 5.
7. Cahill L, McGaugh JL, Weinberger NM (2001) The neurobiology of learning and memory: Some reminders to remember. Trends in Neuroscience 24:578–581.
8. Perez CR, Meira CM Jr., Tani G (2005) Does the contextual interference effect last over extended transfer trials? Perceptual Motor Skills 100:58–60.
9. Shea JB, Morgan R (1979) Contextual interference effects on the acquisition, retention, and transfer of a motor skill.J Exp Psy- chol: Hum Learn Mem 5:179–187.
10. Wright DL, Magnuson CE, Black CB (2005) Programming and reprogramming sequence timing following high and low contextual interference practice. Res Quart Exe Sports 76:258–266.
11. Lin CH, Chiang MC, Knowlton BJ (2012) Interleaved practice enhances skill learning and the functional connectivity of fronto-parietal networks.Human Brain Mapp. 34(7):1542-58
12. Roweis S. (1998) EM algorithms for PCA and SPCA. Neural Inform Process Syst. 10:626–632.
13. Bell AJ, Sejnowski TJ (1995) An information-maximization approach to blind separation and blind deconvolution. Neural Comput. 7:1129–1159.
14. Calhoun VD, Adali T, Pearlson GD et al. (2001) A method for making group inferences from functional MRI data using independent component analysis. Hum Brain Mapp. 14:140–151.
15. Erhardt EB, Rachakonda S, Bedrick EJ et al. (2011) Comparison of multi-subject ICA methods for analysis of fMRI data. Hum Brain Mapp. 32:2075–2095
16. Filippini N, MacIntosh BJ, Hough MG et al. (2009) Distinct patterns of brain activity in young carriers of the APOE-ε4 allele. Proc Natl Acad Sci. 106:7209–7214.
17. Allen EA, Erhardt EB, Wei Y (2012) Capturing inter-subject variability with group independent component analy- sis of fMRI data: a simulation study. Neuroimage. 59:4141–4159.
18. Cordes D, Haughton VM, Arfanakis K et al. (2001) Frequencies contributing to functional connectivity in the cerebral cortex in "resting-state" data. Am J Neuroradiol. 22:1326–1333.

Author: Ho-Ching Yang, Chien-Ho Janice Lin, Ming-Chang Chiang
Institute: Department of Biomedical Engineering
Street: No.155, Sec2, Lining Street
City: Taipei
Country: Taiwan
Email: kawc1034@gmail.com

Computer-Aided Diagnosis of Breast Tumors Using Textures from Intensity Transformed Sonographic Images

C.M. Lo[1], R.F. Chang[1,2], C.S. Huang[3], and W.K. Moon[4]

[1] Department of Computer Science and Information Engineering, National Taiwan University, Taipei, Taiwan
[2] Graduate Institute of Biomedical Electronics and Bioinformatics, National Taiwan University, Taipei, Taiwan
[3] Department of Surgery, National Taiwan University Hospital and National Taiwan University College of Medicine, Taipei, Taiwan
[4] Department of Radiology, Seoul National University Hospital, Seoul, Korea

Abstract— **The malignancy of breast tumors are evaluated via ultrasound images on clinical examination. As a second viewer, a computer-aided diagnosis (CAD) system was developed to classify the breast tumors using texture features to avoid misclassifying carcinomas. A total of 69 cases including 21 malignant and 48 benign masses were acquired. For intensity-invariant texture extraction, the ultrasound images were first transformed into ranklet images to reduce the effect of brightness variability. From the ranklet images, tumor texture and speckle texture were extracted and compared to those from the original ultrasound images for tumor diagnosis. In the trade-offs between sensitivity and specificity, the ranklet-based tumor texture and speckle texture were all significantly better than those of the original US images (Az: 0.83 vs. 0.58, *p*-value=0.0009 and Az=0.80 vs. 0.56, *p*-value=0.02). The proposed CAD system using textures from intensity transformed sonographic images is robust to various gray-scale distributions and is more suitable in clinical use.**

Keywords— **Breast cancer, ultrasound, computer-aided diagnosis, texture.**

I. INTRODUCTION

Breast ultrasound (US) has been used in distinguishing between benign and malignant lesions [1]. The sonographic appearances are interpreted by radiologists for clinical examination and diagnosis. In various computer-aided diagnosis (CAD) systems, the sonographic descriptors were quantified to automatically evaluate the likelihood of malignancy of tumors [2-5]. The quantitative features extracted from the B-mode images included shape, tumor texture, and speckle texture features [4,5]. According to the performance, the CAD system [6] acted as a second reader in classifying benign and malignant tumors collected from different US equipments during a 2-year period. However, the performance of intensity-based texture features was not as good as that of the shape features [6]. The gray-scale intensity variation in images may affect the performance of texture features.

In this study, the ranklet transform [7] was proposed to convert the original US images into ranklet images to extract intensity-invariant texture features. The performance of intensity-invariant texture features was compared with that of the original texture features for the classification of breast tumors.

II. MATERIALS AND METHODS

A. US Acquisition

The institution review board approval was obtained, and informed consent was waived for this retrospective study. The breast US database were collected using an ATL HDI 3000 scanner (Philips, Bothell, WA) or a Medison Voluson 530 scanner (Kretz Technik, Zipf, Austria) and a 5–10 MHz linear transducer during a 2-year period. 69 tumors including 21 malignant and 48 benign masses were collected as the image database in the experiment.

Fig. 1 shows three cases of breast tumor collected in the experiment. The gray-scale distributions of them are various. The possible reasons include that the US images may acquired from different US equipments (ATL HDI 3000 scanner or Medison Voluson 530 scanner). Depend on different operators or scanning settings, more or less difference in image presentation is also unavoidable.

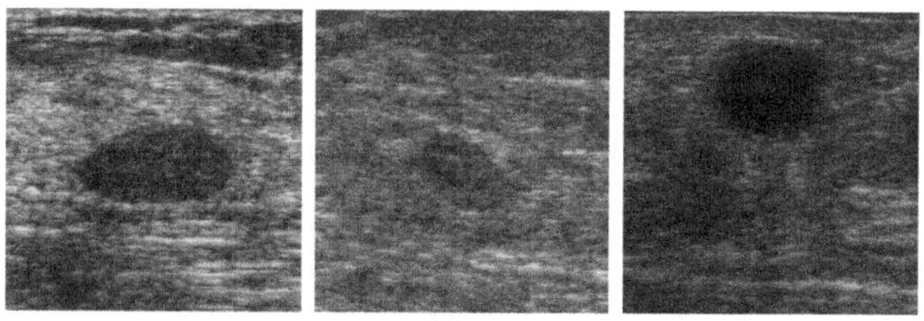

Fig. 1 Gray-scale distributions among ultrasound images are different

B. Tumor Segmentation

Tumor area was delineated first to specify the tissues of interest for further analysis. The automatic level-set segmentation method [8] was used to delineate the tumor contour to reduce operator-dependence. Using the gray-scale gradient in the differential equation, the level-set function evolves the user-defined seeds into a complex shape with changing topology. As a image preprocessing, the sigmoid filter [9] was used to enhance the tumor boundary to deal with weak edges. The gradient magnitude filter [10] was

I. Lackovic (ed.), *1st Global Conference on Biomedical Engineering & 9th Asian-Pacific Conference on Medical and Biological Engineering*,
IFMBE Proceedings 47, DOI: 10.1007/978-3-319-12262-5_35

then applied to generate a gradient image presenting the magnitude between pixels. Using the level-set method on the tumor area in the gradient image achieved the segmentation. Fig. 2(a) shows the tumor contour of the first image in Fig. 1.

C. Texture Features

The texture information in US images was based on the echo pattern presented by gray-scale values. Previous CAD systems [5,11] suggested extracting texture features inside or surrounding tumor for tissue characterization. The texture features can be classified into tumor texture and speckle texture.

Tumor texture is the analysis of pattern inside the tumor area. After tumor segmentation, the tumor area enclosed by the contour is a cluster of similar biological structures shown as gray-scale values. The texture information inside the tumor area can be extracted by analyzing the correlations between pixel values.

Speckle texture is the analyzing of value correlations among speckle pixels. Speckle pattern in B-mode images was demonstrated to have tissue characteristics in breast tumor classification [4,5]. It is generated by microstructure scatterers contained in tissues such as tissue parenchyma. The scatterers scatter US pulses and generate the interference pattern having granular appearances in B-mode images. To extract speckle pixels, the pixel values in a B-mode image were log decompressed to the raw intensity. In the intensity image, pixels have an exponential distribution with a ratio of mean to SD of 0.8-1.0 are speckle pixels. In the experiment, speckle pixels within a distance of 5 to the tumor boundary were gathered to be a speckle map for texture extraction. Fig. 2(b) shows the speckle pixels distributed around tumor area.

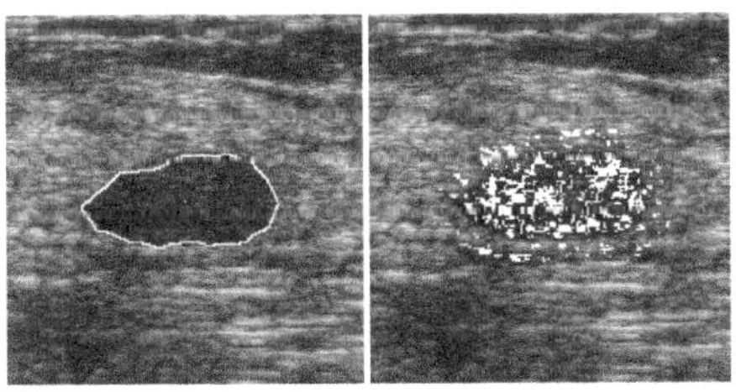

(a) (b)

Fig. 2 Texture features are extracted from (a) tumor area (b) speckle pixels

a) Gray-level co-occurrence matrix:

After specifying the meaningful area for texture extraction, the gray-level co-occurrence matrix (GLCM)[12] was used to analyzing the correlations between pixel values. GLCM is the second-order statistics describing the joint frequencies of pair-wise combinations. Co-occurrence matrices $P=[p(i,j|d,\theta)]$ are constructed by locating each pixel and its surrounding adjacent pixels in a mask. The matrix element $P=[p(i,j|d,\theta)]$ is the frequencies of two adjacent pixels at a distance of d and a direction θ, one with gray-scale i and the other with gray-scale j. The average and standard deviation (SD) of eight GLCM metrics defined below were calculated to be texture features.

$$Energy = \sum_i \sum_j p(i,j|d,\theta)^2 \quad (1)$$

$$Entropy = -\sum_i \sum_j p(i,j|d,\theta)\log(p(i,j|d,\theta)) \quad (2)$$

$$Correlation = \frac{\sum_i \sum_j (i-\mu_x)(j-\mu_y)p(i,j|d,\theta)}{\sigma_x\sigma_y} \quad (3)$$

$$Local\ Homogeneity = \sum_i \sum_j \frac{1}{1+(i-j)^2} p(i,j|d,\theta) \quad (4)$$

$$Inertia = \sum_i \sum_j (i-j)^2 p(i,j|d,\theta) \quad (5)$$

$$Cluster\ Shade = \sum_i \sum_j (i+j-\mu_x-\mu_y)^3 p(i,j|d,\theta \quad (6)$$

$$Cluster\ Prominence = \sum_i \sum_j (i+j-\mu_x-\mu_y)^4 p(i,j|d,\theta \quad (7)$$

$$Haralick's\ Correlation = \frac{\sum_i \sum_j (i\cdot j)p(i,j|d,\theta)-\mu_x\mu_y}{\sigma_x\sigma_y} \quad (8)$$

b) Ranklet transform:

Ranklet transform was used in intensity-based image features for texture extraction [7]. In this study, ranklet transform was applied to the US images for intensity-invariant texture features to reduce the effect of intensity variation. Ranklet transform calculates the relative rank of pixel value rather than original gray-scale pixel value. Using multi-resolution and orientation-selective transformations, ranklet transform considers the characteristics of different scales and angles. Under a resolution value R, a number of overlapping crops with $R\times R$ was extracted by moving a $R\times R$ crop window. For each resolution, a image is separated into two subsets according to the orientations of vertical, horizontal, and diagonal. Then, the number of pixels pairs (P_H, P_L) in each crop is calculated for each resolution and orientation. The derived ranklet transform coefficient R_O is formulated as following:

$$R_O = \frac{\sum_{p \in Y_O} \pi(p) - \frac{C}{4}\left(\frac{C}{2} + 1\right)}{\frac{C^2}{8}} - 1, O = V, H, D \quad (9)$$

where the number in a crop is C. In the subset Y_O, pixels' ranks $\pi(p)$ are summed. The ranklet coefficient of a crop is close to 0 if there is no global variation. After ranklet transform, pixel values are replaced by the ranklet coefficient to express the regularity correlation in neighborhood. As shown in Fig. 3, the gray-scale distributions among different processings are different but the corresponding ranklet images are similar.

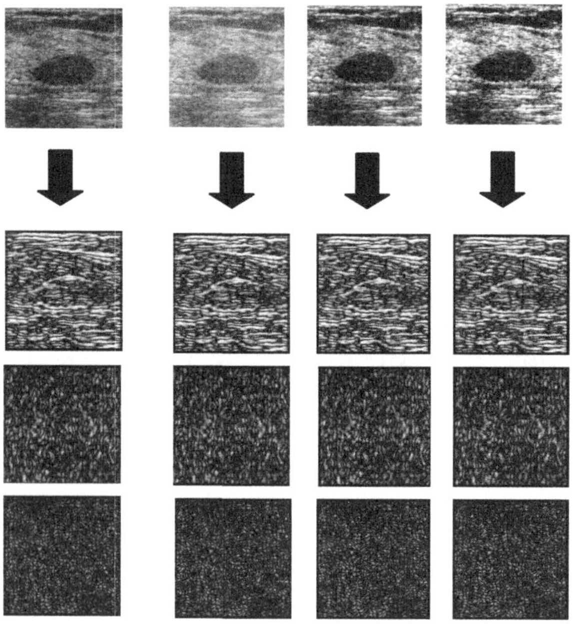

(a) (b) (c) (d)

Fig. 3 The ultrasound images and their corresponding ranklet images in the order of vertical, horizontal, and diagonal orientation for (a) original image (b) gamma filter (c) contrast filter (d) equalization filter

In the experiment, each US image was transformed to ranklet images of five image resolutions (2, 4, 8, 16, and 32) and three orientations (vertical, horizontal, and diagonal). Then, the average and SD of eight GLCM metrics were extracted from the ranklet images for tumor texture and speckle texture. Both feature set has 240 texture features.

c) Classification:

In the classifier of binary logistic regression [13], stepwise backward elimination was used in the evaluation of the texture features. The subset of features with the least error rate was selected to be the most relevant. Leave-one-out cross-validation was then used for the generalization ability. After classification, five performance indices include accuracy, sensitivity, specificity, positive predictive value (PPV), and negative predictive value (NPV) were calculated upon the biopsy-proven pathology. Performance differences were evaluated using chi-square test. Az, area under the receiver operating characteristic (ROC) curve, was used for the trade-offs between sensitivity and specificity.

III. Results

Table 1 shows the performances of texture features extracted from ranklet images compared to the original US images. Most performance indices achieved significant result (p-value>0.05). With respect to Az, both the tumor texure and speckle texture are significantly better than those of the original US images (p-value=0.0009 and 0.02, respectively). The ROC curves are shown in Fig. 4.

Table 1 The performance comparisons of tumor texture and speckle texture with and without ranklet transform using chi-square test

Performance indices	Tumor Texture	Tumor Texture (Ranklet)	p-value	Speckle Texture	Speckle Texture (Ranklet)	p-value
Accuracy	58% (40/69)	80% (55/69)	0.0058*	62% (43/69)	83% (57/69)	0.0076*
Sensitivity	38% (8/21)	76% (16/21)	0.0126*	33% (7/21)	71% (15/21)	0.0134*
Specificity	67% (32/48)	81% (39/48)	0.1035	75% (36/48)	88% (42/48)	0.1167
PPV	33% (8/24)	64% (16/25)	0.0318*	37% (7/19)	71% (15/21)	0.0281*
NPV	71% (32/45)	89% (39/44)	0.0396*	72% (36/50)	88% (42/48)	0.0570
Az	0.58	0.83	0.0009*	0.56	0.80	0.02*

* p-value<0.05 indicates a statistically significant difference.

IV. Discussion

Texture features are widely used in CAD systems for breast tumor classification. However, the performance of the texture features is not consistent in previous studies [5,6]. A reason is that the texture features are easily affected by different gray-scale distribution. In this study, we proposed to use ranklet transform [7] for extracting robust texture features to the intensity variation. The texture features extracted from ranklet images were demonstrated to be intensity-invariant and provide diagnostic information in classifying tumors examined by different US equipments (ATL and Medison). Compared to other existed CAD systems [3,4], our image database composed of different scanner models and settings is similar to the real world situation. Consequently, the result is meaningful in clinical use.

The limitation of this study is the number of cases collected in the experiment. More cases from different scanner models and settings should be included in the future to evaluate the generalization ability.

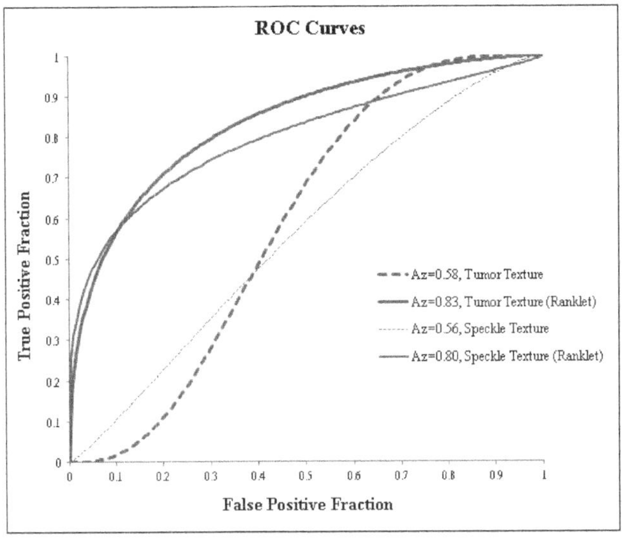

Fig. 4 Roc curves of two texture feature sets with and without ranklet transform

V. CONCLUSIONS

The texture features extracted from ranklet images with multi-resolution and orientations performed significantly better than those from the original US images. The CAD system based on the intensity-invariant texture features would be more reliable to evaluate breast US images acquired from various equipments and settings.

ACKNOWLEDGMENT

The authors thank the National Science Council (NSC 101-2221-E-002-068-MY3), Ministry of Economic Affairs (102-EC-17-A-19-S1-164), and Ministry of Education (AE-00-00-06) of the Republic of China for the financial support. This study was also supported by the grant no. 04-2011-0380 from the SNUH Research Fund.

CONFLICT OF INTEREST

The authors declare that they have no conflict of interest.

REFERENCES

[1] Stavros AT, Thickman D, Rapp CL et al. (1995) Solid breast nodules: Use of sonography to distinguish between benign and malignant lesions. Radiology 196:123-134.
[2] Drukker K, Giger ML, Metz CE. (2005) Robustness of computerized lesion detection and classification scheme across different breast US platforms. Radiology 237:834-840.
[3] Kim KG, Cho SW, Min SJ, Kim JH et al. (2005) Computerized scheme for assessing ultrasonographic features of breast masses. Acad Radiol 12:58-66.
[4] Moon WK, Lo CM, Chang JM et al. (2012) Computer-aided classification of breast masses using speckle features of automated breast ultrasound images. Med Phys 39:6465-6473.
[5] Moon WK, Lo CM, Huang CS et al. (2012) Computer-Aided Diagnosis Based on Speckle Patterns in Ultrasound Images. Ultrasound Med Biol 38:1251-1261.
[6] Moon WK, Lo C-M, Chang JM et al. (2013) Quantitative Ultrasound Analysis for Classification of BI-RADS Category 3 Breast Masses. J Digit Imaging 1-8.
[7] Masotti M, Campanini R. (2008) Texture classification using invariant ranklet features. Pattern Recognit Lett 29:1980-1986.
[8] Moon WK, Chang SC, Huang CS et al. (2011) Breast Tumor Classification Using Fuzzy Clustering for Breast Elastography. Ultrasound Med Biol 37:700-708.
[9] Suri JS. (2008) Advances in diagnostic and therapeutic ultrasound imaging. Artech House, London
[10] Deriche R. (1990) Fast Algorithms for Low-Level Vision. IEEE Trans Pattern Anal Mach Intell 12:78-87.
[11] Lo C-M, Chen R-T, Chang Y-C et al. (2014) Multi-dimensional Tumor Detection in Automated Whole Breast Ultrasound using Topographic Watershed. (in press)
[12] Haralick RM, Shanmuga.K, Dinstein I. (1973) Textural Features for Image Classification. IEEE Trans Syst Man Cybern Smc3:610-621.
[13] Hosmer DW. (2000) Applied logistic regression. 2nd edition. Wiley, New York.

Author: Chung-Ming Lo
Institute: Department of Computer Science and Information Engineering, National Taiwan University
Street: CSIE Building, No. 1, Sec. 4, Roosevelt Rd
City: Taipei
Country: Taiwan
Email: d97001@csie.ntu.edu.tw

A Fast and Accurate Algorithm for Diffeomorphic and Symmetric Non-rigid Registration of Brain Magnetic Resonance Images

Shih-Yen Lin[1], Yong-Sheng Chen[1,2], and Li-Fen Chen[3,4]

[1] Department of Computer Science, National Chiao Tung University, Hsinchu, Taiwan
[2] Institute of Biomedical Engineering, National Chiao Tung University, Hsinchu, Taiwan
[3] Institute of Brain Science, National Yang-Ming University, Taipei, Taiwan
[4] Integrated Brain Research Unit, Department of Medical Research, Taipei Veterans General Hospital, Taipei, Taiwan

Abstract— **This paper proposes a non-rigid, symmetric and diffeomorphic algorithm for the registration of MR images. A log-Euclidean framework was used to model diffeomorphisms. Multiple features were used to enhance the speed of the proposed algorithm, including compactly supported Wendland's basis functions as models of velocity fields, a greedy optimization strategy, and a coarse-to-fine hierarchical framework. Symmetry was ensured through the invertibility of diffeomorphisms and the symmetry of the objective function and optimization algorithm. The proposed algorithm was evaluated using the results of 1560 pairwise registrations of 40 T1-weighted MRIs in the LPBA40 dataset. Our results demonstrated that the proposed algorithm is diffeomorphic with sub-voxel accuracy in terms of symmetry. The proposed algorithm outperforms 14 other registration algorithms in terms of speed (compared with diffeomorphic algorithms) and accuracy.**

Keywords— **Magnetic Resonance Images, diffeomorphisms, non-rigid registration.**

I. INTRODUCTION

Image registration is crucial for spatial normalization of brain magnetic resonance images (MRI). Spatial normalization involves warping multiple images to a single reference frame. This allows researchers to analyze intra-subject and inter-subject anatomical variations on a similar basis.

Among non-rigid registration techniques, diffeomorphic registration algorithms [1-5] can provide a more well-formed solution to overcome the limitations of displacement-based frameworks. This type of framework can ensure a one-to-one relationship of the mapping function, thereby preserving the topology after warping. Nonetheless, the calculation of diffeomorphic mapping functions are computationally intensive comparing to simple displacement-based models.

Another essential property for registration algorithms is symmetry, or inverse-consistency. Symmetric registration algorithms can obtain consistent results when the warped image and reference image are interchanged. It may be a potential solution to avoid bias induced by asymmetric registration algorithms, as reported in [6]. Let $\Phi_{B\to A}$ denote the estimated mapping obtained by registering image A to image B, this inverse consistency can be formulated as:

$$\Phi_{B\to A} = (\Phi_{A\to B})^{-1} \ . \quad (1)$$

The objective of this study is to design a diffeomorphic and symmetric non-rigid registration algorithm that can avoid the heavy computational burdens, usually inevitable in conventional diffeomorphic registration algorithms, and also can surpass other registration algorithms in terms of accuracy.

II. METHODS

A. Model of Diffeomorphism

This study used a log-Euclidean framework [1, 7] to model diffeomorphisms. A diffeomorphic mapping function (Φ) is implicitly parameterized by its projection on the Lie Algebra of the space of diffeomorphisms. This projection is modeled as a time-independent velocity field (V). The conversion between a velocity field and its corresponding mapping function are defined as the *logarithm* and *exponential* operator:

$$V = log\,\Phi\,, \Phi = \exp V \ . \quad (2)$$

Our work used the exponential operator defined in [7], which is the flow of the partial differential equation (PDE) $\dot{x}(t) = V(x)$ at time 1 (denoted as $\varphi_V(\cdot\,,1)$):

$$\exp V = \varphi_V(\cdot\,,1) \ . \quad (3)$$

Through modelling diffeomorphisms by their projection on a Euclidean space of their Lie Algebras, combinations of diffeomorphisms are simplified to linear combinations of velocity fields, and inversions of mapping function is reduced to vector negations. In our work, we used a modified 16-step midpoint method to solve the PDEs.

I. Lackovic (ed.), *1st Global Conference on Biomedical Engineering & 9th Asian-Pacific Conference on Medical and Biological Engineering*, IFMBE Proceedings 47, DOI: 10.1007/978-3-319-12262-5_36

B. Radial Basis Functions

In our work, velocity fields are represented as linear combinations of Wendland Ψ-functions (Ψ) [8] in order to reduce the dimensionality of the optimization problem:

$$V(x) = \sum_i \alpha_i \Psi\left(\frac{\|x-c_i\|}{s_i}\right) , \quad (4)$$

where α is the vector coefficient representing the orientation and magnitude of each basis function, and S specifies the extent of support. Wendland Ψ-functions are piece-wise polynomial and compactly supported radial basis functions(RBFs):

$$\Psi(r) = \begin{cases} (1-r)^4(4r+1), & 0 \leq r < 1 \\ 0, & r \geq 1 \end{cases} . \quad (5)$$

Wendland Ψ-functions yield better computational efficiency when compared with other types of RBFs (e.g. Gaussian function) because of their piecewise-polynomial nature. In addition, their compact support also help to reduce the volume involved when optimizing the coefficients, therefore further increasing the computational efficiency.

C. Optimization

To overcome the curse of dimensionality when searching in the extremely high-dimensional parameter spaces of registration problems, we employed a greedy optimization approach similar to [9, 10]. The coefficient of each RBF is estimated sequentially and individually. We used downhill simplex method [11] to estimate the optimal coefficient of each RBF. A deterministic initialization scheme was imposed to ensure reproducibility and symmetry.

D. The Objective Function

The objective function is the log-likelihood representation of *maximum a posteriori* (MAP) estimates (see [1] for details):

$$E(I_s, I_t, \Phi) = E_1(I_s, I_t, \Phi) + \lambda E_2(\Phi) . \quad (6)$$

In (6), E_1 is the likelihood term, a measure used to indicate the similarity between the warped source image (I_s) and the static target image (I_t). The prior term (E_2) regularizes the warping function (Φ) to conform to given prior knowledge. The regularization parameter (λ) is empirically set to 0.05.

This study used a symmetric version of the correlation ratio (CR) as the likelihood term. CR is a robust measure against variations in the same and different modalities. However, it is not symmetric. This study used a symmetric correlation ratio inspired by [22]:

$$E(I_s, I_t, \Phi) = \frac{1}{2}\left(CR(I_s, I_t, \Phi) + CR(I_t, I_s, \Phi^{-1})\right) . \quad (7)$$

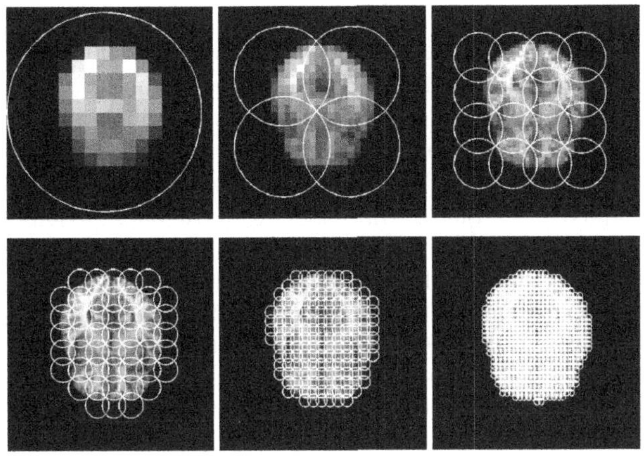

Fig. 1 Illustration of the hierarchical framework. Yellow circles represent the supports of RBFs.

The prior term used in this study was the Laplacian model of the velocity field, which gives a smaller penalty for smoother deformation:

$$E_2(\exp V) = \frac{1}{\Omega}\iiint \left[\left(\frac{\partial V}{\partial x}\right)^2 + \left(\frac{\partial V}{\partial y}\right)^2 + \left(\frac{\partial V}{\partial z}\right)^2\right] dxdydz. \quad (8)$$

In our case, Ω is the support of the current RBF.

E. A Hierarchical Framework

This study used a hierarchical framework similar to that used in [9] in order to increase accuracy and stability. The overall velocity field can be represented as the sum of RBFs with various levels of support extents (or scale level):

$$V = \sum_{j=1}^{L} \sum_{i=1}^{K_j} \alpha_{j,i} \Psi\left(\frac{\|x-c_{j,i}\|}{s_{j,i}}\right) , \quad (9)$$

where L specifies the total number of scale level and K_j denotes the number of RBFs at level j.

The optimization begins with coarse registration using large RBFs and low-resolution images. As the level increases, the mapping is gradually refined through the use of detailed images and smaller RBFs. The RBFs are placed along grid points and the estimation of the coefficient of an RBF is skipped if the evaluation region of this RBF does not contain any brain tissue. This hierarchical framework is illustrated in Fig. 1.

III. RESULTS

A. Data and Registration

Evaluation of the proposed algorithm was performed using the LPBA40 dataset provided by the Laboratory of Neuro Imaging (LONI) at UCLA [12]. LBPA40 contains

256×256×124 T1-wieghted brain MR images (1×1×1 mm resolution) of 40 healthy, normal volunteers with manually delineated labels. The registration process for each image pair comprised 12-parameter affine registration (FLIRT) followed by the proposed non-rigid registration process. The registration of all 1560 source-target pairs was performed on a Linux workstation with 16 Intel Genuine® CPU cores and 48 GB main memory.

An example of the registration result is shown in Fig. 2. The source image (red contours) yields much better correspondence to the target image (gray-scale image) after registration. Quantitative evaluations with regard to various respects are shown in the following sections.

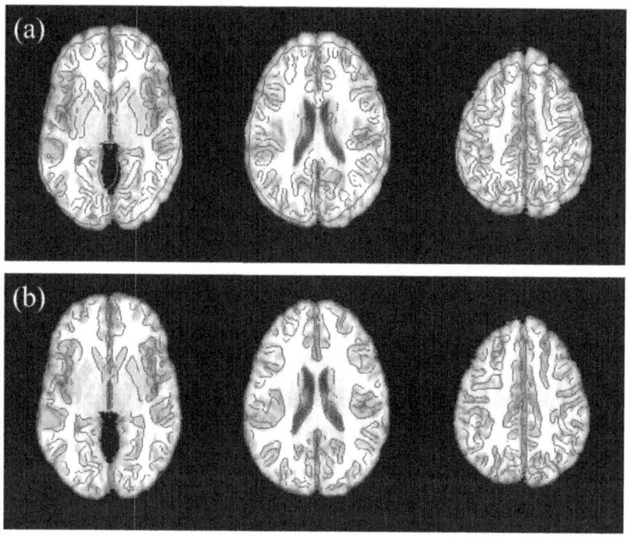

Fig. 2 An example of registration result. The target image is represented with grayscale image superimposed by the contours of the source image (red lines). (a) Before registration. (b) After registration.

B. Evaluation of Diffeomorphism

Evaluation of diffeomorphism was performed using the determinants of the Jacobian matrices of the mapping functions ($\det(\nabla\Phi^{T}\circ x)$). This measure indicates the volume ratio before and after warping. Regions with non-positive determinants indicate lost one-to-one mapping. Our evaluation showed that all voxels off 1560 registrations yield positive determinant values, completely conforming to the property of diffeomorphism.

C. Evaluation of Symmetry

Two types of error measures were designed to evaluate the symmetry: mean residual ($r^{(avg)}$) and mean *inconsistency of velocity fields* ($\mathrm{ICV}^{(avg)}$):

$$r^{(avg)}(A,B) = \mathrm{avg}_{x\in\Omega}\|(\Phi_{A\to B}\circ\Phi_{B\to A} - \mathrm{Id})(x)\|_2 \quad ,(10)$$

$$\mathrm{ICV}^{(avg)}(A,B) = \mathrm{avg}_{x\in\Omega}\|V_{A\to B}(x) + V_{B\to A}(x)\|_2 \quad .(11)$$

Id denotes identity function. The interpretation of error from these two kinds of error measure differs in some respects. While ICV indicates how well the registration algorithm conforms to the properties of symmetry, residuals reflect the actual errors of symmetry of the warped images, which include the numerical errors induced by the finite difference method as well as the discrete representation of velocity field.

All 780 pairs of forward and inverse registrations in LPBA40 dataset were used to evaluate the symmetry of the proposed algorithm. The results are shown in Table 1. It showed that the mean residual is far below the width of the voxels. The largest residual among all results is 0.8503 mm, which is still within the width of the voxels. Furthermore, the ICV is always zero in all registrations. This implies that our algorithm is perfectly symmetric in estimating velocity fields, and the error in residuals is guaranteed to reduce with the use of high-resolution velocity fields or finite difference methods with more number of steps.

Table 1 Error of symmetry for all pairs of forward and inverse registrations in LPBA40 dataset. All 0's are exact values

Number of levels	Mean residual (mm)	Mean. ICA (mm)
1 level	0.0002 (0.0001)	0 (0)
2 levels	0.0004 (0.0001)	0 (0)
3 levels	0.0014 (0.0002)	0 (0)
4 levels	0.0047 (0.0006)	0 (0)
5 levels	0.0125 (0.0011)	0 (0)
6 levels	0.0200 (0.0013)	0 (0)

D. Evaluation of Accuracy

To ensure an objective comparison, we evaluated the accuracy using the procedure proposed in [13] and compared with the result of other 14 registration algorithm listed (6 of which are diffeomorphic). The median target overlap (TO) value for level-5 results and level-6 results were 0.731 and 0.742 respectively. The highest median TO value reported by [13] was approximately 0.725. A more recent study [14] reported a median TO value of 0.753.

E. Evaluation of Speed

100 randomly selected image pairs LPBA40 dataset were registered with parallel computing scheme disabled. The speed comparison with the 6 diffeomorphic algorithms reported in [13] are shown in Table 2.

This comparison is rough but still valid since our experiments were run on similar computing environment to that used in [13]. Lower mean rank, as reported in [13], indicates better accuracy of the algorithm. Our algorithm, when using 5 scale levels, is faster than all other algorithms listed. Although the proposed algorithm using 6 levels is slower than 2 of the 6 algorithms, we must emphasize again that our algorithm, either with 5 or 6 scale levels, yields accuracy higher than all of the listed algorithm.

Table 2 Comparison of speed with other diffeomorphic registration methods.

Algorithm	Mean Rank	Run time (min)
Proposed (level 5)	n/a	~4.5
Proposed (level 6)	n/a	~25
SyN	1.00	77 (15.1)
ART	1.00	20 (1.6)
DARTEL	1.88	71.8 (6.3)
JRD-fluid	2.50	71.1 (1.0)
Diffeomorphic Demons	3.00	8.7 (1.2)
SICLE	> 4	33.5 (6.6)

IV. CONCLUSIONS

In this study we developed an efficient non-rigid registration algorithm, which is symmetric and diffeomorphic. Our evaluation has shown that the proposed algorithm is fully diffeomorphic and has sub-voxel accuracy in terms of symmetry. Also, it outperforms all registration algorithms listed in [13] in term of accuracy, and is faster than the top-ranked diffeomorphic registration algorithm. Future work will include improvements of accuracy and further evaluation based on a variety of datasets and evaluation methods.

ACKNOWLEDGMENT

This work was supported in part by the UST-UCSD International Center of Excellence in Advanced Bioengineering sponsored by the Taiwan Ministry of Science and Technology I-RiCE Program under Grant NSC-102-2911-I-009-101, the Taipei Veterans General Hospital under Grant V102E3-004, and by the Taiwan Ministry of Science and Technology under Grants NSC-102-2220-E-009-040, NSC-102-2629-B-010-001, and NSC-102-2918-I-009-016.

CONFLICT OF INTEREST

The authors declare that they have no conflicts of interest.

REFERENCES

1. Ashburner J (2007) A fast diffeomorphic image registration algorithm. NeuroImage. 38(1):95-113.
2. Beg et al. (2005) Computing large deformation metric mappings via geodesic flows of diffeomorphisms. International Journal of Computer Vision. 61(2):139-157.
3. Vercauteren T et al. (2009) Diffeomorphic demons: Efficient non-parametric image registration. NeuroImage. 45(1):S61-S72.
4. Avants B.B. et al. (2008) Symmetric diffeomorphic image registration with cross-correlation: evaluating automated labeling of elderly and neurodegenerative brain. Medical image analysis. 12(1):26-41.
5. Christensen G.E. et al. (1996) Deformable templates using large deformation kinematics. IEEE Transactions on Image Processing. 5(10):1435-1447.
6. Reuter M. et al. (2010) Highly accurate inverse consistent registration: A robust approach. NeuroImage. 53(4):1181-1196.
7. Arsigny V. et al. (2006) A log-euclidean framework for statistics on diffeomorphisms. in Medical Image Computing and Computer-Assisted Intervention. 924-931.
8. Wendland H. (1995) Piecewise polynomial, positive definite and compactly supported radial functions of minimal degree. Advances in computational Mathematics. 4(1):389-396.
9. Liu J.-X. et al. (2010) Fast and accurate registration techniques for affine and nonrigid alignment of MR brain images. Annals of Biomedical Engineering. 38(1):138-157.
10. Rohde G.K. et al. (2003) The adaptive bases algorithm for intensity-based nonrigid image registration. IEEE Transactions on Medical Imaging. 22(11):1470-1479.
11. Flannery B.P. et al. (1992) Numerical Recipes in C.
12. Shattuck D.W. et al. (2008) Construction of a 3D probabilistic atlas of human cortical structures. NeuroImage. 39(3).1064-1080.
13. Klein A. et al. (2009) Evaluation of 14 nonlinear deformation algorithms applied to human brain MRI registration. NeuroImage. 46(3):786-802.
14. Ashburner J and Friston KJ (2011) Diffeomorphic registration using geodesic shooting and Gauss-Newton optimisation. NeuroImage. 55(3):954-967

Author: Yong-Sheng Chen
Institute: National Chiao Tung University
Street: 1001 University Road
City: Hsinchu
Country: Taiwan
Email: yschen@cs.nctu.edu.tw

Beyond Supporting Pathological Diagnosis: Concept of Support System for Pathologist and Researcher

Takumi Ishikawa[1], Junko Takahashi[1], Hiroshi Takemura[1], Hiroshi Mizoguchi[1], and Takeshi Kuwata[2]

[1] Department of Mechanical Engineering, Tokyo University of Science, Japan
[2] Department of Medical Physics, National Cancer Center Hospital East, Japan

Abstract— **This paper presents the Support System for auto-Pathological Diagnosis (P-SSD) to support pathologists and researchers of auto-pathological diagnosis. P-SSD has two main contributions. First, P-SSD detects cancer area with machine learning methods, and then shows cancer areas to pathologists. The pathologists can make diagnosis with the detected result, which reduce the burden on pathologists. Second, P-SSD is an open software platform for pathological image too. The platform offers some basic functionalities to load and display pathological images, and implement the image-processing methods though plugins. It helps researchers to apply feature calculation and machine leaning techniques to the pathological images effortlessly. In conclusion, P-SSD is the software with potential applications in both of pathological diagnosis and research.**

Keywords— **Auto-pathological diagnosis system, Image-processing.**

I. INTRODUCTION

In Japan, cancer is the most cause of death and killed almost 400,000 people in 2012, which is about 30% in all cause of death. The number of patients suffering from cancer is still increasing every year. On the other hand, the number of pathologists remain almost constant; the shortage of pathologists means that the burden of work each pathologist shoulders gets heavier and heavier, resulting in causing false diagnosis. To prevent those false diagnoses, a support system for auto-pathological diagnosis is needed.

A pathological virtual slide (Fig. 1), which is created when glass slides are digitally scanned, has been increasingly used both for diagnosis and researches, and a lot of methods for auto-pathological diagnosis system have been proposed [1]. Most of them calculate features, learn the features, and then detect cancer by a computer. Takahashi et al. [2] proposed the method that detects cancer area with HLAC and Support Vector Machine (SVM). Ishibashi et al. [3] applied wavelet transformation to calculate frequency features from pathological images. Doyle et al. [4] proposed a multi-resolution Bayesian classifier with AdaBoost and applied that method to the pathological image.

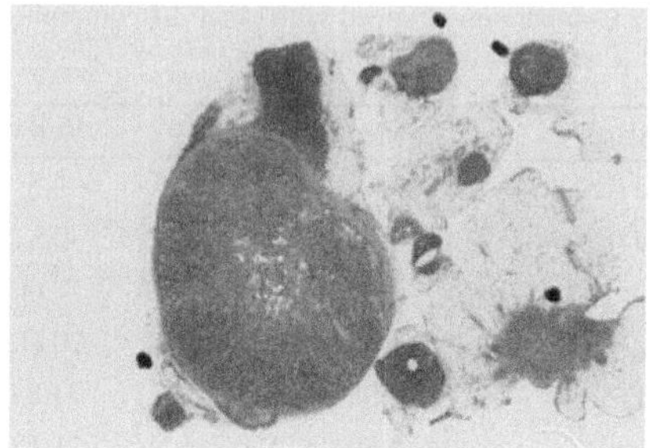

Fig.1 Example of the virtual slide. The tissues in this slide are stained by Hematoxylin and Eosin (HE).

However, the researchers need specific knowledge to work directly on these images, because the virtual slides are usually unique formats. The researchers generally convert the unique format of virtual slide to the normal image format such as JPEG and BMP by the specific viewer, and save the converted images (cvt-image). The cvt-images are still very high resolution, and often occupy several Gigabytes in a computer's memory, which makes it difficult to fully open the saved cvt-images. For example, one 42 x 24 mm slide glass is about 60000 x 52000 pixels image size. To use the cvt-image, the researchers need to save the cvt-image dividing the image into small size images.

There are the other problems in the pathological image-processing research field. In the other image processing research field such as facial recognition [5] and vehicle recognition [6], open standard image database is available. The methods for those fields are assessed correctly because they can be easily compared using that database. On the other hand, the techniques for pathological image processing cannot be assessed correctly since there is no standard database.

There are several open software for bio-image processing research filed. NDP.view is the specific viewer software for "ndpi" format images which is one of the most used slides image format. With NDP.view, pathologists and researchers can convert and save an image on a display such as JPEG and BMP. Resolution of the image is the same as one of the display. The GNU Image Manipulation Program (GIMP) [7] can implement several image-processing methods, and apply them to pathological images after NDP.view convert

I. Lackovic (ed.), *1st Global Conference on Biomedical Engineering & 9th Asian-Pacific Conference on Medical and Biological Engineering*,
IFMBE Proceedings 47, DOI: 10.1007/978-3-319-12262-5_37

virtual slide into processable image format in GIMP and save that image. ImageJ [8] can also apply image-processing methods to pathological images. One of the most interesting characteristics of ImageJ is that it has plugin functionality. C. Deroulers [9] introduced "NDPITools" to ImageJ as the plugin. This plugin enables ImageJ to handle on "ndpi" format image. ImageJ with the plugin firstly converts a virtual slide image to the normal format image, and save these images. Then, ImageJ applies image-processing methods to the pathological images. However, both GIMP and ImageJ don't directly deal with the virtual slides. They need to convert the virtual slide image into processable image format in GIMP or ImageJ, save that image dividing the images into several parts before applying image-processing techniques. It takes more time and computer's memory than directly applying image-processing techniques to the images.

Therefore, we propose and develop the Support System for Pathological Diagnosis (P-SSD). P-SSD consists of several subsystems that make it easy not only for pathologists to double-check their diagnosis but also for researchers to apply image-processing techniques to pathological images. Moreover, the standard pathological database collected by P-SSD is available to researchers.

The rest of this paper is organized as follows. In Section 2, we describe concept of P-SSD. In section 3, we explain recent work on P-SSD and compare it with other software. Some brief conclusions are drawn in the last section.

II. P-SSD

We propose P-SSD to support both pathologists and researchers developing auto-pathological diagnosis system. Fig. 2 shows flow of P-SSD. P-SSD consists of five main subsystems as follows: (i) Converting system, (ii) Supervised database system, (iii) Learning system, (iv) Detection system,(v) Showing system. P-SSD is built with Visual Studio C++, Win32 API and OpenCV. P-SSD has plugin function, which make it easy to apply image-processing to the pathological images.

A. Converting System

This system converts a virtual slide into the proposed original format image. A virtual slide is created as a unique format image when a glass slide is digitally scanned. To deal with the unique format of the virtual slide, P-SSD converts the virtual slide into the proposed format pathological image. It enables researchers to apply image processing to a virtual slide without saving it as other formats. It is easy for researchers with P-SSD to work on the pathological images. Moreover, with P-SSD, time and computer's memory spent to output a virtual slide image as a processable image for researchers are greatly reduced.

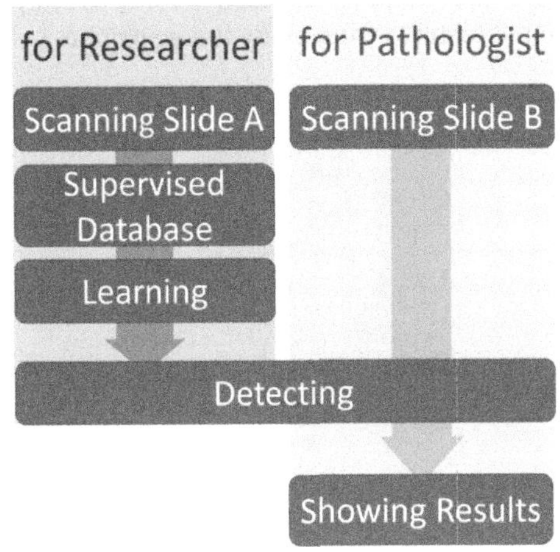

Fig. 2 P-SSD consists of the five processes as follows; (i) converting virtual slide into standard format image, (ii) obtaining supervised database, (iii) learning the feature of cancer cell, (iv) detecting cancer area with learning model, (v) showing the result to pathologists.

B. Supervised Database System

This system obtains supervised database. In P-SSD, in order to obtain the supervised database for researchers, the standardized pathological images are supervised by pathologists marking outlines of cancer areas as shown in Fig. 3, and cancer area is in a blue outline. Pathologists can see a pathological image as a whole because the image is converted into low resolution images with P-SSD. Then the supervised data is outputted as series of points in xml file, and a set of the supervised data and images are stored in the database. Fig. 4 shows the output file; the lines from first to eleventh show first cancer area. Third and seventh lines indicate x-coordinates of points of outline, and fourth and eighth lines indicate one y-coordinate of points of outline. Lines from twelfth to fourteenth shows second cancer area. When that output data is reshown, the series of points are linked to form outlines. By saving the supervised data as text data, not image, computer's memory spent is reduced.

C. Learning System

This system learns the features of cancer and non-cancer. Many methods of cancer detection have been proposed, and the cancer detection method is implemented mostly by the machine learning. The methods calculate features from pathological images supervised by pathologists, and then the learning model is built by machine learning methods.

Usually in researches, the virtual slide is divided into image patches, and the features are then calculated from the image patches. P-SSD can divide the pathological images into the image patches. Those image patches are rectangle images whose size are properly decided by the researchers, and calculate the features from every image patches.

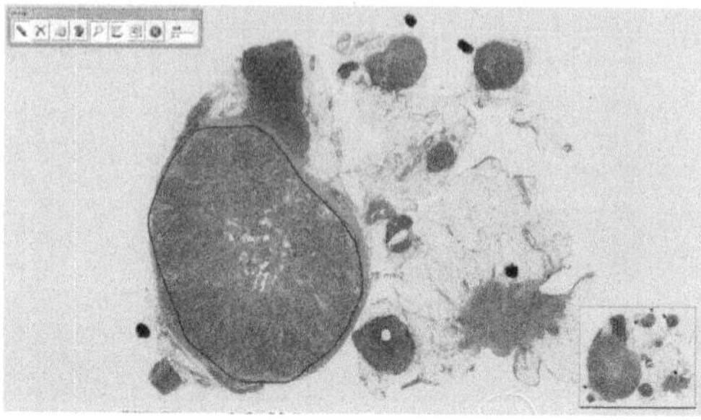

Fig 3 The supervised image. A blue outline indicates the cancer area.

```
<line number="1"> //First cancer area
  <point>
    <x>X1_VALUE</x> //x-coordinate of points
    <y>Y1_VALUE</y> //y-coordinate of points
  </point>
  <point>
    <x>X2_VALUE</x>
    <y>Y2_VALUE</y>
  </point>
...
</line>
<line number="2"> //Second cancer area
...
</line>
```

Fig. 4 Example of the supervised data. From first line to eleventh line show first cancer area. Third and seventh lines indicate x-coordinates of points of outline, and fourth and eighth lines indicate one y-coordinate of points of outline. From twelfth line to fourteenth line shows second cancer area.

The learning model is used in two ways. One way is that it is used for cancer detection in the non-supervised pathological virtual slide, which is explained in the next section. The other way is that the learning model is used for classifying the database into each kind of caner and non-cancer. These classified databases can be used by students majoring in pathology and any other people who are in this field.

D. Detection System

This system detects cancer area. After the virtual slide is divided into image patches, the features are calculated from the image patches on the same way as the learning process. Then, with the applied learning data, cancer area is detected in unsupervised pathological images. Fig. 5 shows an example of xml file P-SSD outputs as result. In the result xml file, the central coordinates of the image patches is shown at the third and the fourth lines. The sixth line shows the detection result. If there is a cancer cell in the interest area, P-SSD outputs TRUE, otherwise, P-SSD outputs FALSE.

```
<brock>
  <point>
    <x>X1_VALUE</x> //x-coordinate
    <y>Y1_VALUE</y> //y-coordinate
  </point>
  <result>TRUE</result> //the result of detection
</brock>
```

Fig. 5 Example of the result xml. The lines from first to seventh show the result of one cancer area. Third and fourth lines indicate a center coordinate of the image patches in the cancer area. Sixth line shows the result of detection.

E. Showing System

This system shows the detected cancer area of a pathological image by painting in red those image patches that includes cancer based on the xml file, each area is shown in a rectangle shape. Pathologists can double-check the cancer area with the result image of detection. Also, P-SSD can screen and sort out the result images with detected cancer from ones without it beforehand, so that pathologists can start the diagnostic work from there.

F. Plugin

There are many features and learning techniques for pathological images in the world. To make it easy to apply those techniques to pathological images, we introduce the plugin function to P-SSD. Also, the techniques for the pathological images such as auto-nuclei segmentation [10] and auto-prediction [11] except for auto-cancer detection are applied to the pathological images.

III. RECENT WORK ON P-SSD

In this paper, P-SSD use "ndpi" format images as the virtual slides image.The existing software such as GIMP and NDPTool need to divide whole virtual slide image which is a 60000 x 52000 pixels image into parts before the pathologists can supervise the images. Table 1 shows the number and the size of the output images from whole virtual slide image. For GIMP, 2336 images of 1920x1024 pixels BMP images, whose resolution depend on the size of display, are saved using NDP.view. For NDPTool, 16 images of 60000 x 52000 pixels TIFF images are saved.

Pathologists mark the outlines using a mouse or a pen tablet, and change some colors of the outlines. Also the pathologists can zoom in and out an interest area with a mouse wheel changing the resolution. Max magnification depends on a scanning machine. After marking the cancer area, the size of the area surrounded by the outlines get calculated, and shown on the image.

In this paper, P-SSD learns and detects cancer after calculating HLAC feature from 128 x128 pathological image patches. The learning model is only used for the cancer detection. The result image of detecting cancer area in that image is painted in red. Each red-painted area is 128 x 128 pixels because the results of cancer detection are outputted in every 128 x 128 pixels.

Table 1 The number and size of images after dividing the virtual slide into the images. NDP.view outputs BMP format images, and ImageJ outputs TIFF format images.

	NDP.view	ImageJ	Our system
The num of images after dividing	2336	16	-
The size of images after dividing	13GB	270MB	-

IV. Conclusions

This paper has presented the Support System for auto-Pathological Diagnosis (P-SSD) to support both the pathologists and the researchers. P-SSD consists of five subsystems: converting system, obtaining supervised database system, learning system, detection system and showing system. Converting system enables researchers to handle the virtual slides directly without outputting them as other format images. In order to obtain the supervised database for researches, with supervised database system, the pathological images are supervised by pathologists marking outlines of cancer areas. Learning system builds leaning model by learning the features of cancer in the pathological images, and then with the learning model, detection system detects cancer areas by distinguishing cancer and non-cancer. Finally, showing system shows the result of cancer detection. We introduce plugin function to P-SSD, which makes it easy to apply feature calculation and leaning techniques.

With P-SSD, the pathologists can double-check the pathological diagnosis, and the researchers can apply their techniques to pathological images more easily. P-SSD can support not only pathologists, but also researchers of auto-pathological diagnosis. Moreover, P-SSD greatly reduces time and computer's memory spent to save the virtual slide image as the normal format.

Conflict of Inteest

The authors declare that they have no conflict of interest.

References

1. Metin N. Gurcan, Laura E. Boucheron, Ali Can, Anant Madabhushi, Nasir M. Rajpoot, Bulent Yener, "Histopathological Image Analysis," Biomedical Engineering, IEEE Reviews, Vol. 2, 2009, pp.147-171.
2. Junko Takahashi, Hiroshi Takemura, Hiroshi Mizoguchi, Takeshi Kuwata,"System to Detect Abnormal Cells in Pathological Images using Higher-order Local Autocorrelation Features and Color Spaces," The 2012 International Conference of Information Science and Computer Applications, 2012, pp.284-288.
3. Yuichi Ishibashi, Atsuko Hara, Isao Okayasu and Koji Kurihara, "DEVELOPMENT OF HISTOPATHOLOGICAL INFORMATION DATABASE SYSTEM WHICH ENABLES IMAGE RETRIEVAL USING IMAGE FEATURES AND TEXT INFORMATION," Journal of the Japanese Society of Computational Statistics, Vol. 24, No.1, 2011, pp.3-21.
4. S. Doyle, M. Feldman, J. Tomaszeweski, and A. Madabhushi, "A boosted Bayesian multiresolution classifier for prostate cancer detection from digitized needle biopsies," IEEE Trans. Biomed. Eng., vol. 59, no. 5, 2012, pp. 1205–1218.
5. Teja G.P., Ravi S., "Face recognition using subspaces techniques," Recent Trends In Information Technology (ICRTIT), 2012 International Conference, 2012, pp. 103-107.
6. Sivaraman S., Trivedi M. M., "A General Active-Learning Framework for On-Road Vehicle Recognition and Tracking," Intelligent Transportation Systems, IEEE Transactions, 2010, Vol. 11, pp. 267-276.
7. Available: http://www.gimp.org/
8. W. Rasband, "ImageJ," U. S. National Institutes of Health, Bethesda, Maryland, USA. [Online]. http://imagej.nih.gov/ij/
9. Duque J. J. Silva L. F., Murta L.O., "Open Architecture Software Platform for Biomedical Signal Analysis," Engineering in Medicine and Biology Society, 2013 35thAnnual International Conference of the IEEE, 2013, pp. 2084-2087.
10. Veta M, van Diest PJ, Kornegoor R, Huisman A, Viergever MA, et al. " Automatic Nuclei Segmentation in H&E Stained Breast Cancer Histopathology Images," 2013, PLoS ONE 8(7): e70221. doi:10.1371/journal.pone.0070221.
11. Banu G. S., Fareeth A., Hudewale N., "Prediction of Breast Cancer in Mammagram image using Support Vector Machine and Fuzzy C-means," Biomedical and Health Informatics (BHI), 2012 IEEE-EMBS International Conference, 2012, pp. 573-576.

Author: Takumi Ishikawa
Institute: Tokyo University of Science
Street: 2641 Yamazaki, Noda
City: Chiba
Country: Japan
Email: 7513606@ed.tus.ac.jp

A Full Digital Design of TCD Ultrasound System Using Normal Pulse and Coded Excitation

Jie Li, Xianfen Diao, Kai Zhan, and Zhengdi Qin

National-Regional Key Technology Engineering Laboratory of China for Medical Ultrasound, Shenzhen University, Shenzhen, P.R.China
Department of Biomedical Engineering, Health Science Center, Shenzhen University, Shenzhen, P.R.China

Abstract— **Transcranial Doppler (TCD) ultrasound is commonly used in some departments to detect blood flow and emboli in the cerebral artery at the forefront of medical technology. Conventional TCD systems expose more and more disadvantages such as inadequate depth information, low sensitivity and poor accuracy in clinical diagnosis. In this study, a full digital design of TCD ultrasound system is introduced, in which raw radiofrequency (RF) is directly converted to digital data with an A/D converter. All signal processors such as digital I/Q demodulator can be achieved by utilizing digital signal processing (DSP) techniques. This design can solve the problems above. In particular, it offers a full-depth intracranial examination, which can be used to locate transcranial windows conveniently so as to make TCD analysis much easier even for an inexperienced person. Furthermore, coded excitation is allowed. In our experimental system, RF signals are collected *in vitro* from a flow phantom using a TCD system, which alternately transmitted 8 wavelengths normal pulse and 4 wavelengths pulse coded by 7-chip Barker code. The *in vitro* results are promising. Qualitatively the blood flow is easier to track using the pulse compressed signal. It is both feasible and beneficial to implement the full digital design in a TCD system.**

Keywords— **Barker, Coded excitation, Digital demodulator, Full-depth, TCD.**

I. INTRODUCTION

Transcranial Doppler (TCD) ultrasound offers a complete array of dedicated studies to address many clinical applications, such as diagnosis of extracranial and intracranial stenosis and occlusion, monitoring during carotid endarterectomy or carotid stenting and detection and counting of emboli [1]. More and more departments in hospitals have outfitted TCD instruments, and some higher quality requirements are claimed at the same time. Currently, most TCDs are analog PC-based systems with bulky and complicated structure whose performances cannot meet doctors' or researches' demands. Furthermore, it will take a considerable time for a freshman to be a TCD technician. So, it is inevitable to develop the next generation of TCD ultrasonography system to cater for clinical diagnosis. The full digital design is one of the promising methods.

In conventional structures of a TCD ultrasound system, RF signal from transducer passes through a T/R (Transmit and Receive) switch (such as MD0101 produced by Supertex inc.), which is designed to protect a low noise receiver from the high voltage transmit pulses in ultrasound applications. And a dual I/Q demodulator and phase shifter (such as AD8333 produced by ADI) demodulates the RF signal after T/R switch. The two channels of I&Q signals are respectively conditioned by amplifiers, dynamic noise reduction systems and filters. Then I/Q signal is depth-sampled, thereby losing most Doppler information except for those in the sample depths. As a result, less depths blood flow information are displayed in conventional TCD systems. Then the depth-sampled signal passes through wall filter previous to analog-to-digital conversion.

To achieve full-depth examination, any depth information should not be lost. When implemented with full digital TCD system introduced in this study, full-depth information can be obtained because A/D converter directly collects RF signal without demodulation and depth-sampling, thereby containing full-depth Doppler information. All depths information in RF signal is processed simultaneously while analog TCD systems cannot support such large-scale data computing. This full-depth examination is similar to power M-mode Doppler (PMD) described in the report by Moehring and Spencer [2]. However, PMD scheme is just a digital-to-be system. Fig. 1 shows the schematics of a conventional system and full digital TCD ultrasound system respectively.

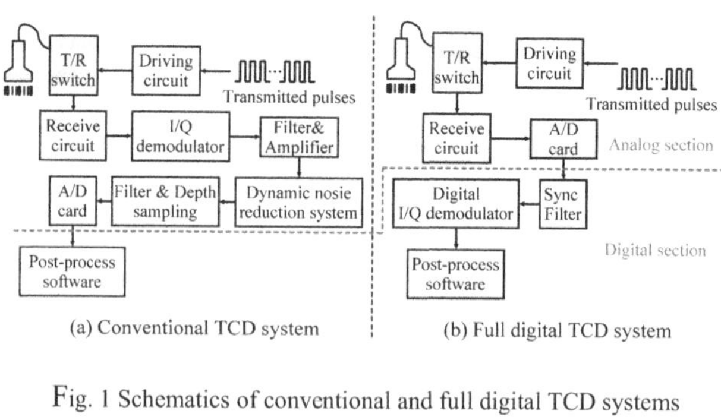

Fig. 1 Schematics of conventional and full digital TCD systems

When executing the full digital design, coded excitation can be used as transmitted pulse. Normal pulse excitation

I. Lackovic (ed.), *1st Global Conference on Biomedical Engineering & 9th Asian-Pacific Conference on Medical and Biological Engineering*,
IFMBE Proceedings 47, DOI: 10.1007/978-3-319-12262-5_38

was seriously limited by the narrow bandwidth of the transmitted pulse which led to poor axial resolution. The axial resolution is inversely proportional to the length of transmitted pulse. Long transmitted pulse is required to obtain an adequate singal-to-noise ratio (SNR). Which means that the tradeoff between axial resolution and SNR in ultrasound system. To improve the resolution, the transmitted pulse length needs to be decreased. In doing so, the pressure amplitude over the duration of the pulse would need to be increased to obtain an adequate SNR. However, increasing the pressure amplitude would increase the mechanical index (MI) and could potentially have an adverse effect on the system safety. Several researches have validated that coded excitation is a feasible and beneficial method to solve the problem [3] [4] [5] [6]. This scheme must be carried out in full digital system.

On the other side, miniaturization and portability are the other trends in the development of medical facilities. Because of the huge signal computing and complicated hardware circuit, most conventional TCD systems are PC-based with giant structures and high power consumption. In full digital TCD design, RF signal is conditioned by T/R switch (such as TL441 produced by TI), then the signal input to a high-speed A/D converter and the data are stored in an onboard buffer. In this case, system can get rid of most analog circuits for signal processing and reduce the demands of signal processor, hence accomplishing miniaturization of TCD system. Moreover, more accuracy and reliability in clinical diagnosis can be achieved using full digital design.

The aim of this study was to validate the viability and benefits of full digital design in TCD ultrasound system. *In vitro* experiments were implemented to perform the promised results in both normal pulse and coded excitation TCD systems. The blood flow signals in different depths can be extracted and displayed at the same time.

II. METHODOLOGY

A. Digital Demodulator

In Doppler ultrasound systems, I/Q demodulation is a common and useful RF signal processing technique since it allows for the direct extraction of amplitude and phase information. Generally, an analog approach to quadrature demodulation shown in Fig. 2 is used under the analog circumstances. I and Q signals are obtained by low-pass filters to remove the sum frequency components generated by the mixing operation. I and Q are digitized by an analog-to-digital (A/D) converter in each channel [7]. When implemented with conventional analog RF components, the demodulator requires the frequency of local carrier to strictly match the frequency of base pulse. While periodic offsets between the local carrier signal and base pulse caused by non-linear characteristics of analog devices, some variations in manufacturing and differences in operation environments lead to mismatch[8]. Besides, a number of inherent errors also degrade the performance of analog I/Q demodulator, including gain balance, DC offsets, impedance match and carrier leakage [9]. As noted above, numerous deficiencies associated current techniques limit the analog demodulator's performance. Techniques for correcting errors in I and Q signals have been proposed in articles by F. E. Churchill et al [10] and D. L. Sharpin et al [11]. However, these techniques for calibrating errors in I and Q signals are nontrivial to implement since the errors must be measured with appropriate test signals and the necessary correction algorithms carried out.

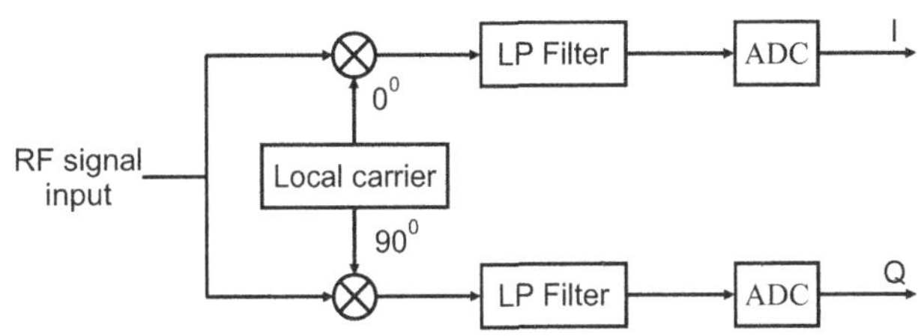

Fig. 2 Conventional I/Q demodulator

Consequently, it would be highly desirable to implement DSP techniques which have several advantages over analog signal processing due to its accuracy, predictability, repeatability and stability. As the full digital design was used in TCD ultrasound system, DSP techniques can be used under the digital circumstances. Recent advances in high-speed analog-to-digital converters allow digital I/Q demodulator to be well implemented, greatly reducing these systematic errors. Fig. 3 shows a design of digital demodulator implementation that inherently improves the performance.

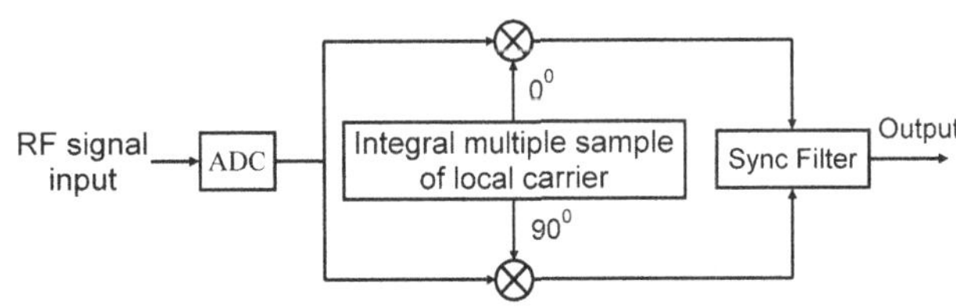

Fig. 3 Digital I/Q demodulator

B. Pulse Generation

To confirm the feasibility of full digital design in both normal pulse and coded excitation TCD ultrasound systems, normal pulse and coded signal were generated by an arbitrary waveform generator. In this experiment, the normal pulse is an 8wavelengths binary sequence which most of energy focused within the transducer bandwidth and the coded transmitted signal is an oversampled 7-chip Barker code demodulated by 4 wavelengths base pulse sequence.

C. Experiment Set-up

In our experimental system, a flow phantom is set up as shown in the schematic in Fig. 4. The depth of the phantom is 10cm. The blood mimicking fluid in it circulates around the flow loop as the flow direction shown in Fig. 4. Flow rate can be controlled by a pump controller. A 2 MHz transducer is used for detecting the blood flow signal while the phantom is run.

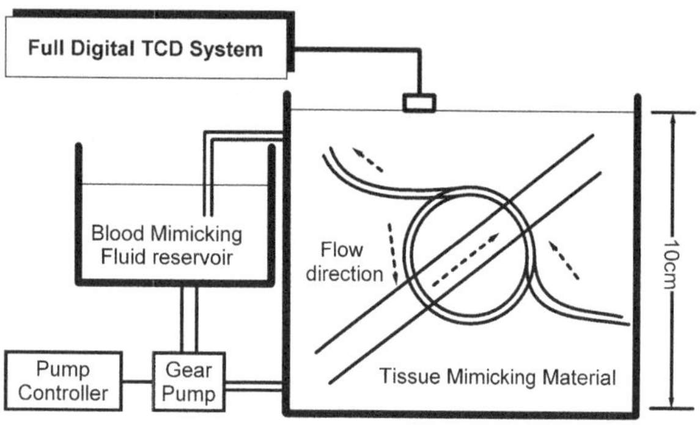

Fig. 4 Schematic of flow phantom

The experimental system is based on a commercially available TCD ultrasound system. The clock source (16 MHz) of the experimental system is connected to an arbitrary waveform generator as external main clock. The arbitrary waveform generator generates 2-channel transmitted signals, trigger signal and 8MHz external clock for A/D converter as sample frequency (f_s). It is flexible to give different transmissions including normal pulse and Barker coded pulses to our experimental system, the trigger signal and 8 MHz clock signal were connected to the PC-housed 16-bit A/D converter. When the RF cable, external 8MHz clock and trigger signal were continuously input to the A/D converter and the data were stored in an on-board buffer. In our experimental system, a single-sensor transducer at 2 MHz was used to insonate the flow phantom at a pulse repetition frequency (PRF) of 7812.5 Hz.

III. Results

After A/D converter, RF data is saved in a variable as row vector in MATLAB. After digital I/Q demodulation, down-sampling and decoding (if coded excitation), the row vector is reshaped as a $M \times N$ dimensional matrix X. M is the number of samples in depth and N is the number of frames in a specified time. Then add a window of W_T in time domain to $X_{M\times N}$ to reduce the Gibbs effect:

$$Y_{M\times N} = X_{M\times N} .* W_T \tag{1}$$

Where $Y_{M\times N}$ is the data after windowing. The following is spectral analysis of $Y_{M\times N}$ based on STFT and appropriate windowing operation in frequency domain:

$$Z = FFT\left[Y_{M\times N}\right] \cdot * W_F \tag{2}$$

Where $FFT[\cdot]$ is STFT operation, W_F is a window in frequency domain. Promising results shown in Fig. 5 can be achieved from matrix Z. Full-depth blood flow information is described in this figure. X-axis is depth and Y-axis is the envelope of frequency shift. Two peaks (P1 and P2 labeled in Fig. 5(a) and Fig. 5(b)) of the line are the blood flow in this depth. Furthermore, as the Y-axis and the width of those two peaks shown, expected effects in both axial resolution and SNR were attained using coded excitation.

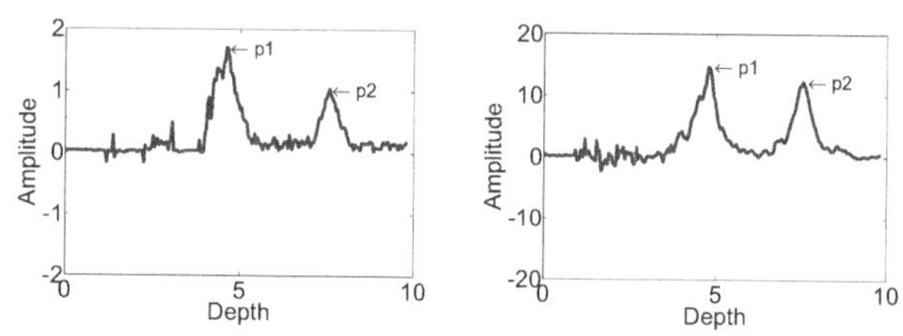

(a) Normal pulse excitation

(b) Barker coded excitation

Fig. 5 Blood flow information in full-depth in vitro is detected by experimental system using normal pulse and coded excitation

According to the image of full-depth blood flow information above shown in the Fig. 5, the depth which has blood flow can be directly found so as to conveniently check the blood flow of the depth and display it. The depths of P1 and P2 are 4.62cm and 7.58cm. Fig. 6(a) (b) and Fig. 7(a) (b) depict the blood flow information in the depth which P1 and P2 located using normal pulse and coded excitation respectively.

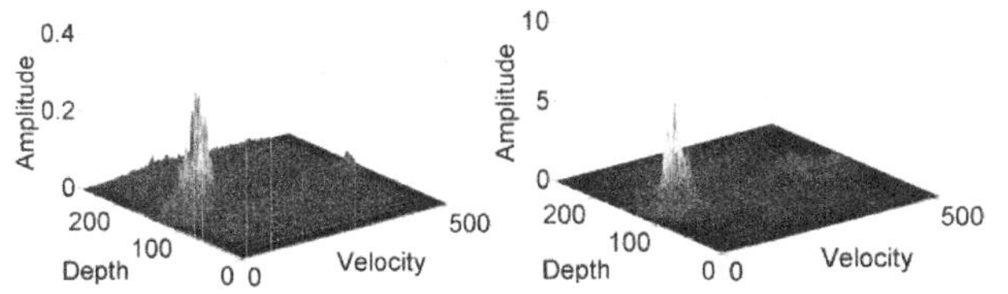

(a) Normal pulse excitation (b) Barker coded excitation

Fig. 6 Blood flow in the depth which P1 located

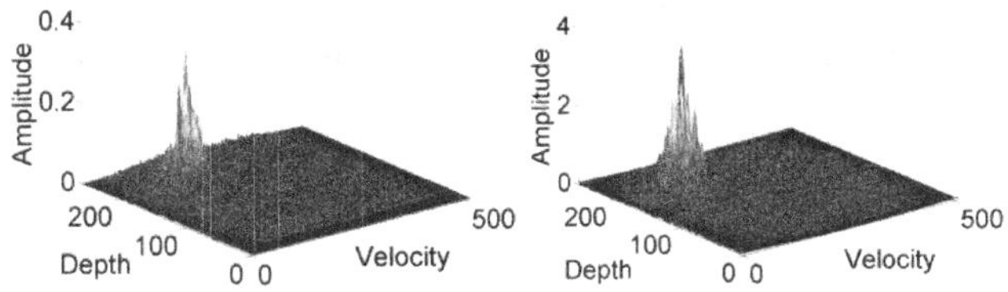

(a) Normal pulse excitation (b) Barker coded excitation

Fig. 7 Blood flow in the depth which P2 located

IV. Conclusions

The results above evidently validate the viability and benefit of the full digital design in TCD ultrasound system using both normal pulse and coded excitation. The full-depth examination from full digital design facilitates vessel identification using depth and direction of flow, and transcranial windows can be easily found and maintained so that it is not necessary to seek a window by changing depth or listening for a Doppler sound. The full digital design of TCD ultrasound system can improve the sensitivity and reliability of detection, but sharp decline the complexity and power consumption.

Restricted by the experimental conditions, there were no vessels within a real cranium with mimic blood flow found in the in vitro experiments. In order to simulate the condition in our experiments, a bone with ultrasound gel was placed between the phantom and transducer. In our future experiments, the study will be extended using better facilities which are closer to reality. Furthermore, clinical experiments will be also conducted using the full digital design.

Acknowledgment

This study was supported by National Nature Science Foundation of China (No.81371637), Natural Basic Research Priorities Program of Shenzhen (No.JC201005280685A), Shenzhen Overseas Innovation Fund Project (No. KQC201105310020A), Improving Project of Shenzhen Key Laboratory (No. CXB201104210003A).

Conflict of Interest

The authors declare that they have no conflict of interest.

References

1. Aaslid R,Markwalder TM, Nornes H. Noninvasive transcranial Doppler ultrasound recording of flow velocity in basal cerebral arteries
2. Moehring MA, Spencer MP. Power M-mode Doppler (PMD) for observing cerebral blood flow and tracking emboli, Ultrasound Med Biol 2002;28:49-57
3. Jie LI etc., Code excitation system for stationary target detection using multi segment coding. IEIT2014, 2014 International Conference on Industrial and Information Technology, p.395-399
4. Qin ZD., Chen SP., Chen X., Coded transmission for ultrasound Doppler detection using truncated long code, Biomedical Engineering and Informatics (BMEI), 2010 3rd International Conference on, vol.1, pp.159-161,16-18 Oct.2010
5. Qin ZD., LIU DQ., Chen SP., Experimental study on the truncated long code sequence for ultrasound Doppler detection, 2012 5th International Conference on Biomedical Engineering and Informatics (BMEI)
6. M. O'Donnell. Coded excitation system for improving the penetration of real-time phased-array imaging systems. IEEE Transactions on Ultrasonics, Ferroelectics, and Frequency Control.1992,39(3):p.341-351
7. Robert J. Inkol, Efficient digital quadrature demodulator, U.S. Patent US5504455 A, April 2, 1995
8. Weon-Ki Yoon, Digital I/Q demodulator for use in wireless networks and on associated method of demodulating an RF signal, U.S. Patent US20060023811 A1, February 2, 2006
9. C. Ziomek and P. Corredoura, Digital I/Q Demodulator, PAC 95
10. F. E. Churchill et al, The Correction of I and Q Errors in a Coherent Processor , IEEE Transactions on Aerospace and Electronic Systems, vol. 17, No. 1, Jan. 1981, pp. 131 to 137
11. D. L. Sharpin, The Effects of Quadrature Sampling Imbalances on a Phase Difference Analysis Technique, the 1990 National Aerospace Electronics Conference in Dayton, Ohio on 21-25 May, 1990, pp. 962 to 968

Author: Jie LI
Institute: Health Science Center, Shenzhen University
Street: Nanhai Ave 3688, Nanshan District
City: Shenzhen
Country: P.R.China
Email: 1989lijie.1989@gmail.com

In Vivo Study of Ischemic Stroke in Mice Brain Using Sodium MRI

Kun-Che Lee[1,3], Yi-Shin Lee[4], Guo-Jen Huang[4], Hsiao-Lung Chan[1], Po-Wen Gu[5], and Jen-Fang Yu[2,3,*]

[1] Department of Electrical Engineering, Chang Gung University, Taoyuan, Taiwan
[2] Graduate Institute of Medical Mechatronics, Chang Gung University, Taoyuan, Taiwan
[3] Taiouan Interdisciplinary Otolaryngology Laboratory, Chang Gung University, Taoyuan, Taiwan
[4] Department of Biomedical Sciences, Chang Gung University, Taoyuan, Taiwan
[5] Department of Laboratory Medicine, Chang Gung Memorial Hospital, Lin-Kou, Taiwan

Abstract— **The purpose of this study is to use sodium magnetic resonance imaging (sodium MRI) to observe the variations in sodium signal intensity in mice brains after ischemic stroke, and to estimate the tissue sodium concentration of the ischemia area in mice brain. Experiments were performed using a 7T MRI system. Before the MRI scan (48 hours), the mice underwent middle cerebral artery occlusion (MCAO) to induce focal brain ischemia. The average signal intensity in the sodium images of mice brains showed a 2.2-fold increase. The average estimated values of the ischemia area and contralateral area in the mice brains were 106.5 mM and 49.9 mM, respectively. This study demonstrates the feasibility of sodium MRI in mice brain of ischemic stroke at 7T MRI. The signal intensity of sodium on the mice brain shows a significant increase in the ischemia area compared to the contralateral brain hemisphere. The estimated values of the sodium concentration exhibited a significant correlation with the biochemical values of the sodium concentrations.**

Keywords— **sodium MRI, ischemic stroke, mice brain, sodium concentration.**

I. INTRODUCTION

Stroke was a serious disease in which the blood supply to the focal brain area was restricted [1]. Although extant clinical imaging methods (such as computed tomography, diffusion MRI, and perfusion MRI) could rapidly and effectively identify the brain regions affected by a stroke. However, the viability of the brain cells in these regions could not be determined. Thus, certain other imaging technologies were required [2].

Apart from proton MRI, use of the sodium MRI in many disease models was a potential method, because of its availability for use as a bio-marker for brain physiology and metabolism [3]. There were many studies have investigated the increase in the tissue sodium concentrations that occurs during stroke using separate animal models of brain ischemia. However, the majority of these studies has been performed on rats, cats, or nonhuman primates; studies involving mice are relatively rare.

Although the signal acquisition of sodium in the mice brain was a challenge due to the volume of mice brain is smaller than other animal models. However, the sodium imaging of mice brain still has the potential to offer the necessary physiological information.

Therefore, the purpose of this study is to use sodium MRI to observe the variations in sodium signal intensity in mice brains after ischemic stroke, and to estimate the tissue sodium concentration of the ischemia area in mice brain.

II. MATERIALS AND METHODS

A. The Animal Models

In vivo MRI was performed on male C57BL/6 mice (≈20 g, n=6). 48 hours before the MRI scan, each mouse underwent middle cerebral artery occlusion (MCAO) to induce focal brain ischemia. The protocol was approved by the Institutional Animal Care and Use Committee of Chang Gung University.

B. Experimental Setup

The experiments were conducted using a 7 Tesla small animal MRI instrument (BioSpec 70/30 USR, Bruker BioSpin GmbH, Germany) equipped with a double-tuned $^{1}H/^{23}Na$ surface coil to excite and receive signals. A surface coil with a 2 cm diameter was placed on the MR imaging instrument. After the mice were anesthetized using a mixture of 1% isoflurane and 100% pure oxygen, they were placed on the supporting platform and connected to external anesthetic machines to manage their anaesthetized state. The supporting platform was connected to a warm water circulation system to maintain the temperature of the mice during the experiment. Furthermore, the mice's respiratory conditions were monitored during the experiment to ensure their safety. The sample side of the surface coil was fixed as close to the brain of the mice as possible for efficient signal acquisition. Subsequently, the supporting platform was moved to the center of the magnetic field before the coil parameters were set. The resonant frequency for hydrogen and sodium nuclides was 300.33 MHz and 79.44 MHz, respectively.

* Corresponding author.

I. Lackovic (ed.), *1st Global Conference on Biomedical Engineering & 9th Asian-Pacific Conference on Medical and Biological Engineering*,
IFMBE Proceedings 47, DOI: 10.1007/978-3-319-12262-5_39

C. MR Imaging of in Vivo Mice

Proton MRI scans were performed using a TurboRARE-T2 pulse sequence. The imaging parameters were as follows: TR = 2500 ms, TE = 33 ms, FOV = 2.5 cm × 2.5 cm, matrix size = 256 × 256, flip angle = 180°, NEX = 4, thickness = 1.5 mm, 7 slices, and scan time = 5 min 20 s.

Sodium MRI scans were performed using a FLASH pulse sequence. The imaging parameters were as follows: TR = 90 ms, TE = 2.5 ms, FOV = 2.5 cm × 2.5 cm, matrix size = 64 × 64, flip angle = 30°, NEX = 300, thickness = 1.5 mm, 3 slices, and scan time = 28 min 48 s.

D. Image Analysis

Image J (National Institutes of Health, USA) was used to analyze the MR images. The inhomogeneous correct method has been described in previous research [4]. The DICOM images were imported into Image J, and the matrix size of the sodium images was made equal to that of the proton images through interpolation. Image analysis was identified and circled the regions of interest (ROIs) in the proton images of the ischemia and contralateral areas of the mice brains. The ROI of the sodium images was defined by referring to the corresponding proton image. Finally, the ROIs were measured for signal intensity. Statistical analysis was performed using the paired Student's t-test and correlation analysis by SPSS software.

E. Estimate of Sodium Concentration

The method of estimation has been described in previous research [5]. The estimated equation is Equation 1. Based on these methods, sodium concentration estimates were obtained directly from the sodium images by measuring the mean signal intensity ($S_{Na(tissue)}$) in circled ROIs in the ischemia and contralateral areas. In addition, the mean signal intensity ($S_{Na(ref)}$) of reference was also measured in the circled ROI in the contralateral area. In our study, the concentration of sodium in the reference was set to 45 mM for normal mice brain tissue concentration ([Na]ref) [6].

$$[Na]_{tissue} = [\frac{S_{Na(tissue)}}{S_{Na(ref)}}] \times [Na]_{ref} \quad (1)$$

Furthermore, after MRI scan, the mice were sacrificed. A part of the cortex tissue from ischemia area and contralateral area of each mouse brain was sampled to measure the biochemical values of sodium concentration in the brain tissue. In this protocol, all efforts were made to minimize suffering. The cortex tissue of the brain was placed in centrifuge tube and diluted with water 10-fold. After the centrifugation process, the clear liquid from the centrifuge tube became the sample. The measure of the biochemical values of sodium concentration was supported by the Department of Laboratory Medicine at Chang Gung Memorial Hospital, Lin-Kou. A biochemical analyzer was used (Lxi725, Beckman, USA).

III. RESULTS AND DISCUSSIONS

Fig. 1 shows the results of the one mouse in vivo measurement. The proton images measured for the mice brains were showed in Fig. 1a. Fig. 1b showed the sodium images of mice brain after inhomogeneous correction. The T2 weighted proton images showed the area of ischemia, defined as the hyperintense areas in the right hemisphere of the mice brain. The sodium image reveals a similar result.

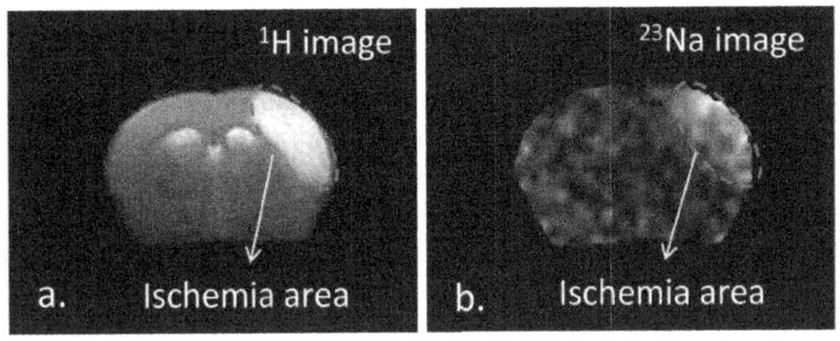

Fig. 1 IFMBE logo Fig. 1. In vivo proton and sodium image of mice brain: (a) proton image, (b) sodium image after approximately correct.

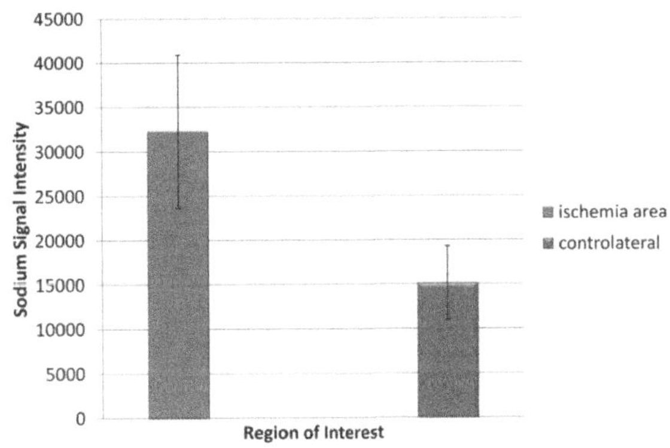

Fig. 2. The average signal intensity of ROI of sodium image six mice brain.

The signal intensity of sodium image was determined for a ROI in the ischemia area and a ROI in the contralateral, as Fig. 2 showed the average signal intensity in the sodium images for 6 mice brain, showing an average 2.2-fold increase in signal intensity. The signal intensity of sodium was significantly increased in the ischemia area compared to the contralateral brain hemisphere (tested with a paired Student's t-test, $P<0.05$). The SNR of sodium image were determined for an ROI in the ischemia area and an ROI in the contralateral from sodium imaging in 6 mice brain. Table 1 shows the average SNR of sodium imaging in 6 mice brain. The average SNR showed a 2.1-fold sodium intensity increase.

Table 1. SNR determined from in vivo measurement

	SNR of sodium imaging
ROI in ischemia area	5.9
ROI in contralateral	2.8

The estimated values of the sodium concentration of the 6 mice brains are presented in Table 2. The average estimated values of the ischemia area and contralateral area in the mice brains were 106.5 mM and 49.9 mM, respectively. The results demonstrated that the estimated value of the sodium concentration was increased in the ischemia area compared to the contralateral brain hemisphere. In addition, the biochemical values of sodium of 6 mice brains are also presented in Table 2. The average biochemical values of the ischemia area and contralateral area in mice brains were 141.3 mM, and 75.6 mM, respectively. The correlation of the estimated values and biochemical values was showed in Fig. 3. The estimated values of the sodium concentration exhibited a significant correlation with the biochemical values of the sodium concentrations (Pearson correlation coefficients R=0.976, explanatory power up to 95.3%, P<0.05).

Table 2. Sodium concentration of mice brain

	Estimate value of sodium concentration of mice brain from sodium MRI		Biochemical value of sodium concentration of mice brain	
	Ischemia area	contralateral	Ischemia area	contralateral
No.1	125.9 mM	53.8 mM	183 mM	88 mM
No.2	115.9 mM	49 mM	154 mM	55 mM
No.3	103.9 mM	54.2 mM	117 mM	62 mM
No.4	78.6 mM	38.6 mM	142 mM	85 mM
No.5	83.4 mM	63.3 mM	90 mM	67 mM
No.6	131.5 mM	40.7 mM	162 mM	97 mM
Average	106.5 mM	49.9 mM	141.3 mM	75.6 mM
Standard deviation	21.9	9.2	33.3	16.6

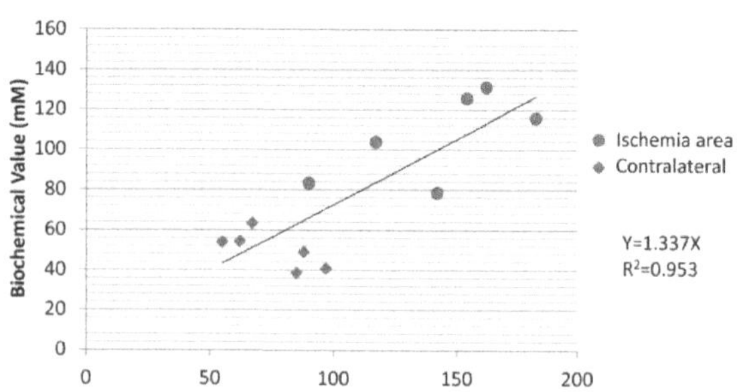

Fig. 3. The correlation of the estimate values and biochemical values.

IV. CONCLUSION

This study demonstrated the feasibility of sodium MRI in mice brain at 7T MRI and to estimate the tissue sodium concentration of the ischemia area in mice brain. The signal intensity of sodium in mouse brain showed significantly increased levels in the ischemia area compared to the contralateral brain hemisphere. The average signal intensity showed a 2.2-fold increase. In addition, the estimated values of sodium concentration exhibited a significant correlation with the biochemical values of the sodium concentrations.

ACKNOWLEDGMENT

The authors wish to thank the Functional Neuroscience Lab at Chang Gung University for animal surgery support, the 7T Animal MRI Core Lab of the Neurobiology and Cognitive Science Center for technical and facility support, and the Instrumentation Center for MRI experiments at National Taiwan University, and the Department of Laboratory Medicine, Chang Gung Memorial Hospital, Lin-Kou for biochemical test support.

CONFLICT OF INTEREST

The authors declare that they have no conflict of interest.

REFERENCES

1. Warren DJ, Musson R, Connolly DJ et al. (2010) Imaging in acute ischaemic stroke: essential for modern stroke care. Postgrad Med J 86: 409-418
2. Boada FE, Qian Y, Nemoto E et al. (2012) Sodium MRI and the Assessment of Irreversible Tissue Damage During Hyper-Acute Stroke. Transl. Stroke Res. 3: 235-245
3. Ouwerkerk R (2011) Sodium MRI. Methods Mol Biol 711: 175-201
4. Axel L, Costantini J, Listerud J (1987) Intensity correction in surface-coil MR imaging. AJR Am J Roentgenol 148: 418-420
5. Constantinides CD, Kraitchman DL, O'Brien KO et al. (2001) Noninvasive quantification of total sodium concentrations in acute reperfused myocardial infarction using 23Na MRI. Magn Reson Med 46: 1144-1151
6. Wetterling F, Tabbert M, Junge S et al. (2010) A double-tuned (1)H/(23)Na dual resonator system for tissue sodium concentration measurements in the rat brain via Na-MRI. Phys Med Biol 55: 7681-7695

Author: Kun-Che Lee
Institute: Department of Electrical Engineering, Chang Gung University
Street: 259 Wen-Hwa 1st Road, Kwei-Shan 333, Taoyuan, Taiwan
City: Taoyuan
Country: Taiwan
Email: feather62j@hotmail.com

Author: Yi-Shin Lee
Institute: Department of Biomedical Sciences, Chang Gung University
Street: 259 Wen-Hwa 1st Road, Kwei-Shan 333, Taoyuan, Taiwan
City: Taoyuan
Country: Taiwan
Email: j3609333@hotmail.com

Author: Guo-Jen Huang
Institute: Department of Biomedical Sciences, Chang Gung University
Street: 259 Wen-Hwa 1st Road, Kwei-Shan 333, Taoyuan, Taiwan
City: Taoyuan
Country: Taiwan
Email: gjh30@mail.cgu.edu.tw

Author: Hsiao-Lung Chan
Institute: Department of Electrical Engineering, Chang Gung University
Street: 259 Wen-Hwa 1st Road, Kwei-Shan 333, Taoyuan, Taiwan
City: Taoyuan
Country: Taiwan
Email: chanhl@mail.cgu.edu.tw

Author: Po-Wen Gu
Institute: Department of Laboratory Medicine, Chang Gung Memorial Hospital, Lin-Kou
Street: 5, Fu-Sing St., Kwei-Shan 333, Taoyuan Taiwan
City: Taoyuan
Country: Taiwan
Email: cooper3892@cgmh.org.tw

Author: Jen-Fang Yu
Institute: Graduate Institute of Medical Mechatronics, Chang Gung University
Street: 259 Wen-Hwa 1st Road, Kwei-Shan 333, Taoyuan, Taiwan
City: Taoyuan
Country: Taiwan
Email: jfyu.phd@gmail.com

Evaluation of Image Quality and Average Glandular Dose Using the Resolution Testing Phantom in Mammography

Y.T. Chao, C.Y. Chen, and S.L. Dong*

School of Medical Imaging and Radiological Sciences/Chung Shan Medical University/Taichung City, ROC

Abstract— **The development of an average glandular dose (AGD) assessment method of the resolution testing phantom is useful in mammographic study. The purpose of this study was the evaluation of image quality and AGD using the resolution testing phantom in mammography. The equivalent thickness of the standard breast phantom with percentage glandular content (PGC) of 50% that would require the same mAs as the resolution testing phantom was calculated. In this study, 2-6 cm resolution testing phantoms were exposed at target/filter/kV combinations of Mo/Mo/27 and 28 kVp. The AGD and spatial resolution of these images were analyzed. Results from this study showed that the equivalent thickness of standard breast linearly increases with increasing thickness of resolution testing phantom. The measured spatial resolutions for different tube voltages were comparable (6-8 lp/mm). The calculated AGDs for the tube voltage of 27 kVp were slightly higher than those of 28 kVp. In conclusion, the equivalent thickness of standard breast phantom (PGC=50%) producing the same exposure factors as resolution testing phantom was developed. As a consequence, both image quality and AGD information can be acquired during the spatial resolution testing in mammography.**

Keywords— **Mammography, dose, image quality, phantom, spatial resolution.**

I. INTRODUCTION

In mammography, it is important to optimize both equipment setting and imaging parameters so that the suitable image quality is obtained at the lowest possible average glandular dose (AGD). Some studies suggested that the AGD to patient and image quality can be estimated by using an appropriate thickness of a breast-tissue-equivalent phantom that requires the same exposure as the breast in mammography [1].

PMMA (polymethyl methacrylate) and BR-12 materials are frequently used for the construction of breast phantom. In the European protocol [2], PMMA slabs with different thicknesses were suggested for the assessments of image quality and the AGD in mammography. In clinical practice, many image testing phantoms are constructed using the image quality testing objects imbedded in a BR-12 slab, such as the resolution testing phantom. These BR-12 based phantoms are not allowed for the assessment of the AGD.

The development of an AGD assessment method of the resolution testing phantom is useful in mammographic study. To achieve this purpose, a simple approach is the determination of equivalent thickness of standard breast phantom with percentage glandular content (PGC) of 50% for the resolution testing phantom. The purpose of this study was the evaluation of image quality and AGD using the resolution testing phantom in mammography.

II. MATERIALS AND METHODS

A digital mammography system (Siemens) was used in this study. A set of the resolution testing phantom (see Fig. 1) was used for the assessments of image quality and the AGD. The standard breast model of a superficial layer of adipose tissue 0.5 cm thick was used in this study. The percentage glandular content (PGC) of each breast, defined as the percentage by mass of glandular tissue in the central region of the standard breast model [3], was used.

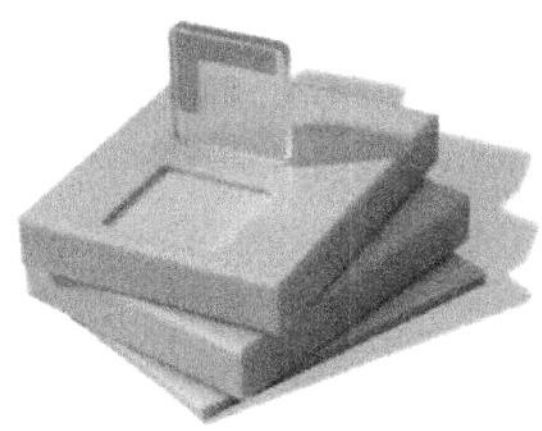

Fig. 1 The resolution testing phantom

The equivalent thickness of the standard breast phantom with PGC of 50% that would require the same mAs as the BR-12 slab was calculated (see Fig. 2). The BR-12 slabs and the standard breast phantom with PGC of 50% at four thicknesses (2, 3, 4, 5, and 6 cm) were exposed at various target/filter/kV combinations of W/Rh/25-32 kVp [4]. The relationship between the equivalent phantom thickness (T) and exposure parameters can be expressed as

$$T = C1 \times \ln(mAs) + C2 \times \ln(kV) + b \qquad (1)$$

where C1, C2 and b are fitted coefficients, and mAs and kV are the tube loading and the tube voltage of each phantom exposure, respectively. A least-squares fit was applied to

* Corresponding author.

I. Lackovic (ed.), *1st Global Conference on Biomedical Engineering & 9th Asian-Pacific Conference on Medical and Biological Engineering*, IFMBE Proceedings 47, DOI: 10.1007/978-3-319-12262-5_40

determine the coefficients (C1, C2 and b) for each calibration data set [5]. These fitted functions were used to calculate the equivalent thickness of the standard breast phantom with PGC of 50%.

To validate the accuracy of the approach used above, the 4.5 cm standard breast phantom with PGC of 50% was exposed with 26-32 kV and target/filter combination of W/Rh. Then, the equivalent BR-12 thicknesses of these exposures were calculated using the fitted functions obtained above. The results obtained were compared with the thickness of the standard breast phantom (4.5 cm).

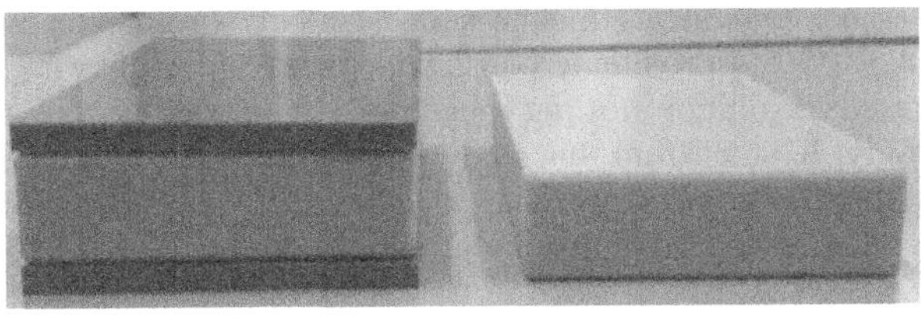

Fig. 2 The standard breast phantom with PGC of 50% (a) and BR-12 phantom (b)

For dosimetry assessment, the method of AGD assessment reported by Dance (1990)[3] was used. The AGD was calculated on the basis of the incident air kerma (Kf) by multiplied a conversion factor *g* [3]. The AGD can be expressed as

$$AGD = Kf \times g \quad (2).$$

Then, the different equivalent-breasts obtained from this study were applied to estimate conversion factor g.

For image quality assessment, 2-6 cm resolution testing phantoms (2, 3, 4, 5, and 6 cm) were exposed at target/filter/kV combinations of Mo/Mo/27 and 28 kVp. The spatial resolution of each image was evaluated.

III. RESULTS

The equivalent thickness of standard breast for each BR-12 slab was estimated using equation (1). The coefficients of determination (R^2) of the fitted functions for all exposures were within 0.999181–0.999973. To validate the accuracy of the fitted functions obtained above, the equivalent thicknesses of the 4.5-cm standard breast (PGC=50%) were estimated for exposures with different tube voltages (see Fig. 3). The average equivalent thickness was 4.43±0.03 cm, which is comparable to the thickness of the standard breast phantom used (4.5 cm).

Figure 4 showed the equivalence between thickness of BR-12 slabs and thickness of the standard breasts (PGC=50%). The equivalent thickness of standard breast linearly increases with the increasing thickness of BR-12 slab.

Table 1 showed the conversion factor g of each BR-12 slab. The conversion factor g decreases with the increasing thickness of BR-12 slab.

Figure 5 and Figure 6 showed the spatial resolution and the AGD of the resolution testing phantoms, respectively. The measured spatial resolutions for different tube voltages were comparable. The calculated AGDs for the tube voltage of 27 kVp were slightly higher than those of 28 kVp.

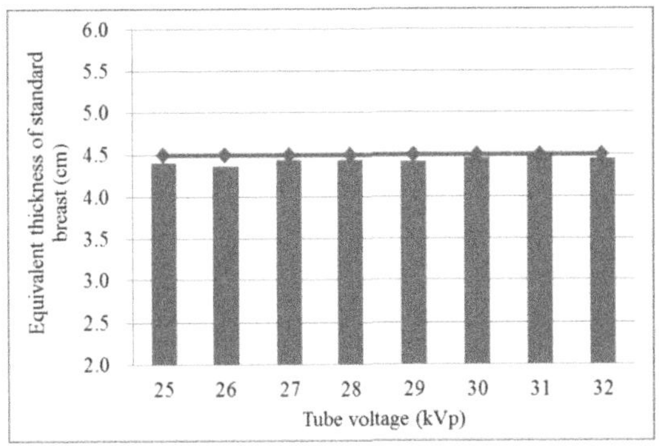

Fig. 3 The equivalent thicknesses of the 4.5-cm standard breast

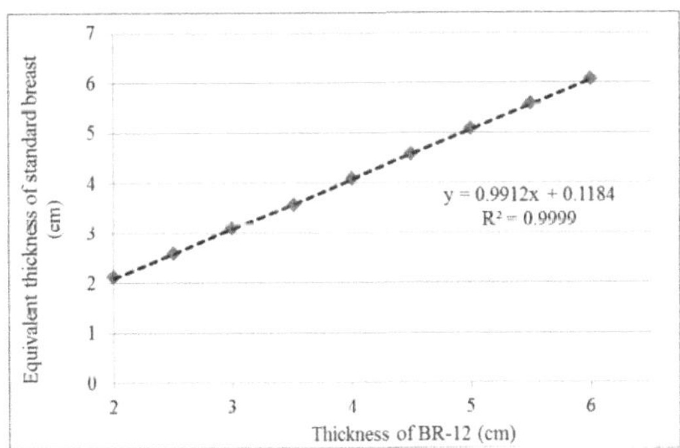

Fig. 4 The equivalent thickness of standard breast for each BR-12 slab

Table 1 The conversion g for 2-6 cm BR-12 slabs

Thickness of BR-12 (cm)	Thickness of standard breast (cm)	HVL (mm Al)						
		0.3	0.35	0.4	0.45	0.5	0.55	0.6
2	2.12	0.376	0.418	0.457	0.493	0.526	0.556	0.572
3	3.09	0.268	0.303	0.335	0.367	0.398	0.429	0.458
4	4.08	0.203	0.231	0.256	0.284	0.313	0.340	0.368
5	5.08	0.162	0.184	0.206	0.229	0.254	0.283	0.306
6	6.07	0.134	0.152	0.170	0.190	0.211	0.234	0.258

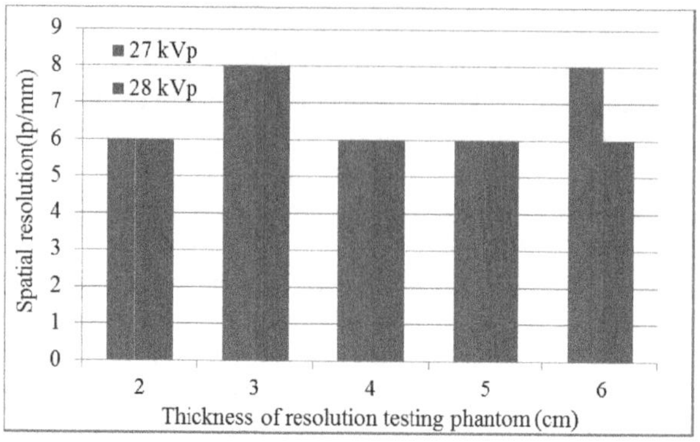

Fig. 5 The spatial resolutions of resolution testing phantoms

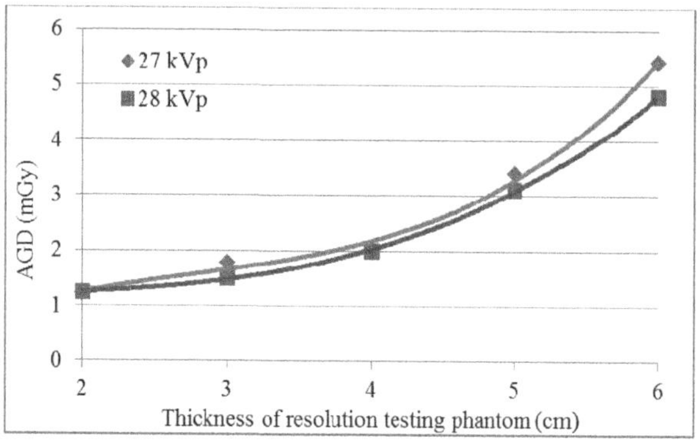

Fig. 6 The average glandular doses of resolution testing phantoms

IV. DISCUSSION

In this study, the equivalent thickness of standard breast is slightly thicker than thickness of the BR-12 slab. The reason of this effect is due to the fact that the standard breast model contents a superficial layer of 0.5 cm adipose tissue. The density of adipose tissue was 0.93 g/cm^3 which is less than the density of BR-12 material (0.98 g/cm^3).

Many protocols recommended that both PMMA and PR-12 slabs can be used for the AEC performance testing. From the the manufacture's document, the PGC of BR-12 material was about 47% which within 0-100%. Therefore, the BR-12 material is suitable for the dosimetry simulation of the breast tissue in mammography.

The conversion factors g for each thickness of BR-12 slab in this study were provided in this study. This allowing for simply calculate the average glandular dose for an exposure acquired from a BR-12 slab. As a result, both image quality and AGD information can be acquired during the spatial resolution testing. Therefore, the results from this study may provide useful information for the estimation of AGD using the resolution testing phantom during the image quality assessments.

V. CONCLUSIONS

The equivalent thickness of standard breast phantom (PGC=50%) producing the same exposure factors as BR-12 based resolution testing phantom was developed in this study. Results from this study show that both image quality and AGD information can be acquired during the spatial resolution testing in mammography.

ACKNOWLEDGMENT

The authors would like to thank radiographers at department of Radiology of Chung Shan Medical University Hospital.

REFERENCES

1. Jamal N, Ng K H, McLean D et al. (2004) Mammographic breast glandularity in Malaysian women: data derived from radiography. Am J Roentgenol 182:713-717
2. Commission of the European Communities (2006) European Guidelines for Quality Assurance in Breast Cancer Screening and Diagnosis. Commission of the European Communities
3. Dance D R. (1990) Monte Carlo calculation of conversion factors for the estimation of mean glandular breast dose. Phys Med Biol 35:1211-1219
4. Kruger R L and Schueler B A. (2001) A survey of clinical factors and patient dose in mammography. Med Phys 28:1449-1454
5. Dong S L, Chu T C, Lin Y C et al. (2011) Determination of equivalent breast phantoms for different age groups of Taiwanese women: An experimental approach. Med Phys 38:4094-4100

Author: Shang-Lung Dong
Institute: School of Medical Imaging and Radiological Sciences/ Chung Shan Medical University
Street: No.110, Sec.1, Jianguo North Rd.
City: Taichung City
Country: Taiwan, ROC
Email: sldong@ms46.hinet.net

Reconstruction of DOI with Geometrical Mismatch between Physical and Computational Models

Liang-Yu Chen[1], Min-Cheng Pan[2], and Min-Chun Pan[1,]*

[1] Graduate Institute of Biomedical Engineering, National Central University, Taoyuan County 320, Taiwan
[2] Department of Electronic Engineering, Tung-Nan University of Technology, New Taipei City 222, Taiwan
pan_minc@cc.ncu.edu.tw

Abstract— **In this paper, preliminary simulated reconstruction results are presented to investigate the effects of geometrical mismatch between the physical and computational models on the reconstructed images. Two types of mismatch are discussed.**

Keywords— **Diffuse Optical Imaging, Inverse Problem, Near Infrared, Breast Tumor Detection.**

I. INTRODUCTION

Diffuse optical imaging (DOI) uses near infrared (NIR) light to interrogate biological tissue such as breast. Functional information like oxy-hemoglobin and deoxy-hemoglobin concentration about breast can be derived for screening [1, 2] and complementary to structural information obtained from X-ray mammography, which is hampered by false positives and negatives [3, 4].

Among the DOI systems investigated recently, some have been physically in conjunction with a commercialized imaging modality such as ultrasound [5], MRI [6] or x-ray mammography [7, 8] for enhancing tumor detection sensitivity and specificity [9]. On the other hand, some stand-alone DOI systems under development have been still drawn attention to avoid limitation by the requirements of the other imaging modality such as metallic compatibility for MRI, and hard breast compression for mammography, etc. With using a stand-alone prostrate DOI imaging system, or even a prostration and compression combined one, the cross-section of breast varies with patient subjects when measurements are performed. In these circumstances, the actual cross-section may be inconsistent with that used in the image reconstruction. This paper aims at investigating and addressing the effect of the geometrical mismatch on image reconstruction.

II. METHOD

Image reconstruction in diffuse optical imaging consists of solving forward and inverse problem. In solving the forward problem, the forward model that usually uses in DOI to predict the distribution of light under condition of presumed optical properties is the diffusion equation:

$$\nabla \cdot \kappa(\mathbf{r})\nabla\Phi(\mathbf{r},\omega) - \left[\mu_a(\mathbf{r}) - \frac{i\omega}{c}\right]\Phi(\mathbf{r},\omega) = -S_0(\mathbf{r},\omega), \quad (1)$$

where $\Phi(\mathbf{r},\omega)$ is the photon density at position $\mathbf{r}$, ω is the light modulation frequency, $S_0(\mathbf{r},\omega)$ is the source term, c is the speed of light in tissue, and μ_a and κ denote the optical absorption and diffusion coefficients, respectively.

In solving the inverse problem, the inverse solution is obtaining by numerical way of iteratively minimizing the difference between the measured diffusion photon density data, Φ^M, around the tissue and the computational model data, Φ^C, from solving the forward problem by finite element method with the current estimated optical properties. This data-model misfit difference is typically defined as:

$$\chi^2 = \sum_{i=1}^{N_M}\left[\Phi_i^C - \Phi_i^M\right]^2, \quad (2)$$

where N_M is the number of measurement data. However, minimizing this defined data-model misfit difference usually runs into difficulty with an ill-conditioned problem, which usually happens in DOI image reconstruction. Therefore, regularization is needed to remedy this problem. In this study, Tikhonov regularization is applied and the inverse solution is obtained by solving the following equation:

$$\left(\mathbf{J}^T\mathbf{J} + \lambda\mathbf{I}\right)\Delta\chi = \mathbf{J}^T\Delta\Phi, \quad (3)$$

where $\Delta\chi$ is the update vector composed of $\Delta\mu_a$ and $\Delta\kappa$, the update length from current estimated optical properties, $\mathbf{J} = \left[\, \partial\Phi^C/\partial\mu_a \quad \partial\Phi^C/\partial\kappa \,\right]$ is the Jacobin matrix, and λ is the regularization parameter.

* Corresponding author.

I. Lackovic (ed.), *1st Global Conference on Biomedical Engineering & 9th Asian-Pacific Conference on Medical and Biological Engineering*,
IFMBE Proceedings 47, DOI: 10.1007/978-3-319-12262-5_41

III. Results

In order to investigate the effect of geometrical mismatch on DOI image reconstruction, the preliminary simulated reconstructions were present. In the simulation, the cross-section of simulated phantom was assumed elliptic to imitate the situation that the cross-section of breast may not be circle when conducting prostrate DOI measurement. This simulated elliptic phantom embedded with one inclusion was employed to generate simulated measurement data for subsequent image reconstruction. Specifically, the simulated measurement data were obtained from solving the diffusion equation Eq. (1) by finite-element method with multiple illuation and measurement positions. But, the cross-section of reconstruction domain was mismatched to be a circle in the simulation.

Two types of simulation conditions were considered here. In the first type, the diameter of circle reconstruction domain is as large as the length of major axis of the simulated elliptic phantom, as illustrated at the left-hand side of Fig. 1. Corresponding reconstructed absorption images are shown at the right-hand side of Fig. 1. As can be seen from the reconstructed images, the reconstructed inclusion suffers from severe distortion although it can still be reconstructed. In the second type, the diameter of circle reconstruction domain is the same as the length of minor axis of the simulated elliptic phantom, as shown in Fig. 2. It can be seen that the inclusion can be well reconstructed; however, serious artifacts in a ring are present around the boundary of reconstruction domain. The degraded ring artifacts result from the compensation of a smaller computation model used which causes extra high absorption coefficients at source and detection positions. It is worth noted that the artifacts near the vertical axis are even worse than those near the horizontal axis due to the degree of mismatch.

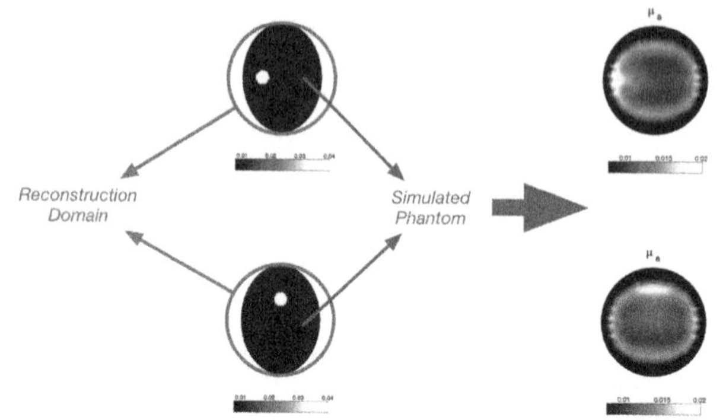

Fig. 1. Simulated reconstruction of absorption images under the condition of geometrical mismatch. Assume round reconstruction domain is larger than the simulated elliptic phantom. Left-hand side: geometry of the test case; right-hand side: reconstructed absorption images corresponding to the synthesized condition.

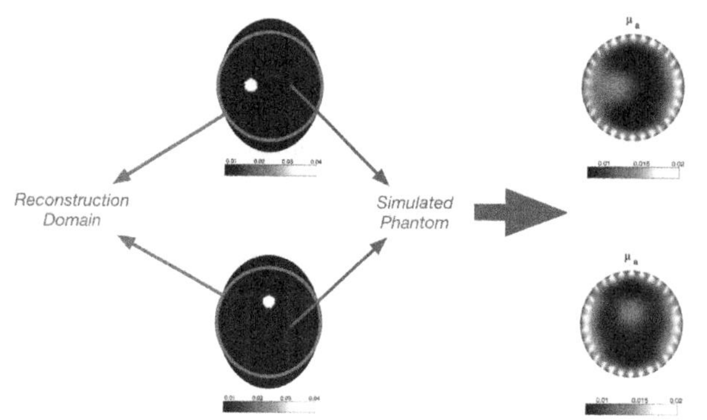

Fig. 2. Simulated reconstructions of absorption images under condition of geometry mismatch. Assume round reconstruction domain is smaller than the simulated elliptic phantom. Left-hand side: geometry of the test case; right-hand side: reconstructed absorption images corresponding to the synthesized condition.

IV. Conclusion

In this paper, we have presented the reconstructed absorption images when the geometry adopted in image reconstruction algorithm is inconsistent with that of physical model. Based on the reconstructed results of Figs.1 and 2, this geometrical mismatch would result in the distortion for the reconstructed inclusion or artifacts around the boundary of reconstruction domain. Some probable interpretations were discussed. Such a geometrical mismatch should be taken into account and minimized when it cannot be prevented during performing measurement with a DOI system.

Acknowledgment

We would like to acknowledge funding from National Science Council through grants 101-2221-E-008-093-MY3 and 101-2221-E-236-014.

CONFLICT OF INTEREST

The authors declare that they have no conflict of interest with presenting this paper.

REFERENCES

[1] Gibson, and H. Dehghani, "Diffuse optical imaging," Phil. Trans. R. Soc. A **367**, 3055–3072 (2009).
[2] D. R. Leff, O. J. Warren, L. C. Enfield, A. Gibson, T. Athanasiou, D. K. Patten, J. Hbden, G. Z. Yang, and A. Darzi, "Diffuse optical imaging of the healthy and diseased breast: A systematic review," Breast Cancer Res. Treat. **108**, 9–22 (2008).
[3] J. G. Elmore, M. B. Barton, V. M. Moceri, S. Polk, P. J. Arena, and S. W. Fletcher, "Ten- year risk of false positive screening mammograms and clinical breast examinations," The New England Journal of Medicine **338**, 1089–1096 (1998).
[4] P. T. Huynh, A. M. Jarolimek, and S. Day, "The false-negative mammogram," Radiographics **18**, 1137–1154 (1998).
[5] Tavakoli, Q. Zhu, "Two-step reconstruction method using global optimization and conjugate gradient for ultrasound-guided diffuse optical tomography," J Biomed Opt, 18(1), 16006 (2013).
[6] CM Carpenter, BW Pogue, S Jiang, H Dehghani, X Wang, KD Paulsen, WA Wells, J Forero, Ch. Kogel, JB Weaver, SP Poplack, PA Kaufman, "Image-guided optical spectroscopy provides molecular-specific information in vivo: MRI-guided spectroscopy of breast cancer hemoglobin, water, and scatterer size," Optics letters, 32(8), 933-935 (2007).
[7] Q. Fang, S.A. Carp, J. Selb, G. Boverman, Q. Zhang, D.B. Kopans, R. H. Moore, E. L. Miller, D. H. Brooks, and D.A. Boas, "Combined optical imaging and mammography of the healthy breast: optical contrast derived from breast structure and compression," IEEE Transactions on Medical Imaging, 28(1), 30-42 (2009).
[8] Jhao-Ming Yu, Liang-Yu Chen, Hung-Chih Chiang, Min-Cheng Pan, Sheng-Yih Sun, and Chia-Cheng Chou, Min-Chun Pan, "Parallel Scanning Architecture for Mammogram-Based Diffuse Optical Imaging," ASME Transactions, Journal of Medical Devices, **7**(2), 020936 (2013).
[9] B.J. Tromberg, B.W. Pogue, K.D. Paulsen, A.G. Yodh, D.A. Boas, A.E. Cerussi, "Assessing the future of diffuse optical imaging technologies for breast cancer management," Medical Physics, **35**(6), 2443-51 (2008).

Corresponding	Author: Min-Chun Pan
Institute:	Graduate Institute of Biomedical Engineering, National Central University
Street:	No. 300, Jhongda Rd.
City:	Jhongli City, Taoyuan County
Country:	Taiwan
Email:	pan_minc@cc.ncu.edu.tw

A Spatial Position Measurement System Using Integral Photography Based 3D Image Markers

Zhencheng Fan[1], Junchen Wang[2], and Hongen Liao[1]

[1] Department of Biomedical Engineering, School of Medicine, Tsinghua University, Beijing, China
[2] Graduate School of Engineering, University of Tokyo, Tokyo, Japan

Abstract— **Stereo tracking systems are used in surgical navigation to measure 3D positions of surgical instruments and patients, including invisible light based tracking systems and image based tracking systems. Optical tracking systems use reflective balls or flat chessboards as markers which can not be used in limited space. This paper introduces a new 3D spatial position measurement system using 3D image markers based on integral photography. This 3D image marker has spatial information encoded into a 2D image. Therefore, it has compact size while providing spatial position measurement. We design 3D image markers for a special probe and display them in 3D space using integral photography. Furthermore, we fulfill the stereo camera calibration, keypoints extraction and 3D position calculation. Experiments were performed to evaluate the accuracy of the system and the application is clarified to express the practicability of integral photography based 3D image markers.**

Keywords— **spatial position measurement, 3D image marker, integral photography, stereo tracking.**

I. Introduction

Tracking systems are used in surgical navigation to obtain positional information, assisting surgeons in confirming the position of surgical instruments and patients.

Current optical tracking systems mainly include near-infrared optical tracking systems as well as image based tracking systems. Both of them use 3-marker probes or 4-marker probes for localizing targets, and the methods to calculate the 3D spatial posture are also both based on computer vision according to keypoints detected on stereoscopic images. Nowadays, various types of tracking systems are commercially available. The NDI (Northern Digital Inc.) Polaris optical tracking system is a near-infrared optical tracking system using reflective balls as markers and near-infrared filter attached lenses to obtain images which only contain the markers [1]. The MicronTracker designed by Claron Technology Inc. is an image based tracking system using 2D-chessboards as markers and visible light instead of near-infrared light for imaging [2]. This technology can combine the environmental information and the positional information, which makes surgical navigation feasible. To sum up, these two types of markers should form the polygon to ensure the spatial degrees of freedom to track and probes can not have the character of small volume of space.

The design of the marker is based on the working environment. Tanaka *et al.* [3] presented a new ArrayMark marker for service robots. Even for the slightest movement, the pattern of this marker will change. In this paper, we recommend a new type of marker based on 3D display technologies to overcome the challenge of the limited space. Integral photography (IP) we used in this study is one of 3D display technologies. Without using any supplementary glasses or instruments, IP [4] can provide 3D images. The main component of IP is an array of tiny lens used to take and display the image or the 3D object [5]. IP possesses varying directional information that every point on the display can be seen from various directions within its viewing angle, as if it appears in the 3D space [6]. Liao and Wang *et al.* [7,8] used an image-rendering algorithm to get a computer-generated image which simulates the multiple rays in the 3D space through a microconvex lens array. In this paper, we get the computer-generated image based on IP, the 3D object is projected to the space and two images with different parallax are captured using a stereo camera. To get the marker's 3D position, this research fulfills the stereo camera calibration, keypoints extraction and 3D reconstruction. Furthermore, we design a new probe based on integral photography 3D image markers which can be used to track the posture of the probe. Different from the traditional one, it can be designed for linear to fit the narrow space, and fulfill the position measurement. Because of these advantages, the 3D position measurement system can be used in surgical navigation and object tracking with both the information of the probe and the environment. Experiments were performed to evaluate the accuracy of the system and the application was clarified to show the practicability of the integral photography based 3D image markers.

II. Methods

A. System Overview

The proposed system consists of a stereo camera, a probe with three 3D image markers and a computer workstation for camera calibration as well as image processing, as illustrated in Fig.1. The stereo camera consists of two cameras

I. Lackovic (ed.), *1st Global Conference on Biomedical Engineering & 9th Asian-Pacific Conference on Medical and Biological Engineering*, IFMBE Proceedings 47, DOI: 10.1007/978-3-319-12262-5_42

(ALLIED guppy pro) is used for tracking patients and instruments. The 3D image marker based on IP is composed of a printed integral photography image and a convex lens hexagonal array placed in front of the image. The 3D marker is captured by the stereo camera and further calculation can get the marker's position in 3D space. Finally, the probe's position can be calculated according to the geometrical relationship. In this system, surgeons can move the probe to the interested area to get the 3D information.

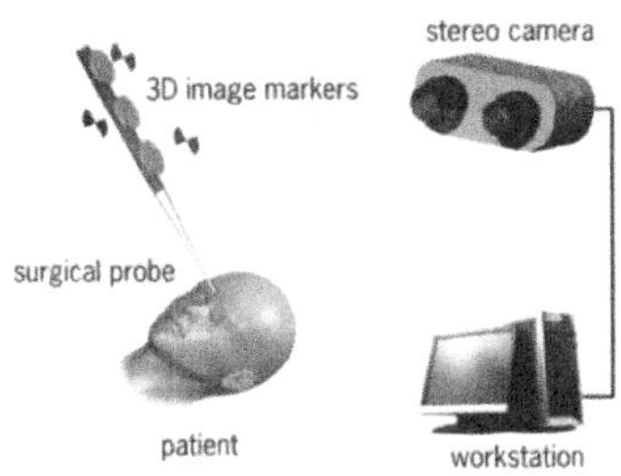

Fig. 1 System configuration.

B. 3D Image Markers

The initial 2D marker was designed to be a chessboard pattern that we can extract its keypoint. Using IP, the 2D marker was processed into 2.5D marker which is a 2D image with the depth information. Fig. 2(a) shows the principle of the 3D image marker. We use an image-rendering algorithm which simulates the ray of light through the micro-convex lens array to get a computer-generated marker. Then we put the lens array whose parameters are the same with the previous one above the generated image to get the 3D marker. Each point in a 3D space is reconstructed by the convergence of rays from pixels on the 2D display through lenses in the array. The 2D display can be a computer display or a printed paper. An observer can see the marker above the lens array from various directions within its viewing angle. Based on the principal above, a new probe is designed which was shown in Fig. 2(b). This probe possesses three collinear 3D image markers whose depth of space can be adjusted according to the demand.

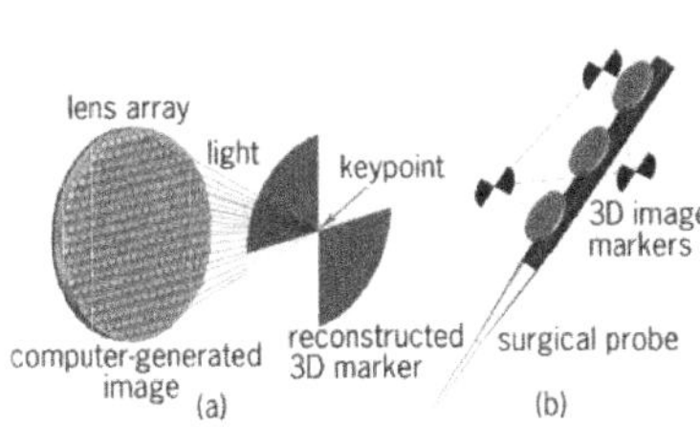

Fig. 2 (a) Principle of 3D image markers; (b) New probe based on three 3D image markers.

In Fig. 2(b), three markers reconstructed by the 3D image markers in the space are configured as a triangle. When people put the tip of probe on surgical instruments or patients, the stereo camera could capture images and the position of the tip would be calculated according to the geometric relationship we designed.

C. Camera Calibration and 3D Reconstruction

The geometrical model of the camera image determines the relationship between the points in 3D space and the 2D points in the 2D images. We regard the camera model as a pinhole one and use a 10×7 chessboard to calibrate the stereo camera based on Zhang's calibration method [9]. According to the parameters of the stereo camera, we can calculate the 3D position of the 3D image marker's keypoint which we designed, as illustrated in Fig. 3. Pl is the keypoint on the left image while pr is the keypoint on the right image. P is the keypoint reconstructed.

We can obtain the formula as follows:

$$\left(T-(x_l-x_r)\right)/(Z-f)=T/Z \tag{1}$$

Simplifying the formula, we get:

$$\begin{aligned} Z &= fT/(x_l-x_r) \\ X &= \left(Z\left((x_l-x_r)/2-c_x\right)\right)/f+T/2 \\ Y &= \left(Z\left((y_l-y_r)/2-c_y\right)\right)/f \end{aligned} \tag{2}$$

We can finally get the 3D position of P.

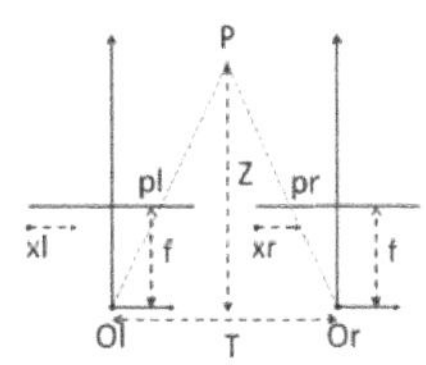

Fig. 3 The geometric image of the calculation.

D. Keypoint Extraction

We use semi-automatic algorithm to fulfill the corner extraction based on OpenCV. Subpixel optimization (SPO) iterates to find the subpixel accurate position of the corner, as shown in Fig.4.

p_i is the adjacent point of the keypoint q which we want to locate. Every vector from q to p_i is orthogonal to the image gradient in p_i. Consider the expression:

$$\varepsilon_i = DI_{pi}^{\ T}\cdot(q-p_i) \tag{3}$$

Where the DI_{pi} is the image gradient in p_i. The value of q can be calculated when ε_i is minimized.

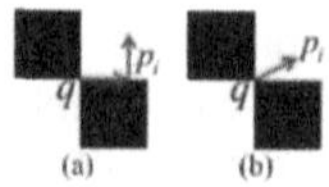

Fig. 4 Subpixel corner extraction.

III. EVALUATION

Fig. 5 shows the evaluation system for 3D position measurement which mainly consists of a stereo camera, 3D image markers, an X-Y platform and a rotation platform. According to the formulas mentioned in the second part, the 3D position of the keypoints can be calculated. The 3D image markers can be moved in the space using the x-y platform and can be rotated using the rotation platform. Fig.6 shows the 3D image marker we designed in detail.

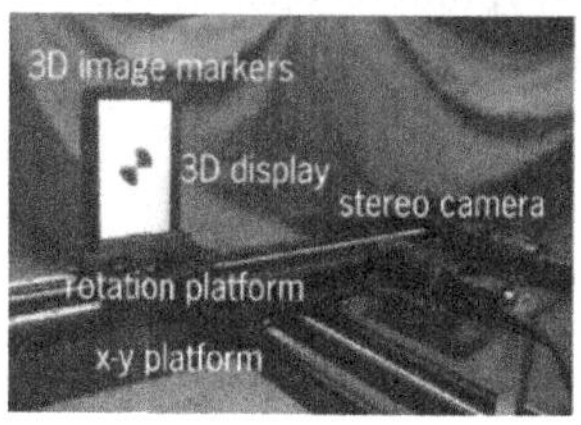

Fig. 5 Evaluation system for 3D position measurement.

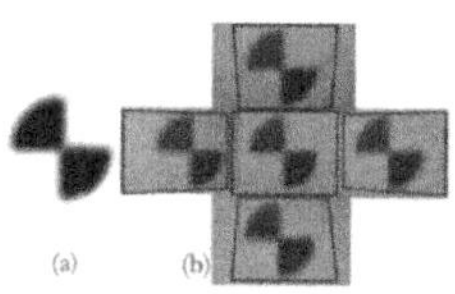

Fig. 6 (a) Computer-generated 2D marker based on IP; (b) 3D image marker in space from different viewpoints.

From the beginning, we made an evaluation to make sure the availability of a single 3D image marker which has only one keypoint. We moved the 3D image marker forward and backward in a step of 10 mm, captured the images using the stereo camera, extracted the keypoint and reconstructed it. Then we moved it right and left, repeating the process. The 3D position of the keypoint can be calculated based on the captured images. Moreover, the relative distance of the keypoints in different 3D position can be calculated. To evaluate the error of the relative distance, the relative distance error was defined as:

$$RD_{err} = |R_d - D| \tag{4}$$

where the R_d is the relative distance we calculated, the D is 10 mm which is the length of each movement. The final data is defined as:

$$RD_{err} \pm \max_{i=0}^{n} \left| RD_{ierr} - \overline{RD_{err}} \right| \tag{5}$$

where the $\overline{RD_{err}}$ is the average of the RD_{err} and n is the number of the experiments.

As a result of a 3D image marker's evaluation, the error of the relative depth distance (RDD) is 1.47±2.19 mm (n=10), the error of the relative depth distance (RDD) using subpixel optimization (SPO) is 1.15±2.51 mm (n=10), the error of relative horizontal distance (RHD) is 0.67±2.16 mm (n=10) and the error of relative horizontal distance (RHD) using subpixel optimization (SPO) is 0.74±1.41 mm (n=10), shown in Table 1.

Table 1 The result of a 3D image marker's evaluation

Parameters	Error	Error(SPO)
RDD/mm	1.47±2.19 (n=10)	1.15±2.51 (n=10)
RHD/mm	0.67±2.16 (n=10)	0.74±1.41 (n=10)

Three markers on the probe can be used to locate the tip of the probe and track the posture of the probe. To measure the accuracy of the probe's movement according to the three 3D image markers which is illustrated in Fig. 2, an extra evaluation was carried out. We used a tablet (nexus 10) to simulate the probe. The geometric space relationship of 3D image markers we designed is shown in Fig. 7(a). Fig. 7(b) is a combination of the images captured by the stereo camera. Keypoint-1 and keypoint-3 were almost 1cm above the tablet owing to the usage of IP. Repeating the procession mentioned above, the 3D position of the tip and the relative distance can be calculated.

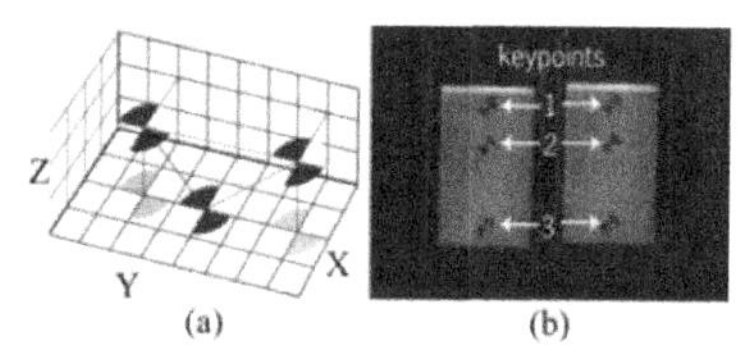

Fig. 7 (a) Geometric information of 3D image markers; (b) Combination of images captured by stereo camera.

As a result of the virtual probe's evaluation, the error of the relative depth distance (RDD) is 1.09±1.44 mm (n=8), the error of the relative depth distance (RDD) using subpixel optimization (SPO) is 0.40±0.31 mm (n=8), the error of relative horizontal distance (RHD) is 0.17±0.16 mm (n=8) and the error of relative horizontal distance (RHD) using subpixel optimization (SPO) is 0.07±0.07 mm (n=8) according to the Table 2.

Different from the traditional probe, 3D image markers on the probe can be designed in line which was shown in

Fig.3 to satisfy the degrees of freedom we need. Therefore, we rotated the pad using the rotation platform to confirm its ability of rotation measurement and got several groups of data. The error of relative rotation (RR) is defined as:

$$RR_{err} = |A_r - A| \quad (6)$$

where the A_r is the angle we calculated and the A is the basic angle which was 4°. We dealt with the data carefully to avoid the influence of other factors. As a result, The average absolute error of rotation is 2.91±2.86° (n=4) and the average absolute error of rotation using subpixel optimization (SPO) is 0.98±1.80° (n=4), shown in Table 2, which means this type of probe can be used for rotation measurement.

Fig. 8 shows a probe we designed and it can be used in spatial position measurement system.

Table 2 Result of virtual probe's evaluation

Parameters	Error	Error(SPO)
RDD/mm	1.09±1.44 (n=8)	0.40±0.31 (n=8)
RHD/mm	0.17±0.16 (n=8)	0.07±.07) (n=8)
RR/°	2.91±2.86 (n=4)	0.98±1.80 (n=4)

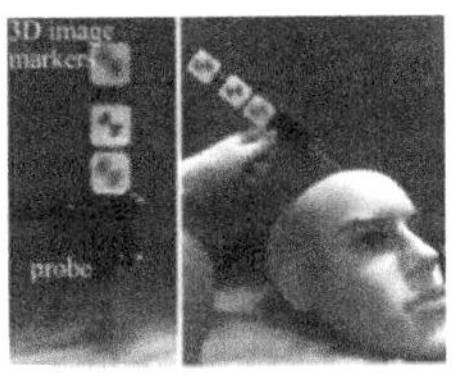

Fig. 8 Evaluation system for 3D position measurement

IV. DISCUSSION AND CONCLUSION

Subpixel optimization (SPO) can improve the accuracy of the result and we will improve the property of the 3D reconstruction algorithm to optimize the results further. Moreover, to reduce the absolute distance error and the absolute error of rotation, we will adopt a better lens array and a higher definition display to get larger view angle and clearer 3D image markers in further study. We also will adopt cameras with high resolution to obtain high quality images. The geometric configuration of the probe consisting of 3D image markers will be further designed to improve the accuracy of the tip's 3D position measurement.

Despite of the error, the probe with 3D image markers holds advantages over the normal one. The 3D image markers on the probe can be designed on a straight line while the normal markers should be designed in the shape of polygon to satisfy the freedom we need in location and posture estimation. Using this type of marker, the space occupied by the probe can be shrunk and the probe can be used in the space-limited environment. Besides, we can get both the environment information as well as the position information because of the stereo camera we used.

Based on the application environment, the 3D image markers can be designed in other forms except for the one mentioned above. Moreover, besides of the IP, other 3D display technologies can be used to design new 3D image markers for tracking. Holding advantages mentioned above, this spatial position measurement system using 3D image markers can be used in location and object tracking.

ACKNOWLEDGMENT

This work was supported in part by National Natural Science Foundation of China (Grant No. 81271735, 61361160417) and Grant-in-Aid of Project 985.

CONFLICT OF INTEREST

The authors declare that they have no conflict of interest.

REFERENCES

1. A. D. Wiles, et al. (2004) Accuracy assessment and interpretation for optical tracking systems[C]//Medical Imaging 2004. International Society for Optics and Photonics, 2004: 421-432.
2. Claron Technology Inc. http://www.clarontech.com/
3. H. Tanaka, et al. (2012) A high-accuracy visual marker based on a microlens array. Intelligent Robots and Systems (IROS), 2012 IEEE/RSJ International Conference on. IEEE, 2012.
4. G. Lippmann. (1908) Epreuves reversibles donnant la sensation du relief. J. Phys. Theor. Appl. 7.1 (1908): 821-825.
5. H. Liao, et al. (2011) Autostereoscopic 3D display with long visualization depth using referential viewing area-based integral photography. Visualization and Computer Graphics, IEEE Transactions on 17.11 (2011): 1690-1701.
6. H. Liao, et al. (2010) 3-D augmented reality for MRI-guided surgery using integral videography autostereoscopic image overlay. Biomedical Engineering, IEEE Transactions on 57.6 (2010): 1476 1486.
7. H. Liao, et al. (2004) High-quality integral videography using a multi-projector. Optics Express 12.6 (2004): 1067-1076.
8. J. Wang, et al. (2013) Augmented Reality Navigation with Automatic Marker-Free Image Registration Using 3D Image Overlay for Dental Surgery. (2013): 1-1.
9. Z. Zhang. (2000) A flexible new technique for camera calibration. Pattern Analysis and Machine Intelligence, IEEE Transactions on 22.11 (2000): 1330-1334.

Author: Hongen Liao
Institute: Department of Biomedical Engineering, School of Medicine, Tsinghua University
Street: Haidian District
City: Beijing 100084
Country: P.R. China
Email: liao@tsinghua.edu.cn

Assessment of Hemodynamic Responses in Cerebral Ischemic Rats Using Near Infrared Spectroscopy

Wan-Chen Shao, Chun-Wei Wu, Chun-Man Yuan, and Jia-Jin Jason Chen

Department of Biomedical Engineering, National Cheng Kung University, Tainan, Taiwan, R.O.C.

Abstract— **Ischemic stroke is a high prevailing and disease in industrialized countries. A valid animal model is essential to develop an extensive research. Among various models, middle cerebral artery occlusion (MCAO) is one of the common used ischemic stroke animal models. In this study, we evaluate the absorption coefficient, reduced scattering coefficient and hemodynamic responses using near infrared spectroscopy (NIRS). The correlation between NIRS signals and the brain infarction volume was measured from histochemical stain. Through the well correlation about reduced scattering coefficient, NIRS can be an effective tool to evaluate ischemic stroke.**

Keywords— **Ischemic stroke, NIRS, histochemical stain.**

I. INTRODUCTION

Ischemic stroke (IS) is the obstruction of blood supply to the brain. Once blood supply is blocked, death of neuron will result. Even though blood flow returns after few hours, the ischemic area will still go on deterioration and eventually cause cell death.

Middle cerebral artery (MCA) is the most common artery involved in human ischemia stroke and the surgery of MCA occlusion can be divided into permanent occlusion or transient ischemia. The transient ischemic model is chosen in this study because it is more compatible to real situation [1]. Near infrared spectroscopy (NIRS) is a noninvasive optical technique which provides the real-time information about dynamic change of oxy-hemoglobin (HbO) and deoxy-hemoglobin (Hb) in cerebral tissue [2]. Because these molecules can absorb specific wavelengths of light, ischemia alters the optical properties of brain tissue. Taking these properties, several studies have investigated brain response during cerebral ischemia using optical methods. Wolf et al. used NIRS to show a decrease in oxyhemoglobin and an increase in deoxyhemoglobin during focal cerebral ischemia in rats [3]. Moreover, Weiguo et al. could locate the cortical ischemia focus of the rats with MCAO by using 760 nm and 850 nm NIR light [4]. In the other hand, near infrared spectroscopy is used widely in the differentiation tissue types. Some results have shown that NIR light in the 700– 850 nm wavelength range is special to tissues as light scattering is more prominent than light absorption [5]. There is a significant difference in light-scattering properties between different tissue types and between healthy and diseased tissues due to their differences in anatomical substructure. In addition, extracellular and intracellular organelles of diseased tissues undergo changes in their density, morphological size, and distribution of scattering [6]. Extracting the mean particle size and number density of scattering particles from the reduced scattering coefficient spectrum in breast tissue was discussed recently [7]. NIR light take a banana-like shape when it goes through high scattering tissue like the brain cortex. Then the transmitted light passes through the thin scalp and skull bone and reaches the detection position. Thus, we can get the brain infarction region through analyzing the parameters of NIRS signals. In addition to NIRS measurement, 2,3,5-triphenyltetrazolium chloride (TTC) as histochemical stain was applied to differentiate between alive and dead neuron [8] as well as to observe the correlation between NIRS signals and infarction volume.

II. MATERIALS AND METHODS

A. Animal Model of Ischemic Stroke

We used male Sprague-Dawley (SD) rats (n=31) weighting 280~330 g (7~9 weeks) in this study. The focal cerebral ischemia was induced by occluding the MCA using the intraluminal suture method. Briefly, rats were anesthetized with Isoflurane by a homemade close loop inhalation system, and nylon filament-tube was used to occlude the origin of the MCA. It was inserted into the internal carotid artery lumen until it met mild resistance, approximately 1.85 cm beyond the common carotid artery bifurcation. After occlusion for 90, 120, or 180 minutes in MCA territory, the filament was removed. Similar procedures were performed in the sham group except no filament in use. During the surgical procedure, the body temperature was maintained at 37.5°C using an electrical heating pad.

B. Measurement of NIRS Signals

To record NIRS signal, the homemade optical probe was placed on skull with its light transmission pathway across the MCA territory along its long axis. The probe contains two light sources and one detector for each hemisphere. Each light source coupling with two laser beams with wavelengths of 690nm and 830nm from Imagent (ISS,Inc). First, absorption coefficient (μ_a), and reduced scattering

I. Lackovic (ed.), *1st Global Conference on Biomedical Engineering & 9th Asian-Pacific Conference on Medical and Biological Engineering*,
IFMBE Proceedings 47, DOI: 10.1007/978-3-319-12262-5_43

coefficient (μ_s') were calculated. Mapping the μ_a at each wavelength with the knowledge of the wavelength-dependent molar extinction (ε) values of the chromophores enables us to calculate tissue chromophore concentration (C) of Hb, HbO separately with Beer Lambert's Law as (1).

$$\mu_a(\lambda) = 2.303[\varepsilon(\lambda)]C \quad (1)$$

where the bracket [ ] represents a matrix and λ is the wavelength. Other studies have shown that the wavelength dependence of scattering in tissue in the near infrared range follows a power-law dependence of the form (Equation 2) [7].

$$\mu_s'(\lambda) = A\lambda^{-sp}, \quad (2)$$

where A is the scattering amplitude, and sp is the scattering power. It has been shown that A and sp are related to geometrical properties; A is related to changes in number density of the scatterers, particle distribution and refractive index. Comparatively, decrease in sp simply reflects an increase in scatterer size and vice versa. The measurements were performed at baseline, during occlusion, immediately after had filament retracted and the 1st, 2nd, 3rd day after acute IS induction in this study.

C. Histochemical Stain

TTC stain is widely used as it is a rapid, easy and economic tool to verify an ischemic stroke model. TTC is colorless in reduced form and oxidized to red color in oxidative form when encountered with vital mitochondrion. In this study, the rats were sacrificed on the 3rd day after MCAO surgery and brain in each rat was rapidly removed after perfusion of saline. Eight, 2 mm coronal sections were made from the olfactory bulb to the cerebellum and then stained with 1% TTC for 30 minutes. Then the mitochondrion in non-ischemia brain parenchyma reacted with TTC and turned to red color. In contrast, loss of mitochondrion in the ischemia area made the reaction impossible and leaves the ischemia territory in white color. The stained brain sections were captured with scanner. The infarction volume of each brain was analyzed by Image J.

D. Statistical Considerations

Correlation between NIRS signals and infarction volume were performed by *Pearson correlation coefficient*. The correlation was considered to be significant at a probability level of less than 0.05 ($p < 0.05$).

III. Results

A. μ_a, μ_s', and Hemodynamic Changes

The changes in μ_a, μ_s' are detected, and oxygen saturation (StO_2), HbO, Hb, total hemoglobin (tHb) in both hemispheres during MCAO compared with baseline and after reperfusion were analyzed and calculated as absolute quantification from Imagent (ISS, Inc) (Fig. 1). Our results show the significant reduction in StO_2, HbO, and tHb during MCAO compared with pre-MCAO and after reperfusion. In addition, μ_s' in two wavelengths increases and scattering power decreases gradually after MCAO surgery.

Compared with sham group, MCAO group including the lesion at cortex and subcortex, as well as subcortex only are presented in Fig. 2. The obvious differences of absorption properties are on the time of MCAO surgery. For example, StO_2 of both MCAO group is obviously lower than that of sham group. However, μ_s' of the lesion at subcortex is closer to sham group, and both differ from the lesion at cortex and subcortex. The sp also has these qualities especially on the third day after MCAO.

B. TTC Stain

The infarction volume is analyzed and compared 90 minutes of reperfusion time with 120 and 180 minutes, as shown in Fig. 3. It seems that the infarct area is equivalent on the occlusion time of 120 and 180 minutes, more than 90 minutes. For this reason, in order to promote the statistical efficacy, we would do the following analysis with these three occlusion times. To explain the variation of the infarct area, Fig. 4 shows the influence of different regions of lesion. The lesion at subcortex only leads to smaller infarction area.

C. Correlation between NIRS Signals and Infarction Volume

According to past studies [9], we assumed that tissue scattering properties is related to tissue structural properties and scattering power (sp) simply reflecting the average size of scatterers. Postoperative day (POD) 3 was chosen because infarction growth is stable from then on. Also, sp and μ_s' (830, 960 nm) of lesion at subcortex only are closer to the sham group and different from the other group on POD 3. In order to investigate the relationship between sp, μ_s' and infarction volume, correlation about them is performed except the group of lesion at subcortex only (Fig. 5). High correlation between μ_s' (830nm) and infarction volume ($r = 0.87$; $p < 0.05$; $n = 8$) can be found. As for the sp, μ_s' (690nm), the r values are -0.51 and 0.44, respectively which are not statistically significant ($p > 0.05$). Additionally, since MCAO group of StO_2 differs from sham group on MCA occlusion time in Fig. 2 (d), correlation is shown in Fig. 6. The r value is -0.14 in the StO_2 which does not reach the significant level.

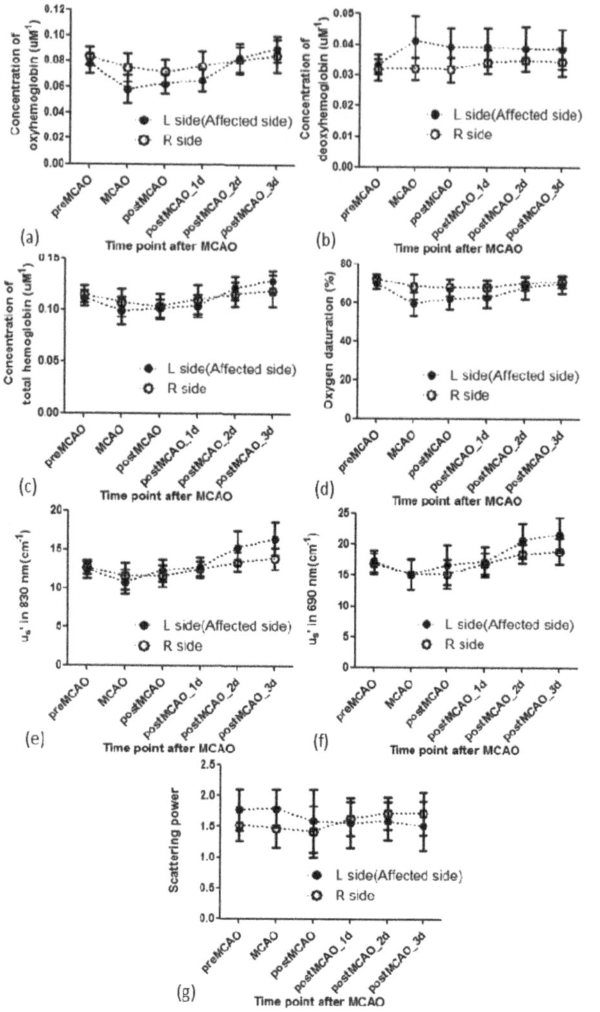

Fig. 1 Measurements of NIRS signals include concentrations of (a) HbO, (b) Hb, (c) tHb, (d) StO_2, and (g) μ_s' in 830 nm, (h) μ_s' in 690 nm, and (i) scattering power are about scattering properties. (n= 16)

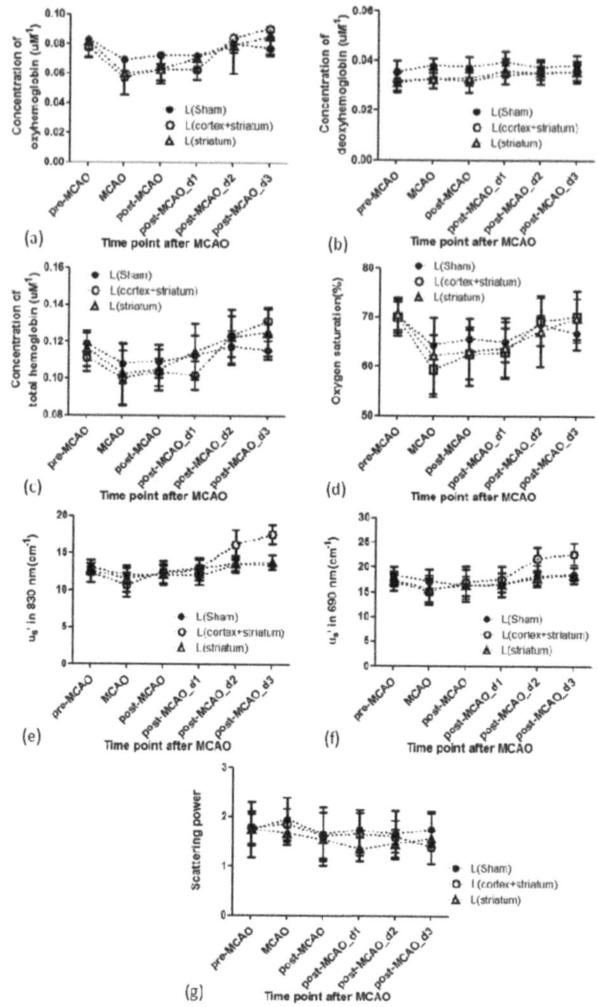

Fig. 2 Measurements on MCAO group including the lesion at cortex, subcortex (n=12), and only subcortex (n=4), compared with sham group (n=7) about concentrations of (a) HbO, (b) Hb, (c) tHb, and (d) StO_2. (e) and (f) are μa in 830 nm and 690 nm, respectively. (g) μs' in 830 nm, (h) μs' in 690 nm, and (i) scattering power are about scattering properties.

IV. DISCUSSION

In Fig. 1, the increases in concentration of Hb, and decrease in concentration of HbO, StO2 apparently occur following MCA occlusion. These changes reflect the pathophysiologic state of the brain and the capability of NIRS to quantify changes in concentration of chromophores with time. We can further compare the difference between both MCAO and sham groups (Fig. 2). Both MCAO groups have the similar absorption properties on occlusion time, but different in scattering properties on the POD 3. It seems that the tissue properties of infarction volume in subcortex cannot be detected by our technique due to the penetration depth of NIR.

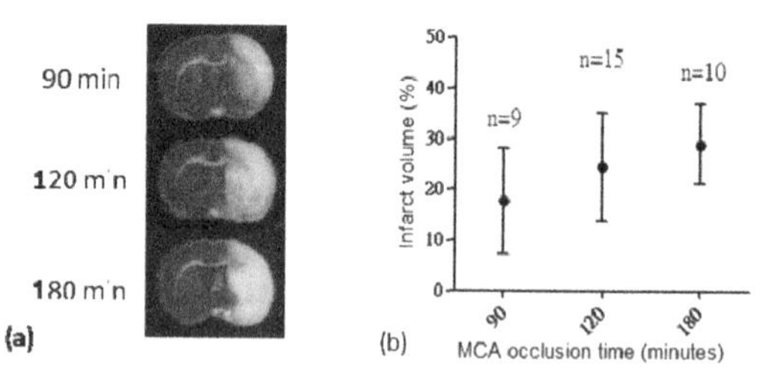

Fig. 3 (a) is an example of the TTC stain with different occlusion time, and (b) is the quantification of infarction volume, including 90, 120, 180 minutes

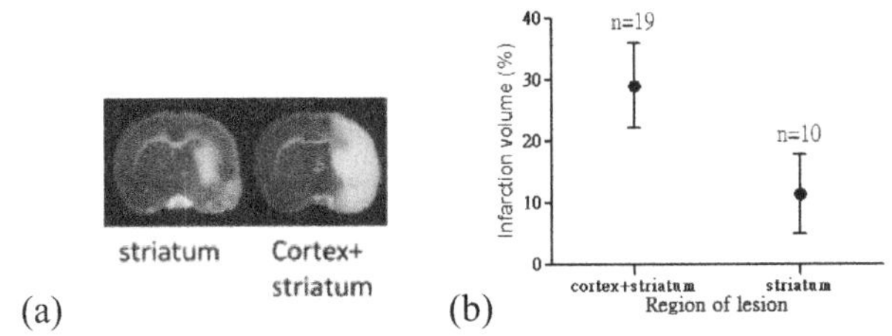

Fig. 4 (a) is an example of TTC stain with different region of lesion. (b) is the quantification of infarction volume at cortex, subcortex and subcortex only

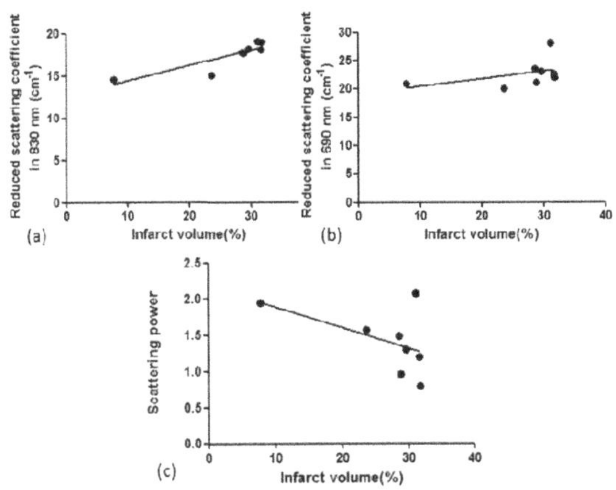

Fig. 5 Correlation of infarction volume with (a) μs' in 830 nm, (b) μs' in 690 nm, (c) scattering power (n=8) are 0.87, 0.44, and -0.51 on POD 3

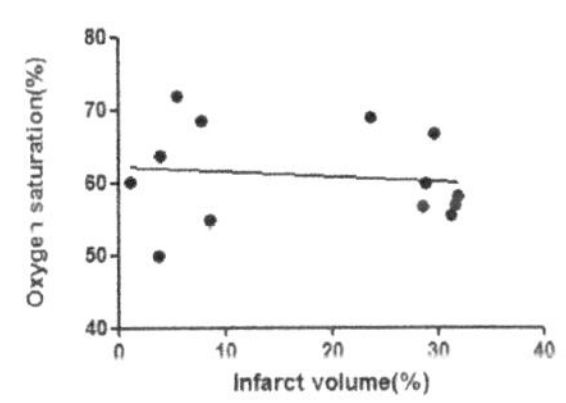

Fig. 6 Correlation of infarction volume with oxygen saturation (n=13) is -0.6838 on MCA occlusion time

For the MCAO group of the lesion at cortex and subcortex, while concentrations of hemoglobin are almost restored, scattering properties differ from the baseline on the POD3 (Fig. 2). It can be inferred that the tissues are destroyed after occlusion, although the vessels are freely flowing. Similarly, the infarction volume of TTC stain corresponds with these phenomena which have higher correlation with scattering parameters than oxygen saturation. Especially, μ_s' (830nm) has high correlation with infarction volume might due to the deeper penetration depth of the larger wavelength, 830 nm. Variation of μs' (690 nm) is relatively higher which probably affected by blood or interference at surface because of the shallower penetration at 690 nm. Thus, the high variation in μs' (690 nm) might influence statistical analysis of both 830 and 690 nm NIR light.

V. CONCLUSIONS

We have investigated the changing tendency of NIRS signals until the third day after stroke and found the irreversible scattering properties. Furthermore, μ_s' in 830nm has high correlation with infarction volume, suggesting that NIRS signals are quite sensitive to tissue alterations.

CONFLICT OF INTEREST

The authors declare that they have no conflict of interest.

REFERENCES

1. Yanamoto H, Nagata I, Niitsu Y et al. (2003) Evaluation of MCAO stroke models in normotensive rats: standardized neocortical infarction by the 3VO technique. Exp Neurol **182**:261-274.
2. Tseng SH, Bargo P, Durkin A et al. (2009) Chromophore concentrations, absorption and scattering properties of human skin in-vivo. Opt Express **17**:14599-14617.
3. Wolf T, Lindauer U, Reuter U et al. (1997) Noninvasive near infrared spectroscopy monitoring of regional cerebral blood oxygenation changes during peri-infarct depolarizations in focal cerebral ischemia in the rat. J Cereb Blood Flow Metab **17**:950-954.
4. Chen W, Lu G, and Lichty W (2002) Localizing the focus of ischemic stroke with near infrared spectroscopy. Chin Med J (Engl) **115**:84-88.
5. Johns M, Giller C, and Liu H (1998) Computational and in vivo investigation of optical reflectance from human brain to assist neurosurgery. J Biomed Opt **3**:437-445.
6. Jacques SL (2013) Optical properties of biological tissues: a review. Phys Med Biol **58**:37-61.
7. Wang X, Pogue BW, Jiang S et al. (2005) Approximation of Mie scattering parameters in near-infrared tomography of normal breast tissue in vivo. J Biomed Opt **10**:051704.
8. Liu F, Schafer DP, and McCullough LD (2009) TTC, fluoro-Jade B and NeuN staining confirm evolving phases of infarction induced by middle cerebral artery occlusion. J Neurosci Methods **179**:1-8.
9. Mourant JR, Fuselier T, Boyer J et al. (1997) Predictions and measurements of scattering and absorption over broad wavelength ranges in tissue phantoms. Appl Opt **36**:949-57.

Author: Jia-Jin Jason Chen
Institute: Department of Biomedical Engineering, National Cheng Kung University
Street: No.1, University Road, Tainan City 701, Taiwan (R.O.C)
City: Tainan
Country: Taiwan
Email: jasonbiolab@gmail.com

The Correlations between Chinese Personality Traits and Cortical Activation

R.S. Luo[1], C.Y. Lee[2], K.Y. Hsu[3], Y.P. Chao[4], J. Hung[5], H.L. Liu[6], C.G. Tsai[7], M.C. Chiu[8], J.H. Chen[9], K.G. Yao[10], and J.F. Yu[1]

[1] Graduate Institute of Medical Mechatronics, Chang Gung University, Taoyuan,Taiwan
[2] Taiouan Interdisciplinary Otolaryngology Laboratory, Chang Gung University, Taoyuan, Taiwan
[3] Department of Psychology, National Chung Cheng University, Chia-yi, Taiwan
[4] Computer Science and information Engineering, Chang Gung University, Taoyuan, Taiwan
[5] Department of Medical Imaging and Radiological Sciences, Chang Gung University, Taoyuan, Taiwan
[6] Graduate Institute of Musicology, National Taiwan University, Taipei, Taiwan
[7] Department of neurology, National Taiwan University Hospital, Taipei, Taiwan
[8] Department of Electrical Engineering, National Taiwan University, Taipei, Taiwan
[9] Department of Psychology, National Taiwan University, Taipei, Taiwan
[10] Department of Neurology, Chang Gung Memorial Hospital, Taipei, Taiwan

Abstract— **The majority of studies investigating correlations between personality and neuroscience have used the Big-Five personality scales developed in Europe and North America. This is the first study to address correlations between Chinese personality traits and cortical activation.**

In this study, we used the Chinese Personality Adjective Rating Scale to analyze the personalities of 23 respondents. We also used functional magnetic resonance imaging to explore the correlations between Chinese personality traits and cortical activation. The results of this study indicated that Optimism/Pessimism, Extraversion/Introversion, and Industriousness/Unindustriousness from the Chinese Personality Adjective Scale were correlated with Neuroticism, Extraversion, and Conscientiousness from the Big Five personality traits. The activation positions were consistent with those identified in earlier studies. Additionally, this study indicated that the clearest position of activation for the dimension of competence vs. impotence was the supplementary motor area. The temporal gyrus and hippocampus were negatively correlated with moral character. The activation of the limbic system was positively correlated with large-mindedness vs. small-mindedness, and the thalamus, temporal lobe, and parietal lobe were positively correlated with flexibility vs. rigidity.

This is the first study to address correlations between Chinese personality traits and cortical activation. The results of this study can serve as an essential reference for research on Chinese personality traits and neuroscience.

Keywords— **fMRI, Brain, Chinese, Personality.**

I. INTRODUCTION

The question of whether environmental or personality factors influence behavior may be the oldest in the field of psychology. A number of neuroscientific methods exist for exploring the correlations between a variety of personality dimensions and neurobiology. In North America and Europe, the NEO-Five Factor Inventory (NEO-FFI) [1] is often used for related research. A number of studies have found relationships between the Big Five personality traits and cortical activity [2]. In Taiwan, the field of psychology often applies the Chinese Personality Adjective Rating Scale to explore Chinese personality traits. Because the Chinese Personality Adjective Rating Scale shares only three dimensions in common with the Big Five personality traits, studies on the Big Five personality traits and neuroscience have been unable to interpret the relationships between the Big Seven personality traits and cortical activity. In this study, we integrated the fields of cognitive neuroscience and personality psychology to investigate the correlations between a variety of Chinese personality traits and cortical activity.

II. METHODS AND MATERIALS

A. Participants

We recruited 23 respondents with normal hearing (10 women and 13 men). Their average age was 26 (*SD* = 4.1), and all were right handed. After all of the respondents signed a written consent form approved by the institutional review board, we ensured that they understood the risks and safety regulations of functional magnetic resonance imaging (fMRI). Then, we performed whole brain scans using fMRI.

B. Personality Assessment

We used the Chinese Personality Adjective Rating Scale to analyze the personalities of the respondents. The version we used was the Simple Chinese Personality Adjective Rating Scale, which had 56 items encompassing 7 personality dimensions: (1) optimistic vs. pessimism; (2) large-mindedness vs. small-mindedness; (3) extravesion vs. introversion; (4) other-orientedness vs. self-centeredness; (5) agreeableness vs. disagreeableness; (6) industriousness vs. unindustriousness; and (7) Competence vs. Impotence. This is a Likert-type

I. Lackovic (ed.), *1st Global Conference on Biomedical Engineering & 9th Asian-Pacific Conference on Medical and Biological Engineering*,
IFMBE Proceedings 47, DOI: 10.1007/978-3-319-12262-5_44

4-point rating scale, with answers ranging from *extremely inconsistent* to *extremely consistent*. Every dimension of the Chinese Personality Adjective Rating Scale has a reliability of at least 0.7, indicating that the dimensions are reliable (optimism vs. pessimism = 0.84; large-mindedness vs. small-mindedness =0.79; extraversion vs. introversion = 0.83; other-orientedness vs. self-centeredness = 0.82; agreeableness vs. disagreeableness = 0.77; industriousness vs. unindustriousness = 0.80; and competence vs. impotence = 0.84).

Table 1 Main demographic and personality measures

Main demographic and personality measures	
Number of subject	23
Men / women	13 vs. 10
Mean age,SD	M=26 , SD=4.1
NEO-FFI scores	
Optimism vs. Pessimism	M=3.84, SD=054
Liberality vs. Stinginess	M=3.66,SD=0.40
Dynamism vs. Passivity	M=3.65,SD=0.44
Moral Character	M=3.71,SD=0.28
Flexibility vs. Rigidity	M=3.65,SD=0.43
Diligence vs. Idleness	M=3.44,SD=0.53
Wisdom vs. Stupidity	M=3.53,SD=0.46

C. fMRI Acquisition

We used block design with echo planar imaging (EPI) to perform 3T fMRI. The method we used to obtain the fMRI images was single-shot T2 weighted EPI. The area scanned included a range from the entire cerebellum to the cerebrum and was divided into 44 slices with a thickness of 3 mm. We obtained the following image parameters: repetition time (TR) = 3000 ms; echo time (TE) = 35 ms; flip angle = 90°; matrix size = 64 * 64; field of view = 192 mm; and dummy scan – 6 s. We simultaneously used case T1 imaging for reference. The T1 imaging parameters were TR/TE/flip angle = 9 ms/4.2 ms/90° and voxel size = 0.86 mm * 0.86 mm * 1.0 mm. In addition, we used E-Prime 2.0 to design the experimental procedure.

D. Statistical Analysis

We used Cronbach's alpha to assess the reliability of the Chinese Personality Adjective Rating Scale (Simple Version). We used MATLAB 8.0 and SPM8 for preprocessing and interpreting the fMRI image data. We used the generalized linear model for analysis.

III. RESULTS

In optimism vs. pessimism, the clearest areas of positively correlated activation were the right superior temporal (T = 4.74, x = 68, y = -26, z = 6) followed by the left supplementary motor area (SMA) (T = 4.61, x = -8, y = -16, z = 62).

In large-mindedness vs. small-mindedness, the clearest areas of positively correlated activation were the right superior precuneus (T = 4.73, x = 6, y = -58, z = 0) followed by the right limbic lobe (T = 4.71, x = 20, y = 2, z = 36).

In extraversion vs. introversion, the clearest areas of positively correlated activation were the right middle cingulum (T = 5.33, x = 12, y = 12, z = 38) followed by the right superior occipital (T = 4.97, x = 28, y = -82, z = 30).

In other-orientedness vs. self-centeredness, the clearest areas of negatively correlated activation were the right middle temporal (T = 4.34, x = 56, y = -2, z = -24) followed by the left parahippocampal (T = 4.04, x = -24, y = -28, z = -22).

In agreeableness vs. disagreeableness, the clearest areas of positively correlated activation were the right thalamus (T = 5.47, x = 10, y = -26, z = 2) followed by the left temporal lobe (T = 4.57, x = -28, y = -64, z = 12).

In industriousness vs. unindustriousness, the clearest areas of positively correlated activation were the right thalamus (T = 4.94, x = 14, y = -30, z = 2) followed by the left middle cingulum (T = 4.35, x = -10, y = 10, z = 40).

In Competence vs. Impotence, the clearest areas of positively correlated activation were the left SMA (T = 5.63, x = -10, y = 2, z = 76) followed by the right SMA (T = 4.95, x = 12, y = 14, z = 56).

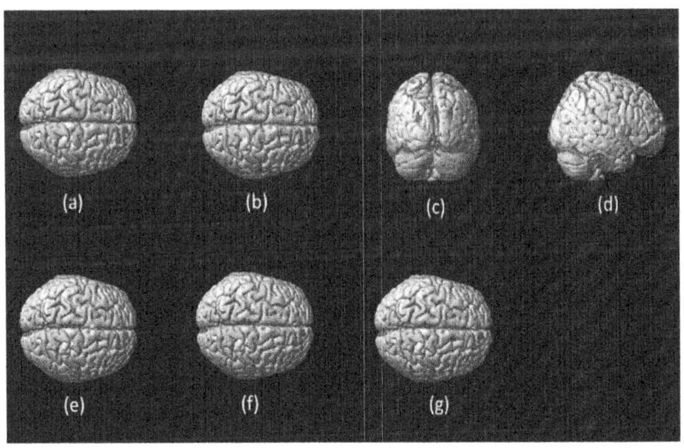

Fig. 1. Point distribution of Chinese personality traits in cortical activation: (a) optimism vs. pessimism; (b) Large-mindedness vs. Small-mindedness; (c) Extraversion vs. Introversion; (d) Other-orientedness vs. Self-centeredness; (e) Agreeableness vs. Disagreeableness; (f) Industriousness vs. Unindustriousness; (g) Competence vs. Impotence.

Table 2. Primary positions of activity in the cerebral cortex for the Chinese personality traits.

Item	Region	T	x	y	z
Optmism vs. Pessimism	R superior temporal	4.74	68	-26	6
	L supplementary motor area	4.61	-8	-16	62
	L rolandic oper	4.27	-48	-12	16
	R postcentral	4.19	58	-12	48
Large-mindedness vs. Small-mindedness	R superior precuneus	4.73	6	-58	0
	R limbic lobe	4.71	20	2	36
	R parietal	4.53	18	-52	72
	R SMA	4.52	12	-8	70
	L angular	3.89	-40	-64	30
Extraversion vs. Introversion	R middle cingulum	5.33	12	12	38
	R superior occipital	4.97	28	-82	30
	L middle occipital	4.53	-36	-72	4
	R SMA	4.33	8	14	54
Other-orientedness vs. Self-centeredness	R middle temporal	4.34	56	-2	-24
	L paraHippocampal	4.04	-24	-28	-22
Agreeableness vs. Disagreeableness	R thalamus	5.47	10	-26	2
	L temporal lobe	4.57	-28	-64	12
	L SMA	4.45	-4	4	62
	R cuneus	4.29	14	-76	38
Industriousness vs. Unindustriousness	R thalamus	4.94	14	-30	2
	L middle cingulum	4.35	-10	10	40
	R cuneus	4.11	8	-78	34
	R postcentral	4	46	26	64
Competence vs. Impotence	L SMA	5.63	-10	2	76
	R SMA	4.95	12	14	56
	R lingual	4.63	8	-72	-10
	R calcarine	4.23	12	-88	8
	L lingual	3.9	-14	-56	-2

IV. DISCUSSIONS

A. Comparison with the Big Five Personality Traits

A study published by Yang et al. [3] indicated that the Chinese Personality Adjective Rating Scale contains three dimensions that are correlated with those in Big Five personality traits. The correlation coefficients between neuroticism and optimism vs. pessimism, extraversion and extraversion vs. introversion, and conscientiousness and industriousness vs. unindustriousness are -0.70, 0.77, and 0.73, respectively However, a 2013 study [4] indicated that neuroticism from the Big Five personality traits is negatively correlated with the upper right parietal cortex. By contrast, in this study, optimism vs. pessimism from the Chinese Personality Adjective Rating Scale was positively correlated with the parietal lobe. Conscientiousness from the Big Five personality traits is positively correlated with the precuneus. We found the same activation position for industriousness vs. unindustriousness in this study. We found positively correlated activity for large-mindedness vs. small-mindedness in the limbic system. The limbic system regulates human emotions. This indicates that people with more straightforward and open personalities than others do show clearer activity in the limbic system. The only negatively correlated personality dimension we found in this study was other-orientedness vs. self-centeredness, which was negatively correlated with both the temporal gyrus and the hippocampus. This indicates that people who are more cunning than others are have clearer activity in these two regions. agreeableness vs. disagreeableness was positively correlated with the thalamus, temporal lobe, and parietal lobe. This indicates that these positions show more activity in people with meek and easygoing personalities. Wisdom vs. stupidity is connected to intelligence. Previous studies have indicated that the motor cortex and prefrontal cortex are connected to intelligence. In this study, we found that the position with the clearest activation for Competence vs. Impotence was the SMA, which is consistent with the findings of previous studies.

B. Research Restrictions

This is the first study to examine the correlations between Chinese personality traits and cortical activation. We adopted the Chinese Personality Adjective Rating Scale. In this scale, liberality vs. stinginess, moral character, flexibility vs. rigidity, and wisdom vs. stupidity cannot be compared with any of the Big Five personality traits. Therefore, no study that can corroborate our findings exist. In addition, this study only involved 23 participants. Because this number is clearly insufficient compared with those in other studies, the validity and reliability of this study may have been reduced.

V. CONCLUSIONS

The results of this study can serve as an essential reference for research on Chinese personality traits and neuroscience. We found correlations between optimistic vs. pessimism, extraversion vs. introversion, and industriousness vs. unindustriousness on the Chinese Personality Adjective Rating Scale and neuroticism, extraversion, and conscientiousness from the Big Five personality traits. The positions of activation were consistent with those identified in previous studies. In addition, the only negatively correlated personality dimension we found in this study was moral character, which was negatively correlated with both the temporal gyrus and the hippocampus. This indicates that people who are more cunning than others have clearer activity in these two regions. We found positively correlated activity for liberality vs. stinginess in the limbic system, which regulates human emotions. This indicates that people with more straightforward and open personalities than others do show clearer activity in the limbic system.

ACKNOWLEDGMENT

We appreciate the sponsorship and funding of the National Science Council Project No. 102-2420-H-182-001.

CONFLICT OF INTEREST

The authors declare that they have no conflict of interest.

REFERENCES

1. COSTA JR, Paul T (1995). Domains and facets: Hierarchical personality assessment using the Revised NEO Personality Inventory. Journal of personality assessment, 64(1) , 21-50.
2. ANDREWS-HANNA, Jessica R., et al.(2010) Functional-anatomic fractionation of the brain's default network. Neuron, 65(4), 550-562.
3. Yang, K. S., Hwang, K. K. (2006). Indigenous and cultural psychology. U. Kim (Ed.). Heidelberg: Springer.
4. SAMPAIO, Adriana, et al. (2013)The Big Five default brain: functional evidence. Brain Structure and Function, 1-10.

Author: Jen-Fang Yu
Institute: Graduate Institute of Medical Mechatronics
Street: 259 Wen-Hwa 1st Road, Kwei-Shan
City: Tao-Yuan
Country: Taiwan
Email: jfyu.phd@gmail.com

The Comparison of Tissue Vibration Signal Extraction Algorithms in Shearwave Dispersion Ultrasound Vibrometry

X. Cai, F. Fan, X.F. Li, B.Q. Pei, H.J. Niu*, and Y.B Fan

Key Laboratory of Ministry of Education for Biomechanics and Mechanobiology,
School of Biological Science and Medical Engineering, Beihang University, Beijing, China

Abstract— **Shearwave Dispersion Ultrasound Vibrometry (SDUV), a method could quantify both tissue elasticity and viscosity has been introduced recently. Vibration extraction is an important step in SDUV. Two vibration extraction algorithms, the quadrature demodulation method (QDM) and the cross-spectrum method (CSM) are usually used in SDUV. However, the extraction quality of QDM and CSM are under appropriate comparison. This study aims at comparing the extraction quality of QDM and CSM based on a parameterized model for various signal-to-noise ratio of ultrasound echoes (SNR_U). Results showed that when $SNR_U \geq 35dB$, the standard deviations of the estimated vibration phase using the vibration extracted by the two methods are close, which has no significant differences on the calculation result of the shear wave speed. The computation efficiency of CSM is lower than that of QDM. As a conclusion, when $SNR_U < 35dB$, the tissue vibration should be extracted by CSM to suppress the estimation error of vibration phase. However, when $SNR_U \geq 35dB$, the tissue vibration should be extracted by QDM to reduce the processing time. The findings in this study may provider some strategy in SDUV, which can optimize the examination protocol and make it more efficient.***

Keywords— **SDUV, QDM, CSM, vibration extraction.**

I. INTRODUCTION

Due to the close relationship with the tissue pathology, the mechanical properties of tissues have a significant value in clinic [1]. Since Ophir supposed an ultrasound elastic imaging method of tissues in 1991, many techniques for tissue elastic measurement have been proposed such as quasi-static elastography, shear wave elasticity imaging, vibro-acoustography and supersonic shear imaging [2]. Although biological tissues are viscoelastic materials, most techniques ignore the viscosity of tissues. Neglecting tissue viscosity may not only cause bias in the estimation of tissue elasticity, but also increase the inaccuracy of diagnosis [3]. To remedy this defect, shearwave dispersion ultrasound vibrometry (SDUV) which can quantify tissue elasticity and viscosity non-invasively was proposed [4].

In SDUV, the estimation accuracy of vibration signal determines the estimation accuracy of viscoelastic parameters. Two vibration extraction algorithms, the quadrature demodulation method (QDM) [5] and the cross-spectrum method (CSM) [6] are usually used in SDUV. QDM shifts the spectrum of the consecutive echoes to be centered at zero Hz, and then remove the high frequency components by a low-pass filter. While CSM extracts the vibration by tracking the phase shifts between consecutive echoes at the frequency where the magnitude of the cross spectrum is maximum. However, the extraction quality for various signal-to-noise ratio of ultrasound echoes (SNR_U), the practical applicable scope and the efficiency of the methods are under appropriate study and comparison.

In this paper, ultrasound echoes based on a parameterized model for various SNR_U were simulated. QDM and CSM were applied to extract the vibration. The vibration phase was estimated to compare the extraction quality of the methods and the computation time was recorded to compare the computational efficiency of the methods.

II. METHOD

A. Quadrature Demodulation

The motion of tissues vibrated by the harmonic force can be represented as [7]:

$$D(t_s) = D_0 \sin(\omega_s t_s + \emptyset_s), \qquad (1)$$

where D_0 is the amplitude of the vibration, t_s is the vibration time of the motion, $\emptyset_s$ is the vibration phase. The spectrum of the vibration can be modeled as a frequency modulated spectrum, when the vibration speed and frequency of tissues are much lower than the propagation velocity and frequency of the interrogating ultrasound echoes [8]. Thus, if the centre frequency of the interrogating ultrasound is ω_f, echoes reflected by vibrating tissues can be modeled as [7]:

$$r(t_f, t_s) = A(t_f, t_s)\cos(\omega_f t_f + \emptyset_f + \beta \sin(\omega_s t_s + \emptyset_s)), \qquad (2)$$

here, t_f is the acquisition time of the echo, $A(t_f, t_s)$ is the complex envelope of $r(t_f, t_s)$, $\emptyset_f$ is the initial phase of the ultrasound signal, β is defined as:

$$\beta = \frac{2D_0\omega_f \cos(\theta)}{c}, \qquad (3)$$

where θ is the Doppler angle and c is the longitudinal sound propagation speed in the medium. The model

---
* Corresponding author.

I. Lackovic (ed.), *1st Global Conference on Biomedical Engineering & 9th Asian-Pacific Conference on Medical and Biological Engineering*,
IFMBE Proceedings 47, DOI: 10.1007/978-3-319-12262-5_45

represented in (2) is quite commonly used in modeling the interrogating ultrasound echoes for vibration tissues in SDUV [5, 9]. Applying a quadrature demodulator to $r(t_f, t_s)$, we can have in-phase and quadrature components [7]:

$$I(t_f, t_s) = |A(t_f, t_s)| \cos(\beta \sin(\omega_s t_s + \emptyset_s) + \emptyset_0), \quad (4)$$

$$Q(t_f, t_s) = |A(t_f, t_s)| \sin(\beta \sin(\omega_s t_s + \emptyset_s) + \emptyset_0), \quad (5)$$

$\emptyset_0$ is a transmitting phase constant. Following Zheng, et al., the complex velocity quantity is defined as [5]:

$$v(t_f, t_s) = X(t_f, t_s) + jY(t_f, t_s) = A(t_f, t_s)A^*(t_f, t_s + T)$$
$$= |A(t_f, t_s)||A(t_f, t_s + T)|e^{j(\emptyset(t_f,t_s)-\emptyset(t_f,t_s+T))}, \quad (6)$$

where $X(t_f, t_s)$ and $Y(t_f, t_s)$ is the real and image part of the complex velocity quantity. Extracting the phase difference, the vibration signal can be represented as:

$$s(t_f, t_s) = \frac{-1}{2\sin(\omega_s T/2)} \tan^{-1}\left(\frac{X(t_f, t_s)}{Y(t_f, t_s)}\right)$$
$$= \frac{-1}{2\sin(\omega_s T/2)} (\emptyset(t_f, t_s) - \emptyset(t_f, t_s + T)), \quad (7)$$
$$= \beta \cos(\omega_s t_s + \emptyset_s + \omega_s T/2)$$

B. Cross-Spectrum

The cross-spectrum method was proposed to solve the displacement of artery-wall using pulse-echo ultrasound [6]. They suggest extracting the displacement at the actual center frequency where the maximum occurs in the magnitude of the cross spectrum [6]. If nth and (n + 1)th echoes were defined as r_n and r_{n+1} and their corresponding frequency spectrums are $R_n(f)$ and $R_{n+1}(f)$, the cross spectrum can be represented as:

$$R_n^*(f)R_{n+1}(f) = |R_n(f)||R_{n+1}(f)|e^{j\Delta\theta_n(f)}, \quad (8)$$

where $\Delta\theta_n(f)$ is the phase shift between consecutive echoes and $*$ is complex conjugation. All echoes should be windowed with a Hann window firstly to ensure a maximum occurs in the magnitude of the spectrum. After that, the phase difference between consecutive echoes at the actual center frequency can be obtained. The vibration velocity of the tissue can be estimated by:

$$v_n = \frac{c\Delta\theta_n(f_0)}{2\omega_f T_{prf}}, \quad (9)$$

f_0 is the actual center frequency, T_{prf} is the pulse repetition period of the pulse-echo interrogation, ω_f is the centre angular frequency of the detecting transducer. The tissue vibration is harmonic at ω_s, thus the displacement of the tissue can be calculated by:

$$D_n = \frac{v_n}{\omega_s}, \quad (10)$$

III. EXPERIMENTS

Under the limitation of FDA ($I_{SPTA} < 720\,mW/cm^2$), the amplitude of tissue vibration usually is on sub-micron level. In this study, the amplitude was set at $1\mu m$, which is a typical value observed in experiments and the other parameters were given in Table 1. Practically, the SNR_U is primarily determined by the electronic noise from the acquisition system [9]. Therefore, the normally distributed noise was added to the simulated ultrasound echoes as:

$$r(t_f, t_s) = A(t_f, t_s) \cos(\omega_f t_f + \emptyset_f + \beta \sin(\omega_s t_s + \emptyset_s)) + n(t_f, t_s), \quad (11)$$

and the SNR_U varied from 20dB to 50dB. There were 100 datasets with different initial noise data added in the ultrasound echoes for the same SNR_U.

Table 1 Parameters of simulated ultrasound echoes

D_0	Vibration amplitude	$1\mu m$
$\emptyset_s$	Vibration phase	45°
N	Cycles of vibration	5
ω_s	Vibration frequency	$2\pi \times 200Hz$
ω_f	Ultrasound frequency	$2\pi \times 9MHz$
F_s	Sampling frequency	100MHz
l_g	Window length	1mm
c	Speed of sound	$1480m/s$

In SDUV, the estimation accuracy of vibration phase determine the estimation accuracy of shear wave speed, which would be used to solve the viscoelasticity of tissues. Thus, we applied QDM and CSM to the simulated echoes to extract the vibration and the SNR of the extracted vibrations were compared. Then, the vibration phase was estimated from the extracted vibration using a Kalman filter [7] to compare the extraction quality of the methods. Parameterized model (11) was used, because it's hard to know the actual vibration phase extracted from real data, so that we cannot quantitatively make the comparison. The analyzed parameters in the follow content and their corresponding meanings were represented by the symbols in Table 2.

Table 2 Symbols for the analyzed parameters in the follow content

SNR_{VD}	The SNR of the vibration extracted by QDM
SNR_{VC}	The SNR of the vibration extracted by CSM
$\emptyset_{VD}$	The estimated vibration phase using the vibration extracted by QDM
$\emptyset_{VC}$	The estimated vibration phase using the vibration extracted by CSM

IV. RESULTS

Fig. 1 illustrates the vibration set up in the experiment and vibrations extracted by QDM and CSM. There are two cycles in the picture. From Figure 1(a), we can see that CSM can extract the vibration reasonably when $SNR_U = 20dB$ and the extraction quality is better than QDM. As illustrated in Fig. 1(b), when $SNR_U = 35dB$, CSM is still better than QDM in the extraction quality. But the difference is smaller than that in Fig. 1(a).

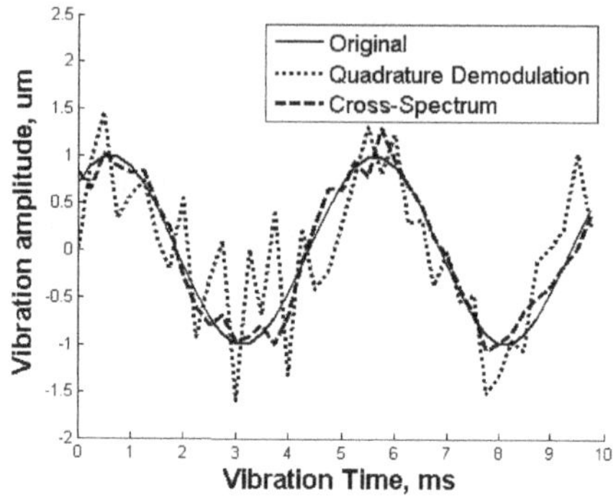

(a) SNR_U=20dB

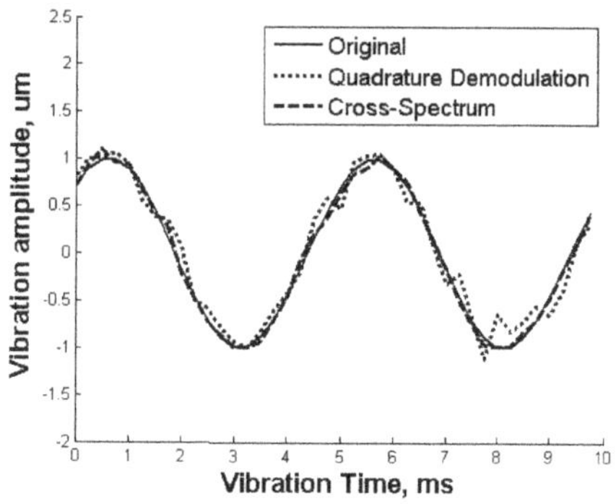

(b) SNR_U=35dB

Fig. 1 The vibration signals extracted by QDM and CSM, solid curve is the vibration set up in the experiment, dotted curve is the vibration extracted by QDM and dashed curve is the vibration extracted by CSM

Table 3 SNR (Mean $\pm$ SD) of the vibration signals extracted by QDM and CSM for various SNR_U

SNR_U	20dB	25dB	30dB	35 dB	40 dB	45 dB	50 dB
SNR_{VD}(dB)	2.80 $\pm$ 0.64	7.75 $\pm$ 0.67	12.79 $\pm$ 0.67	17.75 $\pm$ 0.67	22.72 $\pm$ 0.68	27.86 $\pm$ 0.68	32.67 $\pm$ 0.51
SNR_{VC}(dB)	14.00 $\pm$ 0.64	19.11 $\pm$ 0.67	24.13 $\pm$ 0.64	29.12 $\pm$ 0.60	34.13 $\pm$ 0.64	39.02 $\pm$ 0.67	43.81 $\pm$ 0.64

Table 3 displays the SNR of vibration signal extracted by QDM and CSM. When $SNR_U = 20dB$, the mean and standard deviation (SD) of SNR_{VD} and SNR_{VC} are $2.80 \pm 0.64dB$ and $14.00 \pm 0.64dB$, respectively. When SNR_U varies within $20dB$-$50dB$, SNR_{VC} is about $11dB$ greater than SNR_{VD} for the same SNR_U.

Table 4 illustrates the estimated vibration phase using the vibration extracted by QDM and CSM for various SNR_U. The phase set in the experiment is 45°(Table 1). As SNR_U increases, the standard deviation of $\emptyset_{VD}$ and $\emptyset_{VC}$ decrease and the mean value of the phase approximate to 45°. The SD of $\emptyset_{VC}$ is just 1.00° when $SNR_U = 20dB$, which is much smaller than the figure 3.97° of $\emptyset_{VD}$. When $SNR_U = 35dB$, the mean value of $\emptyset_{VD}$ and $\emptyset_{VC}$ is 45.16° and 45.01°, respectively. The SD of $\emptyset_{VD}$ and $\emptyset_{VC}$, both within 1°, is 0.73° and 0.22°, respectively.

Table 4 The estimated vibration phase (Mean $\pm$ SD) of the vibration extracted by QDM and CSM

SNR_U	20dB	25dB	30dB	35dB	40dB	45dB	50dB
$\emptyset_{VD}$ Degrees	45.05 $\pm$3.97	44.67 $\pm$2.04	45.25 $\pm$1.26	45.16 $\pm$0.73	44.92 $\pm$0.46	45.00 $\pm$0.22	45.00 $\pm$0.13
$\emptyset_{VC}$ Degrees	44.89 $\pm$1.00	45.00 $\pm$0.62	45.02 $\pm$0.34	45.01 $\pm$0.22	44.99 $\pm$0.11	45.00 $\pm$0.06	45.00 $\pm$0.03

V. DISCUSSION

In this paper, ultrasound echoes based on a parameterized model for various SNR_U were simulated. QDM and CSM were applied to the simulated echoes to extract the vibration. The SNR of the extracted vibration was compared and the vibration phase was estimated to compare the extraction quality of the methods. Ultrasound echoes can be modeled as a simple model in this study, because tissues are assumed to be isotropic homogeneous body in SDUV and the window length is usually greater than 0.5mm, which is greater than the pulse duration used in this study in the case of a sound speed of 1480m/s. Although many tissues are inhomogeneous in a macroscopic level, a local homogeneity in 5×5 mm ROIs when using SDUV is suggested [10].

From the results of the extracted vibration signal (Table 3), it is reasonable to conclude that the extraction quality of CSM is better than that of QDM for the same SNR_U. The vibration signal, i.e. the phase of the ultrasound echoes in the fixed center frequency, will be distorted by the noise. QDM extracts the phase of the echoes at the fixed center frequency, which cannot track the actual center frequency after distortion, thus limits its extraction equality. CSM, however, locates the phase shifts according to the actual center frequency and so it is more accurate.

When $SNR_U \geq 35dB$, SNR_{VC} is about $11dB$ greater than SNR_{VD} for the same SNR_U. But the SD of $\emptyset_{VD}$ and $\emptyset_{VC}$ are close ($< 1^{\circ}$), because both SNR_{VC} and SNR_{VD} are greater than $15dB$ when $SNR_U \geq 35dB$ (Table 3, Table 4). This is consistent with the performance of the Kalman filter used in this study, that the SD of the estimated vibration phase $< 1^\circ$ if the SNR of the vibration $> 15dB$. In SDUV, the distance between consecutive measurement points is usually greater than one-tenth of the shear wavelength, i.e. the corresponding phase shift $\geq 36^\circ$. The SD of 1° can be neglected compared to the phase shift between consecutive measurement points, since it has no significant influence on the estimation of the shear wave propagation speed.

In QDM a low-pass filter, which performs Fourier transform and inverse Fourier transform, was implemented on the ultrasound echoes. In CSM, however, ultrasound echoes will be segmented and windowed with a Hann window. The power spectrum and the phase information of the echoes will be calculated. Therefore, CSM is more complex and computational than QDM. In this study, the computation time for extracting the vibration using QDM is 0.081s (Computing Environment: Matlab R2011b, Intel E8200 2.66GHz), while the time consumed by CSM is 0.208s (2.6 times of the former method).

VI. CONCLUSIONS

In summary, the tissue vibration should be extracted using the cross-spectrum method to suppress the estimation error of the vibration phase when $SNR_U < 35dB$. When $SNR_U \geq 35dB$, $\emptyset_{VD}$ and $\emptyset_{VC}$ are close to each other and have no significant influence on the calculation result of the shear wave speed. Meanwhile, the computation efficiency of the cross-spectrum method for vibration extraction is lower than that of the quadrature demodulation method. Therefore, the tissue vibration should be extracted by the quadrature demodulation method to reduce the processing time under this circumstance. The findings in this study suggest a better strategy in SDUV, which may help to optimize the examination protocol and make it more efficient.

In this paper, the differences in the performance of the quadrature demodulation method and the cross-spectrum method in extracting the tissue vibration with normally distributed noise added in simulated ultrasound echoes were discussed. In clinical application, however, a more complex situation may be met in the received ultrasound echoes, which remains further study.

ACKNOWLEDGMENT

This work was supported by the National Natural Science Foundation of China (31170896), Program for New Century Excellent Talents in University (NCET-11-0772)and the National High Technology Research and Development Program of China (863 Program) (2011AA02A102).

CONFLICT OF INTEREST

The authors have no conflicts of interest to disclose.

REFERENCES

1. Sarvazyan A P, Rudenko O V, Swanson S D, et al. (1998) Shear wave elasticity imaging: a new ultrasonic technology of medical diagnostics[J]. Ultrasound in Medicine Biology, 24(9): 1419-1435.
2. Sarvazyan A, Hall T J, Urban M W, et al. (2011) An overview of elastography – an emerging branch of medical imaging[J]. Current Medical Imaging Reviews, 7(4): 255-282.
3. Salameh N, Peeters F, Sinkus R, et al. (2007) Hepatic viscoelastic parameters measured with MR elastography: correlations with quantitative analysis of liver fibrosis in the rat[J]. Journal of Magnetic Resonance Imaging, 26(4): 956-962.
4. Chen S G , Urban M W, Pislaru C, et al. (2009) Shearwave dispersion ultrasound vibrometry (SDUV) for measuring tissue elasticity and viscosity[J]. IEEE Transactions on Ultrasonic Ferroelectrics Frequency Control, 56(1): 55-62.
5. Zheng Y, Greenleaf J F. (1999) Stable and unbiased flow turbulence estimation from pulse echo ultrasound[J]. IEEE Transactions on Ultrasonics Ferroelectrics Frequency Control, 46(5): 1074-1087.
6. Hasegawa H, Kanai H. (2006) Improving accuracy in estimation of artery-wall displacement by referring to center frequency of RF echo[J]. IEEE Transactions on Ultrasonics Ferroelectrics Frequency Control, 53(1): 52-63.
7. Zheng Y, Chen S G, TanW, et al. (2007) Detection of tissue harmonic motion induced by ultrasonic radiation force using pulse-echo ultrasound and kalman filter[J]. IEEE Transactions on Ultrasonics Ferroelectrics Frequency Control, 54(2): 290-300.
8. Huang S R, Lerner R M, Parker K. J. (1990) On estimating the amplitude of harmonic vibration from the Doppler spectrum of reflected signals[J]. Journal of the Acoustical Society of America, 88(6): 2702–2712.
9. Urban M W, Greenleaf J F. (2008) Harmonic pulsed excitation and motion detection of a vibrating reflective target [J]. Journal of the Acoustical Society of America, 123(1): 519-533.
10. Amador C, Urban M W, Chen S G, Greenleaf J F. (2011) Shearwave Dispersion Ultrasound Vibrometry (SDUV) on Swine Kidney [J]. IEEE Transactions on Ultrasonics Ferroelectrics Frequency Control, 58(12), 2608–2619.

Author: NIU Haijun
Institute: Beihang University, ,
Street: No. 37, Xueyuan Road
City: Beijing
Country: China
Email: hjniu@buaa.edu.cn

Evaluating the Sleep Quality Using Multiscale Entropy Analysis

Chih-En Kuo[1], Sheng-Fu Liang[2], Yu-Hsuan Shih[2], and Fu-Zen Shaw[1]

[1] The Institute of Cognitive Science, National Cheng Kung University, Tainan, Taiwan
[2] Department of Computer Science and Information Engineering, National Cheng Kung University, Tainan, Taiwan

Abstract— **Sleep diseases, such as insomnia and obstructive sleep apnea, seriously affect patients' quality of life. For diagnosis, polysomnographic (PSG) recordings are most usually taken to evaluate the sleep quality and efficiency. However, the large amount of wires connections for conventional PSG often cause sleep interference and not self-applicable. In this study, a complexity-measure-based method for evaluating the sleep quality was proposed. We utilize multiscale entropy (MSE) to analyze the 32 all-night sleep polysomnographic (PSG) recordings from 32 adults. The range of the subjects' sleep efficiency was from 56% to 97%. Half of the subjects' sleep efficiencies were equal or higher than to 85% (good sleep) and the other half were lower than 85% (poor sleep). The result shows that the averaged MSE values of poor sleep efficiency group are higher than good sleep efficiency group in each scale factor. This means that the complexity of sleep EEG of poor sleep efficiency group is higher than good sleep efficiency group. This finding may be used to quickly distinguish the subject' sleep efficiency is good or poor.**

Keywords— **Sleep quality, Sleep efficiency, Multiscale entropy, electroencephalogram (EEG).**

I. INTRODUCTION

Human beings spend approximately one third of their lives sleeping. In human physiology, a good deep sleep (SWS) stage can aid physical recovery; in addition, a good rapid eye movement (REM) stage can improve learning ability and memory. Sleep diseases, such as insomnia and obstructive sleep apnea, seriously affect patients' quality of life. These sleep problems may cause daytime sleepiness, irritability, depressive or anxious mood, or even death. For diagnosis of sleep problems, all-night polysomnographic (PSG) recordings including electroencephalogram (EEG), electrooculogram (EOG) and electromyogram (EMG) are usually taken from the patients and scored by a well-trained expert according to Rechtschaffen & Kales (R&K) rules [1].

According to R&K rules, the EEG, EOG, and EMG signals are required for the expert to score the sleep stages. However, the excessive number of wired connections for conventional Polysomnography (PSG) is often a problem that leads to sleep disturbance. In generally, people will have the first night effect if they sleep in hospital [2]. This effect often interferes with sleep quality.

Recently, a new signal analysis method called multiscale entropy (MSE) has been proposed [3, 4] to estimate the complexity associated with the long-range temporal correlation of a time series. Instead of a single scale, it calculates the entropy of a time series over multiple temporal scales. MSE has been applied to analyze the complexity of various biomedical signals such as EEG [5-8], ECG [4], and heart rate [9, 10]. These studies show that MSE values of some biological signals are different between both patients and normal subjects and younger subjects and older subjects. In this study, MSE was applied to analyze the EEG signals of from the people with different sleep quality. Moreover, the MSE values with different sleep stages are also compared between good and poor sleep efficiency groups.

II. METHOD

A. Subjects and Recording

All-night PSG sleep recordings were obtained from 32 healthy subjects (18 males and 14 females) ranging from 18 to 24 years in age. The subjects were interviewed about their sleep quality and medical history. None of them reported any history of neurological or psychological disorders. The PSG recordings of each subject, including six EEG channels (F3-A2, F4-A1, C3-A2, C4-A1, P3-A2, and P4-A1, according to the international 10-20 standard system), two EOG channels (the above right and below left outer canthus), and a chin EMG channel, were acquired through the Siesta 802 PSG (Compumedics, Inc.). The sampling rate was 256 Hz with 16-bit resolution. The filter settings of the cut-off frequencies were 0.5–30 Hz for EEG/EOG and 5–100 Hz for EMG. As suggested by the R&K rules [1], these nine-channel signals were used for manual scoring and only the data of the C3-A2 EEG channel were used for multiscale entropy analysis.

The 32 PSG sleep recordings were visually scored by a sleep specialist using the R&K rules with a 30-s interval (termed the epoch). Each 30-s epoch was classified into one of the five sleep stages, including Wake, rapid eye movement (REM), stage 1 (S1), stage 2 (S2), slow wave sleep (SWS), and movement artifact. In our experiments, only epochs belonging to the five sleep stages were used and movement artifact epochs were rejected.

I. Lackovic (ed.), *1st Global Conference on Biomedical Engineering & 9th Asian-Pacific Conference on Medical and Biological Engineering*,
IFMBE Proceedings 47, DOI: 10.1007/978-3-319-12262-5_46

Sleep efficiency is the ratio of time spent asleep (total sleep time) to the amount of time spent in bed. In clinical diagnosis, people may have a sleep disorder if their sleep efficiencies were lower than 85% [11]. In our experiments, the range of the subjects' sleep efficiency was from 56% to 97%. Half of the subjects' sleep efficiencies were equal or higher than to 85% and the other half were lower than 85%.

B. Multiscale Entropy

Multiscale entropy (MSE) measures the complexity of a time series by taking into account the entropy with respect to multiple temporal scales. MSE can be computed from the different types of entropy with multiple coarse-grained sequences, such as approximate entropy (ApEn) [12] or sample entropy (SampEn) [13]. The sample entropy was utilized as the kernel for entropy calculation in this study.

Given an EEG time sequence with N samples, $x = \{x_1, x_2, ..., x_N\}$, the original times series is divided into non-overlapping windows of length τ, defined as the scale factor. The data points inside each window are then averaged. Each element of the coarse-gained time series $y_\tau(j)$ is calculated by the following equation:

$$y_\tau(j) = \frac{1}{\tau} \sum_{i=(j-1)\tau+1}^{j\tau} x_i,\ 1 \le j \le \frac{N}{\tau}. \tag{1}$$

After obtaining each element of the coarse-gained time series, we calculate the sample entropy [13] for each of the coarse-grained time series. For scale τ, the corresponding coarse-gained time series has N/τ points and is denoted as $Y_\tau = \{y_\tau(1),...,y_\tau(i),...,y_\tau(\frac{N}{\tau})\}$. Defining an m-dimensional sequence vector, $\mu^{(m)}(i) = \{y_\tau(i), y_\tau(i+1),..., y_\tau(i+m-1)\}$, a distance measure for two vectors $\mu^{(m)}(i)$ and $\mu^{(m)}(j)$ with length of m points is defined as $d(i,j) = \max\{|\ y_\tau(i+k) - y_\tau(j+k)\ | : 0 \le k \le m-1\}$. The parameter r is defined as the tolerance for accepting matches, and $\mu^{(m)}(i)$ is similar with $\mu^{(m)}(j)$ when $d(i,j) \le r$. Let $C_i^m(r)$ represent the probability that vector $\mu^{(m)}(j)$ is similar with $\mu^{(m)}(i)$ and can be calculated by the following equation:

$$C_i^m(r) = \frac{\sum_{j=1, j\neq i}^{N/\tau-m-1} \omega_j}{(N/\tau - m - 1)} \tag{2}$$

where ω_j =1 when $d(i,j) \le r$; otherwise, ω_j = 0. In Eq. (2), j ranges from 1 to integer of N/τ, and $j \neq i$ to exclude self-matches. The probability that the two sequences will match for m points can be calculated by the following equation:

$$C^m(r) = \frac{\sum_{i=1}^{N/\tau-m} C_i^m(r)}{(N/\tau - m)} \tag{3}$$

The probability that the two sequences will match for m+1 points is calculated by the following equation:

$$C^{m+1}(r) = \frac{\sum_{i=1}^{N/\tau-m} C_i^{m+1}(r)}{(N/\tau - m)} \tag{4}$$

For the sample entropy, i and j range from 1 to the integer of N/τ for the calculation of both m- and (m+1)-point matching. Finally, the sample entropy for scale τ is calculated by the following equation:

$$SpEn(r, m, \frac{N}{\tau}) = -\ln[C^{m+1}(r)/C^m(r)] \tag{5}$$

Some theoretical and clinical applications have shown that the parameters $m=1$ or 2 and $r = 0.1 - 0.25$ of the standard deviation (SD) of the original time sequence provide good statistical validity for SampEn [14,15]. The parameters $m = 2$ and $r = 0.15 * SD$ were used to calculate MSE values in this study.

III. RESULTS

We calculated the averaged 20 MSE value (the scale factor = 1-20) from good and poor sleep efficiency groups, respectively. Fig. 1 shows the averaged 20 MSE curve of good and poor sleep efficiency groups. We find that the averaged MSE values of poor sleep efficiency group are higher than good sleep efficiency group in each scale factor. Moreover, the averaged MSE values between good and poor sleep efficiency groups are very close when scale factor is 1; the different of the averaged MSE values between good and poor sleep efficiency groups when the scale factor = 2-13 was more obvious than other scale factors. This finding proved that the MSE analysis may be used to quickly distinguish the users sleep efficiency is good or poor.

Then, we compared the MSE curves and the repeated-measure one-way ANOVA of good and poor sleep efficiency groups in five stages, Wake, S1, S2, SWS and REM. Figs. 2 (a)-(e) shows the results of the comparison in Wake, S1, S2, SWS and REM stages, respectively. Some interesting characteristics can be observed from Fig 2.

1) In each stage, the trend of the MSE curve of good sleep efficiency groups is similar with poor sleep efficiency groups.

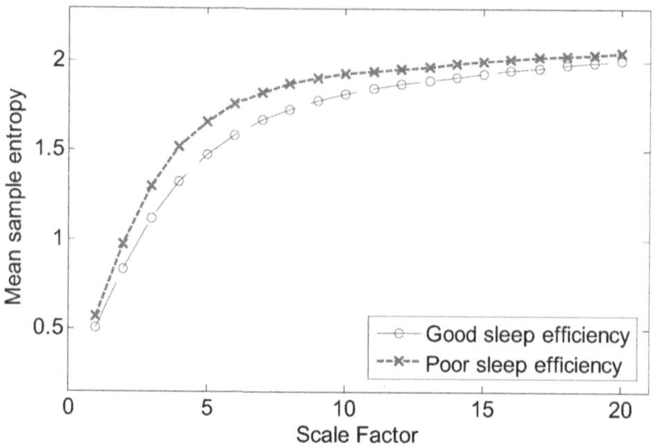

Fig. 1 The averaged 20 MSE curves of the all-night EEG data derived from two groups, good and poor sleep efficiency groups. SampEn was evaluated at 1-20 scale factors. The symbols represent the mean values of SampEn for each group.

2) In addition to Wake, the mean SampEn values of poor sleep efficiency groups are higher than good sleep efficiency groups in other stages.
3) For each scale factor, the entropy values and the levels of sleep depth have negative correlation and the entropy values monotonically decrease from wake to deep sleep (SWS).
4) In addition to Wake and REM, almost all of the MSE values between good and poor sleep efficiency groups have statistical differences.

IV. CONCLUSIONS

In this study, MSE was applied to analyze the EEG signals of from the people with different sleep quality. Moreover, the MSE values with different sleep stages are also compared between good and poor sleep efficiency groups. The result shows that the averaged MSE values of poor sleep efficiency group are higher than good sleep efficiency group in each scale factor. This means that the complexity of sleep EEG of poor sleep efficiency group is higher than good sleep efficiency group. This finding may be used to quickly distinguish the subject' sleep efficiency is good or poor.

From the above results, we concluded that the sleep pattern and the sleep EEG complexity of healthy individual are different from people with low sleep efficiency or patient with sleep diseases. Therefore, we also make some suggestions for improving the performance of most automatic sleep staging methods in the future. Firstly, the averaged MSE value of all night sleep EEG was used to evaluate subject's sleep efficiency is good or poor. Then, the two different classifier-models were utilized to classify the sleep stage of good and poor sleep efficiency groups, respectively. The different classifier-models can enhance the accuracy of the automatic sleep staging system.

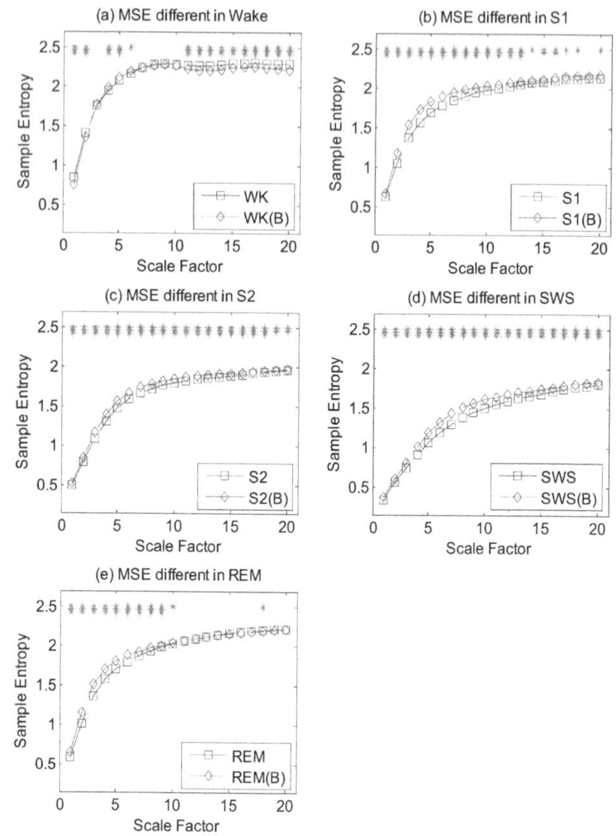

Fig. 2 MSE curves and the repeated-measure one-way ANOVA results of good and poor sleep efficiency groups in five stages. (a) Wake, (b) S1, (c) S2, (d) SWS, (e) REM. (***p<0.001, **p<0.01, *p<0.05)
*The symbol "(B)" denotes the poor sleep efficiency group.

ACKNOWLEDGMENT

This work was supported by the National Science Council of Taiwan under Grants NSC 100-2410-H-006-025-MY3, NSC 103-2811-H-006-006 and Ministry of Science and Technology under Grants MOST 103-2221-E-006 -178 -. This work was partially supported by the "Aim for the Top University Project" of the National Cheng Kung University and Ministry of Education, Taiwan.

CONFLICT OF INTEREST

The authors declare that they have no conflict of interest.

REFERENCES

[1] A. Rechtschaffen and A. Kales, *A manual of standardized terminology, techniques and scoring system for sleep stages of human subjects*: US Government Printing Office, US Public Health Service, 1968.

[2] H. W. Agnew, W. B. Webb, and R. L. Williams, "THE FIRST NIGHT EFFECT: AN EEG STUDYOF SLEEP," *Psychophysiology,* vol. 2, pp. 263-266, 1966.

[3] M. Costa, A. L. Goldberger, and C. K. Peng, "Multiscale entropy analysis of complex physiologic time series," *Phys Rev Lett,* vol. 89, p. 068102, Aug 5 2002.

[4] M. Costa, A. L. Goldberger, and C. K. Peng, "Multiscale entropy analysis of biological signals," *Phys Rev E Stat Nonlin Soft Matter Phys,* vol. 71, p. 021906, Feb 2005.

[5] T. Takahashi, R. Y. Cho, T. Murata, T. Mizuno, M. Kikuchi, K. Mizukami, *et al.*, "Age-related variation in EEG complexity to photic stimulation: a multiscale entropy analysis," *Clin Neurophysiol,* vol. 120, pp. 476-83, Mar 2009.

[6] J.-H. Park, S. Kim, C.-H. Kim, A. Cichocki, and K. Kim, "MULTISCALE ENTROPY ANALYSIS OF EEG FROM PATIENTS UNDER DIFFERENT PATHOLOGICAL CONDITIONS," *Fractals,* vol. 15, pp. 399-404, 2007/12/01 2007.

[7] X. Kang, X. Jia, R. G. Geocadin, N. V. Thakor, and A. Maybhate, "Multiscale entropy analysis of EEG for assessment of post-cardiac arrest neurological recovery under hypothermia in rats," *IEEE Trans Biomed Eng,* vol. 56, pp. 1023-31, Apr 2009.

[8] S.-F. Liang, C.-E. Kuo, Y.-H. Hu, Y.-H. Pan, and Y.-H. Wang, "Automatic Stage Scoring of Single-Channel Sleep EEG by Using Multiscale Entropy and Autoregressive Models," *Instrumentation and Measurement, IEEE Transactions on,* vol. 61, pp. 1649-1657, 2012.

[9] M. Costa, C. K. Peng, A. L. Goldberger, and J. M. Hausdorff, "Multiscale entropy analysis of human gait dynamics," *Physica A: Statistical Mechanics and its Applications,* vol. 330, pp. 53-60, 12/1/ 2003.

[10] P. R. Norris, S. M. Anderson, J. M. Jenkins, A. E. Williams, and J. A. Morris, Jr., "Heart rate multiscale entropy at three hours predicts hospital mortality in 3,154 trauma patients," *Shock,* vol. 30, pp. 17-22, Jul 2008.

[11] H. Danker-Hopfe, P. Anderer, J. Zeitlhofer, M. Boeck, H. Dorn, G. Gruber, *et al.*, "Interrater reliability for sleep scoring according to the Rechtschaffen & Kales and the new AASM standard," *J Sleep Res,* vol. 18, pp. 74-84, Mar 2009.

[12] S. Pincus, "Approximate entropy (ApEn) as a complexity measure," *Chaos: An Interdisciplinary Journal of Nonlinear Science,* vol. 5, pp. 110-117, 03/00/ 1995.

[13] J. S. Richman and J. R. Moorman, "Physiological time-series analysis using approximate entropy and sample entropy," *American Journal of Physiology - Heart and Circulatory Physiology,* vol. 278, pp. H2039-H2049, June 1, 2000 2000.

[14] N. Burioka, M. Miyata, G. Cornelissen, F. Halberg, T. Takeshima, D. T. Kaplan, *et al.*, "Approximate entropy in the electroencephalogram during wake and sleep," *Clin EEG Neurosci,* vol. 36, pp. 21-4, Jan 2005.

[15] D. R. Chialvo, "Physiology: unhealthy surprises," *Nature,* vol. 419, p. 263, Sep 19 2002.

Performance Analysis in a Wavelet-Based Algorithm for Automatic Detection of High-Voltage Spindles in Parkinson's Disease Rat Models

Ramesh Perumal and Hsin Chen

Department of Electrical Engineering, National Tsing Hua University, Hsinchu, Taiwan

Abstract— **The waxing-and-waning high-voltage spindles (HVSs) are the electroencephalographic hallmarks of the abnormalities in the synchronization of oscillatory activities in cortical-basal ganglia networks. The HVSs were observed during waking immobility on lesioned Sprague-Dawley rats by unilateral injection of 6-hydroxydopamine (6-OHDA). The local field potentials (LFPs) collected from the lesioned and control rats were analyzed with continuous wavelet transform using a tunable complex Morlet wavelet function identified with a careful choice of design parameters for the efficient detection of HVSs. In this study, an online detection algorithm optimized with suitable wavelet parameters using a window size of 500 and a constant decision threshold, is verified to detect the HVSs lasting 1.15-3.49 seconds from seven lesioned rats with maximum precision, sensitivity and specificity. These results provide further motivation for the real-time implementation of the automatic HVS detection systems with improved performance for pathophysiological and therapeutic applications to the thalamocortical network dysfunctions like Parkinson's disease.**

Keywords— **HVS, CWT, complex Morlet wavelet, Parkinson's disease, online spindle detection.**

I. INTRODUCTION

High-voltage spindles (HVSs) are characterized as synchronous, immobility-related spike-and-wave patterns of local field potentials (LFPs) and oscillating in the 5-13 Hz frequency band [1]. In general, there are various spindle detection algorithms to detect normal sleep spindles [2] and spike-wave discharges (SWD) [3-4]. There are significant differences between the HVS and normal sleep spindles in terms of physiology and signal dynamics such as: (i) HVS initiates in cortex while sleep spindles in thalamus, (ii) HVSs can occur frequently during passive wakefulness whereas the sleep spindles are prevalent in sleep states, (iii) on contrary to the sleep spindles, the majority of HVSs in experimental models appears to show an increased power in the lower range of theta frequency band (6-7 Hz) [5]. HVSs are found to be associated with spatial memory impairments [1] and Parkinson's disease (PD) [6]. The onset and end of HVSs episodes could occasionally vary across the cortical-basal ganglia structures and thus leads to different morphological features. Besides this, the HVSs are different from the epileptic spike-wave discharges whose dominant frequency lies in the 30 -50 Hz band [3]. Such unique characteristics of HVSs from that of the normal sleep spindles and epileptic SWD demands an existing spindle detection algorithm to be optimized with a suitable choice of wavelet parameters and the thresholding mechanism.

The major findings of our approach are listed as follows. First, a set of complex Morlet wavelets tuned to various bandwidth parameter values (f_b = 9, 10, 11, 12, 13, 14, 15, 16) and centre frequency (f_c = 1 Hz) are used as mother wavelets in continuous wavelet transform (CWT) to detect the characteristic oscillations of HVSs and the detection performance is investigated to obtain the optimal choices. Second, a constant decision threshold is used for the wavelet power to detect HVSs with 100% precision, 100% specificity and 100% sensitivity using the optimal wavelets. Finally, as this algorithm is based mainly on the CWT using the complex Morlet wavelet function whose digital architecture is proved to be time-efficient in Fourier space [7], the proposed algorithm demonstrated with improved performance can be extended further to the FPGA-based real time systems for pathophysiological and therapeutic applications.

II. MATERIALS AND METHODS

A. Data Acquisition

The PD rat models were induced in 3-4 months old Sprague-Dawley rats by unilateral injection (coordinates: AP -4.4 mm, ML +1.2 mm, V -7.8 mm relatively to bregma) of 6-OHDA in the medial forebrain bundle (MFB) at the rate of µl/min using an integrated electrophysiology instrument suitable for deep brain stimulation (DBS) procedure. Four weeks following the unilateral injection of 6-OHDA, the lesioned group of rats were determined as successful PD models through amphetamine-induced rotational behaviour (Amp, 3mg/kg, ip) by measuring the rotational speed of the lesioned rats as 6 turns per minute. The rats were unilaterally implanted bipolar stimulation electrode into the ipsilateral STN with their initial coordinates at AP -3.6 mm and L +2.5 mm. The LFP recordings were collected from a group of twenty four lesioned rats and twenty control rats. The LFPs of the lesioned rats were recorded in both sleeping and waking immobile states in order to study the behaviour of spindling and non-spindling characteristics. The LFPs

I. Lackovic (ed.), *1st Global Conference on Biomedical Engineering & 9th Asian-Pacific Conference on Medical and Biological Engineering*,
IFMBE Proceedings 47, DOI: 10.1007/978-3-319-12262-5_47

without artifacts and with the duration of sixty seconds were considered in the following sections to evaluate the performance of the spindle detection algorithm.

B. Algorithm

The steps involved in the automatic HVS detection algorithm [4] are summarized in Figure 1. The CWT has been used extensively for the analysis of one-dimensional non-stationary signals such as normal sleep spindles and SWD over the two-dimensional time-frequency plane with variable resolutions in both domains [2-4]. Given a specific mother wavelet $\psi(t)$, the wavelet basis function $\psi_{s,\tau}(t)$ is defined as in Eq. (1) and the CWT $W(s,\tau)$ of a 1-D signal $f(t)$ is given by Eq. (2) as shown below.

$$\psi_{s,\tau}(t) = \frac{1}{\sqrt{|s|}}\psi\left(\frac{t-\tau}{s}\right) \quad (1)$$

$$W(s,\tau) = \langle f, \psi_{s,\tau}\rangle = \frac{1}{\sqrt{|s|}}\int f(t)\psi^*\left(\frac{t-\tau}{s}\right)dt \quad (2)$$

In the above equations, the scaling and translation parameters are represented by s and τ. The choice of mother wavelet is critical to determine the detection performance of such wavelet-based spindle detection algorithms. The complex Morlet wavelet has been selected in our approach as they are proved to be successful in automatic spindle detection algorithms [3, 4] and the real part of the wavelet $\psi_r(t)$ is mathematically defined in Eq. (3) where the centre frequency and bandwidth parameters are denoted by f_c and f_b respectively.

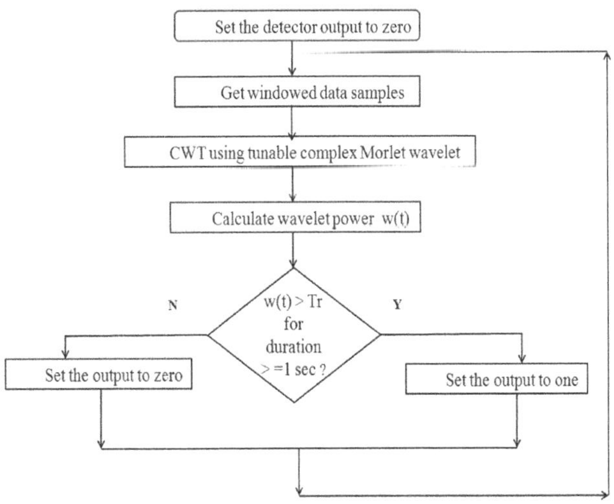

Fig. 1 Flowchart of automatic HVS detection algorithm

$$\psi_r(t) = \frac{1}{\sqrt{\pi f_b}} e^{j2\pi f_c t} e^{-t^2/f_b} \quad (3)$$

The value of f_c is taken as 1 [3, 4] as this choice leads to a simplified relation between the scale s in wavelet domain and the frequency in Fourier space f as summarized in Eq. (4).

$$f = \frac{\omega_c + \sqrt{(2+\omega_c^2)}}{4\pi s} \xrightarrow{\omega_c = 2\pi} f \approx \frac{1}{s} \quad (4)$$

This relation is optimal to have a good frequency resolution in the low frequency range signals such as spindles or neural signals in general.

Next, the bandwidth parameter f_b has to be selected carefully and the effects of this parameter on the performance characteristics of the detection algorithm are evaluated in the present study by tuning its values from 9 to 16. In this context, the complex Morlet wavelet with variable f_b will be denoted by its equivalent MATLAB function cmorf_b-1 in the subsequent sections. The selection of cmorf_b-1 wavelet for the detection of HVS is clearly evident due to its close resemblance to each other as shown in Figure 2. In the present work, the wavelet power $w(t)$ defined as the sum of the square of the CWT coefficients $W(s,\tau)$ in the desired 5-13 frequency band is calculated across the window size T of 500 data points (0.5 sec) for the entire signal as shown in Eq. (5). If the wavelet power is greater than the constant decision threshold (Tr) of 0.5µV^2 [3], then the detector output is set to high to represent the occurrence of HVS, otherwise it is low.

$$w(t) = \int_f |W(t,f)|^2\, df; \qquad f: 5-13\ Hz \quad (5)$$

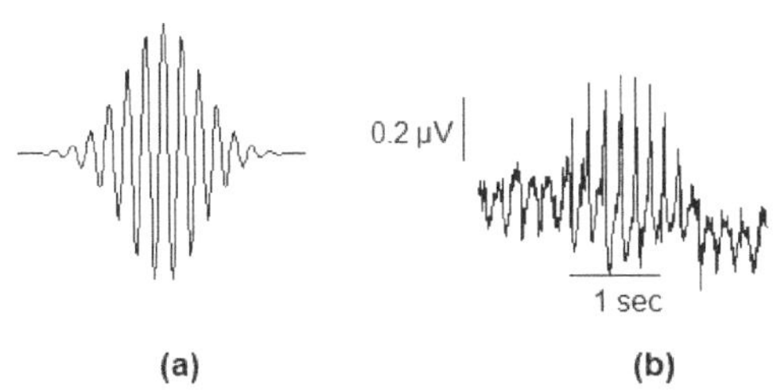

Fig. 2 (a) cmor9-1 wavelet; (b) High-voltage spindle

III. RESULTS AND DISCUSSION

A. Time-Frequency Analysis

The time-frequency distribution obtained from the CWT is used to discriminate the control and PD signals by the energy distribution of the coefficients over the joint time-frequency plane. As shown in Figure 3, the prevalent blue color indicates the lower values of energy distribution in control signal. However in Figure 4, the elevations in the energy distribution corresponding to the occurrence of HVSs in the PD signal are clearly evident where the color map scale is more than twice that of the one in Figure 3.

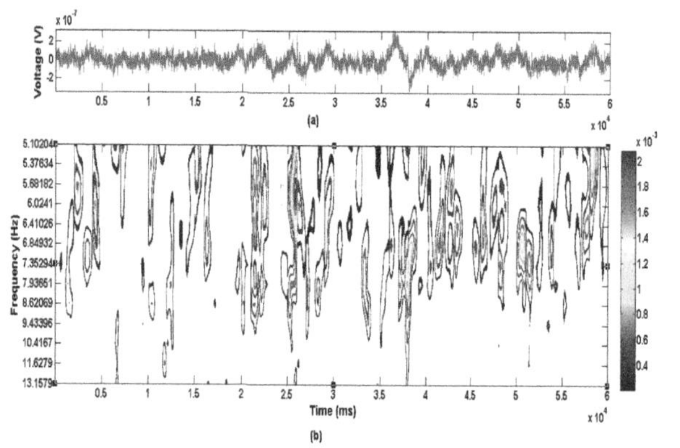

Fig. 3 Time-frequency distribution of a typical control signal. (a) Control signal. (b) Time-frequency distribution of (a) using CWT with cmor9-1 wavelet function.

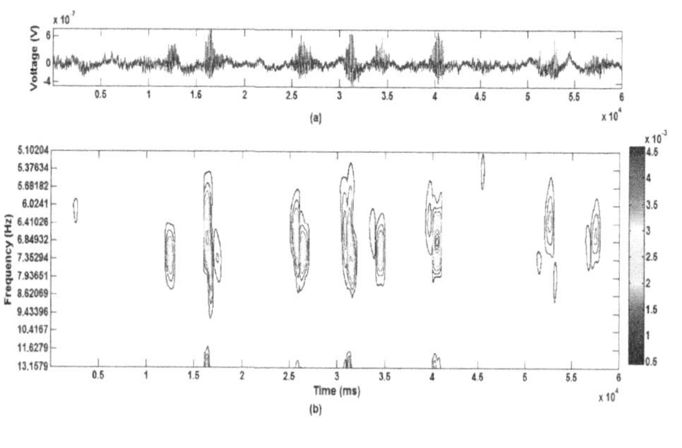

Fig. 4 Time-frequency distribution of a typical PD signal. (a) PD signal. (b) Time-frequency distribution of (a) using CWT with cmor9-1 - wavelet function.

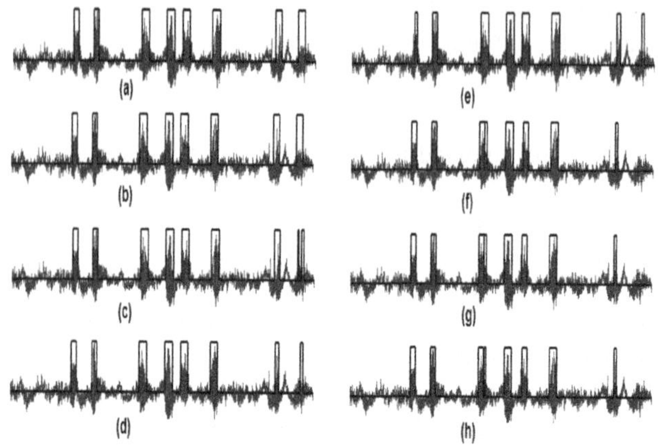

Fig. 5 Response (shown in black color) of the automatic HVS detection algorithm to a typical PD signal (shown in blue color) in Figure 4, for various wavelet functions. (a) cmor9-1, (b) cmor10-1, (c) cmor11-1, (d) cmor12-1, (e) cmor13-1, (f) cmor14-1, (g) cmor15-1 and (h) cmor16-1. Here the amplitude of PD signal and the detector output are normalized to be in the range of 0 to 1.

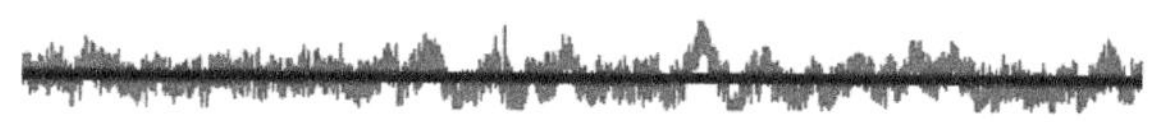

Fig. 6 Response (shown in black color) of the automatic HVS detection algorithm to a typical control signal (shown in red color) in Figure 3, using cmor9-1 wavelet. The response shown here remains same independent of the wavelet functions used in this study. Here the amplitude of control signal and the detector output are normalized to be in the range of 0 to 1.

B. Evaluation of Detection Performance

The response of the algorithm varies with the choice of bandwidth parameters in the cmorf_b-1 wavelet. The values of f_b selected in this study guarantees no false positives (FP) and hence results in 100% specificity for all wavelets as shown in Table 1 and Table 2. The detection performance is characterized by well-defined coverage of the HVS and its corresponding onset and end in time domain by the detector outputs shown in Figure 5. The detector outputs for the cmor9-1 and cmor10-1 wavelets show a prominent performance for all datasets apart from the one shown in Figure 5 (a-b). The spindle duration spanned by the detector outputs for the last spindle in Figure 5 decreases as we progress from cmor11-1 to cmor13-1 wavelets as seen in Figure 5(c-e). As shown in Figure 5 (f-h), for the same spindle, the false negatives (FN) exist in the detector outputs with cmor14-1, cmor15-1 and cmor16-1 wavelets and this reduces the sensitivity significantly. The detection performance of the algorithm shown in Figure 6 for the control signal remains same independent of the choice of wavelets considered in this study due to its very low wavelet power compared to that of the threshold power. The performance metrics shown in Table 1 and Table 2 strongly recommends the choice of cmor9-1 and cmor10-1 as the optimal wavelets for the detection of HVSs using a constant decision threshold with maximum sensitivity, specificity and accuracy.

Table 1 Performance metrics* of the detection algorithm for each spindling PD dataset using cmor9-1 wavelet function with the window size of 500 and a constant threshold power of 0.5μV^2.

S.No.	N_v	TP	FP	FN	Sensitivity %	Accuracy %	Specificity %
1	12	12	0	0	100	100	100
2	12	12	0	0	100	100	100
3	8	8	0	0	100	100	100
4	5	5	0	0	100	100	100
5	14	14	0	0	100	100	100
6	16	16	0	0	100	100	100
7	6	6	0	0	100	100	100
				Mean	100	100	100

*N_v: Number of visual detections; TP: True Positives; FP: False Positives; FN: False Negatives; Sensitivity = (TP / (TP + FN)) x 100; Accuracy = (TP / N_v) x 100; Specificity = (TN / (TN + FP)) x 100;

Table 2 Mean performance metrics* of the detection algorithm for the spindling PD datasets using other cmorf_b-1 wavelet functions with the window size of 500 and a constant threshold power of 0.5μV^2.

S.No.	Wavelet function	Accuracy %	Specificity %
1	cmor10-1	100	100
2	cmor11-1	97.14	100
3	cmor12-1	97.14	100
4	cmor13-1	97.14	100
5	cmor14-1	95.36	100
6	cmor15-1	95.36	100
7	cmor16-1	94.17	100

*Excluding cmor10-1, sensitivity is less than 100% as FN is non-zero in all other cases.

IV. CONCLUSIONS

In this study, the performance of an online HVS detection algorithm is evaluated using CWT with complex Morlet wavelets. The optimal choices of mother wavelets were found to be cmor9-1 and cmor10-1 for a constant threshold wavelet power. Also, the performance metrics were computed for seven PD datasets to verify the detection results for HVSs lasting 1.15-3.49 seconds. As this algorithm uses a window size of 500 to detect the spindles with minimum duration of 1 second, it can be used as an online detection algorithm with minimum latency. Considering the time-efficient FPGA implementation of Morlet CWT [7], the detection algorithm can also be extended to cost effective FPGA-based systems for real time applications.

ACKNOWLEDGMENT

We would like to express our sincere gratitude to Ms. Chi-Fen Chuang and Prof. Yen-Chung Chang of the department of Life Science in National Tsing Hua University for their experimental datasets used in this study.

CONFLICT OF INTEREST

The authors declare that they have no conflict of interest.

REFERENCES

1. Radek R J, Curzon P and Decker M W (1994) Characterization of high voltage spindles and spatial memory in young, mature and aged rats. Brain Research Bulletin 33: 183–188
2. Warby S C et al. (2014) Sleep-spindle detection: crowdsourcing and evaluating performance of experts, non-experts and automated methods. Nature Methods 11: 385–392
3. Sitnikova E et al. (2009) Sleep spindles and spike-wave discharges in EEG: their generic features, similarities and distinctions disclosed with Fourier transform and continuous wavelet analysis. J Neurosci Methods 180: 304–316
4. Ovchinnikov A et al. (2010) An algorithm for real-time detection of spike-wave discharges in rodents. J Neurosci Methods 194: 172–178
5. Leresche N et al. (2012) From sleep spindles of natural sleep to spike and wave discharges of typical absence seizures: is the hypothesis still valid? Pflugers Arch-Eur J Physiol 463: 201–212
6. Shunnan G et al. (2012) Dopamine depletion increases the power and coherence of high-voltage spindles in the globus pallidus and motor cortex of freely moving rats. Brain Research 1465: 66–79
7. Qassim Y T et al. (2012) FPGA Implementation of Morlet Continuous Wavelet Transform for EEG Analysis. Intl. Conf. Computer and Comm. Eng., Kuala Lumpur, Malaysia, 2012

Author: Ramesh Perumal
Institute: National Tsing Hua University, Taiwan
Street: No. 101, Section 2, Kuang-Fu Road
City: Hsinchu
Country: Taiwan
Email: reachtorameshmail@gmail.com

Speech Recognition for Cochlear Implant Users in the Noisy Environment: The Role of Envelope and Fine Structure

Y.C. Lee[1], Y.H. Lee[1], and Charles T.M. Choi[2]

[1] Department of Computer Science, National Taichung University of Education, Taichung, Taiwan, R.O.C.
[2] Department of Electrical and Computer Engineering, National Chiao Tung University, Hsinchu, Taiwan, R.O.C.

Abstract— **Sound signal can be decomposed to a slowly varying envelope cue and a rapidly varying fine structure cue. These cues can help people to sound perception, sound lateralization, speech recognition in noise, and so on. Cochlear implant can help people with hearing loss to hear the sound. However, there are still many restrictions with cochlear implant user and a gap between normal hearing and cochlear implant user. This study investigated the contribution of envelope and fine structure cues with different SNR and simulated cochlear implant in Taiwanese mandarin speech recognition in noise. Ten normal hearing subjects participated in this experiment. Our result shows sentence recognition in noise almost depends on the envelope cues, but the fine structure cues still have limited contributions.**

Keywords— **Envelope, Fine Structure, Cochlear Implant (CI), Normal Hearing Test.**

I. INTRODUCTION

Using *cochlear implant* (*CI*) devices, making patients with hearing loss have the opportunity to hear the sound again. It can provide good speech recognition in quite to CI users. However, even the best performance CI user, there are still many challenges, such as speech recognition in noise and tonal language.

Hilbert in 1912 showed that a signal can be decomposed into a slowly varying *envelope* (*ENV*) and a rapidly varying *fine structure* (*FS*) [1]. Smith *et al.* had investigated the relation of envelope and fine structure for speech reception, melody reception and sound lateralization, and demonstrated that fine structure was the main information carrier for melody and sound localization [2]. The envelope is the loudness contour and the intensity of the sound signal. It is the important part of speech recognition. The fine structure is the detail of the sound signal, that helping to identify the pitch, tonal language and sound lateralization.

The stimulating strategies of cochlear implants, such as *continuous interleaved sampling* (*CIS*), *advanced combination encoder* (*ACE*) and *HiResolution®* (*HiRes*), calculation the intensity of the envelopes from each frequency band, which were used to determine the current of stimulation in each electrode. But the envelope and fine structure of the input sound signals was not clearly delineated in these stimulating strategies of cochlear implants [2]. Only partial fine structure information was conveyed by stimulating strategies to CI users. Thus, the aim of the present study was to investigate the importance and contribution between the envelope and fine structure to recognize the Chinese sentences in noise.

II. METHODS

A. Subjects

10 NH subjects (6 females and 4 males) between the ages of 20 and 28 years old (mean 23.8 years) participated in experimental. All subjects were native speakers of Taiwanese Mandarin. Participants signed an informed consent form and were paid for their participation.

B. Material and Processing

We selected the Mandarin Speech Perception in Noise (MSPIN) proposed in [3] as the speech material. MSPIN is a sentence list which contains 300 Taiwanese Mandarin sentences for speech recognition in noisy environment. Each sentence contains 7~10 words and subjects are asked to recognize the last word after listen the whole sentence. These sentences are evenly classified into two categories: high predictability (HP) and low predictability (LP). A sentence with HP means that it contains 2~3 cues to predict its last word. In contrast, a LP sentence doesn't contain any cue, which means the subject has to recognize the last word directly. The masker used in the experiment was *speech-shaped noise* (*SSN*). SSN is a white noise signal shaped as *long-term average spectrum* (*LTAS*) of target speech. The speech and noise were added at -12 to 12 dB in 6 dB steps. All processing was done digitally via software routines in MATLAB.

The sound source of spatial configurations was simulated using the head-related transfer function (HRTFs) [4]. Fig. 1 shows how we used HRTFs to produce different sound source angle of incidence. Speech source is fixedly originated in the front at 0° azimuth, and noise source is placed at an angle of incidence of 270° (S0N270) azimuth. The distance between source and KEMAR was 1.4 meters.

I. Lackovic (ed.), *1st Global Conference on Biomedical Engineering & 9th Asian-Pacific Conference on Medical and Biological Engineering*,
IFMBE Proceedings 47, DOI: 10.1007/978-3-319-12262-5_48

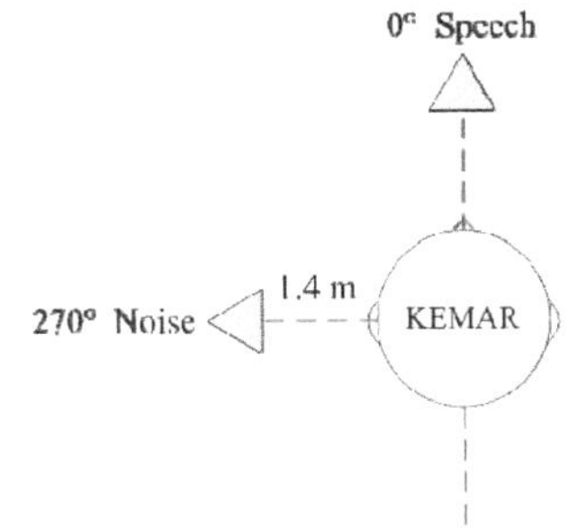

Fig. 1 The source angel of incidence in this experiment. Speech source is in the front at 0° azimuth. Noise source is placed at an angle of incidence of 270° azimuth.

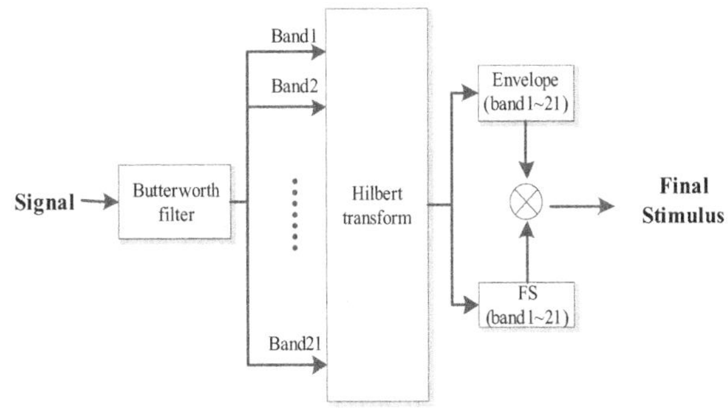

Fig. 2 Schematic of the stimuli production in this experiment.

We take the sound recorded at the left ear of the KEMAR for subsequent evaluation.

Fig. 2 shows how we created the stimuli. Every noisy sentence was divided into 21 critical bands using 12th-order Butterworth filters [5]. Then, the envelope and fine structure were extracted from each band using Hilbert transform [6]. Each extracted envelope was imposed on the fine structure extracted from signals with different SNR.

C. Procedures

Ten normal hearing subjects participate our experiment in a quiet room. All stimuli were presented acoustically with AKG K181DJ headphones. Prior to experiment, subjects were tested in 20 sentences in SNR -5dB to decide whether they can conduct the following experiment. During the experiment, subjects would test in a total 25 conditions, 500 sentences. All of these conditions and sentences were evaluated in random order for each subject. The total duration of experiment was 1.5 hours.

III. RESULTS AND DISCUSSION

Results of the experiment are presented in Fig. 3 and 4. Fig. 3 shows the percent correct of HP sentences, and Fig. 4 shows the percent correct of LP sentences. Upper panels in both Fig. 3 and 4 reported percent correct as a function of SNR_{EVN}, and lower panels reported percent correct as a function of SNR_{FS}. In each panel, a bold line shows the five data points which SNR_{ENV} and SNR_{FS} were identical. It corresponds to baseline performance on speech recognition in noise (i.e., reference function; REF) [7].

A signal with SNR > 0 dB means the sound of speech is greater than the background noise. In this situation, percent correct of HP sentences is greater than LP sentences, which indicates the cues in HP sentences were benefits for recognizing the last word. In contrast, a signal with SNR < 0 dB means the sound of background noise is greater than the speech. According to our experimental results, in this situation the percent corrects are lower than 11% for both HP and LP sentences. That is, whether a sentence contains cues or not, the recognition rate of the last word is not obviously improved under this relatively noisy situation.

In the upper panels of both Fig. 3 and 4, the changes of percent correct along SNR_{ENV} for different SNR_{FS} is similar

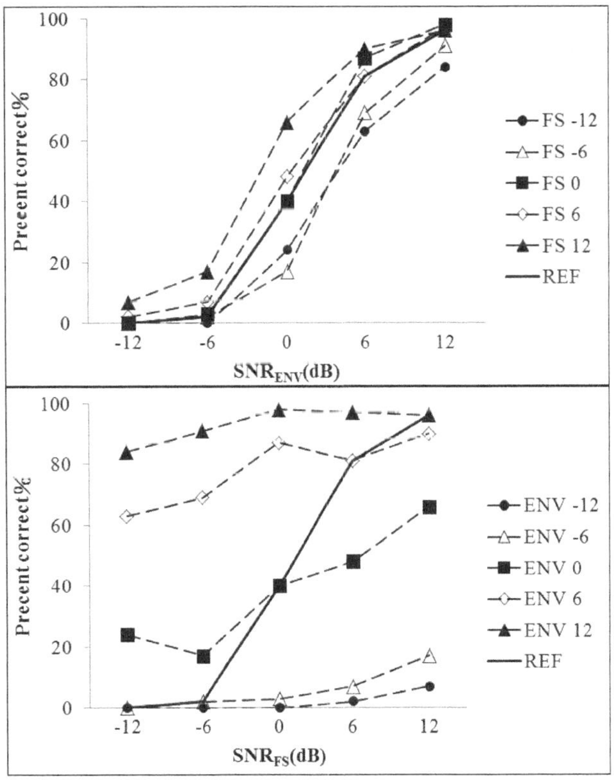

Fig. 3 The high predictability sentences of average sentence recognition rate in speech-shaped noise (SSN) as a function of the SNR of the envelope (upper panel) and as a function of the SNR of the fine structure.

to REF. As the SNR_{ENV} increasing, the percent correct steadily increases for all SNR_{FS} with positive slope. It indicates that the envelope cues influenced the recognition of sentence were large. On the other hand, in the lower panels of both Fig. 3 and 4, the percent correct increases while SNR_{FS} increasing is less obvious. It means the fine structure cues still affect the speech recognition, but the effects were lower than the envelope cues.

The method we have used to evaluate the contribution of envelope and fine structure can be assessed separately. It can avoid a few limitations of the vocoder, which contained the use of a single carrier to carry a mixture of envelopes and a lack of consistency between this single carrier and the mixed envelopes [7]. Forgerty also used similar evaluation approach and found the SNR of envelope and find structure contributed simultaneously [8].

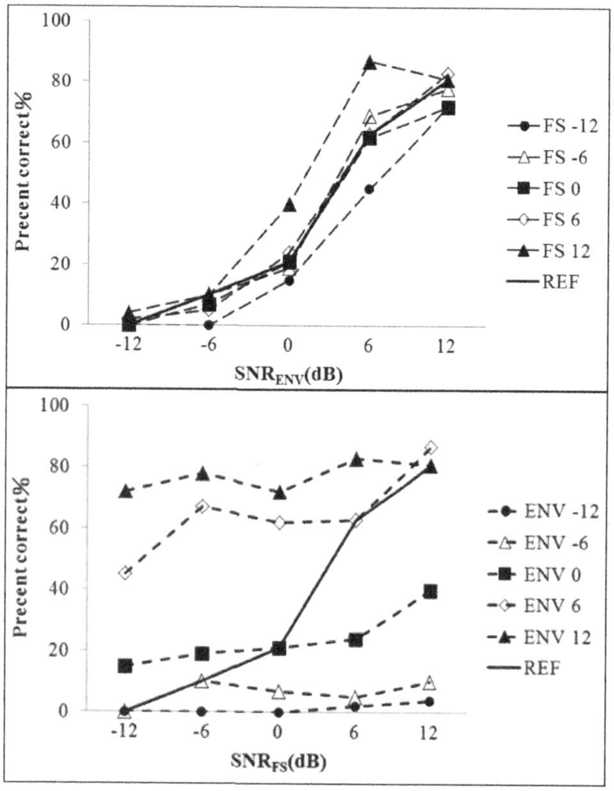

Fig. 4 The low predictability sentences of average sentence recognition in speech-shaped noise (SSN) as a ofunction of the SNR of the envelope (upper panel) and as a function of the SNR of the fine structure.

Furthermore, we consider how the location of speech and noise sources affects the speech recognition. Recall that we assume the speech source is originated in the front at 0° azimuth, and the noise source is placed at an angle of incidence of 270° (S0N270) azimuth. Because we only take the sound recorded at the left ear of the KEMAR for evaluation, the noise is expected to affect the speech recognition critically. Hence, when SNR < 0 dB, the effect of envelope and fine structure were not obvious. On the other hand, when SNR > 0 dB, both envelope and fine structure affected the speech recognition, especially the benefit from envelope cues were very obvious.

IV. CONCLUSIONS

In this study we focus on evaluate the relative contribution of envelope and fine structure cues for speech recognition in noise. The results showed both envelope and fine structure cues helped the speech recognition in noise in Taiwanese mandarin. The benefit from envelope cues apparently influenced the speech recognition, and the contribution of fine structure was less obvious but still helpful. We suggested that to add fine structure cues for cochlear implant may help users to recognize speech in Taiwanese mandarin.

REFERENCES

1. Hilbert D. (1912) Grundzüge einer allgemeinen Theorie der lin- earen Integralgleichungen. Leipzig: Teubner
2. Smith Z.M., Delgutte B and Oxenham A.J. (2002) Chimaeric sounds reveal dichotomies in auditory perception. Nature. 416(4879):87-90
3. Tsai CH, Chen HC (2002) The development of Mandarin speech perception in noise test. Journal of Special Education 23:121-140 (in Traditional Chinese)
4. Gardner B., Martin K. (1995) HRTF measurements of a KEMAR. Journal of the Acoustical Society of America. 97:3907-3908
5. Apoux, F., and Healy, E.W. (2009) On the number of auditory filter outputs needed to understand speech: Further evidence for auditory channel independence. Hearing Research 255:99–108
6. Apoux, F., Millman, R. E., Viemeister, N.F. *et al.* (2011) On the mechanisms involved in the recovery of envelope information from temporal fine structure. Journal of the Acoustical Society of America. 130: 273–282
7. Apoux, F., Sarah E.Y., Carla L.Y. (2013) Role and relative contribution of temporal envelope and fine structure cues in sentence recognition by normal-hearing listeners. Journal of the Acoustical Society of America. 134(3): 2205-2212
8. Fogerty, D. (2011) Perceptual weighting of individual and concurrent cues for sentence intelligibility: Frequency, envelope, and fine structure. Journal of the Acoustical Society of America. 129: 977–98

Author: Yi-Hsuan Lee
Institute: National Taichung University of Education
Street: No. 140, Ming-Sheng Road
City: Taichung
Country: Taiwan
Email: yslee@mail.ntcu.edu.tw

Electrical Impedance Tomography: A Reconstruction Method Based on Neural Networks and Particle Swarm Optimization

Sébastien Martin and Charles T.M. Choi

National Chiao Tung University – Neural Engineering and Interface Laboratory, 1001 University Rd., Hsinchu, 300 Taiwan

Abstract— **Electrical Impedance Tomography (EIT) is a non-invasive image reconstruction technique. Typically, an EIT scheme involves the solution to an inverse problem, which usually gives a poor resolution, due to linearization and ill-posedness of the problem. An alternative approach based on Artificial Neural Networks (ANN) has been used as a replacement of the inverse problem, giving correct results without linearizing the problem. However, training an ANN may be time consuming and usually requires a large amount of iterations before achieving a correct answer to the input stimulation. Several studies focused on training ANNs, and Evolutionary Algorithms (EA) gives a faster global convergence. In this paper, a novel approach based on Artificial Neural Networks and Particle Swarm Optimization (PSO) is proposed to improve the training process. A training method based on PSO algorithm achieves a faster global convergence.**

Keywords— **Electrical impedance tomography, neural network, particle swarm optimization, finite element method, inverse problems.**

I. INTRODUCTION

In Electrical Impedance Tomography (EIT), the main difficulty is to solve an inverse problem while achieving an acceptable accuracy [1]. To do this, the use of Artificial Neural Networks (ANN) as a reconstruction method can generate a correct answer to the inverse problem efficiently [2]1. Since the resulting ANN may have a large number of inputs and outputs, the training process may take a long time before reaching the desired accuracy. This long training time may become problematic in some situations. In this paper, a solution to reduce the number of iterations that occur during the training process is proposed. To find an adaptive solution and quickly adjust the ANN to the problem, it can be interesting to reduce the number of iterations. The global convergence of the Particle Swarm Optimization (PSO) algorithm can be used to train the ANN with a limited number of iterations [3].

This paper introduces an approach based on a PSO algorithm to train the neural network to solve the EIT inverse problem. Evolutionary Algorithms (EA) have been used to train ANNs and their ability to provide a fast convergence has been demonstrated.

II. THEORY

A. Electrical Impedance Tomography

The final goal EIT imaging is to get an accurate map of the electrical conductivities of the different elements contained in the Finite Element (FE) model. The only data available is the electrical voltage or current measured from the boundaries, using a finite number of electrodes [1]. Not only this problem is nonlinear, it is also severely ill-posed, meaning that it does not satisfy the Hadamard's conditions [4].

Several methods have been discussed to solve this problem. These methods can fit into two categories: linear approximations and nonlinear optimization [5]. Linear approximations tend to linearize the problem in order to simplify its resolution while reducing the accuracy of the model (linearization induces smoothness into the underlying mathematical representation). On the other hand, a nonlinear approximation is based on a more complex but correct mathematical model, and therefore on can expect a higher resolution.

B. Artificial Neural Networks

ANNs are computational models based on human brain function. They are capable of approximating the solution of a non-linear problem such as the EIT problem [4].

Typically, an ANN is made of 3 layers of neurons interconnected. From a mathematical point of view, a neuron can be seen as a linear function (here, radial basis and pure linear functions have been chosen) having two variable parameters, called weights and biases, which varies during the training process. Once the neuron calculated the output given a specific input, the result is sent to the next layer of neurons. By passing the information through the different layers of neurons, an ANN is capable of approximating the solution to a non-linear problem.

Before using an ANN, it is required to train it. Typically, this phase is used to determine the different weights and biases used in the network to interconnect the different neurons.

I. Lackovic (ed.), *1st Global Conference on Biomedical Engineering & 9th Asian-Pacific Conference on Medical and Biological Engineering*, IFMBE Proceedings 47, DOI: 10.1007/978-3-319-12262-5_49

C. Particle Swarm Optimization

Evolutionary Algorithms, such as PSO, have been proven to be able to train a neural network with faster global convergence than classical training methods, based on gradient or back-propagation [7]. In facts, an ANN can be trained with a reduced number of training iterations.

PSO, an EA based on the movement of birds in a bird flock, surveys the domain and searches for a global solution to the problem [8]. It is an auto-organized structure capable of training neural networks. In PSO, each particle has its own position X and its own speed V. After iteration k, particles move according to (1). The speed V_{k+1} depends on the previous speed V_k of the particle, its best position P_i and the global best position P_g. The inertia weight ω, and the coefficients b_1 and b_2 depend on the problem and are fixed in advance. Equation (1) is used to update the particle's position in one dimension [8].

$$\begin{aligned} V_{k+1} &= \omega V_k + b_1(P_i - X_k) + b_2(P_g - X_k) \\ X_{k+1} &= X_k + V_{k+1} \end{aligned} \tag{1}$$

When PSO algorithm is used to train a neural network, the weights and biases of the network are adjusted at each iteration of the PSO algorithm. Each particle of the PSO algorithm contains a set of weights and biases (the dimension of the PSO problem is equivalent to the number of weights and biases contained in the network).

After each iteration, the ANN is updated with newly calculated weights and biases. Then, the training data is used to feed the network and calculate an error (Mean Square Error, MSE) on the reconstructed images. The error is transmitted to the PSO algorithm, which updates its particles consequently, according to (1). The goal of the PSO algorithm is to minimize this error by moving the particles in the search space. Eq. (2) defines the MSE function used to compute the error value:

$$MSE = \sum_{elements} abs(targets - outputs)^2 \tag{2}$$

where *targets* and *outputs* are, respectively, the desired outputs and the real outputs values obtained from the ANN.

III. EXPERIMENTS

In this paper, a neural network has been trained to solve the EIT problem. This network was trained using PSO algorithm in order to demonstrate the fast convergence of the PSO algorithm and its possible application in the resolution of ill-posed inverse problems.

The simulations used a FE model of a circular tank of 256 elements, having 16 electrodes at its outer boundary. An electrical current is sent into the simulated tank using two adjacent electrodes, while the other 14 electrodes are used for measurements. Measurements are done using a pair of two adjacent electrodes, allowing a total of 13 measurements per current injection. The same current pattern is sent 16 times, each time using a different couple of adjacent electrodes. By performing 13 measurements for each couple of input electrodes, it is possible to get a total of 208 current measurements from the electrodes

About 200 EIT images were simulated, and their corresponding forward problems were solved to train the ANN. To get a realistic data set, each image contains one circular object having a random size and random conductivity, which can be located anywhere in the tank.

Two different ANN were created and trained with the same data set. One was trained with the PSO algorithm described above, and a second one with the well-known gradient descent back propagation algorithm described in [9].

Finally, another set of EIT images was generated and used to test the efficiency of the neural network. For each reconstructed image, an error was calculated and compared to the error obtained by a linear approximation (Gauss Newton one step).

IV. RESULT

A. Performance

Training neural networks with PSO can achieve a faster convergence. Once the network converges, it can be used to solve the EIT problem without dealing with linear approximations required by linear inverse solvers. With this approach, the number of training samples can be reduced significantly. Since PSO is capable of global convergence, training an ANN with PSO algorithm decreases the error exponentially because the updated weights and bias make the network more accurate.

The two different ANNs were trained to solve the EIT inverse problem and their convergence is plotted in Figure 1 below.

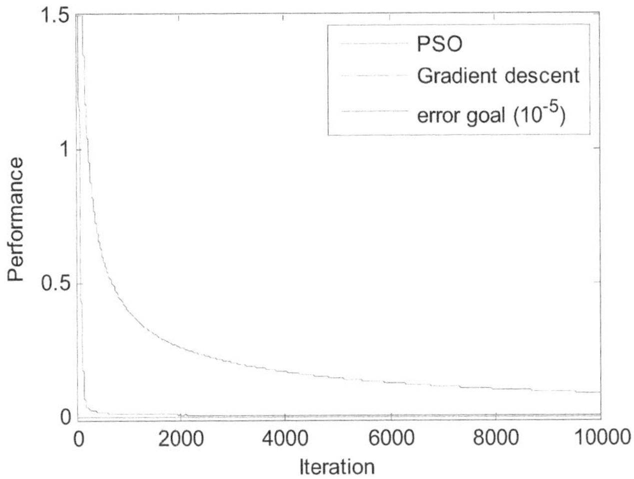

Fig. 1Comparison of training methods. PSO is compared to gradient descent.

Figure 1 clearly shows the positive effects of the global convergence of PSO algorithm during the training process. By training the ANN with EA, the output error is significantly reduced at the beginning of the training process. In the case of the EIT problem, PSO algorithm reached an MSE error of 0.05 with less than 200 iterations, while the gradient descent training algorithm needs more than 10 000 iterations to get the same accuracy.

B. Image Reconstruction

The ANN trained by PSO algorithm has been tested and different EIT images were reconstructed with this neural network. While the linear approximation can give a reconstruction without any training, the nonlinear optimization made by the ANN is expected to give a better result, closer to the original image.

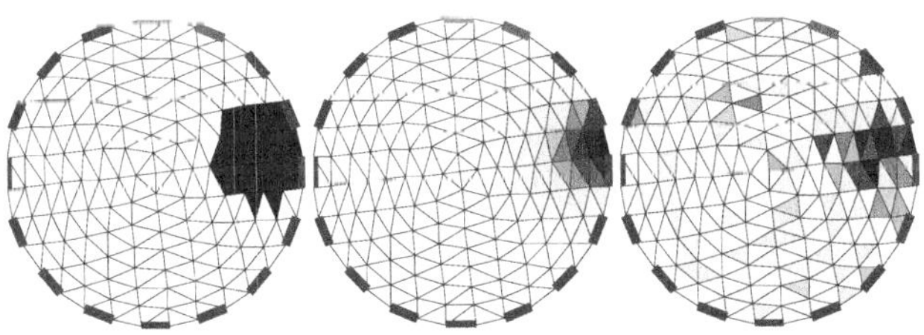

Fig. 2 Comparison of reconstructions using inverse solver (middle) and ANN trained with PSO (right). On the left, the original image.

Fig. 2 shows the EIT image obtained with both inverse solver and the proposed solution, based on artificial neural network and particle swarm optimization. Visually, it can be seen that the solution presented in this paper gives rough boundaries (compared to linear inverse solver). On each reconstruction, an MSE error was calculated. By using a linear inverse solver, an average error of 7.8% is obtained. By using the proposed method, the average error dropped down to 5.5%. Finally, Fig. 2 clearly shows that the proposed method is capable to achieve a higher accuracy than the commonly used linear inverse solvers.

V. CONCLUSION

Solving the EIT with neural networks usually requires fewer resources than linear inverse solvers, and therefore can achieve a good reconstruction in a relatively short time. Using a specific training method, such as PSO, can overcome some limitations of NN in biomedical application. Here, the fast convergence of the PSO algorithm gives a rapid training, by achieving certain accuracy more than 50 times faster than the back propagation algorithm. In addition, due to its mathematical definition, an ANN is capable of solving the inverse problem with a limited smoothness, which usually leads to a closer result of the EIT problem.

CONFLICT OF INTEREST

The authors declare that they have no conflict of interest.

REFERENCES

1. Holder DS (2005) Electrical impedance tomography: methods, history and applications, CRC Press.
2. Mohanna S, Valian E, Tavakoli S (2013) Nondestructive position detection of a metallic target within soil substrate using electromagnetic tomography. Res. Nondestruct. Eval. 24(4): 177–190.
3. Ilonen J, Kamarainen J, Lampinen J (2003) Differential evolution training algorithm for feed-forward neural networks. Neural Processing Letters 17(1): 93–105.
4. Borcea L (2002) Electrical impedance tomography. Inverse problems 18(6): 99–136.
5. Cheney M, Isaacson D, Newell JC (1999) Electrical impedance tomography. SIAM Review 41(1): 85–101.
6. Adler A, Guardo R (1994) A neural network image reconstruction technique for electrical impedance tomography. In: IEEE transactions on medical imaging, 13(4): 594-600.
7. Roy A (2013) Training artificial neural network using particle swarm optimization algorithm. Int. J. Adv. Res. Comput. Sci. Softw. Eng. 3(3): 430–434.
8. Eberhart R, Kennedy J (1995) A new optimizer using particle swarm theory," In: Proceedings of the sixth international symposium on micro machine and human science, 1:39-43.
9. Baldi P (1995) Gradient descent learning algorithm overview: a general dynamical systems perspective, In IEEE transactions on neural networks, 6(1): 182-195.

Author: Sebastien Martin and Charles T. M. Choi
Institute: National Chiao Tung University
Street: 1001 University Rd.
City: Hsinchu, 30010
Country: Taiwan
Email: c.t.choi@ieee.org

Analysis of Post_Movement Event-Related Synchronization (ERS) in Leudoaraiosis Patients Tsing Multivariate Empirical Mode Decomposition

H.T. Hsu, H.C. Chang , F.J. Lin, and P.L. Lee*

[1] Department of Electrical Engineering, National Central University, Jhongli City, Taoyuan County 32001, Taiwan

Abstract— **This study utilized movement-related sensorimotor Mu rhythm to probe EEG abnormalities in leukoaraiosis patients when they were performing self-paced finger movement task. The differences in EEG Mu rhythms between patients and normal subjects were studied and compared. Leukoaraiosis is a descriptive term used to describe neuroimaging findings of diffuse hemispheric white matter abnormalities, mainly characterized by loss of myelin and/or ischemic injury. The leukoaraiosis has been suggested a major risk factor and prognostic factor for stroke. Since EEG signals are weak (μv) and stochastic, the use of traditional digital filter may be unable to well extract the stochastic sensorimotor rhythms which could result in the pitfall of underestimating subject's responses. Accordingly, a novel tool, multivariate empirical mode decomposition (MEMD), was adopted in this study to exact the sensorimotor Mu rhythm in human brain. Our results found the beta event-related synchronization (ERS) of EEG Mu rhythm in Leukoaraiosis patients are significantly lower than those in normal controls using conventional event-related synchronization (conventional beta ERS) (0.44±0.2 uv v.s. 0.84±0.42) (student's t-test, p<0.01). Further analyzing the single-trial beta ERS using MEMD approach, the single-trial beta ERS in Leukoaraiosis patients and normal controls were 2.02±1.68 uv and 1.68±0.73 uv (student's t-test, p<0.05). It can be observed that the standard variation of single-trial beta ERS in Leukoaraiosis patients is larger than that that in normal controls (1.68 uv. v.s. 0.73 uv). The large signal variation in beta ERS could result in the suppression of conventional ERS values in Leukoaraiosis patients.**

Keywords— **Electroencephalograph (EEG), Event-related synchronization (ERS), Multivariate empirical mode decomposition (MEMD).**

I. INTRODUCTION

The Leukoaraiosis a disease which causes changes in the white-matter structure of human brain. Leukoaraiosis is a descriptive term used to describe neuroimaging findings of diffuse hemispheric white matter abnormalities mainly characterized by loss of myelin and/or ischemic injury. Patients suffering from Leukoaraiosis may cause pathologies in myelin loss, sparse perivascular space, neuronal axon loss, gliosis, etc., accompany with clinical symptoms of dementia, handicap, depression, gait instability, and urinary incontinence. Current Leukoaraiosis studies mainly focus on studying the structure changes in MRI images. Lee et al. (2008) found most Leukoaraiosis patients have sever angiosclerosis [1]. Patankar et al. (2006) found high correlateon between atherosclerosiss and Leukoaraiosis [2]. Neurmann-Haefelin et al. (2006) utilized MRI to study the correlateon between Leukoaraiosis and stroke patients [3]. Nevertheless, though some MRI studies on Leukoaraiosis has been reported, only few functional studies were performed in the past.

In this study, we utilized EEG event-related desynchrnoization/ synchronization (ERD/ ERS) as biomarker to probe the abnormality of neural oscillatory activities in Leukoaraiosis patients. Neural oscillatory activities in human brain can be either phase-locked or non-phase-locked reactive to external or internal stimuli. These oscillatory activities usually exist in specific frequency bands and spatial locations [4]. Event-related non-phase-locked neural activities represent power changes, either enhanced or suppressed relative to baseline activities. The power changes in event-related activities can be caused by the decrease or increase in synchrony of the underlying activated neuronal populations. Previous researches have suggested that the event-related power suppression in motor area, serving as physiological meaning of motor planning and movement preparation, called ERD, while the increase of power in the post-movement beta band may reflect deactivation/inhibition during the recovery phase in the movement process, called ERS [5]. Due to fast temporal changes in brain oscillatory activities, Electroencephalogrpahy / Magnetoencephalography (EEG/MEG) are often selected as powerful tools to study ERD and ERS phenomena.

The induced oscillatory activities have been study in many aspects, including somatosensory input response [6], motor functions [5 7-9], cognitive performance [10], level of memory loading [11], etc. Several methods have been developed to quantify the induced oscillatory activities. Pfurtscheller *et al.* developed ERD/ERS technique by simply filtering EEG activities within a fixed frequency band, rectifying the filtered signals, and then averaging over dozens of trials to find an averaged in the primary

* Corresponding author.

I. Lackovic (ed.), *1st Global Conference on Biomedical Engineering & 9th Asian-Pacific Conference on Medical and Biological Engineering*,
IFMBE Proceedings 47, DOI: 10.1007/978-3-319-12262-5_50

sensorimotor cortex [5 12]. Clochon *et al.* utilized amplitude modulation (AM) method based on the Hilbert transform to detect the signal envelope changes [13]. Salmelin *et al.* proposed the temporal-spectral evolution method rectifies and averages filtered MEG signals in pre-defined equi-bandwidth frequency bands [14, 15]. Florian and Pfurtscheller used autoregressive and spectral decomposition methods to extract the significant frequency components in oscillatory signals [16]. However, these approaches presume fixed frequency band and temporal characteristics across trials and require dozens to hundred trials for average which may be too stringent to reflect trial-by-trial dynamics. Since the determination of frequency band for bandpass filtering has been addressed as the most important issue for ERD/ERS detections, the utilization of stereotypical frequency band determined from one or few specified channels may not optimize the extraction of neural oscillatory activities in other channels [5].

To study the inter-trial variation of ERD/ERS, several advanced signal processing techniques have been proposed. Pfurtscheller *et al.* proposed adaptive autoregression and minimum Mahalanobis distance classifier to discriminate EEG oscillatory activities induced from four different motor imagery tasks [7]. Lee *et al.* extracted MEG post-movement beta oscillatory activities using an independent component analysis (ICA)-based approach [17, 18]. Qin and He applied the Morlet wavelet-based time-frequency analysis approach for classifying motor imagery for brain computer interface control [19]. However, the aforementioned methods extract oscillatory activities with assumed basis functions or pre-specified statistical models for signal extraction, which might be not suitable for stochastic signal interpretations. Therefore, considering the non-linearly dynamic and stochastic nature of brain oscillatory activities, the empirical mode decomposition (EMD) has been chosen as a potential tool for extracting event-related oscillatory activities [20-23]. In our previous publications, we had successfully developed an EMD-based approach to extract sensorimotor oscillatory from one single channel in MEG/EEG data [21 22]. Nevertheless, since human brain is a complex system contained intricate neural network, a method for studying inter-trial variations in multichannel EEG/MEG data is needed.

In this study, we detected finger-lifting induced ERD/ERS in Leukoaraiosis patitents, and the detected results were compated with those in normal subjects. To understand inter-trial variability of ERD/ERS in Leukoaraiosis patient, we adopted multivariate empirical mode decomposition (MEMD) to extract movement-induced event-related oscillatory activities in multichannel EEG data [24, 25]. The efficacy of the proposed method has been manifested by the extraction of beta-related oscillatory activities in performing self-paced right and left index-finger lifting tasks. The present approach allows oscillatory activities within the same subband across different channels can be aligned and compared in the same intrinsic mode function (IMF), in which no pre-defined basis or prior information of statistical model is required. The proposed MEMD-based approach also enables the capability of analyzing task-specific frequency band, temporal waveform, and inter-trial variability on a trial-by-trial base, which possibly provides an insightful view on subtle brain dynamics.

II. MATERIALS AND METHODS

Fourteen subjects were recruited in this study. The group 1 was eight right-handed subjects (four males and four females) who were leukoaraiosis patients, aged between 60 and 85 years old. The group 2 was six right-handed healthy subjects (four males and two females) who had no history of nueropathological illness, aged between 23 and 28 years old. Subjects participated in two self-paced finger lifting sessions, one right and one left index-finger lifting tasks. In each session, each subject was requested to perform self-paced index-finger lifting approximately once every 7 s for six-minute EEG recording. Each movement was asked to be performed briskly, while keeping their eyes opened in order to suppress the occipital alpha rhythm. EEG data were acquired by a EEG-recorded device (bandpass, 0.05 – 100 Hz; bandstop, 60Hz; sampling rate, 2000 Hz; V-Amp, Brain Products Co., Munich, Germany), placed in accordance with the International 10 – 20 system. Electrodes were placed the frontal lobe (F3, Fz, F4, FC5, FC1, FC2, FC6) and parietal lobe (C3, Cz, C4, Cp1, Cp2).

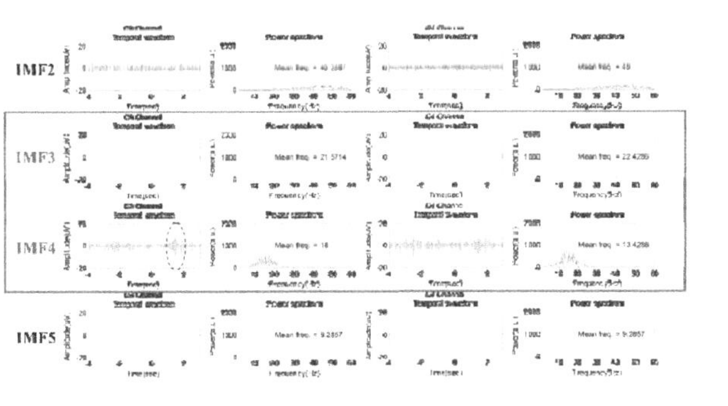

Fig. 1. One example of the MEMD process on C3 and C4 channels from one epoch in subject S1 of the group 2 when he was performing right index-finger movement. The temporal waveforms and power spectra of the decomposed IMFs.

Impedance was kept below 5 kΩ for all electrodes. Bipolar vertical electro-oculograms (EOG) was placed below and above the left eye to detect eye movements and blinks. EEG data were segmented into epochs, ranged from –4 s to 3 s, anchored to movement onsets [12, 19], and artifact-free epochs (EOG < 300μV) were subject to the following MEMD analysis without applying any pre-filtering process.

For multivariate signals, Rehman and Mandic proposed the MEMD by generating multiple N-dimensional envelopes and taking signal projections along different directions in N-dimensional spaces. These projects are then averaged to obtain the local mean [21].

This study manifests the feasibility of using MEMD in extracting oscillatory activities during right and left index-finger lifting task. The mean frequencies (f_{mean}) of IMFs decomposed from each channel were examined, and the IMFs with mean frequencies within beta band (16 – 24Hz), denoted as IMF_{beta}, were chosen and summated to reconstruct the beta-related oscillatory activities.

To achieve trial-by-trial analysis of post-movement beta activities, the beta-related oscillatory activities were extracted in each trial using MEMD. The trial-specific beta bands determined from C3 and C4, denoted as f_{beta_C3} and f_{beta_C4}, were used to extract post-movement beta activities.

Fig. 1 shows an example of the MEMD process on C3 and C4 channels from one epoch in healthy subject S1 when he was performing right index-finger movement. The C3 and C4 channels are listed to observe the sensorimotor responses during the finger movement. The mean frequencies for IMF2s, IMF3s, IMF4s, and IMF5s are 40.29Hz, 21.57Hz, 18Hz, and 9.2857Hz at C3 channel, 49Hz, 22.43Hz, 3.29Hz, and 9.29Hz at C4 channel, respectively. It can be observed that the time course of IMF4 at C3 channel and IMF4 at C4 channel both presented enhanced post-movement beta activity (marked by dashed ellipse) with centralized frequency (18Hz and 21.57Hz, respectively) distribution in beta range. Therefore, the IMF3s and IMF4s (marked by red rectangle) were designated as beta-related IMFs. Other IMFs were considered as beta-unrelated IMFs and should be excluded in the following beta activity reconstruction process to avoid the interference of task-unrelated noise.

III. RESULTS

Fig. 2 shows the whole-head beta-band ERS in S1 of the group 1 (Leukoaraiosis group) obtained from the average of all trials when performing right and left index-finger movements, respectively. The whole-head beta-band ERS in S1 of group 2 (healthy group) in right index-finger movements was shown in Fig. 3. It can observed that the Leukoaraiosis group has suppressed post-movement which

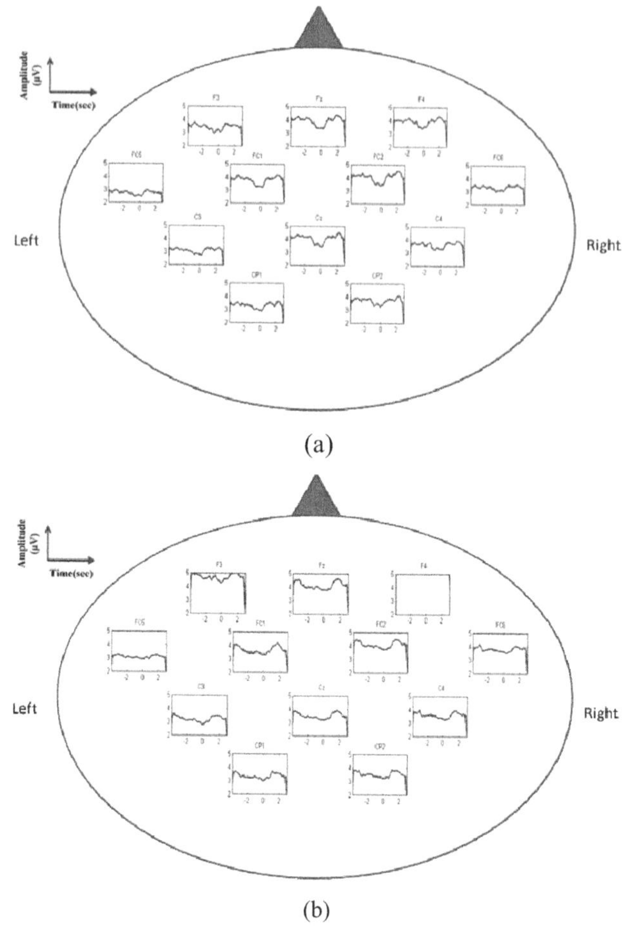

Fig. 2. Whole-head ERS time courses obtained from the average of all trials. (a) The subject S1 of the group 1 lifted the right index-finger. (b) The subject S3 of the group 1 lifted the left index-finger.

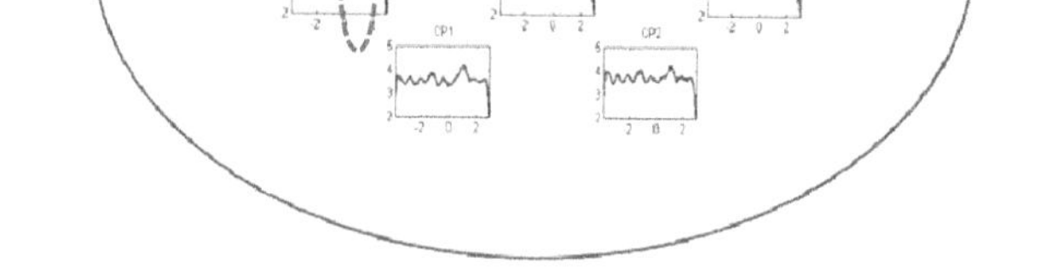

Fig. 3. Whole-head ERS time courses obtained from the average of all trials. The subject S1 of the gropu 2 lifted the right index-finger.

might reflect the difficulty in conducting the finger-lifting movement. Compared with healthy group, clear post-movement ERS (marked by dashed ellipse) was observed. The statistics over all subjects in our study showed that beta ERS of EEG Mu rhythm in Leukoaraiosis patients were significantly lower than those in normal controls using conventional ERS (0.44±0.2 uv v.s. 0.84±0.42) (student's t-test, $p<0.01$).

IV. CONCLUSION

This study presents a MEMD-based approach for extracting neural oscillatory activities in multichannel EEG data. The feasibility of the proposed method has been demonstrated to study the inter-trial dynamics of post-movement beta activities in index-finger lifting tasks. Moreover, this study presents the difference between the normal subject and the Leukoaraiosis patient. The Leukoaraiosis patients' beta-band activity was lower than the healthy subject. The possible reason was that the Leukoaraiosis patients have poorer neural conductivity in initiating a specific movment. The proposed MEMD-based approach might be an effective tool to construct rehabilitative index in future studies.

CONFLICTS OF INTEREST

The arthors declare that they have no conflict of interest in the research.

ACKNOWLEDGMENT

This study was supported by the National Central University, the Center for Dynamical Biomarkers and Translational Medicine (NSC 102-2911-I-008-001),National Science Council (NSC102-2511-S-008-004, 102-2623-E-008-003-D, 102-2221-E-008-086-MY3), and NCU-Landseed Hospital cooperative project (NCU-LSH-101-A-023)

REFERENCES

1. Lee SJ, Kim JS, Lee KS, An JY, Kim WJ, Kim YI, Kim BS and Jung SL (2008) BMC Neurology, 8: 31
2. Patankar T, Widjaja E. Chant H, McCollum C, Baldwin R, Jeffries S, Sutcliffe C, Burns A, and Jackson A (2006) Eur J Neurol 13: 10-16
3. Hakan AY, Arsava E M, Rosand J, Karen L.(2008) Stroke 39: 1409-1413
4. J. Kalcher, and G. Pfurtscheller (1995) Electroencephalogr. Clin. Neurophysiol., vol. 94, no. 5, pp. 381-384
5. G. Pfurtscheller, and F. H. Lopes da Silva (1999) Clin. Neurophysiol., vol. 110, no. 11, pp. 1842-1857
6. E. Houdayer, E. Labyt, F. Cassim, J. L. Bourriez, and P. Derambure (2006) Clin. Neurophysiol., vol. 117, no. 3, pp. 628-636
7. G. Pfurtscheller, C. Brunner, A. Schlogl, and F. H. Lopes da Silva (2006) Neuroimage, vol. 31, no. 1, pp. 153-159
8. C. Dockstader, W. Gaetz, D. Cheyne, F. Wang, F. X. Castellanos, and R. Tannock (2008) Behav. Brain Funct., vol. 4, pp. 8
9. G. Pfurtscheller, K. Pichler-Zalaudek, B. Ortmayr, J. Diez, and F. Reisecker (1998) J. Clin. Neurophysiol., vol. 15, no. 3, pp. 243-250
10. C. Neuper, R. H. Grabner, A. Fink, and A. C. Neubauer (2005) Clin. Neurophysiol., vol. 116, no. 7, pp. 1681-1694
11. P. M. Lahteenmaki, C. M. Krause, L. Sillanmaki, T. T. Salmi, and A. H. Lang (1999) Clin. Neurophysiol., vol. 110, no. 12, pp. 2064-2073
12. C. Neuper, and G. Pfurtscheller (1996) Neurosci Lett., vol. 216, no. 1, pp. 17-20
13. P. Clochon, J. Fontbonne, N. Lebrun, and P. Etevenon (1996) Electroencephalogr. Clin. Neurophysiol., vol. 98, no. 2, pp. 126-129
14. R. Salmelin, and R. Hari (1994) Neuroscience, vol. 60, no. 2, pp. 537-550
15. R. Salmelin, M. Hamalainen, M. Kajola, and R. Hari (1995) Neuroimage, vol. 2, no. 4, pp. 237-243
16. G. Florian, and G. Pfurtscheller (1995) Electroencephalogr. Clin. Neurophysiol., vol. 95, no. 5, pp. 393-396
17. P. L. Lee, Y. T. Wu, L. F. Chen, Y. S. Chen, C. M. Cheng, T. C. Yeh, L. T. Ho, M. S. Chang, and J. C. Hsieh (2003) Neuroimage, vol. 20, no. 4, pp. 2010-2030
18. C. H. Wu, P. L. Lee, Y. T. Wu, and J. C. Hsieh (2008) J. of Medical and Biological. Eng., vol. 28, pp. 155-159
19. L. Qin, and B. He (2005) J. Neural. Eng., vol. 2, no. 4, pp. 65-72
20. W. Huang, Z. Shen, N. E. Huang, and Y. C. Fung (1998) Proc. Natl. Acad. Sci. USA, vol. 95, no. 9, pp. 4816-4821
21. P. L. Lee, L. Z. Shang, Y. T. Wu, C. H. Shu, J. C. Hsieh, Y. Y. Lin, C. H. Wu, Y. L. Liu, C. Y. Yang, C. W. Sun, and K. K. Shyu (2009) Ann. Biomed. Eng., vol. 37, no. 8, pp. 1683-1700
22. C. L. Yeh, H. C. Chang, C. H. Wu, and P. L. Lee (2010) Biomed. Eng. Online, vol. 9, pp. 25
23. C. H. Wu, H. C. Chang, P. L. Lee, K. S. Li, J. J. Sie, C. W. Sun, C. Y. Yang, P. H. Li, H. T. Deng, and K. K. Shyu (2011) J. Neurosci. Methods, vol. 196, no. 1, pp. 170-181
24. N. Rehman, and D. P. Mandic (2010) in Proc. Roy. Soc. A,, vol. 466, no. 2117, pp. 1291-1302

Author: H.T. Hsu
Institute: National Central University
Street: No.300, Jhongda Rd.,
City: Jhongli
Country: Taoyuan County 32001, Taiwan (R.O.C.)
Email: fifaworld91@gmail.com

Author: H.C. Chang
Institute: National Central University
Street: No.300, Jhongda Rd.,
City: Jhongli
Country:Taoyuan County 32001, Taiwan (R.O.C.)
Email: box@cycu.org.tw

Author: F.J. Lin
Institute: National Central University
Street: No.300, Jhongda Rd.,
City: Jhongli
Country: Taoyuan County 32001, Taiwan (R.O.C.)
Email: mosmii333@gmail.com

Author: P.L. Lee
Institute: National Central University
Street: No.300, Jhongda Rd.,
City: Jhongli
Country: Taoyuan County 32001, Taiwan (R.O.C.)
Email: pllee@ee.ncu.edu.tw

One-Step Quantitative Detection of Human Chorionic Gonadotropin by Integrating Immunochromatography Test Strip with Fluorescence Detection of Quantum Qots

Xue Li[1], Yudong Wu[2], Jian Zhang[2], and Jin Chang[1, 2,*]

[1] School of Precision Instruments and Opto-Engineering, Institute of Nanobiotechnology, Tianjin University and Tianjin Key Laboratory of Composites and Functional Materials, Tianjin 300072, P.R. China

[2] School of Materials Science and Engineering, Institute of Nanobiotechnology, Tianjin University and Tianjin Key Laboratory of Composites and Functional Materials, Tianjin 300072, P.R. China

Abstract— **The Immunochromatography test strip (ICTS) is a one step and the commonest commercial point-of-care diagnostic format. Their advantages of convenient and fast testing enable the rapid decisions on diseases. However, the fundamental limitation of quantitative and sensitive analysis severely hampers their application in the field of early detection. Herein, we overcame these limitations by integrating of quantum dots with distinct optical and electronic properties, which were served as the signal reporters for ICTS. Human chorionic gonadotropin (HCG), which has been recognized as a clinic marker of pregnancy, was used as a model analyte to demonstrate the performance of the QDs-based ICTS platform. Under optimized conditions, the detection limit was about 0.24 IU/L. Meanwhile, the concentrations of HCG could be determined within 20 min with high specificity, using only 40 μL of sample. Our data suggests that the QDs-based ICTS platform is a rapid, low-cost, highly sensitive and specific test platform for quantitative point-of-care diagnostics, which holds promise to become part of routine medical testing for other protein markers detections.**

Keywords— **Quantum dots, one step detection, immunochromatography test strip, quantitative detection.**

I. INTRODUCTION

During the past decade, a number of methods have been developed for protein markers detection. Although methodological advances have been achieved, detection methods are still severely restricted [1][2]. For example, conventional methods, such as enzyme-linked immunosorbent assays (ELISA) and chemiluminesc ence immunoassay (CLIA), suffer from the disadvantages of being time-consuming, having low sensitivity and a laborious process. Besides that, these detection methods also require expensive instruments, highly skilled personnel to perform the procedures. Recently, the Immunochromatography test strip (ICTS) has been becoming a powerful tool for detection in a majority of fields for their convenient analysis [3]. However, the limitation of sensitive and quantitative analysis severely hampers their application as a reliable medical testing in early detection of disease. In order to overcome the limitations, more quantitative ICTS has been developed by using various signal reporters, such as colloidal gold [4], up-converting phosphors [5], colored latex particles [6], magnetic nanoparticles[7] and organic fluorophores [8].Quantum dots (QDs) as nano-scaled fluorescent labels, has wildly used in biomedical applications [9]. Their high level of brightness and extraordinary photostability allow ultrasensitive detection, which also provide new opportunities for ICTS.

We herein report on the development of a QDs-based ICTS platform designed to provide fast and portable detection of protein biomarker, using HCG as a model analyte. HCG has been proved as a valuable protein marker for pregnancy. Then the effective reaction time, sensitivity, specificity and capability of quantitative detection of these QD s based ICTS were investigated to display its performance. As expected, our data show the QDs-based ICTS could provide a one step quantitative detection for HCG in a short time with high specificity and sensitivity. Thus the QDs-based ICTS may be widely used for protein markers detection in hospital, community, and even at home, as a first-response point-of-care device.

II. MATERIALS AND CHEMICALS

A. Materials and Chemicals

Selenium powder (99.99%, Aldrich), cadmium oxide (CdO, 99.5%, Aldrich), tri-n-octylphophine (TOP, 90%, Aldrich), tri-n-octylphosphine oxide (TOPO, 90%, Aldrich), octadecylamine(ODA, 90%, ACROS), 1-octadecene (ODE, 90%, ACROS), oleic acid (OA, 90%, Aldrich), sulphur (Aldrich), poly(tert-butyl acrylate-co-ethyl acrylate-co-methacrylic acid) (ABC triblock copolymer) (Aldrich).

* Corresponding author.

I. Lackovic (ed.), *1st Global Conference on Biomedical Engineering & 9th Asian-Pacific Conference on Medical and Biological Engineering*, IFMBE Proceedings 47, DOI: 10.1007/978-3-319-12262-5_51

1-ethyl-3-(3-dimethyl- laminopropyl)-carbodiimide hydrochloride (EDC, GL Biochem(Shanghai) Ltd.). N-hydroxysuccinimide (NHS, GL Biochem (Shanghai) Ltd.). Bovine serum albumin (BSA) and fetal bovine serum (FBS) were supplied by Beijing Dingguo Biotechnology Co., Ltd (China). Mouse monoclonal antibody, goat anti-mouse IgG, nitrocellulose membranes, glass fibers and absorbent pad were obtained from Bioscience (Tianjin) diagnostic technology Co., Ltd. All chemicals were used without further purification.

B. Synthesis of CdSe/CdS/CdxZn$_{1-x}$S/ZnS Nanocrystals

The core/shell QDs CdSe/CdS/CdxZn$_{1-x}$S/ZnS were synthesized based on successive ion layer adsorption and reaction (SILAR) method. First, CdSe nanocrystals were made by a typical synthetic procedure, 0.0386 g of CdO, 0.4 mL of OA, and 4 mL of DOE were added to a three-necked flask and heated to 260°C under argon until complete dissolution of CdO. After cooling to room temperature, 2.5 g of ODA and 0.5 g of TOPO were added into the flask. The solution was heated to 300°C. The solution containing 0.14 g of selenium, 2 mL of TOP was injected into the solution quickly. Then the growth temperature was set to 250 °C for 10 min. After that time, the heating mantle was removed and the products were isolated using at least three times hexane-methanol extractions.

Next, for shell growth, a tipical procedure reported previously was slightly modified. The solution containing the CdSe were mixed with 1.5 g of ODA and 5.0 g of ODE in a new three-neck flask, and the system was kept at 100 °C under argon flow for 15 min to remove the undesired materials. Subsequently, the system was heated to 240 °C for shells growing. The amount of the injection solution for each monolayer was determined by calculating the number of the surface atoms of a given size of a nanocrystal, and the Cd precursor (0.4 M) solutions, Zn precursor (0.4 M) solutions, sulfur precursor (0.4 M) solution were previous prepared, The final product was diluted by hexane after a methanol extraction at least three times.

C. Preparation of Biocompatible QDs and QD-Antibody Conjugats

To prepare biocompatible QDs, the QDs and 2 mg of octadecylamine (ODA) grafted poly(tert-butyl acrylate-co-ethyl acrylate-co-methacrylic acid) (ABC-g-ODA) was mixed with 960 μL of dichlormethane to form the organic phase. Then 10mL of de-ionized (DI) water was slowly added into the organic phase under an ultrasonicator at 200 W for 5 min. Then the mixture was stirred magnetically until the organic phase was totally removal. Then the products were washed 3 times with DI water and centrifuged to collect.

The QD-antibody conjugates were prepared as followed. The biocompatibie QDs, mouse monoclonal antibody and EDC were mixed in PBS buffer solution (0.01 M, pH=7.4) at a QDs/antibody/EDC molar ratio of 1:8:4000. After reacting for 2 h, the final products were purified by centrifugation and stored in PBS buffer solution (0.01 M, pH 7.4, 0.5% BSA) overnight at 4°C.

D. Test Strip Preparation and Fluorescence Assay Procedure

The test strip consists of sample pad, conjugate release pad, reaction membrane, absorbent pad, and backing card. QD-antibody conjugates were diluted 20 times with blocking buffer (pH 7.4), which containing 0.01 M PBS, 3% (w/v) BSA, 5% (w/v) sucrose, 2% (w/v) PEG4000, 0.1% (w/v) Tween-20). After that, the solutions were dispensed onto the conjugate pads. The pads were dried at 37°C for 2 h. The T zone and C zone of the strips were prepared by dispensing a certain volume of 2 mg/mL mouse monoclonal antibody solution and goat anti-mouse IgG respectively with the dispenser XYZ-3050 BioJet Quanti 3000 onto a reaction membrane. After 2 h of drying at 37 °C, the membrane was blocked with 1% BSA at room temperature for 1 h, dried under vacuum for 30 min, and then stored at 4 °C. Then the parts were assembled on a plastic adhesive backing card. Each part overlapped 2 mm to ensure the solution migrating through the strip during the assay. Then the whole assembled plate was cut into 4mm strips and stored at room temperature.

40 μL of samples containing a desired concentration of HCG in Fetal bovine serum (FBS) was dropped onto the sample pad and flowed through the reaction membrane under capillary action. Control experiment was performed by FBS samples without any analyte. After the completion of immunoreactions, the strip in a cassette was inserted into laboratory-built test strip reader [10] to read fluorescence intensity of the test zone and the control zone to quantify the analytes. The results were got by reading the fluorescent response with the strip reader after appropriate time.

III. RESULTS AND DISCUSSION

A. Principle of the Method

As schematically illustrated in Fig.1, a strip usually realized with five components, a sample pad, a conjugate pad, a reaction membrane, an absorbent pad and a backing card [11]. The principle of protein biomarkers detection was based on the sandwich assays. Sample was added on the sample pad and migrated to the conjugate pad driven by the capillary action, then the analyte in the sample interacted with the QD-antibody conjugates and form the immune complex, after that, the immune complex migrated to the reaction membrane, where the immune complex was recognized by capture antibodies immobilized onto reaction membrane surfaces to form test zone and the control zone. Then, excess reagents moved past the capture lines and were entrapped in the absorbent pad. Results were interpreted on the reaction membrane as the presence or absence of test zone, read either by naked eye with excited by a handheld ultraviolet lamp or using a strip reader. Fluorescence intensity of the T zone and C zone were related to the amount of analyte in the sample and reflected validity of the strip.

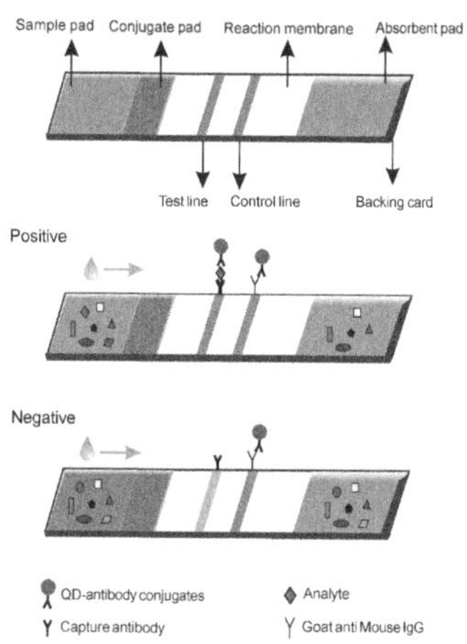

Fig. 1 Schematic illustration of ICTS detection of protein markers.

Herein, quantitative analysis was carried out by recording fluorescence intensity in the T zone and the C zone respectively by the test strip reader. Fluorescence intensity ratio between the T zone and the C zone was recorded as fluorescence signal (T/C). The signal to noise ratio (S/N) was defined as fluorescence peak area ratio between the target and the blank control samples. Detection results of the strips were analyzed by test strip reader for three times and the average values were plotted as a function of analyte's concentration.

B. Effective Reaction Time of the QDs-Based ICTS

Figure2A displays the signal response (T/C) of the ICTS under different reaction time ranging from 5min to 30min using 50 IU/L HCG, and the responses of FBS were set as the blank control group. Fig. 2B revealed the corresponding signal to noise ratio (S/N). As shown in the figure, the detectable signal emerged at the first 5 min after samples were applied, and either the T/C or S/N reached a constant at 20 min. The standard error was based on three duplicated measurements of analytes. These results indicated the short immunoreaction time of this biosensor. Thus, signals for quantitative analysis were measured at 20 min after the sample addition in all the succeeding studies.

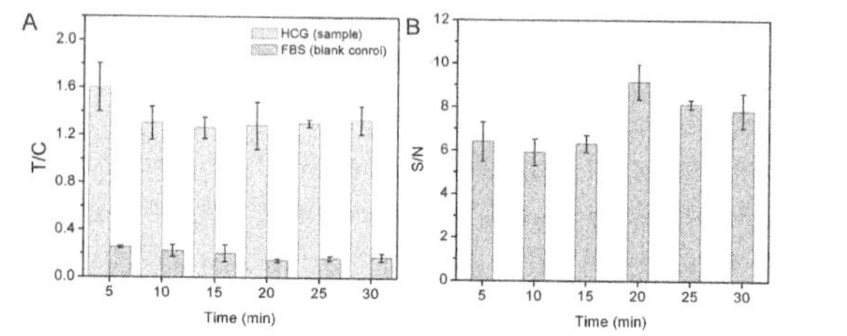

Fig. 2 Effect of immunoreactions time on the fluorescent responses of ICTS

C. Specificity of the QDs-Based ICTS

To recognize the ability of targets selectively, we prepared another 4 type of proteins marker including CA199, CEA, HCG and AFP, FBS was set as the blank control group to further test the strip specificity. When the non-specific binding existed, the non-target proteins marker would be captured by capture antibody on test zone. Consequently, strong signal response of the T zone would be detected with CA199, CEA, HCG, AFP and FBS. As a result, a clear distinction could be observed between the strips added HCG and the strip added FBS, CA199, CEA, AFP and PSA (Figure 3). Both the T/C and the S/N of the strips added HCG antigen were obvious higher than the strips added non-targeted antigens and FBS. We did not observe any crosstalk or interference with either CA199, CEA, AFP, PSA or FBS. From these measurements, we conclude that the test strips featured very high specificity.

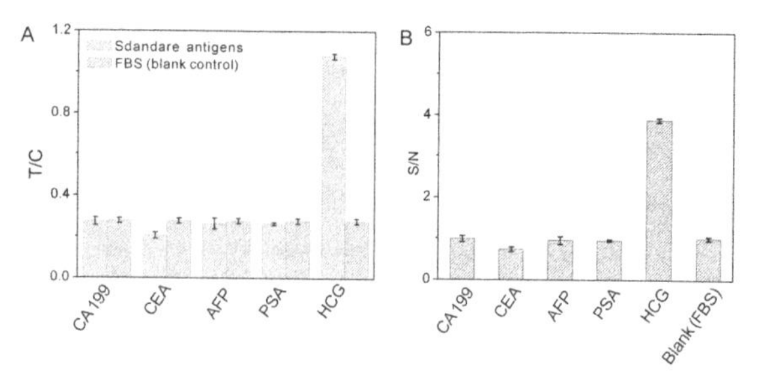

Fig. 3 Characterization of ICTS specificity.

D. Sensitivity and quantitative analysis of the QDs-based ICTS

To explore the feasibility for clinical application, the ability of quantitative detection of the QDs-based ICTS was characterized by analyzing standard HCG samples at a concentration gradient of 0~1000 IU/ml diluted in FBS. Fig. 2 revealed the fluorescence imaging of the ICTS excited by the ultraviolet lamp. As seen in the Fig. 2 the brightness of the fluorescence band could be easily observed by naked eyes. This result indicated that we can easily judge the existence or not of target proteins by observing the fluorescence band directly. For quantitative detection, there was a significant linear relationship between HCG concentration and fluorescence signal in the log-log plot with R^2=0.994, (y=0.427x-1.051). The detection limit was 0.24 IU/L (S/N=3), which was calculated as the concentration corresponding to 3 times the standard deviation of the blank control. Error bars are based on three duplicated measurements of HCG at different concentrations.

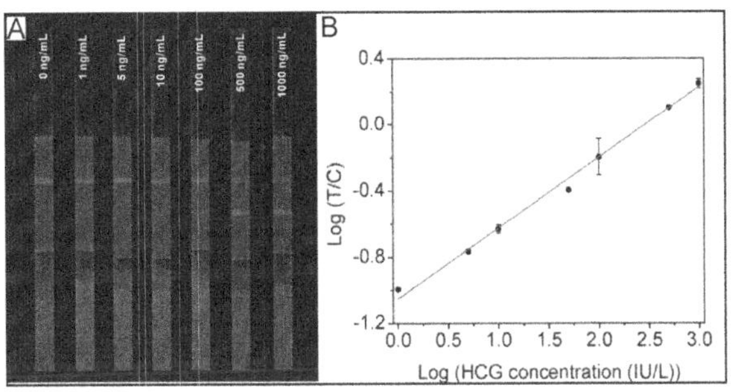

Fig. 4 Fluorescence imaging of the QDs-based ICTS added different concentrations HCG (A) and calibration curve of the quantitative detection (B)

IV. CONCLUSIONS

A well-performing biosensor was designed by combining the ICTS with QDs for the quantitative detection of protein biomarkers. The integration enabled the ICTS to sensitively and specifically determine the concentration of HCG in 20 min. Under the optimized conditions, the detection limit was about 0.24IU/L. There was a significant linear relationship between HCG concentration and fluorescence signal in the log-log plot with R^2=0.994. These results demonstrated the QDs-based ICTS was a rapid, sensitive, specific and low cost point-of-care diagnostic format. In view of its advantages, the new biosensors may be a nascent sensing technology that opens up new opportunities for the early detection of diseases at the site of patient care.

ACKNOWLEDGMENT

The authors gratefully acknowledge the National High Technology Program of China (863 Program) (2012AA022603), the Natural Science Foundation of China (51373117 and 81171372), the Key Project of the Tianjin Applied Basic Research Program (13JCZDJC33200), and the Doctoral Base Foundation of the Educational Ministry of China (20120032110027).

CONFLICT OF INTEREST

The authors declare that they have no conflict of interest.

REFERENCES

1. Rissin D M, Kan C W, Campbell T G et al. (2010) Nat. Biotechno l28:595–599.
2. Ramanaviciene A, German N, Kausaite-Minkstimiene A et al. (2012) Biosens Bioelectron 36:48–55.
3. Gubala V, Harris L F, Ricco A J et al. (2011) Anal Chem 84:487–515.
4. Zhou Y, Pan F G, Li Y S (2009) Biosens Bioelectron 24:2744–2747.
5. Corstjens P L, van Lieshout L, Zuiderwijk M et al. (2008) Clin Microbiol 46:171–176.
6. Karakus C, Salih B A. (2013) Immunol. Methods 396:8–14.
7. Wang D B, Tian B, Zhang Z P et al. (2013) Biosens Bioelectron 42:661–667.
8. Khreich N, Lamourette P, Boutal H et al. (2008) Anal Biochem 377:182–188.
9. Rosi N L, Mirkin C A. (2005) Chem Rev 105:1547–1562.
10. Yang Q, Gong X., Song T et al. (2011) Biosens Bioelectron 30:145–150.
11. Holland C A., Kiechle F L. (2005) Curr Opin Microbiol 8:504-509.

Author: Xue Li[1], Yudong Wu[2], Jian Zhang[2] and Jin Chang[1, 2]
Institute: Institute of Nanobiotechnology
Street: No.92, Weijin Road, Nankai District
City: Tianjin
Country: China
Email: jinchang@tju.edu.cn

Electrically Assessing the Effect of TGF-β1 on MDA-MB-231 Cells

C.-I. Lai[1], W.-T. Chen[1], Y.-T. Lai[2], and C.-M. Lo[2]

[1] Taipei Municipal Jianguo High School, Taipei, Taiwan
[2] National Yang-Ming University/Department of Biomedical Engineering, Taipei, Taiwan

Abstract— **We investigated the effect of transforming growth factor-beta1 (TGF-β1) on cell micromotion and wound healing migration of breast adenocarcinoma cells, MDA-MB-231. Central to this work was the use of electric cell-substrate impedance sensing (ECIS), a cell-based biosensor that monitors motility and other morphology changes of cells adherent on small gold electrodes. To detect the alternation of cell micromotion in response to 10 ng/ml of TGF-β1 challenge, time-series impedance fluctuations of cell-covered electrodes were monitored and the values of variance, power slope, and Hurst coefficient were calculated to verify the difference. These measures describe the motile and persistent behavior of these cells in culture. Furthermore, ECIS wounding assay was used to wound and monitor the healing process of TGF-β1 treated cell layers. Our data indicated that TGF-β1 treated MDA-MB-231 cells, in comparison to control cells, demonstrated higher fluctuation amplitude and unreduced long-term correlation for about 20 hours long. In addition, the wound healing rate of MDA-MB-231 cells significantly increased after cells were treated with 10 ng/ml of TGF-β1 though the effect decreased along with time. The results suggest that treatment of MDA-MB-231 cells with TGF-β1 facilitates their scattering behavior.**

Keywords— **ECIS, TGF-β1, MDA-MB-231, impedance fluctuations, wound healing.**

I. INTRODUCTION

The motility of cancer cells has been widely studied and considered as an intrinsic component of the metastasis process. Metastatic tumor cells generally migrate at a faster rate than normal cells or non-metastatic tumor cells do [1,2]. Previous studies indicate that TGF-β can activate downstream signaling pathways of breast cancer cells and facilitate their invasion and metastasis in vivo [3]. The conventional methods to detect cell motion, however, are often qualitative and require human judgment or involve the acquisition of video images and subsequent processing of large amounts of data. We have been involved in developing an electrical method that readily detects changes in cell-substratum interactions in tissue culture and hence cell motility. The electric cell-substrate impedance sensor (ECIS) is a device that monitors the impedance of a small gold electrode used as a substratum for cells in culture. As cells attach and spread on the sensing electrode, they restrict the current flow and hence cause the increase of electrical impedance. Furthermore, cell motion may reveal itself as a fluctuation in the measured impedance, which is always resulted from living cells and continues even when the cells grow into a confluent layer. The impedance fluctuations are mainly due to a change in the size of the cell-substrate space as cells persistently rearrange their cell-substrate adhesion sites. The magnitude of this sort of vertical motion detected by ECIS is of the order of nanometers and referred to as micromotion. Fluctuations in impedance measured with the ECIS have been experimentally related to cell motility [4-8]. Here we applied ECIS to monitor the effect of TGF-β1 on cell micromotion of breast adenocarcinoma cells, MDA-MB-231. We also tested the feasibility of utilizing the ECIS wound healing assay to obtain data that is correlated with the conventional measurements and can be used in quantitating metastatic abilities of cancer cells [9]. Because the measurement is relatively simple, quantitative in nature, and highly sensitive, it should have great potential for a general research tool.

II. MATERIALS AND METHODS

A. Cell Culture

Human breast cancer cells, MDA-MB 231, were obtained from the Bioresource Collection and Research Center (BCRC; Taiwan). These cells were cultured at 37°C humidified incubator with 5% CO_2 in Dulbecco's Modified Eagle's Medium (DMEM) supplemented with 10% fetal bovine serum (FBS), 100 U/ml penicillin, 100 μg/ml streptomycin and 250 ng/ml amphotericin B. Cells were subculture when they were 80% confluent, and the medium was changed every 72 hours thereafter.

B. Experimental Approach

Electrode arrays, relay bank, lock-in amplifier and software for the ECIS measurement and data analysis were obtained from Applied BioPhysics (Troy, NY). Each 8W1E electrode array consisted of eight wells which was 1 cm in height and 0.8 cm^2 in bottom area; each well contained a 250 μm diameter gold electrode (area ~ 5×10^{-4} cm^2) and a much larger gold counter electrode. The large electrode and one of the small electrodes were connected via the relay bank to a phase-sensitive lock-in amplifier. A 1 volt AC signal at 4 kHz was applied to the sample through a 1 MΩ resistor to maintain a constant current of 1 microampere through the sample (Fig. 1). For impedance measurement of the MDA-MB-231 cell layers upon addition of TGF-β1,

I. Lackovic (ed.), *1st Global Conference on Biomedical Engineering & 9th Asian-Pacific Conference on Medical and Biological Engineering*,
IFMBE Proceedings 47, DOI: 10.1007/978-3-319-12262-5_52

cells were allowed to attach and spread at 10^5 cells/cm^2 density for at least 24 hrs before impedance was measured. After 24 hours in culture, the confluency and viability of the cell monolayer was confirmed by light microscopy and electrically by the resistance values.

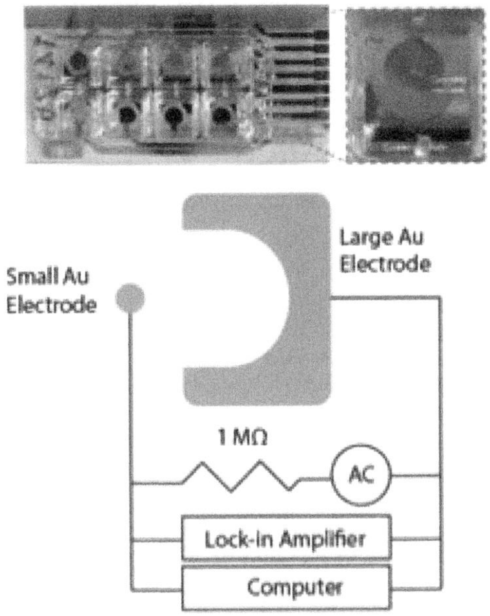

Fig. 1 A schematic of the ECIS setup.

Before stimulation with TGF-β1, MDA-MB-231 cells were gently rinsed twice with serum-free DMEM and then serum-starved with DMEM supplemented with 1% FBS. After starvation for 6 hours, cells in the ECIS electrode-containing wells were treated with 10 ng/ml of TGF-β1 and measured immediately. For detection of cell micromotion, impedance data of each well were taken every 2 sec and up to four individual wells were followed successively for 20 hrs. The time series data were normalized and numerically analyzed by calculating variance (the square of the standard deviation), power slope, and Hurst coefficient as we previously described [8]. For measuring wound healing time course, the wounding parameters were set as 20 sec of wound time, 2000 microamperes of wound current, and 40 kHz of AC frequency. The impedance data was recorded for 30 minutes as baseline prior to wounding the cells on the small sensing electrodes, and continuously monitored for 24 hours after 20-sec electrical wounding [9].

III. RESULTS AND DISCUSSION

Because of the selection of 4 kHz AC signal for the micromotion measurement, the fluctuations in the resistance were much larger than those in the capacitive reactance. Thus, we focused on the resistance time course for data analysis. Fig. 2 shows typical 20-hr resistance time series data measured from MDA-MB-231 cell-covered electrodes in response to the exposure of TGF-β1 or DMEM only (n = 16). Although fluctuations were observed on each curve, an initial rise in resistance (~30%) was observed almost immediately following TGF-β1 addition. This was followed by a slow decline and stabilized at the similar level of the initial resistance value. As for the control group, a gradual decrease in resistance without any evident rise was generally observed (n = 16).

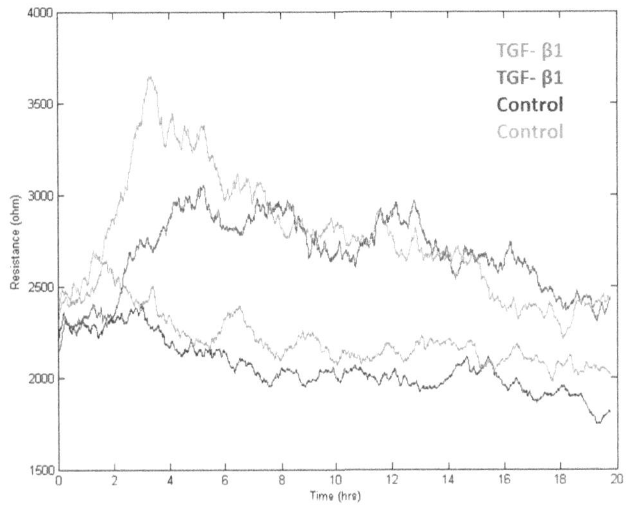

Fig. 2 Resistance time series data of MDA-MB-231 cell-covered electrodes upon addition of TGF-β1 or DMEM only as controls.

In order to quantitate the fluctuations in resistance series, the normalized variance method [4] was used to distinguish the difference between the TGF-β1 treated cells and controls. Since we measured the impedance data of each well every 2 sec for 20 hrs, 4500 points had been obtained every 2.5 hrs, and we analyzed the first 4096 points of them. We then split every 4096 point data set into 256 subsets of 16 points each. The variance was calculated and averaged for all sets. The calculated value was then divided by the square of the average resistance of the 4096 point data set to get the normalized variance. Fig. 3 shows the profile of micromotion changes over 20 hrs for TGF-β1 treated cells and controls. The increased variance values of the resistance fluctuations for the TGF-β1 treated cells, as compared with controls, indicated increased cell micromotion. Note that resistance time series and normalized variance at different time periods had similar profiles (Figs. 2 and 3) though they implied different cell behaviors. These data suggest that TGF-β1 stimulation on MDA-MB-231 cells is a time-dependent process; it caused the change of cell morphology (higher resistance) and the increase of cell micromotion (higher variance of resistance time series) for 10 hours (5 to 15 hr).

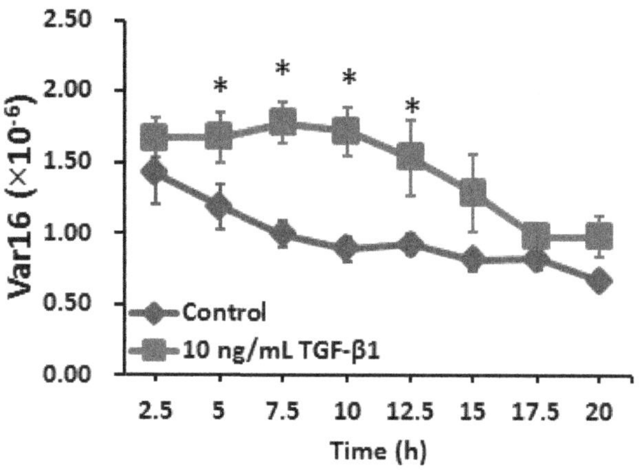

Fig. 3 Variance analysis of the resistance time series implying increased micromotion for TGF-β1 treated cells as compared with controls. Each point represents an average variance value over a 2.5-hr interval (n =16, *$p < 0.05$).

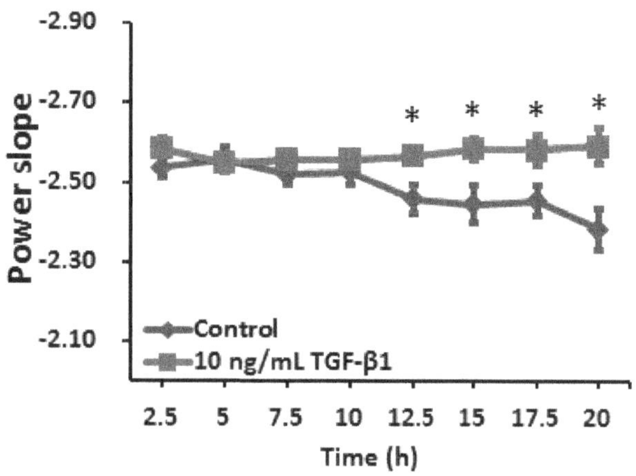

Fig. 4 Power slope analysis of the resistance time series implying unreduced long-term correlation for TGF-β1 treated cells as compared with controls. Each point represents an average variance value over a 2.5-hr interval (n =16, *$p < 0.05$).

We also characterized the long-term correlations in the resistance time series by calculating power slope (Fig. 4) and Hurst exponent (Fig. 5). A log–log plot of spectral density against frequency f indicates an intensity varying as $f^{-\beta}$. Brownian noise displays an f^{-2} power law and a nonzero β shows signs of long-term correlations. The power spectrum for the TGF-β1 treated MDA-MB-231 cells varied as $f^{-2.6}$ (β value ~ 2.6) while the control cells displayed a gradually drop of the β value, from 2.5 to 2.4. The higher β value implies a stronger temporal correlation in the MDA-MB-231 cells' activities affected by TGF-β1. Both power slope and Hurst exponent measures show that the long-term correlation of control cells decreases along with the time while the TGF-β1 treated cells maintain similar long-term correlation.

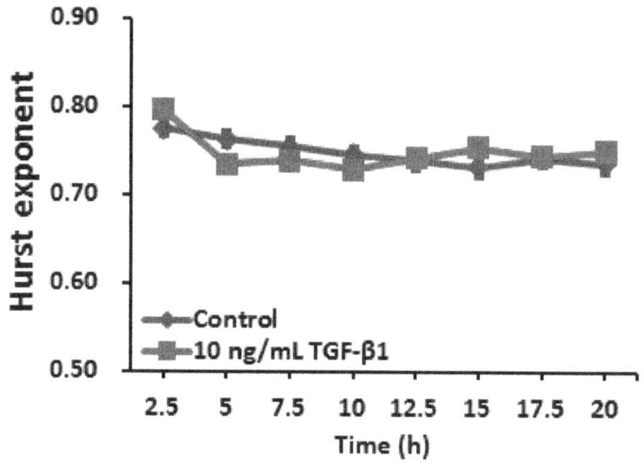

Fig. 5 Hurst exponent analysis of the resistance time series implying unreduced long-term correlation for TGF-β1 treated cells as compared with controls (n =16).

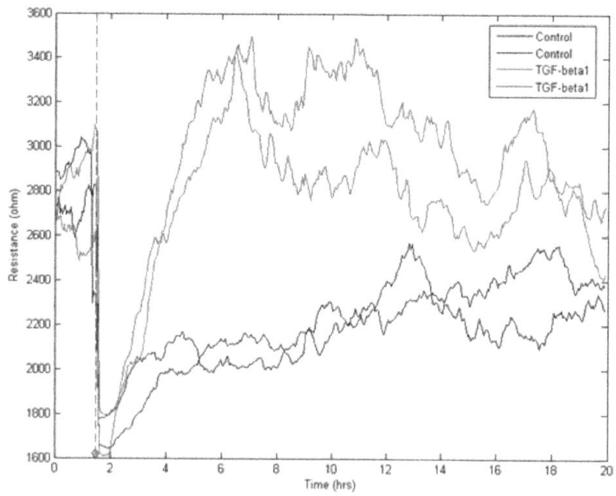

Fig. 6 ECIS wound healing data for TGF-β1 treated MDA-MB-231 cells and controls.

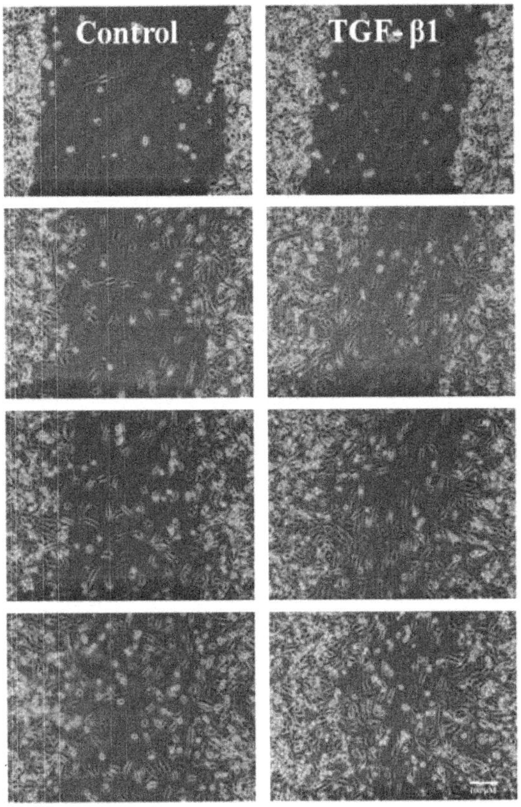

Fig. 7 Scratch wound healing assay of MDA-MB 231 cell layers in the absence or presence of TGF-β1 for different periods of time.

To investigate the wound healing migration of MDA-MB 231 cells in response to TGF-β1 treatment, cells cultured on the ECIS electrodes were applied with elevated field pulse at 40 kHz to cause cell death and the resistance alterations were continuously monitored by ECIS at 4 kHz (Fig. 6). The resistance values of cell-covered electrodes after onset of the wound immediately dropped to about 1700 Ω which is the resistance of a cell-free electrode. The resistance of TGF-β treated cells recovered within 4 hrs while control cells took more than 20 hrs for recovery.

To compare with ECIS wound healing measurement, the traditional scratch wound healing assay was carried out in our study. MDA-MB 231 cells were cultured in the 6-cm culture dishes until forming a confluent cell layer prior to scratch wound. Six hours after serum starvation, TGF-β1 was added into the medium. A pipet tip was used to make the wounding gap on the cell layer. By using inverted light microscope with 100x magnification, images of MDA-MB 231 (Fig. 7) were taken at the indicated time points (0, 4, 8, and 12 hours after 10 ng/ml of TGF-β1 was added).

In summary, these data suggest that the invasive breast carcinoma cells, MDA-MB-231, promotes cell migration and micromotion in response to TGF-β1 stimulation. These responses are time-dependent processes and may facilitate scattering behavior and play an important role in metastasis.

ACKNOWLEDGMENT

This work was supported by the Ministry of Science and Technology, Taiwan. (Grant number: NSC 102-2628-B-010-010-MY3).

CONFLICT OF INTEREST

The authors declare that they have no conflict of interest.

REFERENCES

1. Condeelis J, Segall J (2003) Intravital imaging of cell movement in tumours. Nat Rev Cancer 3:921-930.
2. Gupta G, Massague J (2006) Cancer metastasis: building a framework. Cell 127:679-695.
3. Felding-Habermann B (2001) Integrin activation controls metastasis in human breast cancer. PNAS 98:1853-1858.
4. Lo C, Keese C, Giaever I (1993) Monitoring motion of confluent cells in tissue culture. Exp. Cell Res. 204:102-109.
5. Lo C, Keese C, Giaever I (1994) pH changes in pulsed CO_2 incubator cause periodic changes in cell morphology. Exp. Cell Res. 213:391-397.
6. Giaver I, Keese C (1993) A morphological biosensor for mammalian cells. Nature 366:591-592.
7. Giaever I, Keese C (1991) Micromotion of mammalian cells measured electrically. PNAS 88:7896-7900.
8. Opp D, Wafula B, Lim J. et al. (2009) Use of electric cell-substrate impedance sensing to assess in vitro cytotoxicity. Biosens Bioelectron. 24:2625-2629..
9. Keese C, Wegener J, Walker S et al. (2004) Electrical wound-healing assay for cells in vitro. PNAS 101:1554-1559.

Author: Cheng I Lai, Wei-Tse Chen
Institute: Taipei Municipal Jianguo High School
Street: Nan Hai Road
City: Taipei
Country: Taiwan
Email: jefflai108@gmail.com, chenweitse123@gmail.com

Author: Yi-Ting Lai, Chun-Min Lo
Institute: National Yang-Ming University
Street: Linong Street
City: Taipei
Country: Taiwan
Email: g39904002@ym.edu.tw, cmlo@ym.edu.tw

Initial Design of the Capacitive Micromachined Ultrasonic Transducers (CMUT) with Helmholtz Resonance Aperture

Xue Wen Cao[1], Bo Jin[1], Yuan Yu Yu[1,2], Jiu Jiang Wang[1,2], Sio Hang Pun[2], Mang I. Vai[1,2], and Peng Un Mak[1]

[1] Department of Electrical and Computer Engineering, Faculty of Science and Technology, University of Macau, Macau, China
[2] State Key Laboratory of Analog and Mixed-Signal VLSI, University of Macau, Macau, China

Abstract— **In this paper, we have demonstrated the performance improvement of the air-borne Capacitive Micromachined Ultrasonic Transducers (CMUT) in transmit mode using the Helmholtz resonance principles. The natural frequency of the resonance cavity, and the Helmholtz resonance frequency of the aperture which is formed in the center of membrane, were matched for resonance during the design. In order to verify the theoretical concept, Finite Element Analysis (FEA) simulation was performed using COMSOL software. Through the simulation comparison with the traditional CMUT, the proposed CMUT demonstrates the feasibility to improve the output acoustic pressure and SPL of the air-borne CMUT in transmit mode by combining the mechanical resonance theory with Helmholtz resonance principle.**

Keywords— **Capacitive Micromachined Ultrasonic Transducers (CMUT), Helmholtz resonance, FEA simulation.**

I. INTRODUCTION

Ultrasound plays an important role in many industry and medical fields, such as Non-Destructive Evaluation (NDE), SONAR identification, ultrasound imaging[1]. Piezoelectric ultrasound transducers are widely used for a long time, especially in medical imaging [2]. However, limited by the properties of Piezoelectric crystal, it is hard to achieve a better performance (sensitivity, resolution, etc). The technology of CMUT has recently emerged as an alternative substitute for traditional transducers.

In comparison with the traditional PZT, CMUT is not only a simple replacement of the piezoelectric transducer in potential low cost if volume production, but also owns many advantages, especially in the integration with the electronics using the MEMS technology[3]. But the output pressure of the traditional CMUT is lower than the PZT [4]. For getting a high-quality image, a higher output acoustic pressure is usually desired.

The aim of this paper is to increase the acoustic output pressure of the air-borne CMUT in transmit mode by using the Helmholtz resonance principles. An aperture was made in the center of the top plate. So the air in the cavity can be coupled with the outside ambient medium through the aperture. When the CMUT works, it will combine the mechanical vibrating mode with the Helmholtz resonance mode together at a condition with a constant ambient pressure. So the radiation acoustic waves from both plate and the air in the aperture can be superimposed[5]. This will enhance the acoustic output pressure. Finite Element Analysis (FEA) was used to verify this theoretical concept and to show the possibility of the higher acoustic output pressure.

II. PRINCIPLE OF CMUT WITH HELMHOLTZ RESONANCE APERTURE

A. Mechanical Vibrating Resonance Mode

The membrane of basic CMUT, shown in Figure 1 a), is actuated by a driven voltage and generates the ultrasound waves in the air. It is worthy of note that mechanical vibration caused by the stimulation mostly occurs at the 1st resonance frequency of the CMUT. The top plate of CMUT in this work was designed to be in the clamped boundary condition at the edge[6]. The natural frequency of the plate is defined as the following equation[7]:

$$f_c = 0.47\sqrt{\frac{Y_0}{\rho(1-\gamma^2)}}\frac{t}{a^2} \qquad (1)$$

where t is membrane thickness, a is membrane radius, ρ is the density of membrane, Y_0 and γ are the Young's modulus and Poisson's Ratio of membrane material, respectively.

From the equation we know that the resonance frequency of CMUT depends on both the material properties and the geometry of membrane.

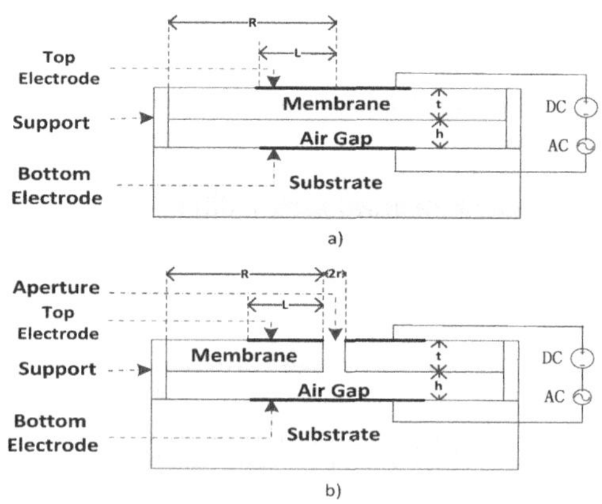

Fig. 1 Schematic structure of a CMUT cell a) basic CMUT b) CMUT with an aperture

I. Lackovic (ed.), *1st Global Conference on Biomedical Engineering & 9th Asian-Pacific Conference on Medical and Biological Engineering*, IFMBE Proceedings 47, DOI: 10.1007/978-3-319-12262-5_53

B. Helmholtz Resonance Mode

Helmholtz resonance is a phenomenon that air in the neck (the aperture), as shown in Figure 1 b), oscillates as a mass- spring system at a resonance frequency. Because of the compressing or expanding air in the cavity, the air in the open aperture will oscillate at one certain frequency which is defined as the Helmholtz resonance frequency, f_h. The formula of this frequency f_h is given as follows:

$$f_h = \frac{c}{2\pi}\sqrt{\frac{S}{V(l+\delta)}} \tag{2}$$

where c is velocity of sound; S is surface area of aperture; V is the volume of cavity; l is the length of aperture; δ is the end-correction factor which depends on the dimension of the aperture [8]:

$$\delta = 0.96\sqrt{S} \tag{3}$$

The Helmholtz resonance frequency depends on the dimension of the system, so the size of aperture should be designed carefully.

Assuming the working frequency of the system is the natural resonance frequency, f_c, the radiation acoustic wave generated by the membrane is in phase with that from the acoustic aperture when the Helmholtz resonance frequency f_h is approximate equal to the f_c. In this situation, the two radiation ultrasound wave will be enhanced. So the value of f_h should be equal to the natural frequency f_c in order to couple the two resonance modes as the Figure 2 shown:

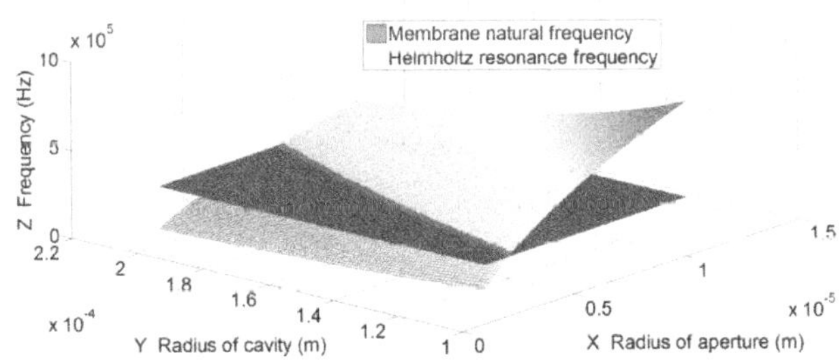

Fig. 2 Interception of Helmholtz frequency for the cavity as a function of radius of aperture and membrane

The radius and thickness of membrane were set to be 150um and 2um, respectively; the radius of acoustic aperture was selected from Figure 2 when the cavity radius was 150um. Above all, the physical dimensions of the CMUT cell with aperture are given as follows in Table 1:

Table 1 Dimensions of CMUT cell

Parameter	***Value***
Membrane radius (R) [um]	150
Electrode radius (L) [um]	75
Cavity radius (H) [um]	150
Aperture radius (r) [um]	4
Cavity height (h) [um]	2
Thickness of membrane (t) [um]	2
Natural frequency (f_c) [MHz]	0.34

III. FEA SIMULATION METHODOLOGY

FEA is a fast way to simulate the characteristics of the CMUT, Comsol Multiphysics (Comsol Inc., Burlington, MA, USA) is chosen in our simulation and analysis because it contains the coupling of multiple physics. With circular structured membrane, cavity and aperture in the center, and spherical air domain, a 2D-axisymmetrical model was built (shown in Figure 3).

CMUT cell was assigned using Electromechanical (emi) physics and its edges were set with the Fixed Constraint nodes. For purpose of calculating the acoustic pressure in the surrounding medium, the air domain of a sphere shape was built around the cell using the Pressure Acoustic, Frequency Domain (acpr) physics. Spherical Wave Radiation [9] was chosen around outside of the surrounding medium to eliminate the acoustic wave reflections. The air mass was modeled by using acpr physics in the aperture, the same with air, to simulate the radiation from the aperture. In the Mesh step, the minimum element size of the Mesh size should be smaller than 10% of the wavelength. The material of the CMUT was chosen the single-crystal silicon and the material parameters in COMSOL setting were listed in Table 2:

Table 2 Material properties used in COMSOL

Parameter	***Value***
Young's modulus [GPa]	150
Poisson Ratio	0.17
Density [kg/m^3]	2330
Dielectric constant	11

Due to the viscosity of the fluid (air), squeeze-film gas damping should be considered in many MEMS transducers, especially the devices with a narrow gap and an aperture. So after mesh, Thin-Film Damping was added on the bottom of the membrane.

To couple the two physics solvers, the normal acceleration was applied on the upper edge of the membrane. Then the acceleration makes the membrane generate acoustic pressure. And a boundary load needs to be set on the membrane due to the acoustic wave generating [10].

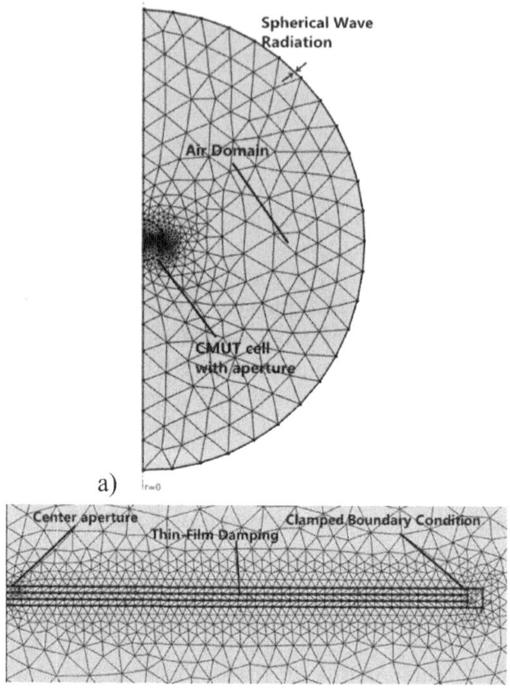

Fig. 3 a) 2D axisymmetric model of CMUT cell and medium. b) Details of the CMUT cell with an aperture

IV. RESULT

A. Plate Displacement

In the simulation, the CMUT cell was biased at 54.3V DC voltage and driven by 1V amplitude harmonic perturbation. Figure 4 shows the displacement comparison between traditional CMUT cell and the one with an aperture at the center of plate in simulation. The peak value of displacement occurs at the working frequency, 0.32MHz, which has a frequency shift from the theory value (0.34MHz) due to the spring- softening effect[11]:

$$k_{soft} = k - \frac{\varepsilon S V_{DC}^2}{d_0^3} \tag{4}$$

where k is the spring constant, ε is electric permittivity, S is area of membrane, d_0 is gap height.

Thus, a frequency drop has been seen as V_{DC} is increased. From the result it is observed that the Helmholtz resonance frequency couples well with the natural frequency of plate in one working frequency, the displacement combined the two frequencies is 9.2% higher than the traditional surface one. The difference between two structures is due to the effect of air-cushion in the CMUT cavity. With the aperture, the air-cushion effect will weaken, and the membrane can get a larger displacement.

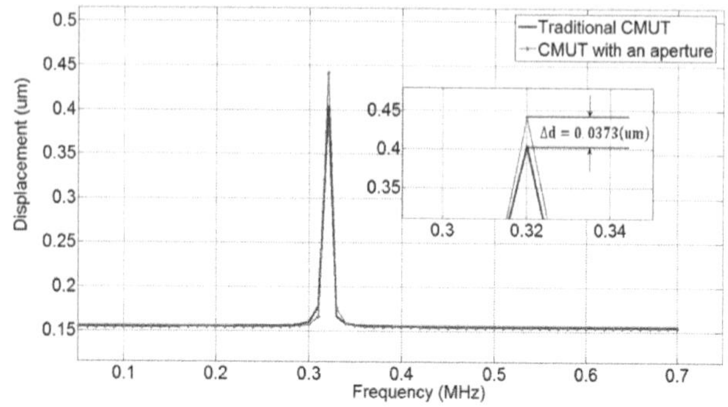

Fig. 4 The displacement of two kinds of CMUT cell as a function of frequency in response to a 54.3V (70% collapse voltage) and 1V amplitude harmonic perturbation voltage.

B. Acoustic Output Pressure

A circular CMUT cell can be treated roughly as a circular piston source in the infinite baffle in ultrasound radiation analysis. Due to the uniform acoustic pressure, radiation superposition should be observed in the far-field region which beyond the last local maximum energy at z_m, where $z_m = \frac{8a^2}{\lambda}$ for the engineering purposes[12], a is the radius of source, λ is the wavelength at resonance frequency. In this region, the pressure amplitude drops monotonously at a rate inversely proportional to the distance from the sound source.

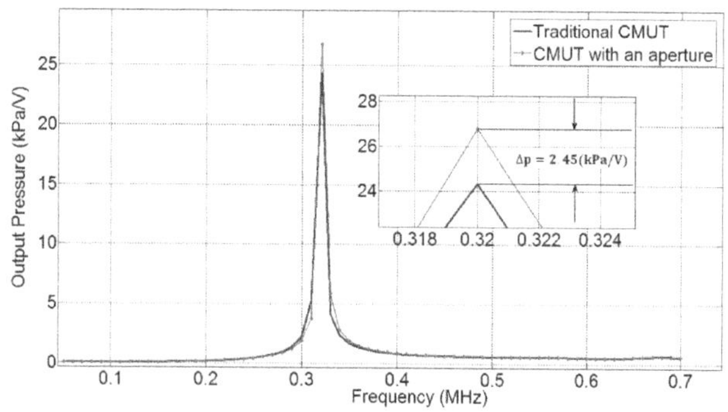

Fig. 5 Far-field acoustic pressure of basic CMUT and the CMUT with aperture as a function of frequency

The acoustic output pressure comparison of the CMUT with aperture and the traditional CMUT is shown in Figure 5. With the calculation of the size of the aperture and the cell cavity, the radiation waves from both the aperture and the plate are superimposed and enhanced when the CMUT combines with the Helmholtz resonator. The acoustic output pressure is calculated at the point z_m from center of membrane under this condition. The increased acoustic pressure is about 2.45 kPa/V, 10.1% higher than that of the traditional one.

C. Sound Pressure Level (SPL)

Figure 6 shows the Sound Pressure Level (SPL) of the proposed CMUT cell with aperture and the traditional one. The SPL values of both cells were evaluated at z_m from center of each membrane in order to reduce the near-field effects. The CMUT cell with aperture has a peak SPL value of 117.4 dB, 0.8dB higher than the traditional one.

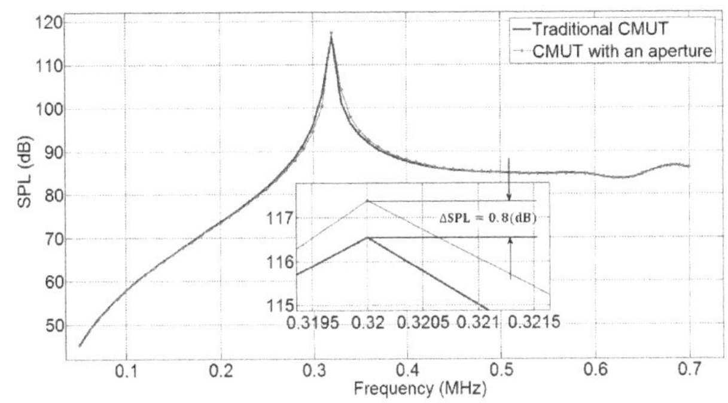

Fig. 6 SPL of two kinds of CMUT cell as a function of frequency

V. CONCLUSIONS

An improved proposal of CMUT-cell based on Helmholtz resonance has been presented in this work. FEA simulation using COMSOL has been performed to check the performance of CMUTs. Based on this design, the superposition of the radiation from the Helmholtz resonance aperture and the radiation from the membrane enhance the acoustic pressure in the far-field region. Through the comparison between the CMUT cell with an aperture and the traditional one, it can be found that the acoustic output pressure, displacement of membrane and the sound pressure level of transducer are all improved by using the technique of Helmholtz resonance by 9.2%, 10.1%, and 0.8dB, respectively. The results indicate that it is feasible to improve the performance of the air-borne CMUT in transmit mode using this method.

CONFLICT OF INTERESTS

The authors declare that there is no conflict of interests regarding the publication of this paper.

ACKNOWLEDGMENT

This work was supported by The Science and Technology Development Fund of Macau (FDCT) under Grants 024/2009/A1, 087/2012/A3, & 047/2013/A2; The Research Committee of the University of Macau under Grants RG072/09-1OS/MPS/FST, MYRG076(Y1-L2)-FST12-MPU, MYRG079(Y1-L2)-FST12-VMI, MYRG103(Y1-L3)-FST13-VMI , MRG014/MPU/2014 /FST, & MYRG2014-00010-AMSV.

REFERENCES

1. Muhammed Sabri Salim, M.F. Abd Malek, R.B.W. Heng, K.M. Juni, Naseer Sabri 'Capacitive Micromachined Ultrasonic Transducers: Technology and Application', Journal of Medical Ultrasound (2012) 20, pp 8-31
2. Alessandro Caronti, G. Caliano, R, Carotenuto, A. Savoia, M. Pappalardo, E. Cianci, V. Foglietti, 'Capacitive micromachined ultrasonic transducer(CMUT) arrays for medical imaging', Microelectronics Journal 37 (2006) pp.770-777
3. Omer Oralkan, A. Sanh Ergun, Jeremy A. Johnson, Mustafa Karaman, Utkan Demirci, Kambiz Kaviani, Thomas H. Lee, Butrus T. Khuri-Yakub, 'Capacitive Micromachined Ultrasonic Transducers: Next-Generation Arrays for Acoustic Imaging?' ,IEEE Transaction on Ultrasonics, Ferroelectrics, and Frequency Control, Vol. 49, NO. 11, November 2002, pp.1596-1608
4. D. M. Mills and L. S. Smith, "Real-time in-vivo imaging with capacitive micromachined ultrasound transducer (cMUT) linear arrays," in Proc. IEEE Ultrasonics Symp., 2003, pp. 568–571
5. A. Octavio Manzanares, F. Montero De Espinosa Freijo, 'Ultrasonic transducers with resonant cavities as emitters for air-borne applications' Bol. Soc.Esp. Ceram.V. 48,4, (2009),pp.205-209
6. Dale Ensminger, Foster B. Stulen, Ultrasonics: Data, Equations and Their Practical Uses, CRC Press (December 17, 2008), pp. 97-98
7. Kwan Kyu Park, Hyunjoo Lee, Mario Kupnik, Omer Oralkan, Jean-Pierre Ramseyer, Han Peter Lang, Martin Hegner, Christoph Gerber, Butrus T. Khuri-Yakub,'Capacitive micromachined ultrasonic transducer (CMUT) as a chemical sensor for DMMP detection', Sensors and Actuators B: Chemical, Volume 160, Issue 1, 15 December 2011, pp. 1120 1127
8. U.Ingard, On the theory and design of acoustic resonator, The Journal of the Acoustical Society of America 25(1953) 1037-1061
9. COMSOL Multiphysics 4.3a User Guide—The Pressure Acoustic, Frequency Domain Interface, Plane, Spherical, and Cylindrical radiation Boundary Conditions, pp. 681-688
10. Wei You, Edmond Cretu, Robert Rohling, 'Analytical Modeling of CMUTs in Coupled Eletro-Mechano-Acoustic Domains Using Plate Vibration Theory', IEEE Sensors Journal, Vol.11, NO. 9, September 2011, pp.2159-2168
11. Igal Ladabaum I, Jin X, Soh HT, Atalar A, and Khuri-Yakub BT, "Surface Micromachined Capacitive Ultrasonic Transducers," *IEEE Transactions on Ultrasonics, Ferroelectrics and Frequency Control*, vol. 45, May 1998, pp. 678-690
12. COMSOL Multiphysics 4.3a, COMSOL Documentation-Acoustic Module-Modeling with the Acoustic Module-Fundamentals of Acoustic Modeling-Evaluating the Acoustic Field in the Far-Field Region

Address of the corresponding author:
Author: XueWen Cao
Institute: Faculty of Science and Technology, University of Macau
Street: Avenida da Universidade, Taipa, Macau, China
City: Macau
Country: China
Email: ascxw2008@gmail.com

A Prototype System for Using Eye Control on a New Type of Hospital Beds

Min-Ru Tsai and Chia-Yen Yang

Department of Biomedical Engineering, Ming Chuan University, Taoyuan, Taiwan

Abstract— **Normally, bedridden patients need nurses to help moving their body or changing lying positions. However, to patients, changing lying positions by others may cause two problems: One is the timing and frequency of movement may not be adequate and the other is the cozy position of the movement may not be perfect for patients. Therefore, in this study, we tried to build up a handy system which can help bedridden patients to control hospital beds in several lying positions that match their preferences closely by only moving their eyes. In the results, we have already built up an eye-controlled equipment which allowed user to control hospital beds by themselves. This equipment had advantages of light and handy. Besides, we also constructed a model of our home-made hospital bed with six specific bed boards. This new type may help users to change their lying positions in left right tilt. Although there still have some tests to be conducted, the system of using eye control on our new type of hospital bed is possible. In the future, we expect that this handy system can help bedridden patients to appropriately control hospital beds in several lying positions that match their preferences closely by only moving their eyes.**

Keywords— **Eye control, Hospital bed, Left right tilt, Simulink, Visible light image of pupil.**

I. INTRODUCTION

As the International NPUAP-EPUAP Pressure Ulcer Definition: A pressure ulcer is localized injury to the skin or underlying tissue usually over a bony prominence, as a result of pressure, or pressure in combination with shear [1]. Normally, bedridden patients need nurses to help moving their body or changing lying positions which could be a big work load and occupational injury on nurses [2]. To solve that problem, some advanced hospital beds have been designed to help nurses taking care of patients, who have pressure ulcers, with automatic control to move their bodies [3-5]. However, to patients, changing lying positions by others may cause two problems. One is the timing and frequency of movement may not be adequate and the other is the cozy position of the movement may not be perfect for patients. In that case, a better way to take care the bedridden patients which can help them to change their positions as what they want and whenever they want as possible should be important for clinical applications.

Now day, most of the modern hospital beds are control by electric button switches or crank handles. However, some needed users of those hospital beds may be the patients who are paralytic (and hence cannot feel potentially harmful seating pressure-points) or are unable to move within the hospital by themselves. It means that those bedridden patients cannot move their hand to control switches or handles for adjustment of beds. Fortunately, although they are unable to move their body appropriately, many of them can still move their eye. Hence, eye control is an alternative and complementary method to using own hands for those kind of patients. By using a head-mounted eye tracking equipment, patients only need to wear on a camera non-invasively to capture images of eyes and then sent the command to the computer to control the back-end device.

Therefore, in this study, we tried to build up a handy system which can help bedridden patients to control hospital beds in several lying positions that match their preferences closely by only moving their eyes. This system included two parts: One was a new type of hospital bed with six specific bed boards which had functions to change users' lying positions in left right tilt. The other one was an eye-controlled equipment which allowed user to control our hospital bed by themselves.

Generally, there are three basic types of eye trackers. First is eye-attached tracking which uses a special contact lens attached to an eye and measures the movement. Second is optical tracking which uses a video camera to get the light reflected from an eye and analyzes the information. The last one is electric potential measurement which places electrodes around an eye and measures the electric potentials [6]. In nowadays, optical methods (particularly those based on camera recording) are widely used for eye tracking studies of being non-invasive and inexpensive which is adopted in our study. Notably, in the visible light photography, the color of the pupil and that of the iris are really similar so it is difficult to distinguish between pupil and iris. But in the infrared photography, the color of pupil is dark black and the color of iris is light gray, which can be distinguished very easily. Because of these characteristics, using infrared images to find the pupil center should be easier and also more accurate for determining eye movements [7].

II. MATERIAL AND METHODS

Figure 1 shows the control procedures for our homemade bed by using eye movements. To move or to stop depended

I. Lackovic (ed.), *1st Global Conference on Biomedical Engineering & 9th Asian-Pacific Conference on Medical and Biological Engineering*,
IFMBE Proceedings 47, DOI: 10.1007/978-3-319-12262-5_54

on a switch which control by winks. If user winked three times in 3 seconds, condition would be changed. Details were described as followings.

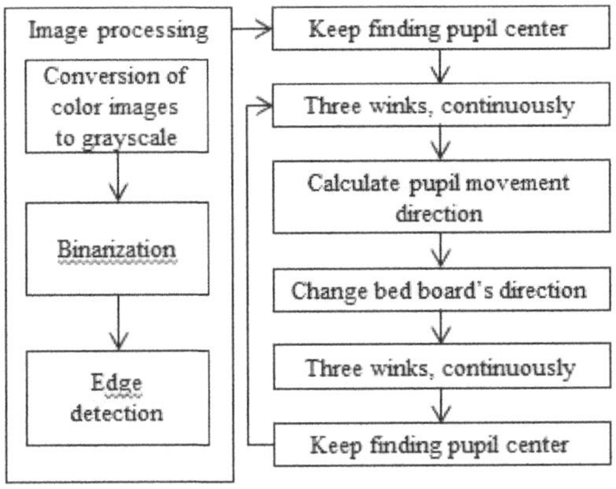

Fig. 1 Flow chart of the control procedures for our homemade bed by using eye movements.

A. Head-mounted Image Capture Equipment

In order to get a clear infrared image of pupils in a cheaper and more convenient way, using web camera is a possible choose in that situation. Although the camera is for visible light image, it can get an infrared image by replacing infrared cut filter (ICF) with infrared (IR) filter. Hence, the use of webcam in this study was USB2.0 CAM-02 with a sampling rate of 30 Hz and the IR filter was 25mm R760.

The support frame has to be lightweight and easy to wear on but hard enough to carry a camera. So we used a glasses frame and added two bars at the right side to fix the web camera. The mounted way, as shown in Figure 2, allowed the camera lens to focus on the pupil.

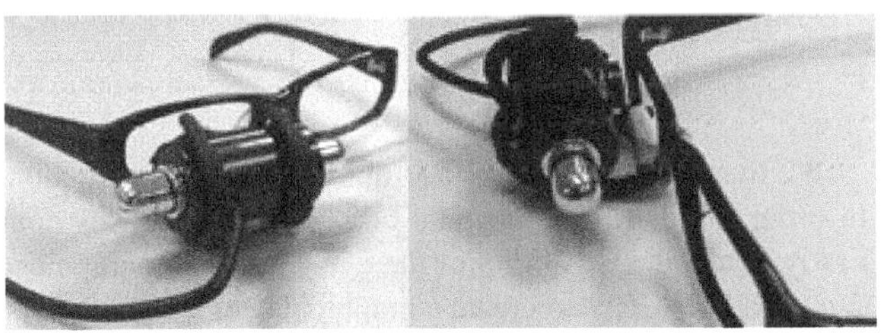

Fig. 2 The head-mounted equipment.

B. Image Processing

MATLAB is a high-level language and interactive environment for numerical computation, visualization, and programming. By using Simulink, an extension of MATLAB, it could easily connect software and hardware to construct an interactive system [8].

The captured consecutive images were processed in the following steps: conversion of color images to grayscale, binarization and edge detection.

(1) Conversion of color images to grayscale: Because the output image was in YUV color space which included too many information that we may not need (i.e., we only want to know which part is the darkest in the image), converting color images to grayscale could remove those data which is not important and make further analysis more efficient and simple (Figure 3).

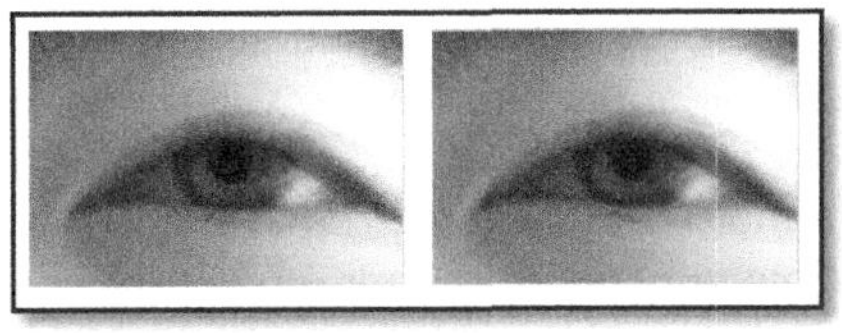

Fig. 3 An infrared image (left) and its grayscale image (right).

(2) Binarization: Image binarization is typically treated as simply a segmentation operation on a grayscale image. A binary image is a digital image that has only two possible colors, black and white. The separation process of pixel values into two groups (i.e. 0 and 1) needs a threshold. The threshold in this study was the grayscale of the first peak in the histogram of the grayscale image, as shown in Figure 4. We did not use zero as threshold although the pupil should be the darkest area in the image, because of some noises, especially the light refraction from corneal. By this way, it could make sure that the black color in the binary image was a pupil or part of pupil while the white one was the other parts of eyes or face. After that, it would be easier to find out the pupil center.

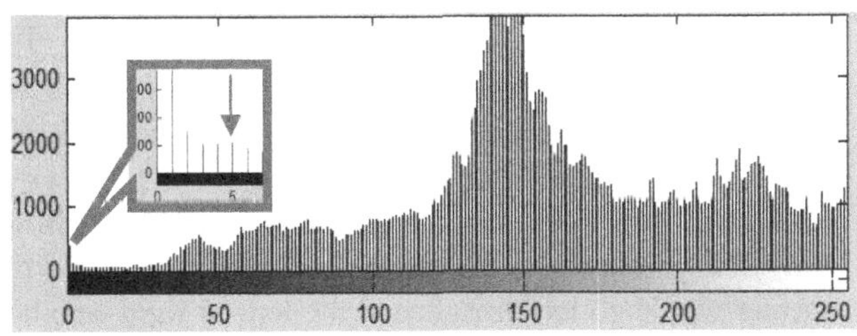

Fig. 4 The histogram of the grayscale image (1st peak is at 5).

(3) Edge detection: One of the easiest ways to find out the edge of pupil is to use Sobel operator in the binary image. However, the edge should be like a circle or a part of circle but usually not in practice. Because of this problem, we used ellipse fitting to fix it to the ellipse most similar to the pupil [9]. After that, the pupil center could be found as shown in Figure 5.

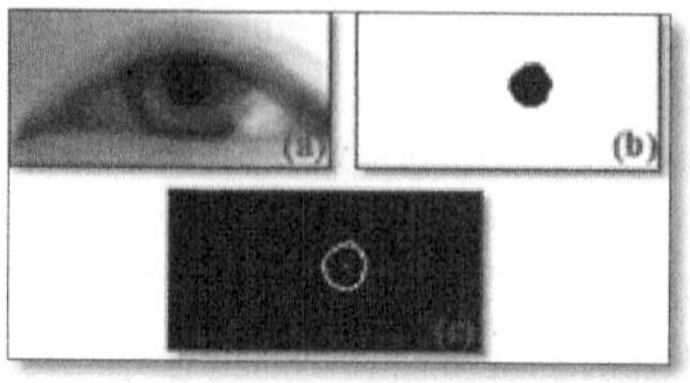

Fig. 5 A grayscale image (a)and its binary image (b) with edge and pupil center (c) found in it. The white points indicate the edge and the red point indicate the center of the pupil after calculation.

After getting the coordinate of pupil centres, we classified them into six different instructions, as shown in Figure 6. The locations in the red, orange, yellow, green, blue and purple areas mean “hold on”, “sit up”, “lie down”, “turn right”, “turn left” and “winks”, respectively. Because in the eye-closed condition (as a part of wink motion), ellipse fitting was done only for lower eyelid, the pupil center would be located outside the eye.

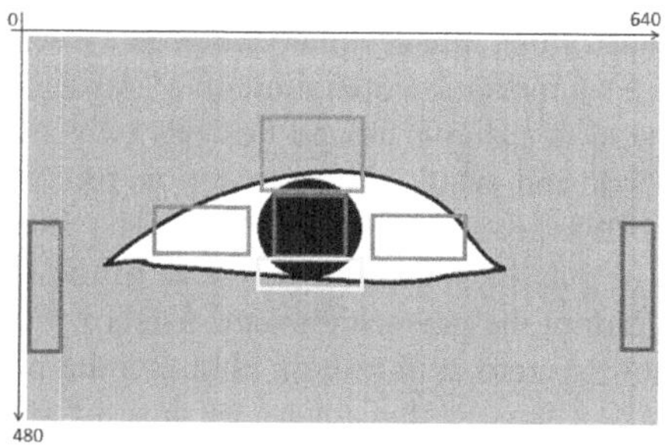

Fig. 6 The classification clusters of different pupil centers.

C. *Production of the Homemade Hospital Bed*

A digital model was built firstly by using AutoCAD. This 3D hospital bed model was then put into SHOWCASE to set up materials and to simulate its boards turning (If the user looked up, the pupil center would go up and the head board would rise up and make the user in a sit position. If the user looked down, the pupil center would go down and the head board would lie down and make the user in a lie position. Similarly, if the user looked left or right, the pupil center would go left or right and the left- or right-side board would rise up and make the user in a lateral recumbent position. To prevent the user from falling down, action of turning left or right could not be done in the sitting position. Finally, if the preview conform our design, an actual hospital bed would be built in a size with only one tenth to the real one which would be 21cm (length) *9cm (width)*10cm (height). After that, a real hospital bed should be built in the further future.

III. Results

A. *Detection of Pupil Center*

The head-mounted equipment could successfully get the pupil centers as eyes looking up, looking down, looking left, looking right and looking front (Figure 7) in the table 1.

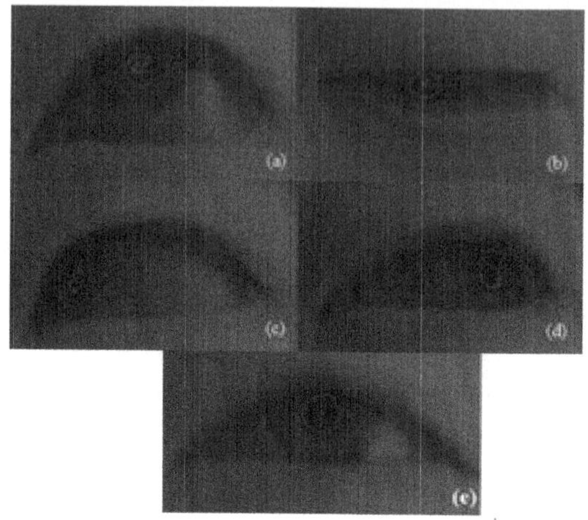

Fig. 7 Detections of pupil centers as (a) looking up, (b) looking down, (c) looking left, (d) looking right and (e)looking front.

Table 1. Pupil center coordinates in pixel

	X	Y
Look front	219	319
Look up	99	234
Look down	451	321
Look left	213	550
Look right	242	180

We then calculated these coordinates into the instructions. In order to control the hospital bed, a simulation was done firstly to test the feasibility of the eye-controlled equipment. We used LabVIEW to create a graphical user interface (GUI) which has four lights on it (Figure 8) and tried to light the lights by eye movements. A user worn on the camera and moved his eye. Images were captured to one computer with analysis program. After calculating the orientation of eye movements, an instruction message was sent to another computer via DAQ card and lighted the light corresponding to the instruction finally.

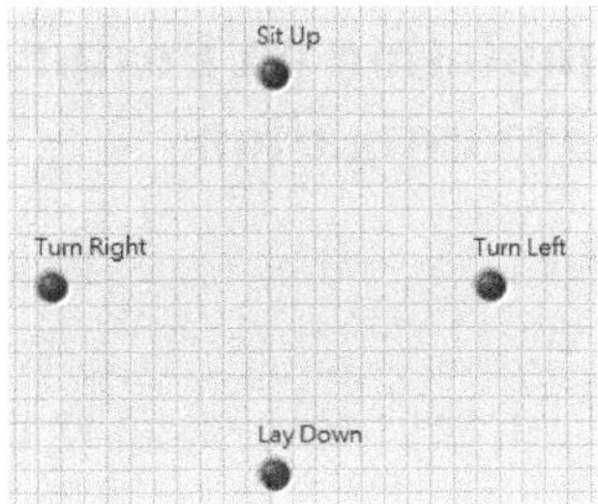

Fig. 8 The GUI for a simulation test of the eye-controlled equipment.

Notably, no matter in the light room or in the dark (but not all black) room, the pupil centres could be found robustly. However, since we did not want to irradiate user's eye by other light source, a weak light environment may still be necessary in order to get a clear enough image.

B. Production of the Homemade Hospital Bed

Our preliminary model is shown in Figure 9. A perfect preview on SHOWCASE could be implemented for actual one. However, it may be hard to make the bed in such small size. Hence, some problems were needed to be solved.

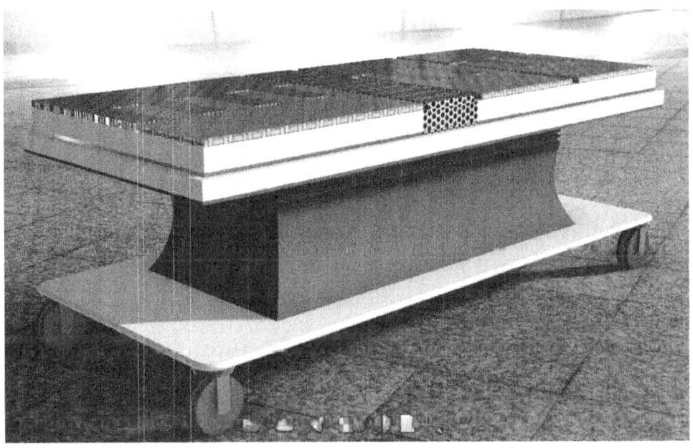

Fig. 9 Model of the homemade hospital bed

IV. CONCLUSION

In this study, we have already built up an eye-controlled equipment which allowed user to control hospital beds by themselves. This equipment had advantages of light and handy. Besides, we also constructed a model of our homemade hospital bed. This new type may help users to change their lying positions in left right tilt. Although there still have some tests to be conducted, the system of using eye control on our new type of hospital bed is possible. In the future, we expect that this handy system can help bedridden patients to appropriately control hospital beds in several lying positions that match their preferences closely by only moving their eyes.

ACKNOWLEDGMENT

This study was supported in part by research grants from National Science Council (NSC 101-2632-E-130-001-MY3, MOST 103-2221-E-130 -005-MY2), Taiwan.

CONFLICT OF INTEREST

The authors declare that they have no conflict of interest.

REFERENCES

1. NPUAP at http://www.npuap.org
2. Trinkoff A, Brady B, Nielsen K (2003) Workplace Prevention and Musculoskeletal Injuries in Nurses. JONA 33: 153-158
3. Hsieh CH (2007) Innovative design of sickbed for decubitus ulcer free : Force analysis of muscles and joints. National Central University, Zhongli City
4. Lee TH (2008) An innovative sickbed design for pressure ulcer prevention: Human muscles' tension analysis and preliminary support system design. National Central University, Zhongli City
5. Stephen M (1997) A hybrid bed/chair system for bedridden patients ± elimination of transfer between a bed and wheelchair. ASME D DSCD 61: 29-31
6. wiki at http://en.wikipedia.org/wiki/Eye_tracking
7. Wang KP (2008) Mobile eye tracker construction and gaze path analysis. National Chengchi University, Taipei City
8. MathWorks at http://www.mathworks.com/
9. Yu LC (2009) Gaze-based human-computer interaction. National Chengchi University, Taipei City

Author: Tsai, Min-Ru and Yang, Chia-Yen
Institute: Department of Biomedical Engineering, Ming Chuan University
Street: 5 De Ming Rd
City: Taoyuan
Country: Taiwan
Email: mike711330@gmail.com;

Effects of Different Noise-Enhanced Vibrotactile Stimulation on Postural Control in Upright Standing: A Preliminary Investigation

C.K. Chien[1], L.Y. Guo[2], and C.H. Yang[1]

[1] Department of Physical Therapy, College of Medicine Tzu-Chi University, Hualien, Taiwan
[2] Faculty of Sports Medicine, College of Medicine, Kaohsiung Medical University, Kaohsiung, Taiwan

Abstract— **Stochastic resonance (SR) has been regarded as improving functions of sensory and motor in human via noise input, and increasing feedback of somatosensory may improve ability of posture control in upright standing. To date, regardless of previous literature has reported its efficacy of improving postural control, whether optimal noise can be used remains largely unknown. Present studies examined whether there was effect on postural control in upright standing using two types of interference waves: white noise (WN) with sinusoid signal and Gaussian noise (GN) with sinusoid signal. The finding suggests a promising setup for its application to increase postural control in upright standing. This study is aimed to examine the different effect on postural control in upright standing using two types of interference waves.**

Keywords— **White noise, Gaussian noise, Vibration, Postural control, Stochastic resonance.**

I. INTRODUCTION

Improving posture control with vibration under the plantar sole is a popular issue for the recent research. Previous literature has used various types of vibration, included different frequency, amplitude and wave shape, to enhance the capability of postural control [1-5]. The mechanism by which signal detection is improved by noise is called stochastic resonance (SR). Stochastic resonance is described as sinusoid signal in combination with noise, and the wave shape was described by Hijmans [3]. Stochastic resonance is usually regarded as stimulation for sensory nerve, the mechanism of firing up nerve was described by Moss [5].

Input noise can enhance sensory and motor function, via a mechanism known as stochastic resonance [1-3]. In this present study, we employed 3V, 100-300Hz sinusoid signal in combination with 3V, 100Hz noise (white noise or Gaussian noise) as a wave form of stochastic resonance to examine its effects on posture control. White noise (WN) and Gaussian noise (GN) are two common noises for stochastic resonance, which has been used in previous research.

In this present study, we aimed to examine the effect of sinusoid signal in combination with white noise and sinusoid signal in combination with Gaussian noise in different frequencies to identify which type of stochastic resonance has the better effect for the capability of posture control in upright standing.

II. MATERIALS AND METHODS

A. Subjects

We have recruited subjects without a history of neurological disease, diabetes, flat foot, open wound on foot, infectious dermatosis or lower limb had been injuried within three months. Each subject performed his or her standing balance with eyes closed over one minute prior to the participation in the experiment. A total of seven healthy collegiate students (7 males, aged 21.5±0.5 years, height 171.5±8.5 cm, and weight 60.5±6.5 kg) was participated this study. These subjects were divided into two different type of stochastic resonance groups: sinusoid signal in combination with white noise (white noise group, WN) and sinusoid signal in combination with Gaussian noise (Gaussian noise group, GN). Four subjects were randomly selected in the white noise group and three subjects in Gaussian noise group.

B. Materials

We have developed one customized miniature vibration actuator as shown in Figures 1 and 2. Three vibration actuators were inserted into a plastic plate, to provide the stimulation under the plantar sole.

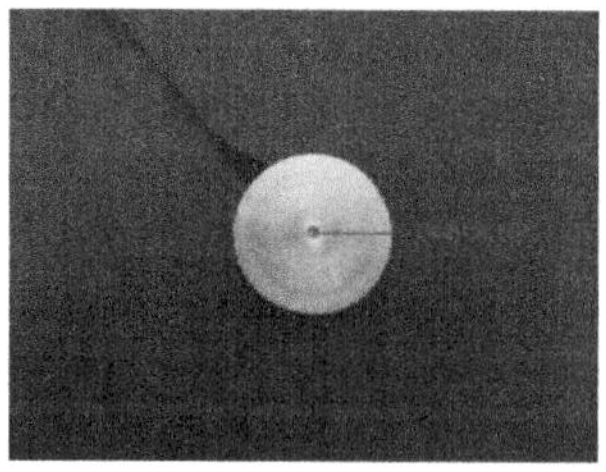

Fig. 1 Superior view of vibration actuator

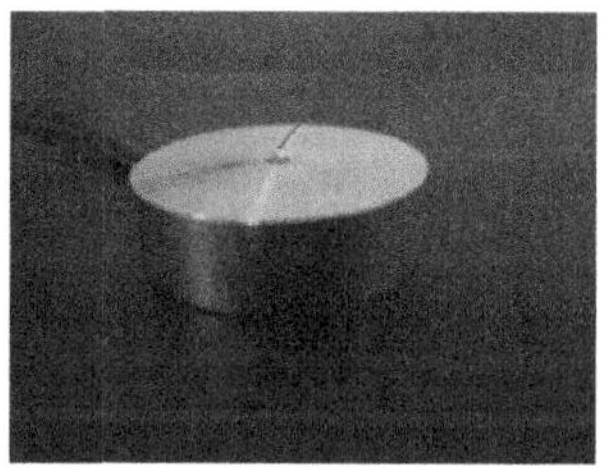

Fig. 2 Lateral view of vibration actuator

Three specific areas of foot plantar sole were selected, including the head of 1st metatarsal bone, the head of 5th metatarsal bone and calcaneus of the dominant foot.

A multiprocessor (DDS-3X25 USB, Hentek, China) was used to generate white noise or Gaussian noise with amplitude of 3V and frequency at 100Hz. A signal generator (PASCO, USA) was used to generate sinusoid signal

I. Lackovic (ed.), *1st Global Conference on Biomedical Engineering & 9th Asian-Pacific Conference on Medical and Biological Engineering*,
IFMBE Proceedings 47, DOI: 10.1007/978-3-319-12262-5_55

amplitude of 3V and frequencies at 100, 200 and 300Hz. The multiprocessor and the signal generator were connected with an oscilloscope (HITACHI, Japan) to monitor the wave form of mixed signal (Stochastic Resonance, SR vibrotactile wave) before transferring to vibration actuators.

An electromagnetic motion capture system with MotionMonitor™ Software (Innovative Sports Training, Inc., USA) and one forceplate (Bertec, USA) to used to record the kinematics and ground reactions during upright standing tasks.

C. Methods

Each subject was instructed to stand on one plastic plate with three vibration actuators with his dominant foot at a preferred standing posture with eyes-closed and eyes-open conditions. Two different wave forms (White noise and Gaussian noise) of vibrotactile stimulation in 0Hz, 100 Hz, 200 Hz and 300Hz were employed in white noise (WN) group and Gaussian noise (GN) group, respectively. Eight conditions were recorded for each in a randomized order with an interval of one-minute rest.

The raw data, the excursion of center of mass (COM), were calculated by MotionMonitor software. The variables of the excursion of COM were selected to examine the change in postural control of upright standing: root-mean-square (RMS) of displacement of COM in anterior-posterior (RMSCMap) and medial-lateral (RMSCMml) directions. RMS values of COM displacement in anterior-posterior (ap) and medial-lateral (ml) directions at all conditions were calculated by a custom-made program (MATLAB R2007b, Mathwork, Inc. USA). RMS describes dimensions of COM displacement from the mean position during a time interval.

III. Results

There were eight tables showed RMS of COM displacement of anterior-posterior and medial-lateral directions in WN group and GN group with eyes-closed and eye-open conditions. A forceplate recorded the location of COM at every record point, data collection frequency of the forceplate was 100Hz, for one minute. RMS was the root of the mean of the sum of the square for COM displacement of all record points. COM was relation to the ability of posture control in upright standing, and the greater value of RMS of COM displacement indicated poorer ability of posture control in upright standing.

The Tables 1-4 exhibited RMS of COM displacement in anterior-posterior direction.

Table 1 RMSCMap at 0Hz, 100Hz, 200Hz and 300Hz (WN group, EC)

Subject	0Hz	100Hz	200Hz	300Hz
Subject 1	23.23	8.27	6.03	13.24
Subject 2	77.92	84.08	79.47	81.59
Subject 3	74.13	70.36	69.74	69.30
Subject 4	91.68	93.86	92.39	88.64
Mean	66.74	64.14	61.91	63.19

Table 2 RMSCMapat 0Hz, 100Hz, 200Hz and 300Hz (WN group, EO)

Subject	0Hz	100Hz	200Hz	300Hz
Subject 1	36.80	22.02	12.79	15.26
Subject 2	77.38	84.83	84.23	83.87
Subject 3	73.33	69.98	73.07	70.65
Subject 4	92.67	94.57	92.37	90.18
Mean	70.04	67.85	65.61	64.99

Table 3 RMSCMap at 0Hz, 100Hz, 200Hz and 300Hz (GN group, EC)

Subject	0Hz	100Hz	200Hz	300Hz
Subject 5	82.58	83.44	82.75	81.10
Subject 6	70.66	68.89	69.96	71.65
Subject 7	50.66	51.46	50.97	49.51
Mean	67.97	67.93	67.89	67.42

Table 4 RMSCMap at 0Hz, 100Hz, 200Hz and 300Hz (GN group, EO)

Subject	0Hz	100Hz	200Hz	300Hz
Subject 5	86.35	83.47	81.98	82.50
Subject 6	70.18	73.63	70.73	72.22
Subject 7	51.12	52.02	50.33	52.67
Mean	69.22	69.71	67.68	69.13

The Tables 5-8 demonstrated RMS of COM displacement in medial-lateral direction as shown in the following,

Table 5 RMSCMml at 0Hz, 100Hz, 200Hz and 300Hz (WN group, EC)

Subject	0Hz	100Hz	200Hz	300Hz
Subject 1	99.31	96.08	95.14	97.95
Subject 2	174.55	176.04	172.44	167.61
Subject 3	158.42	163.07	161.10	159.67
Subject 4	134.63	134.50	131.87	128.07
Mean	141.72	142.42	140.14	138.33

Table 6 RMSCMml at 0Hz, 100Hz, 200Hz and 300Hz (WN group, EO)

Subject	0Hz	100Hz	200Hz	300Hz
Subject 1	101.48	94.08	96.17	97.98
Subject 2	170.39	175.69	170.19	170.33
Subject 3	158.67	161.75	161.88	165.82
Subject 4	133.87	134.79	129.43	128.67
Mean	141.10	141.58	139.42	140.70

Table 7 RMSCMml at 0Hz, 100Hz, 200Hz and 300Hz (GN group, EC)

Subject	0Hz	100Hz	200Hz	300Hz
Subject 5	189.45	187.06	182.66	185.10
Subject 6	107.57	109.18	108.76	110.51
Subject 7	79.54	75.31	75.40	76.40
Mean	125.52	123.85	122.27	124.00

Table 8 RMSCMml at 0Hz, 100Hz, 200Hz and 300Hz (GN group, EO)

Subject	0Hz	100Hz	200Hz	300Hz
Subject 5	190.70	186.17	188.26	186.06
Subject 6	111.40	116.78	111.89	110.60
Subject 7	79.99	78.24	78.10	78.58
Mean	127.36	127.06	126.08	125.08

IV. DISCUSSION

Small changes in postural control between white noise group and Gaussian noise group with various frequencies were found in this preliminary investigation. We cannot conclude which noise may be optimal used for improving postural control in upright standing.

Interestingly, the results have shown that the lower mean values in each variables appear in a wave form with sampling frequency at 200Hz. This trend may imply an optimal frequency of signal wave form is 200Hz.

In addition, white noise group demonstrate better postural control in anterior-posterior direction of COM displacement. This finding may provide a good reference to setup an optimal vibrotactile stimulation from a defined stochastic resonance signal. The limitation of this study is a small sample size and a large sample population is warranted in future research.

V. CONCLUSIONS

This preliminary result may not confirm the effect of noise-enhanced vibrotactlie stimulation for improving postural control in upright standing due to small sample of subjects. However, noise-enhanced stochastic resonance signal (200Hz, white noise) may be an optimal protocol for increasing postural control in upright standing.

CONFLICT OF INTEREST

The authors declare that they have no conflict of interest.

REFERENCES

1. Priplata A, Niemi J, Harry J et al. (2003) Vibrating insoles and balance control in elderly people. Lancet 362:1123–1124
2. Priplata A, Niemi J, Salen M et al. (2002) Noise-enhanced human balance control. Phys Rev Lett 89:238101
3. Hijmans J, Geertzen J, Zijlstra W et al. (2008) Effects of vibrating insoles on standing balance in diabetic neuropathy. JRRD 45:1441-1450
4. McDonnell M, Abbott D (2009) What is stochastic resonance? Definitions, misconceptions, debates, and its relevance to biology. PLoS Comput Biol 5:e1000348
5. Moss F, Ward L, Sannita W (2004) Stochastic resonance and sensory information processing: a tutorial and review of application. Clin Neurophysiol 115:267-281

Author: Chen-Kai Chien; Lan-Yuen Guo; Chich-Haung Yang
Institute: Tzu-Chi University
Street: No.701, Sec. 3, Jhongyang Rd., Hualien City
City: Hualien County 97004
Country: Taiwan
Email: C5826@ms18.hinet.net; r.chyang@mail.tcu.edu.tw

Measurements of Compressed Thickness of Compression Paddle Using a Bolus Phantom in Digital Mammography

Y.H. Chen[1] and S.L. Dong[2,*]

[1] Department of Biomedical Sciences/Chung Shan Medical University/Taichung City, ROC
[2] School of Medical Imaging and Radiological Sciences/Chung Shan Medical University/Taichung City, ROC

Abstract— **The purpose of this study is the investigation of compressed thickness of the fix and flexible compression paddles using a Bolus phantom in digital mammography. A 5-cm-tihck Bolus phantom and a 5-cm-tihck PMMA phantom were used for the assessments of compressed thickness. The compression forces of 0-200 N and 0-140 N were applied to the Bolus phantom and the PMMA phantom, respectively. Results from this study show that the displayed thickness of the PMMA phantom was greater than the displayed thickness of the Bolus phantom for the same compression force. The difference of displayed thickness was increased with increasing compression force and the maximum value was 0.4 cm. In conclusion, the Bolus phantom is suitable for the measurements of compressed thickness during mammographic compression procedure.**

Keywords—**Mammography, compression force, compression paddle, compressed thickness, bolus.**

I. INTRODUCTION

Many women have been experienced discomfort during compression procedure in mammography. The flexible compression paddle was therefore designed for reducing this discomfort during imaging procedure. In recent years, modern digital mammographic systems are equipped with the flexible compression paddle.

In digital mammography, the imaging settings of each patient are determined by the automatic exposure control (AEC) system depending on the compressed breast thickness (CBT) measured. In clinical practice, there is a +/- 0.5 cm tolerance on actual and displayed compressed breast thickness. Therefore, a correction for compressed breast thickness was required [1].

Most of testing phantoms used in mammography are designed to rigid configuration. Therefore, these phantoms cannot be deformed during the compression procedure. Bolus phantom is a soft-tissue equivalent material used in radiation therapy. The density of Bolus material is 1.03 g/cm^3 which is similar to the density of breast tissues 0.93~1.04 g/cm^3. Therefore, Bolus material may be a good candidate for simulating breast tissue in mammography.

* Corresponding author.

The purpose of this study is the investigation of compressed thickness of the fix and flexible compression paddles using a Bolus phantom in mammography.

II. MATERIALS AND METHODS

A digital mammography system (Siemens) with a flexible compression paddle and fix compression paddle was used in this study. A 5-cm-tihck Bolus phantom and a 5-cm-tihck PMMA phantom were used for the assessments of compressed thickness (see Fig. 1). The compression forces of 0-200 N and 0-140 N were applied to the Bolus phantom and the PMMA phantom, respectively. The applied compression forces and displayed thickness were recorded. The thicknesses of both phantoms for various compression forces were analyzed and compared.

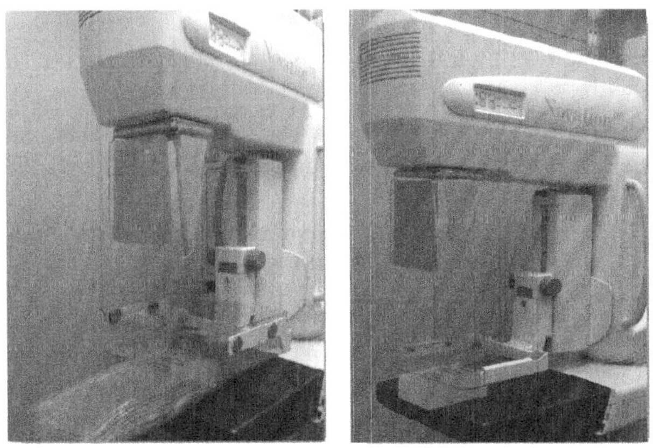

Fig. 1 Bolus and PMMA phantoms compressed with the compression paddle

III. RESULTS

Figure 2 shows the compressed thickness of fix compression paddle for different compression forces. The displayed thicknesses ranged from 4.7 to 3.6 cm and from 5.0 to 2.6 cm for PMMA and Bolus phantom, respectively.

I. Lackovic (ed.), *1st Global Conference on Biomedical Engineering & 9th Asian-Pacific Conference on Medical and Biological Engineering*,
IFMBE Proceedings 47, DOI: 10.1007/978-3-319-12262-5_56

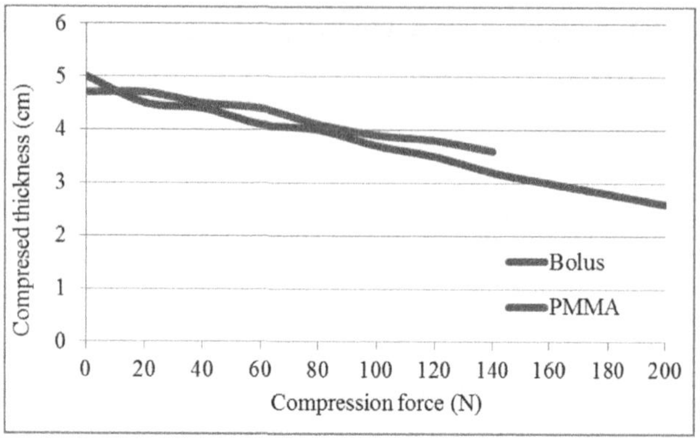

Fig. 2 The compressed thickness of fix compression paddle for different compression forces

Figure 3 shows the compressed thickness of flexible compression paddle for different compression forces. The displayed thicknesses ranged from 5.2 to 4.3 cm for the PMMA phantom and ranged from 5.4 to 3.4 cm for the Bolus phantom.

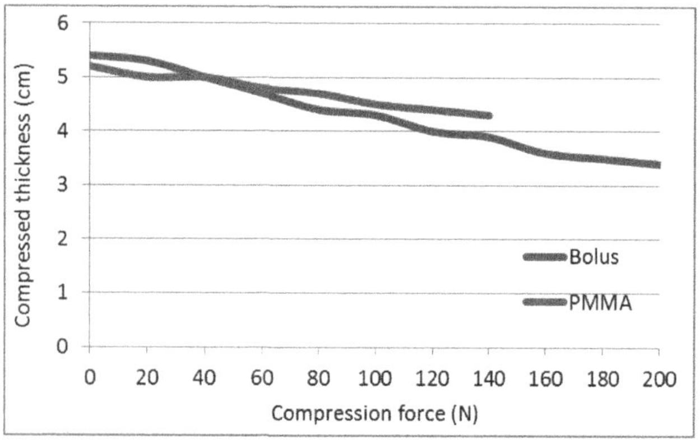

Fig. 3 The compressed thickness of flexible compression paddle for different compression forces

Figure 4 shows the difference of compressed thickness between PMMA and Bolus phantom. For the same compression force, the displayed thickness of the PMMA phantom was greater than the displayed thickness of the Bolus phantom. The difference of displayed thickness was increased with increasing compression force and the maximum value was 0.4 cm.

IV. DISCUSSION

For the compression forces used in clinical mammographic procedure (about 100 N), the thickness of Bolus phantom is thinner than that of PMMA phantom for both fix and flexible compression paddles. Since it is difficult to analysis the variation of compression thicknesses of breast in patients, the results obtained in this study is important.

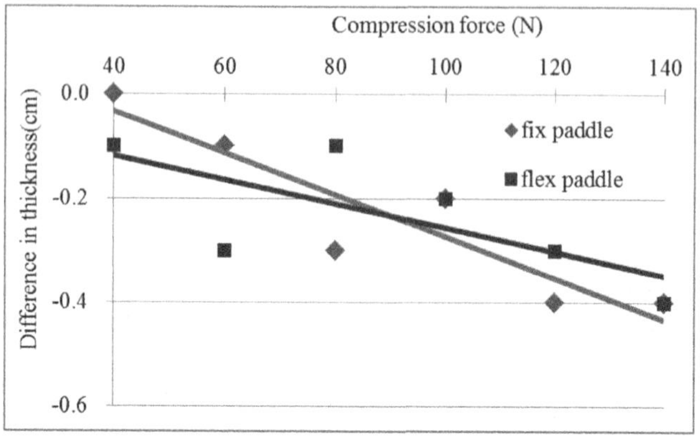

Fig. 4 The difference of compressed thickness between Bolus and PMMA phantom (Bolus-PMMA)

Many studies [2,3] have developed CBT correction techniques in mammography. The most convenient approach is the use of a rigid phantom with fixed thickness. By using different forces to compress the phantom, the differences between displayed thicknesses and phantom thickness can be applied to correct the recorded CBT of each exposure according to the compression force applied in the imaging procedure.

In our previous study [4], the CBT correction was measured using a 6-cm BR-12 phantom (rigid) and a fix compression paddle. An additional 0.4, 0.5, 0.6, and 0.7 cm were added for the applied forces of 100–119, 120–139, 140–159, and 160–179 N, respectively. These compressed breast thickness correction factors were used to adjust the compressed breast thickness from the patient records. Results from this study show that the correction factors obtained in our previous study [4] and other similar studies [1,5] may be insufficient due to the fact that the difference of compressed thickness between PMMA and Bolus phantom is significant.

For the 4.5-cm standard breast phantom, an error of 0.1 cm in the CBT correction resulted in a 7% difference in the percentage glandular content [6]. The CBT correction error obtained from this study was up to 0.4 cm for the compression force > 100 N. Therefore, the CBT correction uncertainty may be important for extremely thin breasts.

V. CONCLUSIONS

Results from this study demonstrated that the Bolus phantom is suitable for the measurements of compressed thickness of the fix and flexible compression paddles during mammographic compression procedure.

ACKNOWLEDGMENT

The authors would like to thank radiographers at department of Radiology of Chung Shan Medical University Hospital.

REFERENCES

1. Kruger R L and Schueler B A. (2001) A survey of clinical factors and patient dose in mammography. Med Phys 28:1449–1454
2. Tyson A H, Mawdsley G E, Yaffe M J. (2009) Measurement of compressed breast thickness by optical stereoscopic photogrammetry. Med Phys 36:569-576
3. Mawdsley G E, Tyson A H, Peressotti C L et al. (2009) Accurate estimation of compressed breast thickness in mammography. Med Phys 36:577-586
4. Jamal N, Ng K H, McLean D et al. (2004) Mammographic breast glandularity in Malaysian women: data derived from radiography. Am J Roentgenol 182:713-717
5. Dong S L, Chu T C, Lan G Y et al. (2011) Development of an adjustable model breast for mammographic dosimetry assessment in Taiwanese women. Am J Roentgenol; 196:W476-481
6. Dong S L, Chu T C, Lin Y C et al. (2011) Determination of equivalent breast phantoms for different age groups of Taiwanese women: An experimental approach. Med Phys 38:4094-4100

Author: Shang-Lung Dong
Institute: School of Medical Imaging and Radiological Sciences /Chung Shan Medical University
Street: No.110, Sec.1, Jianguo North Rd.
City: Taichung City
Country: Taiwan, ROC
Email: sldong@ms46.hinet.net

Inpatient Meal Booking System

M.H. Yang[1], M.M. Lo[1], T. Chou[1], J.H. Lin[2], and S.T. Tang[1,*]

[1] Department of Biomedical Engineering, Ming Chuan University, Taoyuan, Taiwan
[2] Department of Electronic Engineering, Kun Shan University, Tainan, Taiwan

Abstract— **In the hospital the inpatients' meal is not only for patient's hungry, is also for the treatment assistant. The meal is designed and ordered by the nutritionists, which are basing on the physician's advice. But in a hospital a nutritionist usually cares dozens patients, results in the heavy loading. In the meal order process, this involves departmental data transferring and manpower, and then needs lots of time. As a result, the first meal of the inpatient or the first modified meal would miss. For the purpose of providing the inpatients a in time nutritional care, so we proposed the inpatient meal booking system. Our system developed the electronic forms of meal booking based on the interactive Web technology. The physician's advises are ordered via the web page, which are then directly transferred to the nutritionist. As a result, the nutritionist could get the inpatient's data in time, and then assesses the nutritional requirements, issues the meal order.**

Keywords— **Electronic forms, Interactive web, Booking system.**

I. INTRODUCTION

An important factor to keep the human healthy is proper nutrition. Particular, the prevalence of domestic chronic diseases rises in every year. In disease treatment or surgery, the nutritional therapy (including nutritional supplements and diet control) has been considered as a part of the treatment of disease. Therefore in medical profession, the concepts about "Nutrition Medical" have been increasing emphasis. [1, 2] Providing good patient meal service and thus enhance the quality of care, which has been become the concerning topics. [3] If the hospital meal service can match with the nutritional requirements of a variety of clinical disease, then the patients can correctly intake nutrient, and to improve the malnutrition problems, which will have a positive impact. Generally the hospital diet service is based on physician's recipes, and then nutritionists design the meal detail then issue the meal order. The ward nurse also assesses the patient's conditions, and then suggests the patient's diet. In the hospital every nurse has to care about eight patients, and nutrition should care about the dozens patients, it is too overloaded. The data transfer and the input process of the entire meal booking operation needs to consume a long time, which cannot immediately provide diet for inpatient. As a result, the first meal of the inpatient or the first modified meal would miss.

* Corresponding author.

Hospital provides inpatient the meal service that is a part of the treatment, which accords the patient's individual physical condition as a basis to set the intake of nutrients. Generally, the inpatient's meal booking process is as following. The first step is the doctor's determinant of patient's hospitalization, and then the patient books the meals according with the doctor's orders. After confirmation of the nutritionist, this accomplishes the meal order. The whole process is shown in Fig. 1.

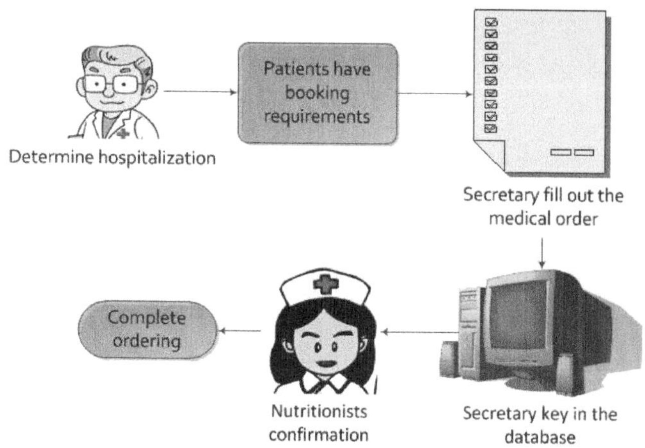

Fig. 1 Current meal booking process

This process was cumbersome. The inpatient's first meal usually must be waited for a long time even the next day. It takes too much human resources and time. Additionally, the data key-in and transmission easily lead to errors happen.

In order to shorten the time spend in booking and human resources, let the inpatient can eat meals in the right time. This study designed a meal booking system to provide easy meal booking and errors preventable.

II. METHODS

A. *Workflow*

This study aimed to develop an electronic form system. Design a new operating procedure to meet the needs of nutritionist. After the patient's hospitalization, doctors can use the system to book patient's meals. And through the proposed system, the nutritionist could immediately achieve

I. Lackovic (ed.), *1st Global Conference on Biomedical Engineering & 9th Asian-Pacific Conference on Medical and Biological Engineering*, IFMBE Proceedings 47, DOI: 10.1007/978-3-319-12262-5_57

the information of patient's meals. Ward nurse would also immediately receive patient's meal information. As then the inpatients would have their meal in time. The full process is a collaborative model, composed by physician, nurse and nutritionist, which is shown in Fig. 2. [4, 5]

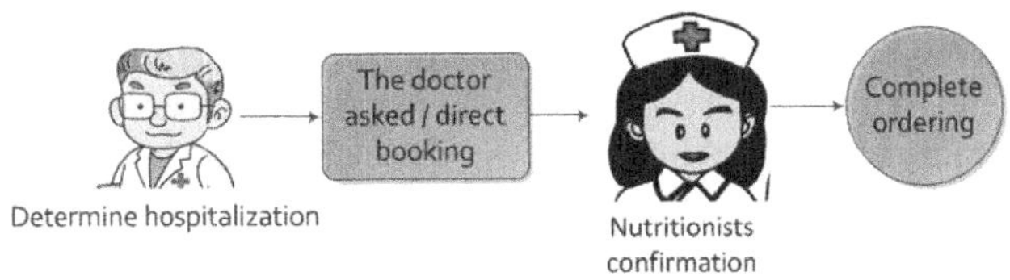

Fig. 2 Proposed meal booking process

B. Form System Architecture

We refer the hospital diet category to establish the electronic form. There are the following features: (1) input patient information from the HIS (Hospital Information System), LIS (Laboratory Information System), and other information systems. (2) Provides the prescription diet options. (3) Share information to the nutritionist, ward nurse, and kitchen worker system. (4) Output data to a database for long term storage. The system structure is shown in Fig. 3. [6, 7]

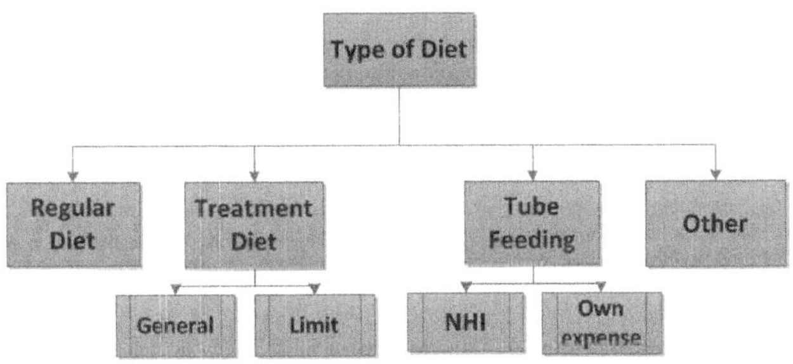

Fig. 3 Proposed meal booking process

C. Form Content

The completed meal booking forms include the Diet Category, Regular Diet, Treatment Diet, Tube Feeding, and Other note items, as shown in Fig. 4. When doctors in interrogation, who could achieve the patient's complete information from HIS, or LIS, and then issue the meal booking basing on the patient's conditions. The form design is fully according with physician's recipe. [8]

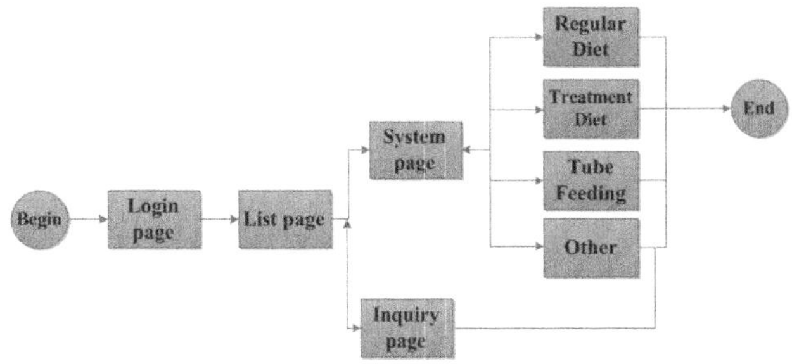

Fig. 4 Working flowchart of the system

D. Use of Tools - RIA (Rich Internet Application)

This study used Visual Studio 2010 C# in an ASP.NET system to implement the interactive web pages of the electronic meal booking forms. ASP.NET is the NET Framework part. In writing an ASP.NET application, the .NET Framework classes can be accessed. Any of the CLR (Common Language Runtime) compliant language is also can be deployed for writing applications, including Microsoft Visual Studio 2010 C#.

The implemented database is developed via the Microsoft Access. It has the basic database functions range from input, query, modifies, reported. Its characteristics are easy to implement and use. We integrated the MS Access and ASP.NET to develop the proposed system.

The booking forms have the following features: facilitates doctor's meal booking, providing the patient's meal archive, quick check to the nutritionist, and the ward nurses can fulfill the patient's needs in time.

III. RESULTS

This system is divided into four pages. First page is the home page, shown in Fig. 5, which provide the system login. Second page is the dietary page, shown in Fig. 6. This is the most important user interface, the user only need to use mouse click, and then complete the patient data entry, and stored in a database. Third page is a query interface, shown in Fig. 7, which is for checking the patients' diet information, user can specify a range of data and query certain period of time for the all patients.

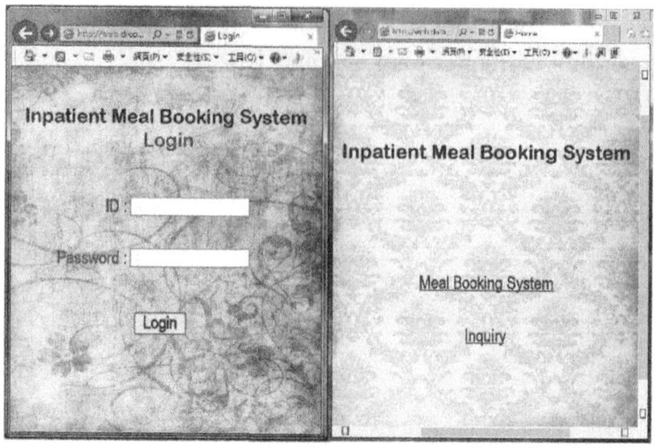

Fig. 5 System home page

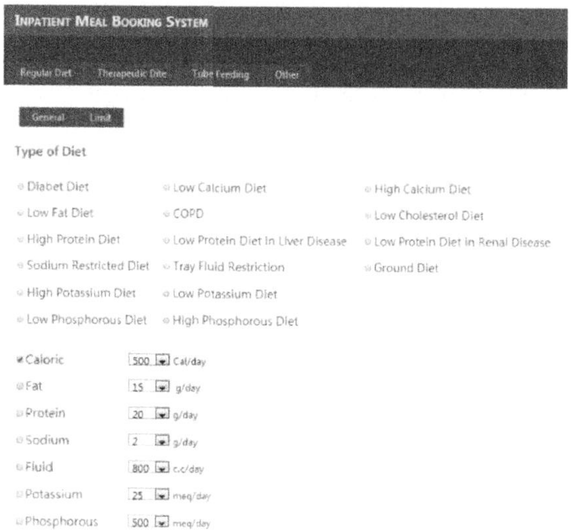

Fig. 6 Meal booking system interface

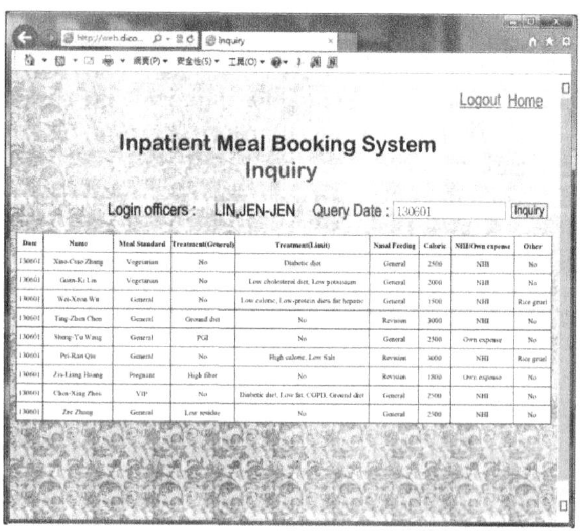

Fig. 7 Query page

IV. CONCLUSION

Generally the hospital's meal ordering process needs a lot of processes. In the lengthy procedure, the patients usually have to omit the first meal when they are just hospitalization or meal modified. Additionally, during the convenient meal booking process, it is easy in data errors or booking the wrong meals our proposed system provides doctors directly entering the meal data in the interrogation. The patient meal information would directly enter the database, the booking meals abnormal rate would decreased significantly. And reduce personnel (nutritionist, nurse, secretary) operating hours, enhance the quality of patient care.

REFERENCES

1. Husain W, Wei LJ, Cheng SL, and Zakaria N (2011) Application of Data Mining Techniques in a Personalized Diet Recommendation System for Cancer Patients, IEEE Colloquium on Humanities, Science and Engineering Research, Penang, Malaysia, 2011, pp 239–244
2. Bantle JB, Wylie-Rosett J, Albright AL, Apovian CM, Clark NG, Franz MJ, Hoogwerf BJ, Lichtenstein AH, Mayer-Davis E, Mooradian AD and Wheeler ML (2008) Nutrition recommendations and interventions for diabetes, A position statement of the American Diabetes Association, Diabetes Care 31 :61–78
3. Weekes CE, Elia M and Emery PW (2004) The development: validation and reliability of a nutrition screening tool based on the recommendations of the British Association for Parenteral and Enteral Nutrition (BAPEN), Clinical Nutrition 23:1104–1112
4. Johns N, Hartwell H and Morgan M (2010) Improving the provision of meals in hospital. The patients' viewpoint, Appetite 54:181–185
5. Stanga Z, Zurflüh Y, Roselli M, Sterchi AB , Tanner B and Knecht G (2003) Hospital food: a survey of patients' perceptions, Clin Nutr. 22:241–246
6. Saisunee J, Sudajai L and Tidanuch P (2012) Nutrition Therapy System for elderly with Diabetes, Procedia - Social and Behavioral Scienes 40:220–224.
7. Hong SM, Cho JY, Lee JH, Kim G and Kim MC (2008) NutriSonic web expert system for meal management and nutrition counseling with nutrient time-series analysis, e-food exchange and easy data transition, Nutrition Research and Practice 2(2):121–129
8. Huang SH, Chen PR, Chang CJ, Lai HS, Cheng CP, Liu HY and Yang RS (2005) The Effects of Nutritional Status and Gastrointestinal Complications on the Nutrient Intake Among the Inpatients with Tube Feeding, Journal of the Formosan Medical Association 9:467–474

Author: Shih-Tsang Tang
Institute: Ming Chuan University
Street: 5 De Ming Rd., Gui Shan District
City: Taoyuan
Country: Taiwan
Email: sttang@mail.mcu.edu.tw

A Wireless Electrocardiogram System-on-a-Chip with Reed–Solomon Coding and Frequency-Shift-Keying Transmitter for Healthcare Application

Tsung-Yen Chen[1], Yul-Lung Chang[2], and Shuenn-Yuh Lee[3]

[1] Department of Electrical Engineering, National Chung Cheng University, Chiayi, Taiwan
[2] Automotive Research & Testing Center, No.6, Lugong S. 7th Rd., Lukang, Changhua, Taiwan
[3] Department of Electrical Engineering, National Cheng Kung University, Tainan, Taiwan

Abstract— **This paper presents a wireless electrocardiogram (ECG) acquisition and monitoring system for healthcare application. This system consists of three parts, namely, an analog front end, a Reed–Solomon (RS) encoder, and a frequency-shift-keying (FSK) transmitter. The analog front-end circuit acquires and digitizes the ECG signal. The RS encoder encrypts the digitized data before being sent to the FSK transmitter. The encrypted data are then up-converted to radio frequency for wireless communication. The integrated system is implemented in TSMC 0.18 μm standard CMOS process and demonstrated on a printed circuit board to verify its capability to acquire the ECG signal from the human body.**

Keywords— **electrocardiogram, frequency shift keying, Reed–Solomon, radio frequency transmitter, acquisition system.**

I. INTRODUCTION

The tenseness of daily life has increased in recent years as a result of rapid economic growth and industrial development. Negative emotions, such as anxiety, nervousness, and melancholy, are aggravated by increased tenseness [1]. Such emotions and fast-paced lifestyle could cause mental stress, which could lead to ischemic heart disease, the top cause of death worldwide [2].

With the development of very large-scale integration (VLSI) and modern wireless communication technologies, an integrated multi-functionality system with mixed-mode, digital, and radio-frequency circuits can be easily achieved. Moreover, a system-on-a-chip (SoC) that integrates an entire system into a single piece of silicon, thereby facilitating device minimization, has become popular in recent years. Features of the proposed SoC include low power consumption, low cost, and small size, which are advantageous characteristics for wearable or implantable applications.

Body sensor networks (BSNs) are an important healthcare technology. To achieve safety, a high-privacy and convenient BSN with a well-integrated SoC device has been recently developed [3]. With the SoC device, bio information can be easily collected, processed, and monitored. Moreover, modern wireless communication technology can be adopted in the device to achieve real-time application anytime and anywhere.

A wireless bio-signal acquisition SoC for BSN is proposed in this paper. The rest of this paper is organized as follows. Section II describes the architecture of the proposed system. The circuit diagrams and design consideration of the proposed system are presented in Section III. Section IV provides the measurement results. Finally, Section V presents the conclusion.

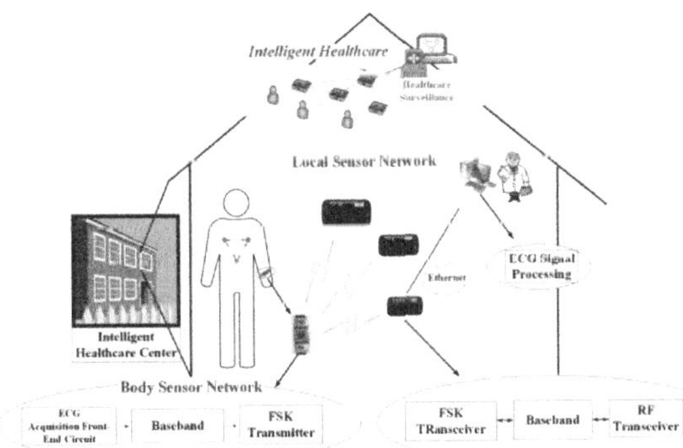

Fig. 1 Intelligent healthcare and monitoring system [6]

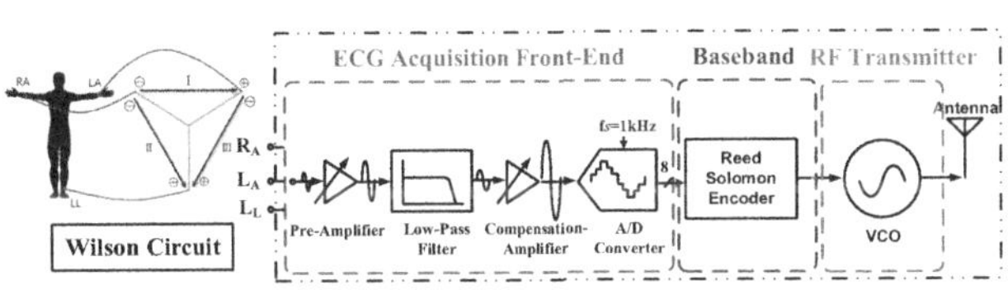

I. Lackovic (ed.), *1st Global Conference on Biomedical Engineering & 9th Asian-Pacific Conference on Medical and Biological Engineering*, IFMBE Proceedings 47, DOI: 10.1007/978-3-319-12262-5_58

Fig. 2 Circuit diagrams of the proposed wireless bio-signal acquisition SoC device

II. SYSTEM ARCHITECTURE OF HEALTHCARE MONITORING

Recent economic troubles may have emotional impacts on everyone, causing heightened levels of stress. Stress can cause a long-term burden on the human body, particularly on the heart. Patients with risks of heart disease should not be allowed to self-diagnose or self-medicate. Therefore, a warning and monitoring device with a home telecare system (HTS) function can be adopted. This device can transmit bio-signals from the patient to the medical center or hospital through the Internet or wireless communication systems [4] [5]. However, the HTS was not designed for patient use anytime and anywhere. To solve this problem, an Interactive Intelligent Healthcare and Monitoring System (IIHMS) should be built [5]. Fig. 1 shows an IIHMS with heterogeneous networks. The system consists of two major parts: a BSN and a local sensor network (LSN) [6]. The BSN is the network between the wearable device, which acquires the bio-signal, and the portable device, which performs data analysis, processing, and display. The LSN is the network between the portable device and the medical center for healthcare and treatment issues.

III. CIRCUIT DIAGRAMS AND DESIGN CONSIDERATION

Fig. 2 shows the circuit diagrams of the proposed SoC with a frequency-shift-keying (FSK) transmitter. This system has three major parts: an ECG acquisition front-end, which includes a programmable pre-amplifier, a low-pass filter (LPF), a compensation amplifier, and an analog-to-digital converter (ADC). To reduce the bit error rate caused by the interference of radio frequency (RF) communication, a Reed–Solomon encoder is implemented behind the ECG acquisition front-end. The output data is carried with 2.4 GHz by the RF circuits and transmitted by wireless communication. The detailed circuits are described in the following subsection.

A. ECG Acquisition Front-End

The programmable pre-amplifier is implemented by a differential difference amplifier (DDA) and a programmable gain stage (PGA) [7]. The DDA can simultaneously realize both negative feedback and differential input to implement the function of instrumentation amplifiers, which are widely used in biomedical systems. The output gain of PGA is designed by using a capacitor array. The total gain can be programmed between 30 and 40 dB.

To obtain the magnitude of R wave and T wave for the detection of cardiac disease, the LPF is adopted to filter the out-of-band noise. The filter with a double-terminated RLC-ladder prototype can be replaced by operational transconductance amplifiers and capacitor [8] in the integrated circuits.

The post-amplifier is designed to compensate the gain attenuation of LPF and to fit with the amplitude requirement of ADC. In addition, the post-amplifier can act as buffer between LPF and ADC. A low-power 8-bit successive approximation with sampling frequency of 1 kHz is adopted to digitize the ECG signal, because the bandwidth of the bio-signal is below 250 Hz.

B. Baseband Circuit

To attain privacy and error correction, a RS encoder is designed as baseband circuit in this system. A RS code can be described as (n, k), where n is the block length in symbols and k is the number of information symbols in the message. According to RS code (n, k), the required generator polynomial $g(x)$ and the message $m(x)$ can be illustrated as Equations (1) and (2), respectively.

$$g(x) = g_0 + g_1x + g_2x^2 + \cdots + g_{n-k-1}x^{n-k-1} + x^{n-k} \quad (1)$$

$$m(x) = m_0 + m_1x + m_2x^2 + \cdots + m_{k-1}x^{k-1} \quad (2)$$

Equations (1) and (2) can be used to calculate the RS code word C(x) in Equation (3) and the remainder in Equation (4), respectively.

$$C(x) = x^{n-k} \cdot m(x) + \frac{x^{n-k} \cdot m(x)}{g(x)} \Big| (\text{mod} g(x)) \quad (3)$$

$$\frac{x^{n-k} \cdot m(x)}{g(x)} = r(x) \quad (4)$$

For wireless communication protocol, an 8-bit header is added to the 8-bit binary output of ADC to serve as input to the RS encoder. The 16-bit data is further encoded by the RS encoder as a 31-bit code word for error correction.

C. RF Transmitter

The FSK RF transmitter is adopted to convert the baseband data to RF signal for wireless communication. A complementary cross-coupled differential structure is adopted to implement the required voltage control oscillator (VCO) for FSK modulation [7]. Compared with in-phase and quadrature-phase (I/Q) modulation, the FSK is simpler and has lower power consumption, which are suitable characteristics for wearable applications.

IV. MEASUREMENT RESULTS

The proposed FSK SoC with an ECG acquisition front-end, a RS encoder, and an FSK transmitter is fabricated in TSMC 0.18-μm standard CMOS process with chip area of 3 mm^2. Figs. 3(a) and 3(b) show the chip photo and the test board, respectively.

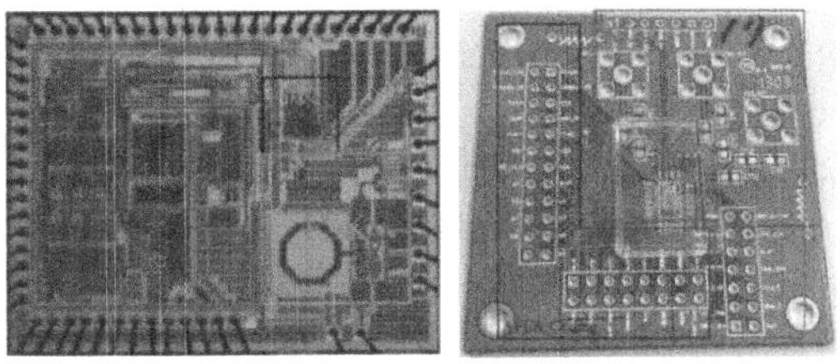

(a) (b)

Fig. 3 (a) The chip photo of proposed FSK SoC and (b) test board of the system

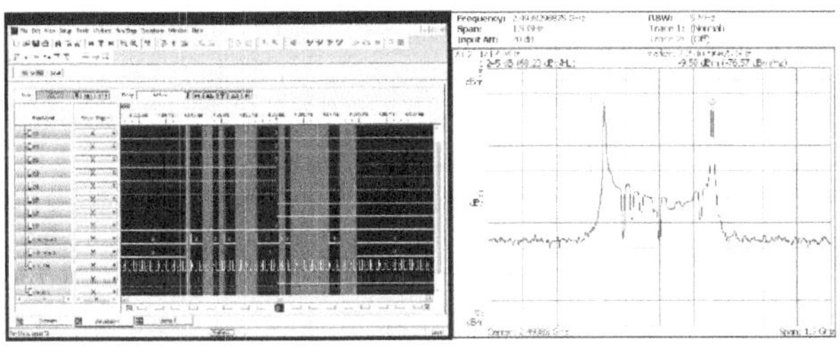

(a) (b)

Fig. 4 (a) Measurement result of RS encoder (b) Output spectrum of FSK transmitter

Fig. 4(a) shows the measurement result of the RS encoder. The message $m(x)$ is [1001101001111000], and the measured code word C(x) based on Equations (3) and (4) is [10011010011110000101111111100111]. The code word is consistent with the format of the RS encoder. Fig. 4(b) shows the measured output spectrum of the FSK transmitter. The mark frequency represented 1 is 2.725 GHz, whereas the space frequency represented 0 is 2.251 GHz.

V. CONCLUSION

An IIHMS system consisting of a BSN and a LSN is proposed for healthcare application. The proposed system, which includes an ECG acquisition front end, a RS encoder, and an FSK transmitter, is implemented on a single chip to verify the circuits. Measured results of the proposed SoC revealed the function work, and the system platform will be developed in future works.

CONFLICT OF INTEREST

The authors declare that they have no conflict of interest

ACKNOWLEDGMENT

The authors would like to thank the Chip Implementation Center and the Ministry of Science and Technology of Taiwan, R.O.C. under Grant Nos. NSC102-2221-E-006-289-MY3, and NSC102-2622-E-006- 038-CC1 for supporting this work.

REFERENCES

1. C. Gullette, J. A. Blumenthal, M. Babyak, W. Jiang, R. A. Waugh, D. J. Frid, C. M. O'Connor, J. J. Morris, and D. S. Krantz (1997) Effects of mental stress on myocardial ischemia during daily life. JAMA 277(19):1521-1526
2. World Health Organization, "The top 10 causes of death," at http://www.who.int/mediacentre/factsheets/fs310/en/
3. G. Yang, L. Xie, M. Mantysalo, J. Chen, H. Tenhunen, and L. R. Zheng (2012) Bio-patch design and implementation based on a low-power system-on-chip and paper-based inkjet printing technology. T-ITB 1043-1050
4. K. Lorincz, D. J. Malan, T. R. F. Fulford-Jones, A. Nawoj, A. Clavel, V. Shnayder, G. Mainland, M. Welsh and S. Moulton (2004) Sensor networks for emergency response: challenges and opportunities. Pervasive Computing 16-23
5. S. Y. Lee, L. H. Wang, and Q. Fang (2010) A Low Power RFID Integrated Circuits for Intelligent Healthcare Systems. T-ITB 1387-1396
6. L. H. Wang, T. T. Chen, K. H. Lin, and S. Y. Lee (2014) A low-power super-regenerative BFSK transceiver for intelligent healthcare monitoring system, ISBB Proc. Chung Yuan Christian University, Taoyuan, Taiwan, 2014, pp. 1-4.
7. S. Y. Lee, C. J. Cheng, and M. C. Liang (2011) A low-power bidirectional telemetry device with a near-field charging feature for a cardiac microstimulator. TBCAS 357–367
8. P. Corbishley and E. Rodriguez-Villegas (2007) A nanopower bandpass filter for detection of an acoustic signal in a wearable breathing detector. TBCAS 163-171

Authors: Tsung-Yen Chen[1], Yul-lung Chang[2], Shuenn-Yuh Lee[3]
Institute: CCU[1], ARTC[2], NCKU[3]
Street: No. 1 University Road
City: Tainan
Country: Taiwan
Email: 98yancy@cbic.ee.ncku.edu.tw, maxchang@artc.org.tw, ieesyl@mail.ncku.edu.tw

Young's Modulus Estimation of Soft Tissues by Video Tactile Pneumatic Sensor

M.M. Gubenko[1], I.G. Goryacheva[1], M.Z. Dosayev[2], A.V. Morozov[1], A.N. Lyubicheva[1], F.-C. Su[3], C.-H. Yeh[3], and M.-S. Ju[4]

[1] Institute for Problems in Mechanics of Russian Academy of Sciences, Moscow, Russia
[2] Institute of Mechanics of Lomonosov Moscow State University, Moscow, Russia
[3] Department of Biomedical Engineering of National Cheng Kung University, Tainan, Taiwan
[4] Department of Mechanical Engineering of National Cheng Kung University, Tainan, Taiwan

Abstract— **An indentation technique is one of effective methods to determine the elastic modulus of materials using information about contact geometry, indenter shape and applied load. This paper presents a device and a method that allow us to estimate elastic modulus of soft materials through indentation by video tactile pneumatic sensor. The device is a sealed metal cylinder ending with a soft silicone shell of a semispherical shape with 5 mm radius. During penetration by the silicone tip into investigated material the measured parameters are contact radius and displacement of the central point of the shell.**

The contact interaction between hollow elastic semisphere and a sample is modeled using finite element method. The axisymmetric contact problem was solved in geometrically nonlinear formulation, as the large strains were observed in the tests. The linear elastic model was used to describe mechanical properties of the sensor head and the sample. The Young's modulus of the soft tissue was estimated based on the experimental results and numerical calculations.

Keywords— **minimally invasive surgery, soft tissue, Young's modulus, indentation, tactile sensor.**

I. INTRODUCTION

The mechanical properties identification of soft biological tissues is one of the important objectives of the contact mechanics in the area of bioresearch. An indentation technique is widely used method for definition of elastic characteristics which is based on information about contact geometry, indenter shape and applied load. From the other hand, palpation of human organs through skin was a prototype for development of an innovation device that will be discussed further. During palpation the characteristics that can be analyzed by tactile and muscular sense of surgeon are stress and deformation under his fingertips. But sometimes it is not possible to palpate tissues directly by hands. In such situation like laparoscopic surgery operation there are different devices that are made for estimating the elastic properties of internal tissues. One of them is a tactile sensor for detection lumps in liver tissue using pressure distribution map in the area of contact [1]. The other is aspiration device that can determine Young's modulus of tissue at the contact point [2]. Making "elasticity map" of internal organ at different stages of the disease progression allows doing earlier and more precise diagnostics (e.g. liver fibrosis). Moreover, knowing Young's modulus in a certain area of points permits us to improve detection of tumors and to define its size and location. This paper describes another method of estimating the elastic properties of internal organs, which is based on indentation technique.

The procedure of elastic modulus evaluation relies firstly at the experimental measurements of contact characteristics and secondly at a theoretical model calculating stress-strain state of interacting bodies. A miniature pneumatic video tactile sensor with semi sphere pneumatic shell (as a sensor head) was designed for contact tests with soft biological tissue.

This paper presents experimental results for series of indentation tests for different contact pairs: silicone sensor head, interacting with rigid body, silicone sample or soft tissue, which is simulated by gelatin. A comparison of experimental and calculation results are shown as well.

II. THE EXPERIMENTAL TECHNIQUE

To determine the characteristics of the contact interaction, a miniature video tactile pneumatic sensor was designed. Photo of the device is shown in Fig. 1.

Video tactile pneumatic sensor mounted in the tribometer UMT-3M consists of a sealed metal cylinder (3) fixed by one of its endings to the load cell (1). Another side of cylinder ends with a soft silicone shell (5), which has semispherical shape of 5 mm radius. Video camera, an optical proximity sensor and a LED are located under this shell. The proximity sensor allows to measure displacement of the central point of the shell and the LED permits regulating the illumination in the chamber to provide better visualization of contact area by the video camera. It is necessary to use a "reflector" for correct work of the proximity sensor, so there is a miniature mirror of 1.5 mm diameter in the center of the silicone shell (5).

I. Lackovic (ed.), *1st Global Conference on Biomedical Engineering & 9th Asian-Pacific Conference on Medical and Biological Engineering*,
IFMBE Proceedings 47, DOI: 10.1007/978-3-319-12262-5_59

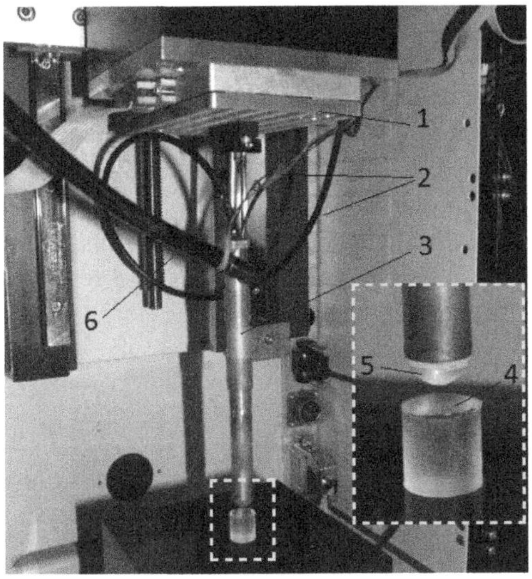

Fig. 1. Photo of video tactile pneumatic sensor mounted in the tribometer UMT-3M: (1) – load cell, (2) – wires of built-in camcorder, LED and optical proximity sensor, (3) – cylindrical tube of the sensor, (4) – the sample, (5) – silicone shell of the sensor head, (6) – compressed air supply

It was observed in experiments and confirmed in calculations that central part of the silicone head bends inwardly during indentation. So the contact area becomes a ring instead of a circle. To avoid this bending and to ensure a convex contact area an additional air pressure inside the cylinder can be applied in the range from 6 to 15 kPa. The pressure in the system is measured by a sensitive air-gauge and can be adjusted by a pressure regulator. Furthermore, it allows to vary stiffness of the sensor and to investigate various materials with significantly different elastic modulus.

During penetration of the transparent shell into the investigated material video camera captures the images of the contact area, and after that the contact radius can be measured. The boundary of the contact area is well determined on the image by the reflected light on the bended shell surface. The dependences of the contact area radius vs. the displacement of the central point of the shell were obtained by applying the developed experimental method to different contact pairs, contact surface conditions and values of the internal pressure.

Diagram of the contact interaction is shown in Fig. 2. To calibrate the optical proximity sensor indentation tests of rigid sample were produced thus data received from the optical proximity sensor – u_S – had to be equal to the displacement h of the moving cylinder in stationary reference system. Calibration procedures for different values of air pressure inside the sensor head were carried out.

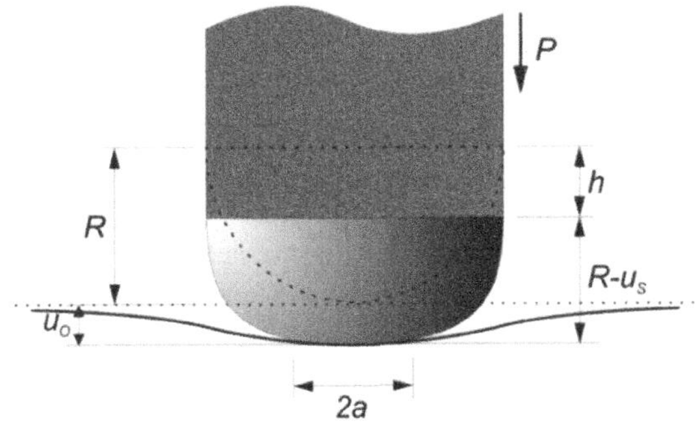

Fig. 2.Contact interaction of silicone shell of the sensor with surface of the sample, where R is a radius of the semispherical shell; h – vertical displacement of the cylinder; u_S – normal displacement of the central point of the shell, u_O – displacement of the sample surface, a – radius of the contact area. Dotted lines indicate the undeformed state at the initial moment of contact.

The sensitivity of the developed method is illustrated in Fig.3 which shows dependences of the applied normal load P vs. displacement of the central point of the silicone shell u_S. The graph indicates that changing of the air pressure inside the sensor (that is changing its stiffness) adjusts the sensitivity of the device.

For measurement the contact area radius a camcorder, built-in the sensor, is used. The camera captures image of the visible area during the process of loading the sample surface by the transparent shell. The area of contact between the shell and the sample is fixed by the well distinguishable glare on the bending of the silicone shell surface.

To calibrate a built-in camcorder an external reference camera was used, working synchronously with the first one. For better identification of the contact area the fluid was added into the contact. The boundary of the liquid meniscus is visible through both of cameras.

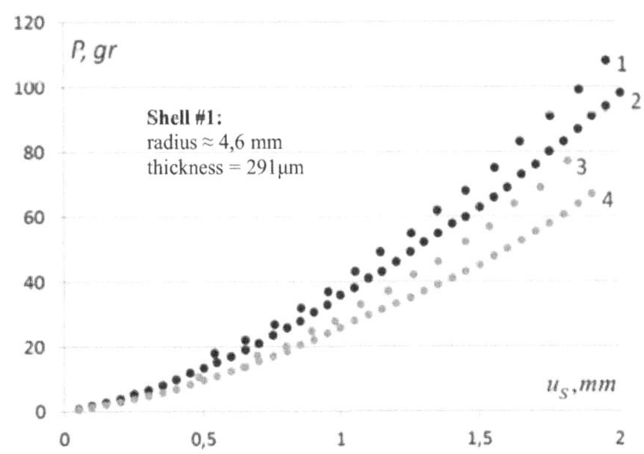

Fig. 3. Dependence of applied normal load vs. displacement for testing samples with different stiffness (1, 3 – for rigid sample, 2, 4 – for soft silicone) and different values of the pressure under the shell (black markers for 15 kPa, grey ones for 6 kPa).

A mechanical model of contact interaction between the sensor head and the sample is proposed [3]. The sensor head is modeled by a linear elastic hollow semisphere with specified mechanical characteristics. The counterbody is modeled by cylinder with linear elastic mechanical properties. To solve the contact problem the finite element method was applied. Geometrical and mechanical characteristics of proposed tactile sensor were taken into account during calculations.

An axisymmetric contact problem for linear elastic bodies was considered. The problem was solved with geometrically nonlinear formulation, as the large strains were expected. Specified mesh consisted of higher order 2-D elements 8-node or 6-node. Representative mesh size for the sensor head was about 0,06 mm. The amount of elements did not exceed fifteen thousand for all the models. Contact interaction was modeled using asymmetric augmented Lagrange method with sample as a target surface and sensor head as a contact surface.

The boundary conditions reproduced the experimental conditions as close as it's possible. The base of the investigated sample was fixed in normal direction, symmetric boundary conditions were set on the axis of symmetry. Load conditions are defined as normal displacements on edge of semisphere. Contact friction coefficient and sample's material properties were varied from one contact pair to another (silicone shell either with rigid body, or with silicone, or with gelatin).

A method of Young's modulus determination of soft biological tissues is based on test results and on the solution of the reverse contact mechanical problem for indentation of the sample by the silicone shell.

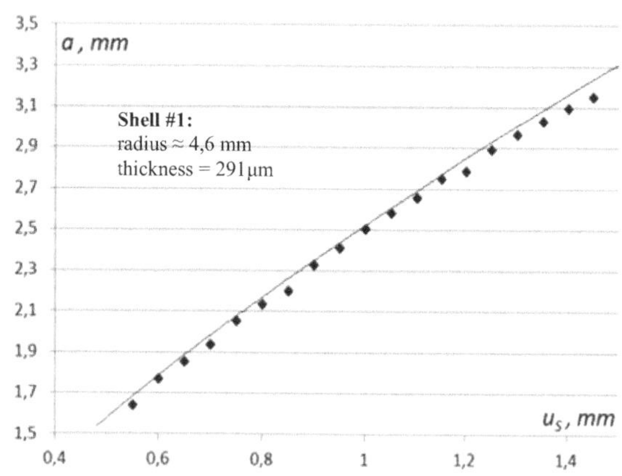

Fig. 4. Dependence of the contact area radius a vs. u_S. Comparison of the theoretical calculation and experimental data obtained during indentation of rigid sample with pressure inside the sensor of 6 kPa.

By applying the developed experimental method of the contact characteristics determination the dependences of a vs. u_S were obtained during tests of samples with different stiffness values. Comparison of the theoretical calculation and experimental data for tests with rigid body is shown on Fig. 4. As it can be seen from the graph, the developed model is in good agreement with experiments.

Fig. 5 shows the comparison of test results for rigid body, silicone and gelatin samples.

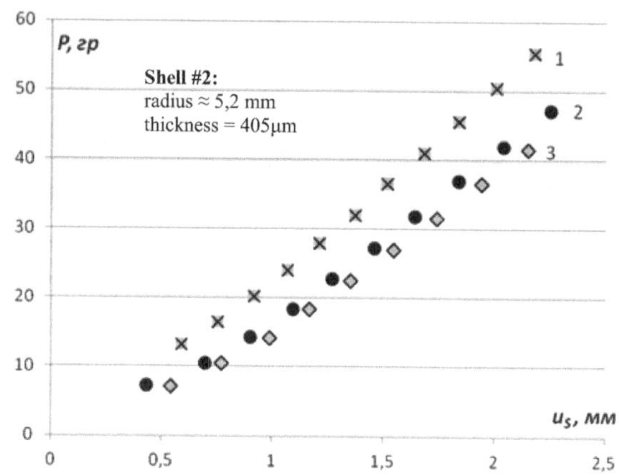

Fig. 5. Dependence of the applied normal force P vs. displacement u_S for tests of gelatin sample (1), silicone sample (2) and rigid body (3). Pressure inside the sensor is 6 kPa.

III. CONCLUSIONS

As a result a new method and a device are proposed to define the contact characteristics during indentation of soft biological materials by video tactile pneumatic sensor, which can be applicable in laparoscopy. Measured parameters are contact area and deformation of the silicone sensor head. Presented results, obtained during series of tests with rigid body and silicone samples, were used for calibration the sensor. An elastic modulus of testing material can be obtained from the experimental data by using the mathematical modeling. A comparison of experiments and theory model is made and it shows a good agreement of test results for rigid sample. Studying the elastic properties of soft tissues (for example, porcine liver) and making the "Young's modulus map" is the subject of the further research.

ACKNOWLEDGMENT

The work is supported by Russian Foundation Basic Research Grant № 12-08-92005 and Program of the RAS #25.

CONFLICT OF INTEREST

The authors have no conflict of interest.

REFERENCES

1. Beccani M., Di Natali C., Sliker L.J., Schoen J., Rentschler M.E., Valdastri P. (2014) Wireless Tissue Palpation for Intraoperative Detection of Lumps in Soft Tissue. IEEE Transactions on Biomedical Engineering.61(2): 353-361
2. Hollenstein M., Bajka M., Rhrnbauer B., Badir S., MazzaE. (2012) Measuring the in vivo behavior of soft tissue and organs using the aspiration device. Soft Tissue Biomechanical Modeling for Computer Assisted Surgery. Heidelberg, 11: 201-228.
3. Goryacheva I.G., Martynenko Yu.G., Fong-Chin Su, Ryazantseva M.Yu., Antonov F.K. (2013) Analysis of contact interaction between artificial video-tactile sensor and soft biological tissue. Russian Journal of Biomechanics. Vol. 17, No. 1 (59): 5–17.

Author: M.M. Gubenko
Institute: Institute for Problems in Mechanics of Russian Academy of Sciences
Street: prosp. Vernadskogo 101, block 1
City: Moscow
Country: Russia
Email: maxgubenko@mail.ru

Author: I.G. Goryacheva
Institute: Institute for Problems in Mechanics of Russian Academy of Sciences
Street: prosp. Vernadskogo 101, block 1
City: Moscow
Country: Russia
Email: goryache@ipmnet.ru

Author: M.Z. Dosayev
Institute: Institute of Mechanics Lomonosov Moscow State University
Street: Michurinskiy prospekt, 1
City: Moscow
Country: Russia
Email: dosayev@imec.msu.ru

Author: A.V. Morozov
Institute: Institute for Problems in Mechanics of Russian Academy of Sciences
Street: prosp. Vernadskogo 101, block 1
City: Moscow
Country: Russia
Email: morozovalexei@mail.ru

Author: A.N. Lyubicheva
Institute: Institute for Problems in Mechanics of Russian Academy of Sciences
Street: prosp. Vernadskogo 101, block 1
City: Moscow
Country: Russia
Email: lyubicheva@mail.ru

Author: F.-C. Su
Institute: Department of Biomedical Engineering of National Cheng Kung University
Street: №1, University Road
City: Tainan
Country: Taiwan
Email: nckubme@gmail.com

Author: C.-H. Yeh
Institute: Department of Biomedical Engineering of National Cheng Kung University
Street: №1, University Road
City: Tainan
Country: Taiwan
Email: csyeh@itri.org.tw

Author: M.-S. Ju
Institute: Department of Mechanical Engineering of National Cheng Kung University
Street: No.1, Ta-Hsueh Road
City: Tainan
Country: Taiwan
Email: msju@mail.ncku.edu.tw

Risk Management of the New Dynamic Spinal Stabilization System

R.F. Kuo[1], C.J. Yang[1,*], R.M. Lin[2] and C.H. Weng[1]

[1] Medical Device Innovation Center, National Cheng Kung University, Tainan, Taiwan
[2] Orthopedics Department, National Cheng Jung University Hospital, Tainan, Taiwan

Abstract— **A risk management report is an important part of the technical documentation of any medical device since it contains the risks and hazards linked to use and how the manufacturer handled them for the purposes of performance and safety. For devices sold in Europe, EN ISO 14971 provides methods and tools for manufacturers to analyze and manage the risks associated with their devices. This study analyzes a new dynamic spinal stabilization system based on ISO 14971 to optimize the performances and safety of the new design.**

Keywords— **Dynamic Spinal Stabilization System, Risk Analysis, Risk Management, ISO14971.**

I. INTRODUCTION

The inherently risky nature of medical devices, especially those that come into contact with critical systems, means that manufacturers must thoroughly analyze their device risks against many factors. Risk management will help manufacturers identify hazards, prevent misuse, and estimate the risks for each hazard to better control and minimize these hazards [1].

A spinal stabilization system is usually used in the clinical treatment of degenerative spinal diseases and deformities, such as disc herniation, spinal fractures, and spondylolisthesis [2]. A growing number of clinical studies have indicated that the traditional spinal fusion surgery spinal fixation system unduly restricts vertebrae activity, resulting in concentration of stress on adjacent vertebrae, thus accelerating the degradation of adjacent vertebrae [3-4]. To remedy this situation, a dynamic stabilization system [5-7] with a non-fusion vertebral fixation device was developed. This provides better stability, and allows the affected vertebrae to have slight mobility to avoid stress concentration and consequent adjacent vertebrae degradation. This study aims to show the result of risk management in our new developed dynamic spinal stabilization system.

II. MATERIALS AND METHODS

On the following section including text and diagram is directly referenced from ISO 14971 [8]. The manufacturer shall establish, document and maintain throughout the life-cycle an ongoing process for identifying hazards associated with a medical device, estimating and evaluating the associated risks, controlling these risks, and monitoring the effectiveness of the controls. This process shall include the four main elements: risk analysis; risk evaluation; risk control; production and post-production information. A schematic representation of the risk management process is shown in Figure 1. Depending on the specific life-cycle phase, indi-vidual elements of risk management can have varying em-phasis. Also, risk management activities can be performed iteratively or in multiple steps as appropriate to the medical device.

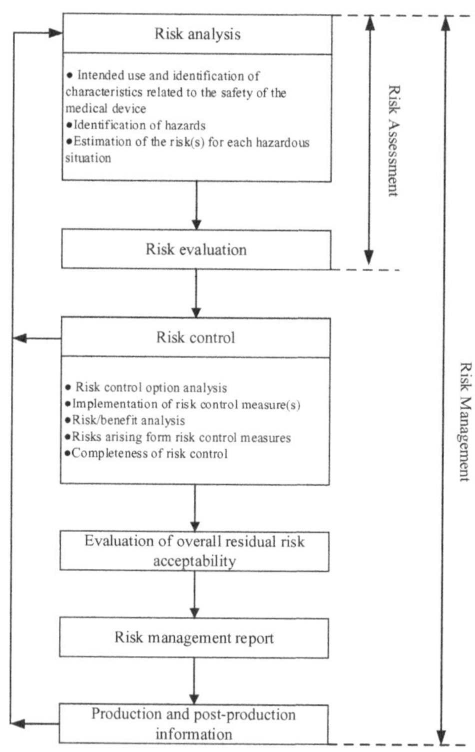

Fig. 1 A schematic representation of the risk management process

A. *Risk Analysis*

Risk analysis shall be performed for the particular medical device as described in step (a) to step (c). The implementation of the planned risk analysis activities and the results of the risk analysis shall be recorded in the risk management file.

[*] Corresponding author.

I. Lackovic (ed.), *1st Global Conference on Biomedical Engineering & 9th Asian-Pacific Conference on Medical and Biological Engineering*,
IFMBE Proceedings 47, DOI: 10.1007/978-3-319-12262-5_60

a) Intended Use and Identification of Characteristics Related to the Safety of the Medical

Identify and document those qualitative and quantitative characteristics that could affect the safety of the medical device and, where appropriate, their defined limits.

b) *Identification of Hazards*

Compile documentation on known and foreseeable hazards associated with the medical device in both normal and fault conditions.

c) *Estimation of the Risk(s) for Each Hazardous Situation*

Reasonably foreseeable sequences or combinations of events that can result in a hazardous situation shall be considered and the resulting hazardous situations shall be recorded.

B. Risk Evaluation

For each identified hazardous situation, the manufacturer shall decide, using the criteria defined in the risk management plan, if risk reduction is required. If risk reduction is not required, the requirements given in step (a) to step (e) do not apply for this hazardous situation (i.e., proceed to step (f)).

a) *Risk Control Option Analysis*

The manufacturer shall use one or more of the following risk control options in the priority order listed: (1) inherent safety by design; (2) protective measures in the medical device itself or in the manufacturing process; (3) information for safety.

b) *Implementation of Risk Control Measures*

The manufacturer shall implement the risk control measures selected in step (a). Implementation of each risk control measure shall be verified. The effectiveness of the risk control measures shall be verified.

c) *Residual Risk Evaluation*

After the risk control measures are applied, any residual risk shall be evaluated using the criteria defined in the risk management plan. If the residual risk is not judged acceptable using these criteria, further risk control measures shall be applied (see step (a)).

For residual risks that are judged acceptable, the manufacturer shall decide which residual risks to disclose and what information is necessary to include in the accompanying documents in order to disclose those residual risks.

d) *Risk/Benefit Analysis*

If the residual risk is not judged acceptable using the criteria established in the risk management plan and further risk control is not practicable, the manufacturer may gather and review data and literature to determine if the medical benefits of the intended use outweigh the residual risk. If this evidence does not support the conclusion that the medical benefits outweigh the residual risk, then the risk remains unacceptable. If the medical benefits outweigh the residual risk, then proceed to step (e).

For risks that are demonstrated to be outweighed by the benefits, the manufacturer shall decide which information for safety is necessary to disclose the residual risk.

e) *Risks Arising from Risk Control Measures*

The effects of the risk control measures shall be reviewed with regard to: (1) the introduction of new hazards or hazardous situations; (2) whether the estimated risks for previously identified hazardous situations are affected by the introduction of the risk control measures.

f) *Completeness of Risk Control*

Ensure that the risks from all identified hazardous situations have been considered. Compliance is checked by inspection of the risk management file.

C. Production and Post-production Information

Establish, document and maintain a system to collect and review information about the medical device or similar devices in the production and the post-production phases.

This study follows ISO 17971:2007 for risk assessment of the new dynamic spinal stabilization system. The process begins from identifying safety features, deciding impacts on safety and scoring the probability (Table 1) and qualitative severity levels (Table 2).

III. RESULTS AND DISCUSSION

A. Results

Table 1 Example of semi-quantitative probability levels

Common terms	Example of probability range	Scope
Frequent	$>10^{-3}$	5
Probable	10^{-3}~10^{-4}	4
Occasional	10^{-4}~10^{-5}	3
Remote	10^{-5}~10^{-6}	2
Improbable	$<10^{-3}$	1

Table 2 Example of five qualitative severity levels

Common terms	Possible description	Scope
Catastrophic	Results in patient death	5
Critical	Results in permanent impairment or life-threatening injury	4
Serious	Results in injury or impairment requiring professional medical intervention	3
Minor	Results in temporary injury or impairment not requiring professional medical intervention	2
Negligible	Inconvenience or temporary discomfort	1

a) Questionnaire Used to Identify the New Design Characteristics that could Impact on Safety:

Following ISO 14971:2007, the detailed safety assessment of the new design is listed in Table 3.

Table 3 The assessment of the new design characteristics

Num.	Question	Answer
1	What is the intended use and how is the medical device to be used?	(1) Recovery spinal stability, support, rotation and bending.
2	Is the medical device intended to be implant-ed?	Yes, implanted onto patients spine.
3	Is the medical device intended to be in contact with the patient or other persons?	(1) Implantation: Permanent contact with the spine implants (more than 30 days) (2) Tool: Invasive surgical equipment, short exposure (less than 24 hours)
4	What materials or components are utilized in the medical device or are used with, or are in contact with, the medical device?	Ultra-high-molecular-weight polyeth-ylene (UHMWPE) and Ti alloy
5	Is energy delivered to or extracted from the patient?	Not applicable
6	Are substances delivered to or extracted from the patient?	Not applicable
7	Are biological materials processed by the medical device for subsequent re-use, transfu-sion or transplantation?	Not applicable
8	Is the medical device supplied sterile or intended to be sterilized by the user, or are other microbiological controls applicable?	(1) Sterile implants following EN556-1 and EN552 standards (2) Non-sterile tools: manual should show the steps of removing contami-nants, cleaning and steam sterilization. (3) Implants: labeled instructions "Single use." (4) Tools: After cleaning and disinfec-tion, sterilization before use, manual should provide steam sterilization methods.
9	Is the medical device intended to be routinely cleaned and disinfected by the user?	Tools should be cleaned and disinfected before and after use every time, manual contains the explanatory of cleaned and disinfected; cleaning and disinfection methods have been confirmed.
10	Is the medical device intended to modify the patient environment?	Not applicable
11	Are measurements taken?	Not applicable
12	Is the medical device interpretative?	Not applicable
13	Is the medical device intended for use in conjunction with other medical devices, medicines or other medical technologies?	Only interaction between tools and implants, tools and implants supply together
14	Are there unwanted outputs of energy or substances?	Not applicable
15	Is the medical device susceptible to environ-mental influences?	Use the implant in an aseptic environ-ment. The implant is not affected by the environmental like temperature, light and vibration.
16	Does the medical device influence the environment?	Not applicable
17	Are there essential consumables or accessories associated with the medical device?	Only implants and tools
18	Is maintenance or calibration necessary?	Tools should be checked before use, and properly disassembled, cleaned and assembled
19	Does the medical device contain software?	No
20	Does the medical device have a restricted shelf-life?	Sterile Implants: Four years shelf life after the sterilization; the expiration date is marked on the packaging
21	Are there any delayed or long-term use effects?	The implant is planned for long-term use and not removed
22	To what mechanical forces will the medical device be subjected?	Consider the positive pressure force, positive tension force, torsion force in accordance with ASTM 1717.
23	What determines the lifetime of the medical device?	(1)Implant: long-term use and not removed (2) Tool: Multi frequency of use will gradually wear and loss of function; Multi frequency of sterilization will gradually corrode
24	Is the medical device intended for single use?	(1) Implant: Yes (2) Tool: It can be reused after removing the pollution and sterilizing. It takes steam way for sterilization.
25	Is safe decommissioning or disposal of the medical device necessary?	No
26	Does installation or use of the medical device require special training or special skills?	Use by a professional surgeons, including carefully selects the suitable sizes
27	How will information for safe use be provid-ed?	From the manual
28	Will new manufacturing processes need to be established or introduced?	Not applicable
29	Is successful application of the medical device critically dependent on human factors such as the user interface?	Not applicable
30	Does the medical device use an alarm system?	Not applicable
31	In what way(s) might the medical device be deliberately misused?	Not applicable
32	Does the medical device hold data critical to patient care?	Not applicable
33	Is the medical device intended to be mobile or portable?	Not mobile or portable
34	Does the use of the medical device depend on essential performance?	Not applicable

b) New Design Assessment Procedure

The assessment procedure entails: Defining the functional requirements of the implant spine; simulating the failure mode in accordance with the functions; assessing its probability of occurrence and severity; and performing risk control. The risk level is a function of the probability and severity. User should maintain all risk levels to fall under level C (Scope: 15~11).

c) Identify Failure Modes and Risk Control Functions of the New Design

The new design uses a metal balls arc linkage to provide universal rotation function. The patient's spine can do rotation, flexion, and lateral movements after surgery. Additionally, it can be fitted in patients with different lordosis angle to provide multi-selection of spinal implants. The new design uses outer cladding metal sleeve and uses ultra-high-molecular-weight polyethylene (UHMWPE) for elasticity. This can accelerate bone cell growth, increase the fixative effects and prevent the phenomenon of accelerated degradation. The outer cladding metal sleeve prevents exposure of internal parts, reducing risk to the patient. Tables 4 and 5 are the evaluation results of the functions in accordance with the requirements specification for risk analysis of the new dynamic spinal stabilization system.

Table 4 Function failure of the spinal system

Failure mode	Fixed Function	Buffering function	Spin function	Buckling function	Cover function
Severity	5	3	3	2	5
Probability	3	2	2	2	4
Risk Level	15	6	6	4	20
Risk Assess-ment	Loose screws	Elastic fatigue of UHMWPE	The coefficient of friction of metal balls is too high	Too rigid of the link rod	Metal sleeve embrittlement
Risk Control	Design anti-loose torque mechanism	The stiffness of materials are consistent with the standard	The coefficient of friction of materials are consistent with the standard	The Rigid of materials are consistent with the standard	Material properties are consistent with the standard
Phase	Design	Manufacturing	Manufacturing	Manufacturing	Manufacturing
Acceptable level of residual risk	5	3	3	2	5

Table 5 Equipment characteristics of the hazard sources

Failure mode	(Implantation) (Side effects) (Complications)	Physiological suited of patients Loss of clinical effective and safety	Incompatibility of the biological material
Severity	5	5	5
Probability	4	3	3
Risk Level	20	15	15
Risk Assess-ment	Surgery performed by a doctor; Each step should have a safety alert to help the doctor to evaluate	After implantation, probably loss the clinical effective due to personal exercise habits	The Sources of material and components should confirm
Risk Control	Doctors assess the risk of the patient in by the instructions	There are a variety of implant sizes, according to patient characteristics, carefully evaluate the types of specifi-cations	Material properties are consistent with the standard
Phase	Surgical stage	Usage phase	Manufacturing phase
Acceptable level of residual risk	5	10	5

B. Discussion

All potential hazards have been identified and analyzed for risk analysis. The risk levels of each hazard with unacceptable range have been remediated and to reduce risk to an acceptable range. The benefits of a new dynamic spinal stabilization system would be greater than the risks that may arise.

IV. CONCLUSIONS

The new dynamic spinal stabilization system should ensure that the design and manufacture under expected conditions of use will not harm patients. The manufacturer is required to follow these principles: (1) identify known hazards, estimate the risks arising from expected use or misuse; (2) minimize the risk by safety design and manufacturing; (3) take appropriate steps to reduce the residual risk as much as possible; (4) inform users of the residual risk.

ACKNOWLEDGMENT

This work is supported by the Southern Taiwan Science Park, Taiwan, under grant numbers: BZ-22-15-42-102.

CONFLICT OF INTEREST

The authors declare that they have no conflict of interest.

REFERENCES

1. Ciarkowski A (2006) Management for Medical Devices. Wiley Encyclopedia of Biomedical Engineering.
2. Panjabi, Manohar M (1992) The Stabilizing System of the Spine. Part I. Function, Dysfunction, Adaptation, and Enhancement, Vol. 5, No. 4.
3. Schlegel, J D, Smith, J A, Schleusener, R L, (1996) Lumbar Motion Segment Pathology Adjacent to Thoracolumbar, Lumbar, and Lumbosacral Fusions, Spine, Vol.21, No.8, pp.970-981.
4. Kumar M N, Baklanov A, Chopin D, (2001) Correlation between sagittal plane changes and adjacent segment degeneration following lumbar spine fusion, European spine journal, Vol. 10, pp.314-319.
5. Welch W C, Cheng B C, Awad T E et al. (2007) Clinical outcomes of the Dynesys dynamic neutralization system: 1-year preliminary results, Neurosurg Focus, Vol. 22, No.1.
6. Wilke H J, Heuer F, Schmidt H, (2009) Prospective design delineation and subsequent in vitro evaluation of a new posterior dynamic stabilization system, Spine, Vol.34 ,No.3, pp. 255–261.
7. Barrey C, Perrin G, Champain S, (2013) Pedicle-Screw-Based Dynamic Systems and Degenerative Lumbar Diseases: Biomechanical and Clinical Experiences of Dynamic Fusion with Iso-bar TTL, ISRN Orthopedics, 2013.
8. ISO 14971, (2000) Medical devices - Application of risk management to medical devices.

Author:	Rong-Fu, Kuo
Institute:	Medical Device Innovation Center
	Street: No.1, University Road
City:	Tainan City
Country:	Taiwan
Email:	wankuo@gmail.com
Author:	Cheng-Jung, Yang
Institute:	Medical Device Innovation Center
	Street: No.1, University Road
City:	Tainan City
Country:	Taiwan
Email:	benyang0521@gmail.com
Author:	Ruey-Mo, Lin
Institute:	National Cheng Jung University Hospital
	Street: No.1, University Road
City:	Tainan City
Country:	Taiwan
Email:	wechiu@ortho.clmed.ncku.edu.tw
Author:	Chen-Hsun, Weng
Institute:	Medical Device Innovation Center
	Street: No.1, University Road
City:	Tainan City
Country:	Taiwan
Email:	b88501113@gmail.com

One Piece Dental Implant Development

R.F. Kuo[1], C.J. Yang[1,*], and Z.S. Lin[2]

[1] Medical Device Innovation Center, National Cheng Kung University, Tainan, Taiwan
[2] ComMed Technologies Co., Ltd., Taipei, Taiwan

Abstract— **There are three common types of single tooth dental implant surgery. Bone level implant was first developed in 1965, and evolved to a simpler tissue level implant, which in turn, evolved into a one piece implant type. The structure of the one piece implant type combines the abutment and the fixture of an artificial tooth together. This study describes the current characteristics, surgical procedure, and issues of the one piece implant system, and explains how to resolve issues in the future.**

Keywords— **Artificial teeth, one piece implant, dental implant.**

I. INTRODUCTION

For single tooth implant surgery, bone level implant is the safest. Because after first surgery, the implant is completely buried under the gingival margin suture and the implant is completely isolated from external forces. Three to six months later when the implant and jawbone has fused together, the second surgery cuts the gums and affixes the abutment section by screw. Though this is the safest approach; patients have to do endure two surgeries, which is a burden on patients [1].

The tissue level implant type was developed after several years for better performance of the fixture part of an artificial tooth. The fixture part can be exposed a little above the gums. The exposed part can directly be used to connect the abutment without a second surgery. Even though this is simpler than bone level, it still uses a screw mechanism to lock the abutment to the fixture. Unfortunately, the screw mechanism is one of the biggest single point of failure for implants. The interaction between the two parts causes the screw mechanism to loosen from day life activities [1].

The greatest advantage of the one piece implant type is the integration the fixture and abutment. It does not require a screw mechanism so it is free from the loosening effect. This type of implant only needs one surgery. However, due to the base being directly exposed to the oral cavity, it is susceptible to external forces. It is difficult to guarantee the internal implant retainer completely rests in conjunction with bone tissue after a certain time. Infection occurs easily because of the direct contact with periodontal bone tissue. and is not conducive to the healing of the implant to the bone tissue and gum tissue interface. The success rate is not as good as Tissue level implant type [2]. Figure 1 shows the three types of single artificial tooth implant.

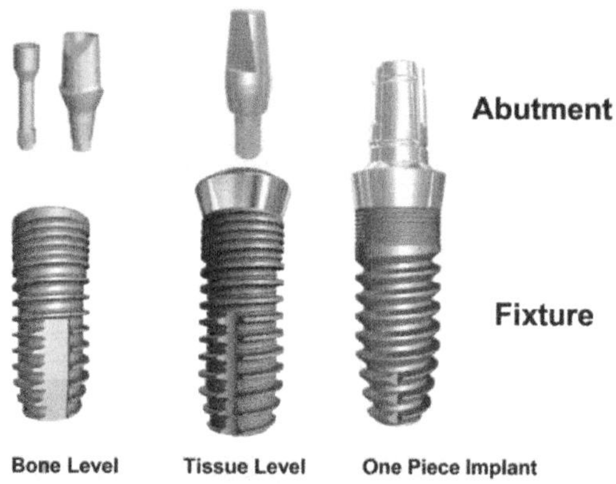

Fig. 1 Three types of single artificial teeth implant

II. MATERIALS AND METHODS

A. The Characteristics of the One Piece Dental Implant

The basic characteristics of one piece implants encompass the solid groove part, the solid segment part, the root part of the neck, fine thread fixed part, implant segment part, implant thread part, point end part of the implant thread and the chip occlusal grooves part. Tables 1 to 9 show the comparative characteristics of three systems from Biodenta, ComMed and OCO, B.M. [3-5].

Table 1 The side view drawing of the three products [3-5]

Biodenta	ComMed	OCO B.M.
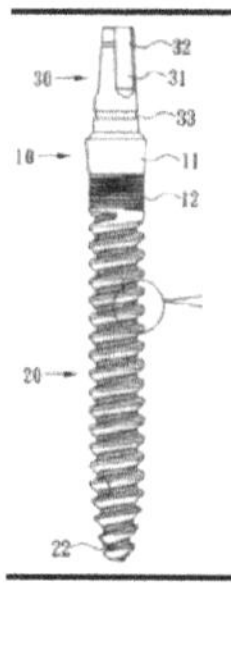	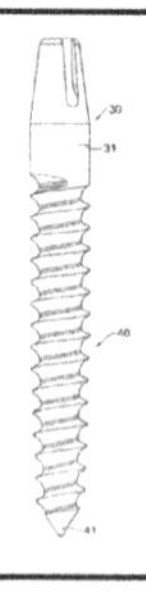	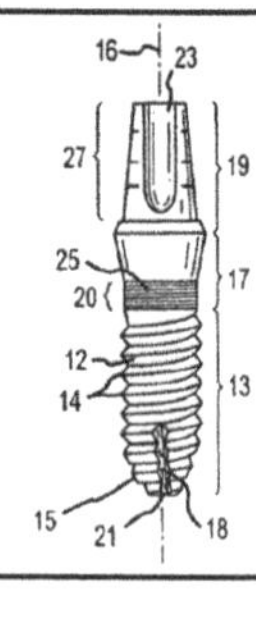

* Corresponding author.

I. Lackovic (ed.), *1st Global Conference on Biomedical Engineering & 9th Asian-Pacific Conference on Medical and Biological Engineering*,
IFMBE Proceedings 47, DOI: 10.1007/978-3-319-12262-5_61

Table 2 The solid groove part of the three products [3-5]

Biodenta	ComMed	OCO B.M.
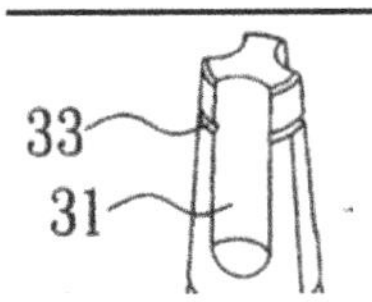	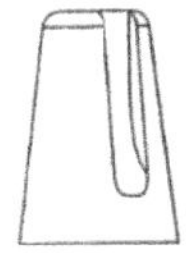	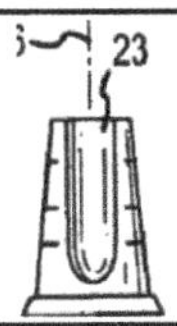
▪Spaced every 120 degrees ▪Length: at least 1.5 mm ▪Groove depth: 0.5 mm	▪Spaced every120 degrees	▪Spaced at 90 and 135 degrees

Table 3 The solid segment part of the three products [3-5]

Biodenta	ComMed	OCO B.M.
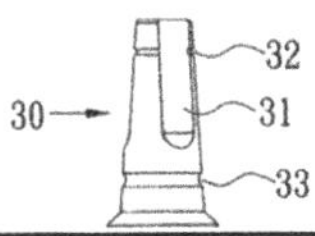	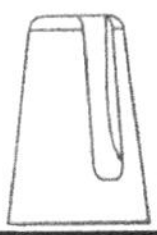	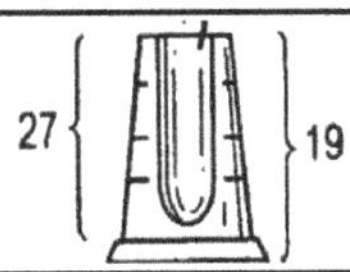
▪Outer diameter is reduce toward the back ▪A slot on the solid segment part ▪A solid impression groove between the solid segment and the end part	▪A abutment between the top and the neck of the solid segment part	▪Some slots on the solid segment part

Table 4 The root part of the neck of the three products [3-5]

Biodenta	ComMed	OCO B.M.
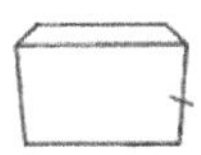	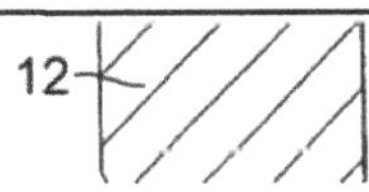	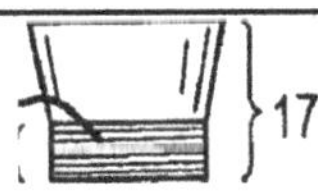
▪Spread shape ▪High polished surface ▪5 to 10 degrees inclination	▪Non spread shape	▪Continuously axial extension between the base and the main part

Table 5 The fine thread fixed part of the three products [3-5]

Biodenta	ComMed	OCO B.M.
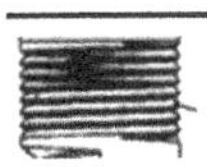	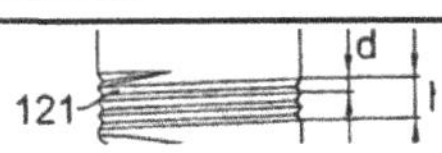	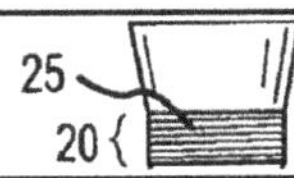
▪Fine Thread	▪Pitch ranged is from 0.22 to 0.27 mm; height is about 1.0 mm	▪Under the bulk collar ▪ 0.1 mm for the height; 0.2 mm for the pitch ▪Surface micro roughness process

Table 6 The implant segment part of the three products [3-5]

Biodenta	ComMed	OCO B.M.
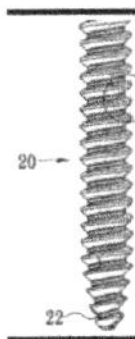	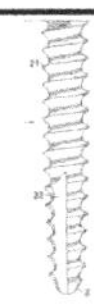	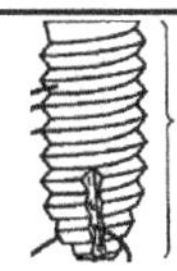
▪The sum length of the implant segment and the root neck of the implant segment is 22 mm ▪ 1 to 1.5 degrees roughly tilt tapered	▪Standard V shape thread ▪Rod diameter is 3.5 mm or 4.5 mm; length is 22 mm ▪Rod diameter is 5.6 mm; length is 18 mm	▪Diameter decreases by the distance ▪Obtuse is non-cutting end

Table 7 The implant thread part of the three products [3-5]

Biodenta	ComMed	OCO B.M.
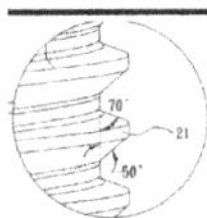	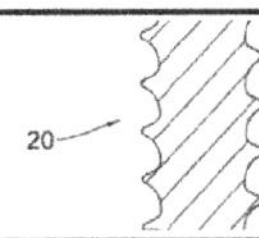	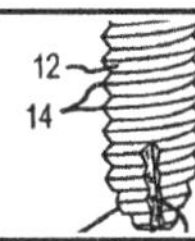
▪Trapezoidal thread ▪The angle between the front section and longitudinal axis is 50 degrees ▪The angle between the end section and longitudinal axis is 70 degrees	▪Standard V-thread ▪Rod diameter is 3.5 mm or 4.5 mm; length is prefer 22 mm ▪Rod diameter is 5.6 mm; length is prefer 18 mm ▪Extending away from the base body	▪Helical thread ▪The diameter range of outer thread is from 1.8 to 6 mm ▪Preferred length range of the threaded body is from 6 to 20 mm ▪Rough surface process

Table 8 The point end part of the implant thread of the three products [3-5]

Biodenta	ComMed	OCO B.M.
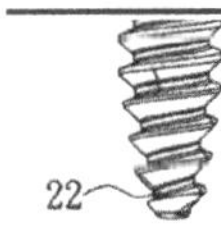	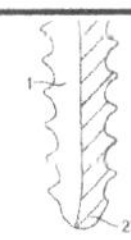	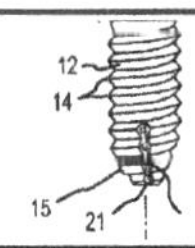
▪ Round slow end face ▪Occlusal grooves of complex chip	▪Blunt shape ▪Occlusal grooves of single chip	▪Obtuse is non-cutting end ▪Occlusal grooves of complex chip

Table 9 The chip occlusal grooves part of the three products [3-5]

Biodenta	ComMed	OCO B.M.
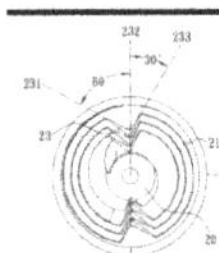	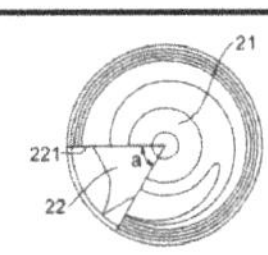	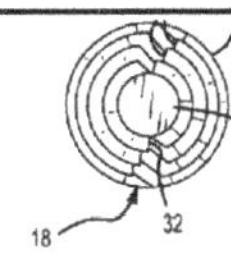
▪90 degrees of the side section ▪Two grooves	▪Side angle of the axially adjacent plane is between 59.5 and 60.5 degree ▪One groove	▪Two grooves ▪Two opposite longitudinal grooves

B. Surgical Procedure

The implant surgical procedure follows these five stages:

a) Make an incision for the dental implant

Incise along the top of the alveolar ridge under local anesthesia. Peel and fixate periosteal flap flips to fully expose bone surface and protect nerves.

b) Prepare the implant hole

Follow the pre-designed template; select a suitable length for the dental implant and the corresponding series of drills according to the amount of alveolar. Use fast speed drilling and flush with plenty of physiological saline. For positioning and drilling, use Round Burr. Gradually expand the implant hole by split diamond and navigation drilling, then expand the size of upper hole and wash the wound.

c) Introduce implant into the implant hole

Switch to slow drilling, flush with plenty of physiological saline to reduce temperature of the surrounding tissues. Use tap equipment to plant the screw on the bone wall of the implant hole.

d) Planting dental implant

Use the provided special tool to slowly and carefully tighten the dental implant into the prepared implant hole; . Make sure the top edge of the dental implant is flat with the bone surface.

e) Suture wounds

Use mattress suture for the mucoperiosteal flap. Make sure the periosteal layer is inside when performing the suture. Completely cover the top of dental implant without tension. Patients can wear temporary dentures after the stitches. After 4-6 weeks until implant stability, take the module and complete the final restoration.

III. RESULTS AND DISCUSSION

The structure of the one piece implant type combines the abutment and the fixture of an artificial tooth together without using screws so it does not require a second surgery. However, the implant faces forces in the oral cavity during the healing time for jawbone interface. This may reduce the success rate. Another drawback is the one piece dental implant cannot provide custom implant angles or special abutments.

IV. CONCLUSIONS

Although the three types of surgical implants has their own advantages and disadvantages, the trend of implant technology is going towards simplicity. The next trend for a one piece implant system will be to focus on designing a variety of abutment angles for use in canines and incisors. Another idea is to develop an easy method for positioning and placing the dental implant at correct height and rotational angle.

ACKNOWLEDGMENT

This work is supported by the ComMed Technologies Co., Ltd.

CONFLICT OF INTEREST

The authors declare that they have no conflict of interest.

REFERENCES

1. Consumer guide to dentistry at http://www.yourdentistryguide.com/implant-types/
2. Biodenta Swiss Ag, at http://www.biodenta.com/index.php? option=com_content&view=article&id=137&Itemid=128&lang=en-GB
3. Biodenta Swiss Ag, (2012) Dental implant, WO2012027879 A1.
4. ComMed Technologies Co., Ltd. (2012) Taiwan implant, Inventive Patent, Number: 098118524.
5. OCO Biomedical Inc., (2012) Screw-type dental implant, US8277218 B2.

Author: Rong-Fu, Kuo
Institute: Medical Device Innovation Center
Street: No.1, University Road
City: Tainan City
Country: Taiwan
Email: wankuo@gmail.com

Author: Cheng-Jung, Yang
Institute: Medical Device Innovation Center
Street: No.1, University Road
City: Tainan City
Country: Taiwan
Email: benyang0521@gmail.com

Author: Zhi-Sheng, Lin
Institute: ComMed Technologies Co., Ltd.
Street: 6F., No.48, Sec. 2, Ren'ai Road
City: Taipei
Country: Taiwan
Email: susan@commed.com.tw

A Laser Ablation End-Effector with Multiple Degrees of Freedom for Minimally Invasive Surgery

Baiquan Su, Zhan Shi, and Hongen Liao

Department of Biomedical Engineering/School of Medicine, Tsinghua University, Beijing, China

Abstract— **A surgical tool with multiple degrees of freedom is designed, working as a laser ablation end-effector for minimally invasive surgery. The end-effector mainly consists of four springs which provide multiple degrees of freedom and four flexible shafts which contracts or extends four springs. The mechanical configuration of the designed end-effector is detailed presented and the mathematical model is formulated. The prototype of the end-effector is built and its motion performance is tested.**

Keywords— **Minimally Invasive Surgery, End-effector, Laser Ablation.**

I. INTRODUCTION

Laser ablation is one of the promising methods removing tumor or cancer, such as colorectal cancer [1], brain cancer [2], for the reason that lesion can be coagulated by laser's high power energy in a restricted area. Some researchers devoted their effort to develop some laser ablations modules or systems for open or minimally invasively surgical applications. Su et al designed a micro laser ablation system integrated with image sensor for minimally invasive surgery [3]. Ben-Yakar designed a micro laser module which integrated several optical lens into a module with the overall diameter of 4 mm [4]. Theisen-Kunde et al designed a new laser scalpel for laparoscopic surgery [5]. Yamashita et al developed a miniature bending manipulator for fetoscopic intrauterine laser therapy to treat twin-to-twin transfusion syndrome [6]. However, the optical and mechanical configuration of the abovementioned modules and systems are fixed, i.e., the optical axis is motionless with respect to the module or system. It is not convenient for the modules and systems to perform laser ablation in irregular inner organ channel.

To overcome this disadvantage, several researchers targeted to develop modules and systems which are with multiple degree of freedom. Liao et al designed an automatic focusing and robotic scanning mechanism for precision laser ablation in neurosurgery [2]. However, the laser ablation system is not appropriate for minimally invasively surgeries due to its larger size, although the system is with multiple degree of freedom. Thus, it is necessary to reduce the size of the laser ablation module and keep multiple degree of freedom. In other words, for the sake of flexible operation in confined space, including inner organ or tissue, it is necessary to design a laser ablation end-effector with small size and multiple degree of freedom.

On the other hand, operation failure and malfunction of surgical tools, especially failures of the end-effector of surgical apparatuses, may severely hurt organ or tissue, if all the joints of the surgical tools and apparatus are rigid. It is convenient and preferable for surgical tools and apparatus to have both flexibility and elasticity which can protect organ and tissue. Spring can flexibly transfer force and torque, also it can change directions of force and torque. Furthermore, when it contact object, it can deform and reduced the shock on the object. The advantages of spring is its passive deformation under external force. The characteristics of spring are beneficial to protect soft organ and tissue when spring is used to interact with them. Simultaneously, omni-direction bending motion of spring is beneficial for providing multiple degrees of freedom. Researchers take the advantage of spring in surgical device designs [7], [8], [9], [10].

In this paper, we design a new laser ablation module whose system configuration is different to that in [3] to overcome the lack of degree of freedom of the existing laser ablation modules. We mainly use four springs to realize the multiple degree of freedom of the system and four flexible shafts to change positions of the springs.

The rest of the paper is organized as follows. The mechanical configuration of the designed end-effector is presented in detailed in the section II. The mathematical model of the proposed system is derived under some assumptions in section III. The prototype of the end-effector is built and its basic motion performance is tested in section IV. Concluding remarks and future work are given in the last section.

II. SYSTEM CONFIGURATION

The end-effector consists of four springs and the auxiliary mechanical components. There are seven typical components in the proposed end-effector shown in figure 1, i.e., the outer-cover, the front table, the four springs, the four drawing bars, the bottom table, the fixture bolt, and the four flexible shafts. There exists one-to-one correspondence between every pair of drawing bar and spring, and that between every pair of drawing bar and flexible shaft. The optical fiber which transfer laser beam is not shown in figure 1.

I. Lackovic (ed.), *1st Global Conference on Biomedical Engineering & 9th Asian-Pacific Conference on Medical and Biological Engineering*,
IFMBE Proceedings 47, DOI: 10.1007/978-3-319-12262-5_62

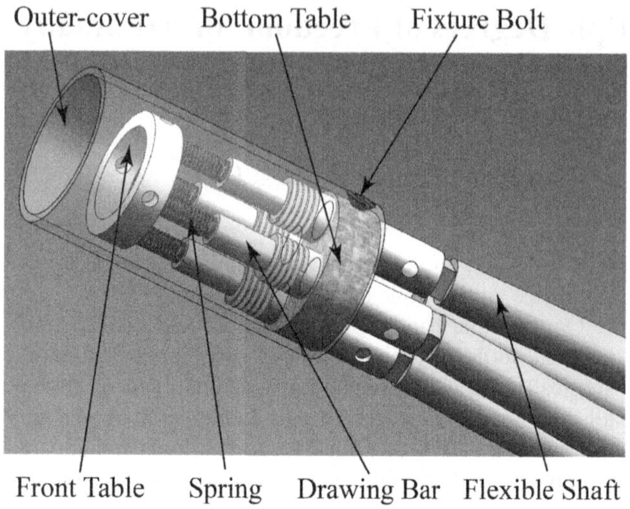

Fig. 1 System configuration.

The general motion procedure of the laser ablation module is stated as follows:

1) The flexible shafts are moved according to a prescribed gait,
2) the drawing bars extend or retract with the lengths determined by the prescribed gait in the first step,
3) each spring will move under the force of its corresponding drawing bar and front table, and
4) the front table will be in a preferred posture, i.e., position and orientation, due to the force transferred by the springs.

The Hooke's coefficient of springs is chosen based on the tool-tissue interaction of the organ where the proposed end-effector are operated.

III. MATHEMATICAL MODEL

Assume that the motion of the springs is slow, thus the dynamic effect of the springs are neglected. We analyze the model of the module in this section. The origin O of the coordinate $O\text{-}XYZ$ is at the intersection point between the axis of fiber and the plane Γ.

The bottom ends of the four springs are B_1, B_2, B_3 and B_4, and the front ends of the four springs are U_1, U_2, U_3 and U_4, respectively. The x-axis and y-axis of coordinate frame $O\text{-}XYZ$ are parallel to vector $\overrightarrow{B_2B_1}$ and $\overrightarrow{B_1B_3}$, respectively. The translational distances of the springs are δ_1, δ_2, δ_3 and δ_4, respectively. The schematic diagram of the module is shown in figure 2.

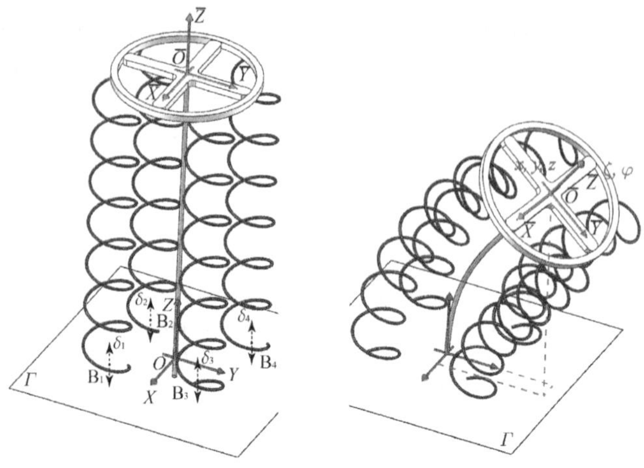

Fig. 2 Schematic for mathematical modeling.

To determine the orientation of the front table, we allocate a local coordinate $\overline{O}\text{-}\overline{XYZ}$ to it. The origin of $\overline{O}\text{-}\overline{XYZ}$ is at center of the front table, and the axes are parallel and with same positive directions to that of the coordinate $O\text{-}XYZ$ i.e., when the springs are at initial states and the translational distances of the drawing bars are all zero. The position of the center of the front table is $\{x; y; z\}$ and the yaw and pitch angles of the plane of the front table with respect to the horizontal plane Γ are $\{\phi; \theta; \psi\}$, respectively.

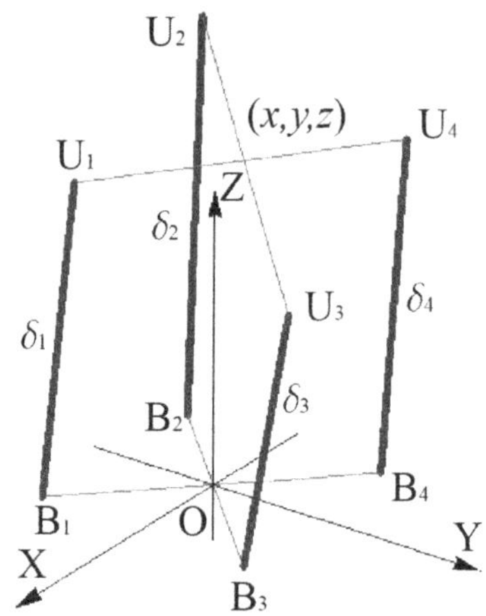

Fig. 3 Analysis of force and torque of spring deformation.

To drive the front table to a pair of desired position and orientation, the control inputs $U = \{u_1; u_2; u_3; u_4\}$ are the position of B_1, B_2, B_3 and B_4. The coordinates of the bottom ends of the springs are $B_1 = \{\bar{d}; -\bar{d}; u_1\}$, $B_2 = \{-\bar{d}; -\bar{d}; u_2\}$, $B_3 = \{-\bar{d}; \bar{d}; u_3\}$ and $B_4 = \{\bar{d}; \bar{d}; u_4\}$, where $\bar{d}$ is a constant distance which is determined by mechanical design. At the initial state, the coordinates of the upper ends of the springs are

$\overline{U}_1 = \{d, -d, \overline{H}\}$, $\overline{U}_2 = \{-d, -d, \overline{H}\}$, $\overline{U}_3 = \{-d, d, \overline{H}\}$ and $\overline{U}_4 = \{d, d, \overline{H}\}$, where $\overline{H}$ is the natural length of the springs. Assume there only exists axial deformation of springs as shown in figure 3.

By using the position $\{x, y, z\}$ and the orientation $\{\phi, \theta, \psi\}$ of the front table, we can obtain the positions of the upper ends of the springs as follows, i.e.,

U_1, U_2, U_3, U_4

$$U_1 = \begin{pmatrix} d\sin\phi\cos\psi - d\cos\theta\sin\phi\sin\psi + d\cos\phi(\cos\psi + \cos\theta\sin\psi) + \overline{h}_x \\ -d\cos\theta\cos\psi(\cos\phi - \sin\phi) + d\cos\phi\sin\psi + d\sin\phi\sin\psi + \overline{h}_y \\ -d\cos\phi\sin\theta + d\sin\theta\sin\phi + \overline{h}_z \end{pmatrix} \quad (1)$$

$$U_2 = \begin{pmatrix} d\sin\phi\cos\psi + d\cos\theta\sin\phi\sin\psi + \overline{h}_x + d\cos\phi(\cos\theta\sin\psi - \cos\psi) \\ -d\cos\theta\cos\psi(\cos\phi + \sin\phi) - d\cos\phi\sin\psi + d\sin\phi\sin\psi + \overline{h}_y \\ -d\cos\phi\sin\theta - d\sin\theta\sin\phi + \overline{h}_z \end{pmatrix} \quad (2)$$

$$U_3 = \begin{pmatrix} -d\cos\psi\sin\phi + d\cos\theta\sin\phi\sin\psi - d\cos\phi(\cos\psi + \cos\theta\sin\psi) + \overline{h}_x \\ d\cos\theta\cos\psi(\cos\phi - \sin\phi) - d\cos\phi\sin\psi - d\sin\phi\sin\psi + \overline{h}_y \\ d(\sin\theta)(\cos\phi) - d(\sin\theta)(\sin\phi) + \overline{h}_z \end{pmatrix} \quad (3)$$

$$U_4 = \begin{pmatrix} -d\cos\psi\sin\phi - d\cos\theta\sin\phi\sin\psi + d\cos\phi(\cos\psi - \cos\theta\sin\psi) + \overline{h}_x \\ d\cos\theta\cos\psi(\cos\phi + \sin\phi) + d\cos\phi\sin\psi - d\sin\phi\sin\psi + \overline{h}_y \\ d\sin\theta\cos\phi + d\sin\theta\sin\phi + \overline{h}_z \end{pmatrix} \quad (4)$$

where, U_1, U_2, U_3 and U_4 are the coordinates of the upper ends of the springs, and $\overline{H} = \{\overline{h}_x, \overline{h}_y, \overline{h}_z\}$. Thus, the distances between the upper ends and the bottom ends of the four springs are

$$\delta_i = \|B_i U_i\|, i = 1, 2, 3, 4 \quad (5)$$

The detailed formulae in equation (5) are omitted here for space consideration.

Next, we analyze the force and torque condition of the module. The force and torque relationships should also be guaranteed for a static system. We neglect the elastic coefficient of the optical fiber and the lateral deformation due to springs bending. The Hooke's coefficient of the springs is k_i, $i = 1, 2, 3, 4$. We derive the equation of the module model in the following. According to Hooke's law, the forces of springs are $-k_i\delta_i$, $i = 1, 2, 3, 4$. The directions of the forces of the springs are $\overrightarrow{B_iU_i}$, $i = 1, 2, 3, 4$. According to the formulae of distance between two skew lines

$$l = \overrightarrow{MN} \cdot \frac{u \times v}{|u \times v|} \quad (6)$$

where M and N are arbitrary points on the skew lines respectively, and u and v are arbitrary vectors along the skew lines respectively. Thus, the equilibrium equations for torques with respect to axes OX, OY and OZ are respectively

$$\sum_{i=1}^{4} k_i\delta_i l_{x_i} = 0, \quad \sum_{i=1}^{4} k_i\delta_i l_{y_i} = 0 \text{ and } \sum_{i=1}^{4} k_i\delta_i l_{z_i} = 0 \quad (7)$$

where l_{x_i}, l_{y_i} and l_{z_i}, $i = 1, 2, 3, 4$ are torque arms of spring force with respect to axes OX, OY and OZ, respectively. The equilibrium conditions for spring forces are

$$\begin{cases} \sum_{i=1}^{n} k_i\delta_i(\overrightarrow{U_iB_i} \cdot \vec{i}) = 0 \\ \sum_{i=1}^{n} k_i\delta_i(\overrightarrow{U_iB_i} \cdot \vec{j}) = 0 \\ \sum_{i=1}^{n} k_i\delta_i(\overrightarrow{U_iB_i} \cdot \vec{k}) = 0 \end{cases} \quad (8)$$

where $\vec{i}$, $\vec{j}$ and $\vec{k}$ are unit vectors along axes OX, OY and OZ, respectively. Thus, given a group of control inputs U, we will obtain $\{x, y, z\}$ and $\{\phi, \theta, \psi\}$ of the front table by solving equation (7) and (8). The detailed formulae of $\{x, y, z\}$ and $\{\phi, \theta, \psi\}$ are omitted here for space consideration.

IV. PROTOTYPIC VERIFICATION

A simplified experimental prototype of the laser ablation module is built to check its basic motion performance and verify its feasibility of multiple degrees of freedom. The prototype of the laser ablation module is shown in figure 4, where α represents the bending angle of the module.

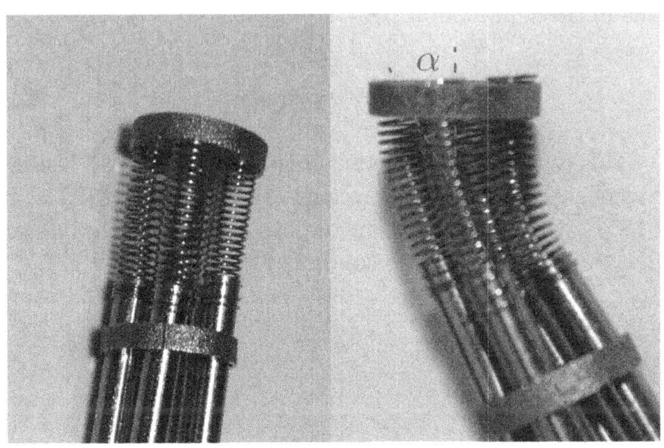

Fig. 4 Simplified prototype of the proposed end-effector.

The overall diameter of the prototypic end-effector is 10 millimeters, and the outer diameter of the springs are 6 millimeters. It should be mentioned that the sizes of the experimental module could be further minimized by using smaller springs. The spring is with length is 10 millimeters and the diameter of the spring is 2.93 millimeters. The maximum of the inclined angle ® is 55± shown in table 1. From the results in table I, the pitch and yaw angles of the proposed module are both 55±. Thus, the module is with multiple rotational degrees of freedom, and the overall angle of the module is 110 ± which can cover 61% (=110±/180±) of the front space of the laser ablation module. The workspace of the module is the inner of the cone with the apex angle 110±.

Table 1 Experimental Results

Workspace	Size
Diameter	6 millimeters
Length	12 millimeters
Pitch Angle	55±
Yaw Angle	55±

V. CONCLUSIONS

The snake robot surgical end-effector designed is with multiple degree of freedom for minimally invasive surgery. It is demonstrated the effectiveness of the multiple degrees of freedom laser ablation module proposed. The bending angle could be enlarged by using longer springs. The prototype of the module is with the maximal bending angle 55±.

In future, we will analyze the tool-tissue interaction force exerted to the organ and tissue. Moreover, we will check the feasibility of the proposed design which employs three, five or more springs and implement performance analysis which is similar to that developed in this paper. We implement more detailed experiments which are neglected in this paper due to space limitation.

ACKNOWLEDGMENT

This work was supported in part by National Natural Science Foundation of China (Grant No. 81271735, 61361160417) and Grant-in-Aid of Project 985. The authors declare that they have no conflict of interest.

REFERENCES

1. Puls R, Langner S, Rosenberg C, et al (2009) Laser ablation of liver metastases from colorectal cancer with MR thermometry: 5-year survival. J Vasc Interv Radiol, 20(2):225–234
2. Liao H, Noguchi M, Maruyama T, et al (2010) Automatic focusing and robotic scanning mechanism for precision laser ablation in neurosurgery. In IEEE/RSJ International Conference on Intelligent Robots and Systems (IROS), 2010, pp 325–330
3. Su B, Shi Z, Liao H (2014) A novel laser ablation module for minimally invasive surgery, IROS2014, accepted
4. Ben-Yakar A (2013) Image-guided ultrafast laser scalpel for precise and minimally invasive surgery. in CLEO: 2013. Optical Society of America, 2013, p. CM4H.3.
5. Theisen-Kunde D, Ott V, Brinkmann R, et al (2007) Potential of a new cw 2um laser scalpel for laparoscopic surgery. Med Laser Appl, vol. 22(2):139–145
6. Yamashita H, Matsumiya K, Masamune K, et al (2008) Miniature bending manipulator for fetoscopic intrauterine laser therapy to treat twin-to-twin transfusion syndrome. Surgical Endoscopy, 22(2): 430–435
7. Misra S, Ramesh K, and Okamura A (2008) Modeling of tool-tissue interactions for computer-based surgical simulation: A literature review, Presence: Teleoper. Virtual Environ 17(5): 463–491
8. Cianchetti M, Ranzani T, Gerboni G, et al (2013) Stiff-flop surgical manipulator: Mechanical design and experimental characterization of the single module, in Intelligent Robots and Systems (IROS), 2013 IEEE/RSJ International Conference on, Nov 2013, pp. 3576–3581.
9. Kota S, Lu K, Kreiner Z, et al (2005) Design and Application of Compliant Mechanisms for Surgical Tools, Journal of Biomechanical Engineering, 127(6):981–989
10. Tantanawat T and Kota S (2006) Design of Compliant Mechanisms for Minimizing Input Power in Dynamic Applications," Journal of Mechanical Design, 129(10):1064–1075

Author: Baiquan Su, Zhan Shi, [Hongen. Liao]
Institute: Department of Biomedical Engineering/School of Medicine, Tsinghua University
Street: South Street, Haidian District
City: Beijing
Country: China
Email: baiquansu@tsinghua.edu.cn, liao@tsinghua.edu.cn

A Home Rehabilitation Platform for Child Articulation Disorder

M.M. Lo[1], T. Chou[1], M.H. Yang[1], H.Y. Ho[2], E.K. Lee[2], J.H. Lin[3], and S.T. Tang[1,*]

[1]Department of Biomedical Engineering, Ming Chuan University, Taoyuan, Taiwan
[2] Division of Rehabilitation Medicine, Tao Yuan General Hospital, Taoyuan, Taiwan
[3] Department of Electronic Engineering, Kun Shan University, Tainan, Taiwan

Abstract— **I Speech therapy is usually treated in the hospital by language therapist, but the home practice is also very important. The cooperation of parents and therapists would help children have a better effect. In this study, a home-practice platform is developed, which provides a collection of the correct pronunciations, practice methods and pronounce evaluations. As a result, the platform could enhance the progress of treatment and provide home exercises more resources for parents and children.**

Keywords— **Articulation disorder, Speech therapy, Home rehabilitation.**

I. INTRODUCTION

The Articulation disorder for the children is about 50% to 70%. According to the normal development process, the children of 3.5 to 4 years old can pronounce the most of the words, but the individual differences still exist. If the children of 3.5 years old are found that speak with lisp problem, which should be concerned. If kids are more than four years old still inarticulate phenomenon that should accept the language assessment and treatment. If parent find child has a lisp situation can go to ENT (Ear, Nose, and Throat) or plastic surgery to check for organ defects. The organ problems should be treated by surgery, and then speech rehabilitation is necessary. The most appropriate age for language therapy is in the age of 4–6. In order to avoid the inarticulate problems cause child suffering from inferiority complex and classmates ridiculed, that will affect children's mental health, relationships, and may even affect learning [1].

Speech Therapy is a highly personalized and time-consuming treatment process. Speech therapists should arrange the treatment course according to the individual situation. To effectively treat speech disorder, the first condition is a large number of language therapists. Next is the rich of the treat materials, and accompanied by a high efficiency personalized treatment planning, and followed effectively tracking and evaluating. However, the insufficient of the language therapists is a common situation [2]. Enderby and Pickstone was assessed at least 26.2 speech therapists is needed for every 100,000 population [3]. But in Taiwan, which is much lower than that. There is only about 1.6 language therapists per 100,000 population, and the distribution of these therapists are very uneven. Most of the therapists are concentrated in the medical center and language rehabilitation institutes. Speech therapy is severely limited in time and place. Therefore, the treatment, follow-up monitoring, and evaluation are quite limited. In addition, although the speech therapist can teach patients to help their child, but the effectiveness is deeply depending on whether the patient could consistently carry out home practice. According to the present way of speech therapy, whether regularly home practice or the practice way is correct? There are still unknown before the next hospital visiting. As a result, the effectiveness of treatment has its blind spots. Therefore, speech therapy after the treatment course, the patient must help their children for long-term home practice in order to continuously improve the pronouncement.

In summary, the problems of the treatment for children with articulation disorder is shown in Fig.1, and the purpose of this study is to propose solutions for overcoming these problems; shown the yellow arrows.

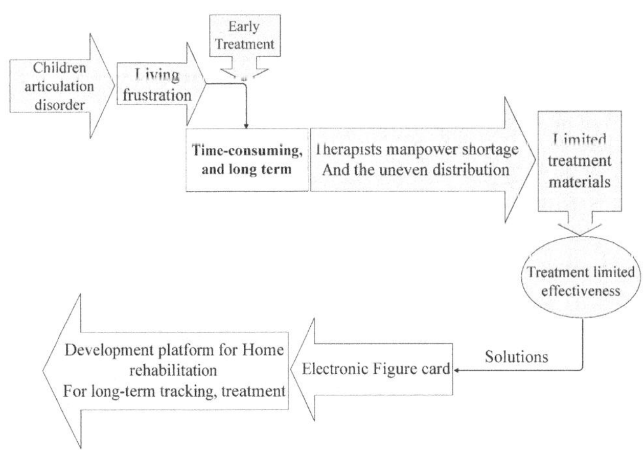

Fig. 1 Children dysarthria problems and proposed solutions.

For speech therapy, in addition to the hospital treatment weekly, the home practice is also necessary. Therefore, we focused on improving the home practice, to develop a platform for home assistant to effectively in home practice.

* Corresponding author.

I. Lackovic (ed.), *1st Global Conference on Biomedical Engineering & 9th Asian-Pacific Conference on Medical and Biological Engineering*,
IFMBE Proceedings 47, DOI: 10.1007/978-3-319-12262-5_63

This platform contains the correct pronunciations and practice methods, which is implemented in a tablet accessible computer.

II. METHODS

First we would describe the design of the speech rehabilitation processes, next is the proposed architecture and user interface; including the verbal rehabilitation platform, accessible computer and application software (APP), and finally addresses the treatment materials, treatment assessment, and the clinical trials.

Generally the dysarthria child needs speech therapy. Speech language therapist (SLT) would teach the patient children to practice and arrange home practice materials. Regularly the patient's revisit of hospital weekly. So that the SLT could understand the effectiveness of practice and would adjust the home practice course. Basically the patient's home practice is the key to improve the dysarthria. As a result, the developed speech rehabilitation platform is designed to help in home practice, which would provide the practice course and record the progress of home practice, then the SLT would realize the status of home practice. Fig.2 shows the whole processes.

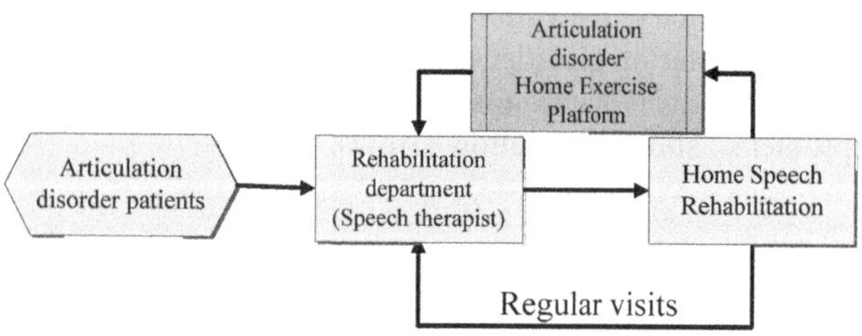

Fig. 2 Patients with dysarthria speech rehabilitation processes.

To help patients in effectively home practice, the basic requirements of the speech rehabilitation platform are as follows:

- The convenience of use: The eBook form of the treatment materials would easy update content and modify the user interface.
- With learning feedback: integrating the perceptual evaluation of speech quality (PESQ) method to evaluate the intelligibility and the APP interactive voice technology that would interest the patient children. In the past, the patient who practice by himself in home. Because of unknown the effectiveness of practice, that would decrease the motivation of practice. Learning feedback allows the patient to immediately understand practice effectiveness, which would be very progressive and strengthened. It can motivate patients to proactively practice [4].
- Record practice progresses and storage functions: As home practice is the key of speech rehabilitation, thus recording practice progress can understood the home practice situations: such as the number of practice, each practice time, practice effects. When patient is in practice, the entire progress will be recorded and stored in the tablet computer. And then the SLT would realize the practice circumstances when the patient backs to the hospital. The SLT could modify the home practice course according with to records.

On-line treatment materials updateable: In fact, each patient's home practice situation would not the same. Some people practice well, but others do not. If the treatment materials don't suit to the patient, the materials can be updated on-line to avoid the practice dela

A. Home Rehabilitation Processes

The process of the home speech rehabilitation is shown in Fig.3. After the program's initialization, firstly the home environment background noise is determined. (Currently speech therapist suggested 50dB of threshold). If the background noise is too large, it will advise the patient to choose another room for practice. If the background noise is in the acceptable range, you will enter the "MENU" screen; the practice options include oral motion exercises [5], tone exercises, words practice, idioms practice, sentences practice, practice review and ending the program. The default option is the Tones exercises, which includes volume practice and intelligibility practice.

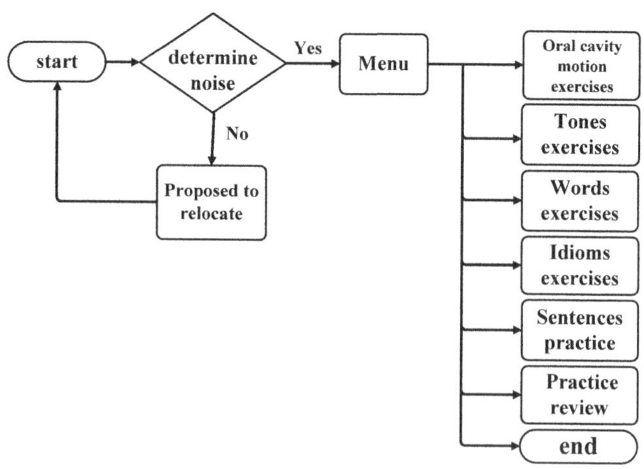

Fig. 3 Home Exercises speech rehabilitation of processes.

B. Speech Rehabilitation Information Platform

The whole system is in a typical architecture of the Android environment, the application is developed by Android APP tools. There is a database in the platform, where stores the patient demographic data, process records, treatment corpus, and statistical reports. Patient demographic data are entered by the SLT or directly linked the hospital information system. Primarily the SLT would determine the abnormal pronounces of the patient children, and then prepares the treatment corpus that would download to the platform database.

C. Accessible Hardware Interface

At the beginning, the personal computer (PC) was operated by the keyboard, which are with high learning barriers. As a result, the graphical user interface and mouse were introduced. Even the mouse that is still difficult to the people who firstly used it. Microsoft Windows operating system associated with the games of "Solitaire" and "Step to the Radar" are for training the mouse skills of click, double click, drag, etc. But for the younger children, the mouse is still an obstacle. The traditional PC is not suitable to the dysarthria children. This research proposed the tablet PC to develop the home rehabilitation platform, which is easy use and without training. The tablet computer does not need the keyboard or mouse, and have not complex signal lines, power lines. The tablet computer is an interactive gesture-based screen interface. Using the tablet computer only need the finger or fingers, which are very friendly to the children. This study used the Android tablet computer to develop the rehabilitation platform for the younger dysarthria children.

III. RESULT

The screen of the system main menu is shown in Fig. 4. "Oral motion exercises" is for presenting the SLT pre-recorded videos, which would show the mouth and tongue positions according with pronunciation. The patient can continue self-review at home by these videos. "Tone Exercise" is for the practices of some special pronounces, which provides the pronounce tips and the associated voice files and the system would evaluate the patient's pronunciation providing the feedback to the patient. "Word Exercises (Fig.5)" is for mono tone exercise, which as well provides patients with the right pronunciation and feedback. "Idiom Exercises (Fig.6)" and "Sentence Exercises," "Tone Exercises" and "Word Exercises" are the advance course for practice. "Exercise Review" is to realize the statuses of the past practice. In the next hospital visit, the records of the patient's home exercises can be inspected by the SLT, and the treatment course would be adjusted.

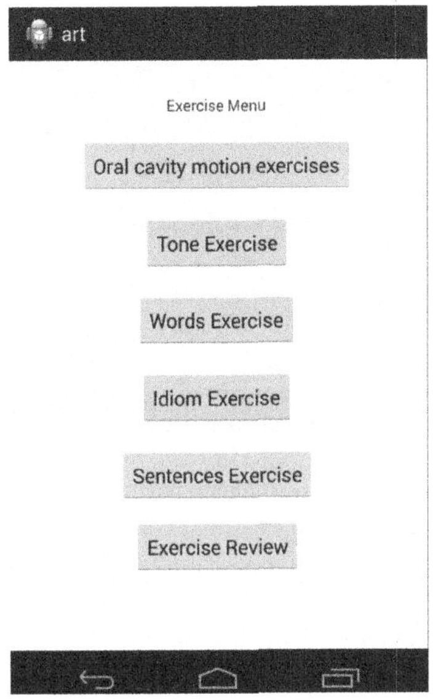

Fig. 4 Exercise Menu

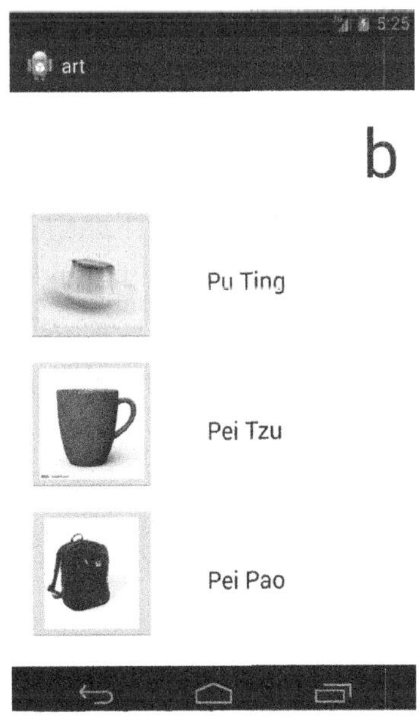

Fig. 5 Words exercise.

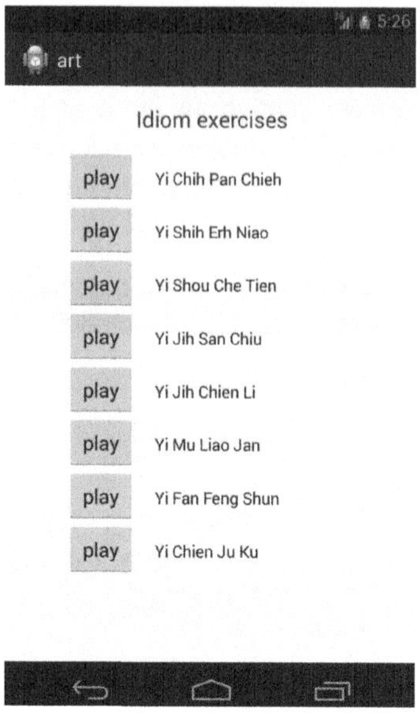

Fig. 6 Idioms practice.

IV. CONCLUSIONS

There are already other pronunciation exercises platforms [6, 7, 8], but they are all lack of feedback and progress records or convenience usage. Therefore, this study focused on that, which. Would encourage patient to continuously practice and record the full home practice progress. The developed platform provides more resources for patient children and the parents, and the effectiveness of the home exercises.

Articulation disorder is very negative factor on the child's development, which also affect the patient's mental and physical state. This developed platform for home speech rehabilitation acts as an auxiliary tool. This would improve and strengthen the home practice. The SLT is thus can keep track of the patient's home practice quality and quantity. For the end of the hospital treatment course, the developed platform can provide persistent practice to maintain the effectiveness. Therefore, improving the quality of life for the patient will be meaningful.

CONFLICT OF INTEREST

The authors declare that they have no conflict of interest

REFERENCES

1. Wang HM, Wu JM and Lee CT (2012) The study of caregiver of late talker on construction of language interactive distress and asking for help experiences. Taiwan Journal of Chang Gung Institute of Technology 17:75–92
2. Glykas M and Chytas P (2004) Technology assisted speech and language therapy. Greece Intnational Journal of Medical Informatics 73(6):529–541
3. Enderby P and Pickstone C (2005) How many people have communication disorders and why does it matter? N Engl International Journal of Speech-Language Pathology 7(1):8–13
4. Rahman MM, Ferdous SM and Ahmed SI (2010) Increasing Intelligibility in the Speech of the Autistic Children by an Interactive Computer Game, Multimedia (ISM), 2010 IEEE International Symposium on, Taichung, Taiwan, 2010, pp 383–387
5. Morawej A and McLeod RD (1997) Fonetix-Speech Articulation & Hearing Perception Software, WESCANEX 97: Communications, Power and Computing. Conference Proceedings.IEEE, Winnipeg, man, Canada, 1997, pp 153–156
6. Cagatay M, Ege P, Tokdemir G and Cagiltay NE (2012) A SERIOUS GAME FOR SPEECH DISORDER CHILDREN THERAPY. Health Informatics and Bioinformatics (HIBIT), 2012 7th International Symposium on, Nevsehir, Turkish, 2012, pp 18–23
7. Awad SS, Curless MW, and Merson R (1999) Computer Assisted Treated for Motor Speech Disorders. Instrumentation and Measurement Technology Conference, 1999. IMTC/99. Proceedings of the 16th IEEE, Venice, Italian, 1999, pp 595–600
8. Chen YJ, Huang JW, Yang HM, Lin YH, and Wu JL (2007) Development of Articulation Assessment and Training System with Speech Recognition and Articulation Training Strategies Selection. Acoustics, Speech and Signal Processing, 2007. ICASSP 2007. IEEE International Conference on, Honolulu, HI, Hawaii, 2007, pp 209–212

Author: Shih-Tsang Tang
Institute: Ming Chuan University
Street: 5 De Ming Rd., Gui Shan District
City: Taoyuan
Country: Taiwan
Email: sttang@mail.mcu.edu.tw

Therapeutic Time Window for rt-PA Thrombolysis in a Rat Photothrombotic Ischemic Stroke Model

Aishwarya Bandla[1,2], Ji Min Ling[1,3], Yu-Hang Liu[1,4], Hsin-Yi Lai[5], You-Yin Chen[6], Nitish V. Thakor[1,2,4,7], and Lun-De Liao[1,*]

[1] Singapore Institute for Neurotechnology (SINAPSE), Singapore
[2] Department of Biomedical Engineering, National University of Singapore, Singapore
[3] Department of Neurosurgery, National Neuroscience Institute, Singapore
[4] Department of Electrical and Computer Engineering, National University of Singapore, Singapore
[5] Department of Physical Medicine, Chang Gung Memorial Hospital and Chang Gung University, Taiwan
[6] Department of Biomedical Engineering, National Yang Ming University, Taiwan
[7] Department of Biomedical Engineering, Johns Hopkins University, USA
gs336.tw@gmail.com

Abstract— **The narrow 3h therapeutic time window for recombinant tissue-type plasminogen activator (rt-PA) thrombolysis is a challenging limitation in acute ischemic stroke treatment. Intense research focus is being laid on developing novel therapeutic interventions for extending the thrombolysis time window using animal stroke models. However, these animal models are anatomically and physiologically different. Here, we assess the effective time window of rt-PA thrombolysis in the photothrombotic ischemic (PTI) stroke model using the electrocorticography (ECoG) system and histology study. Our results indicate that rt-PA provides effective thrombolysis when administered in the initial 1 to 3 hours post-ischemia, beyond which it does not facilitate recovery. This complements the FDA-approved rt-PA time window in humans. However, it is interesting to note that the trend of neural activity did not strictly correspond to infarct volume changes, indicating the importance of multimodal imaging for holistic assessment of therapeutic efficacy. Therefore, in the future, this ECoG setup will be integrated with the functional photoacoustic microscopy (fPAM) system to jointly evaluate neural activity and cerebral hemodynamics to probe neurovascular function changes effective with thrombolysis.**

Keywords— **Acute ischemic stroke, recombinant tissue-type plasminogen activator (rt-PA), Electrocorticography (ECoG), Photothrombotic ischemia (PTI), Thrombolysis time window.**

I. INTRODUCTION

Recanalization by means of recombinant tissue-type plasminogen activator (rt-PA) is currently the only approved treatment for acute ischemic stroke, a leading cause of death and disability worldwide [1]. Hemorrhagic transformation, incomplete reperfusion, neurotoxicity, and the short treatment time window comprise major challenges for thrombolytic therapy [2]. Improving rt-PA therapy has become one of highest priorities in the stroke field [3, 4]. Intense research has been directed towards developing novel therapeutic interventions targeting extension of the limited therapeutic time window for rt-PA thrombolysis [5, 6]. In this direction, several animal stroke models have been utilized to study and validate the effects of therapeutic interventions [7, 8]. Of the numerous existing animal models, photothrombotic ischemic (PTI) model offers a highly reliable and focal ischemic stroke in the desired cortical region [9]. Thus, we used this model for determining the effective therapeutic time window of the rt-PA. With the advantage of using electrocorticography (ECoG) (i.e., to evaluate the neuronal integrity as a marker of recanalization) combined with histology (i.e., to evaluate the infarct volume), we proposed a model to study the effective thrombolysis time window specific to the PTI rat model in this study.

II. MATERIALS AND METHODS

A. Animal Preparation

All experimental protocols presented herein were evaluated and approved by the Institutional Animal Care and Use Committee (IACUC) of the National University of Singapore. Twelve male Wistar rats weighing 250 – 300 g (InVivos Pte Ltd, Singapore) were used in this study and divided into six groups (a control group and 5 experimental groups), including two animals in each of the groups. The animals were maintained anesthetized with pentobarbital (50 mg/kg bolus and 15 mg/kg/h maintenance i.p.) throughout the experiment. The anesthetized rats were mounted on a stereotaxic frame to reduce motion artifacts during the experiment, and the skin was excised to expose the bregma landmark. The body temperature was measured using a rectal probe and was maintained at 37 ± 0.5°C using a self-regulating thermal plate (TCAT-2 Temperature Controller, Physitemp Instruments, Inc., Clifton, NJ, USA).

Six stainless steel epidural electrodes were secured to the skull bilaterally over the primary motor cortex regions (M1: anterior–posterior (AP) = +4.2 mm, medial–lateral

[*] Corresponding author.

I. Lackovic (ed.), *1st Global Conference on Biomedical Engineering & 9th Asian-Pacific Conference on Medical and Biological Engineering*,
IFMBE Proceedings 47, DOI: 10.1007/978-3-319-12262-5_64

(ML) = ±3 mm; Ch1 and Ch2) and the forelimb primary somatosensory cortex regions (S1FL: Ch3/Ch4 and Ch5/Ch6, AP = +1.7 mm and -0.8 mm, respectively; ML = ±4.5 mm) for resting-state ECoG and somatosensory evoked potential (SSEP) recordings (Figure 1). One reference electrode was positioned at 3 mm to the right of the lambda landmark. The electrodes, connected with silver wires, were interfaced with the data acquisition system through a ZIF-Clip headstage (Tucker-Davis Technologies, Inc., Alachua, FL, USA). Next, a cranial window of approximately 3 mm (AP) × 4 mm (ML) (indicated by black box in Figure 1) for photothrombotic stroke induction, centered at the bregma, was produced with a high-speed drill, with care taken to maintain the dura intact.

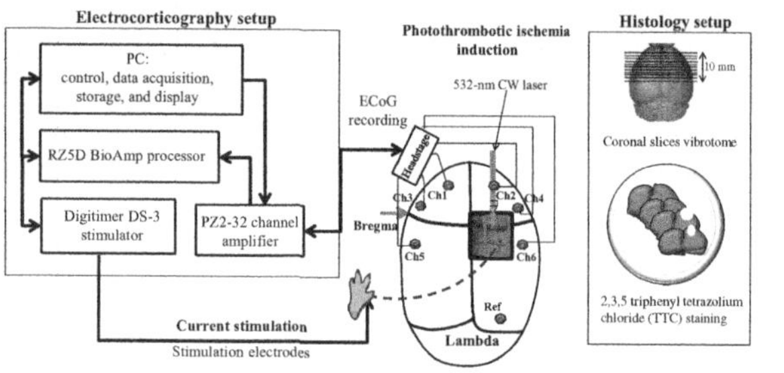

Fig. 1 Illustration of experimental setup with ECoG system, photothrombotic focal ischemia induction and histology setup for qualitative and quantitative analysis.

B. Photothrombosis Technique for Focal Ischemic Stroke Induction

The photothrombosis method was employed to devise a highly reliable, focal ischemic model, targeting a selected cerebral arteriole, which is a distal branch of the middle cerebral artery (MCA) located in the right hemisphere S1FL cortical region [9]. The photosensitizer Rose Bengal (Na+ salt, R3877; Sigma-Aldrich, Singapore), diluted to 10 mg/ml in HEPES-buffered saline, was injected into the tail vein at 0.2 ml/100 g rat body weight by infusion over 2 min. The cortical blood vessel selected for occlusion was subsequently illuminated with a 10-mW, 532-nm continuous wave (CW) laser light (MGM-20; Beta Electronics, Columbus, Ohio, USA) [10]. The CW laser light, as illustrated in Figure 1, was focused on the selected cerebral vessel located in the right S1FL region for 15 min until a stable clot was formed.

C. Forepaw Electrical Stimulation Protocol

Forepaw electrical stimulation was applied to evoke neural activity response (SSEP). A monophasic constant current of 2 mA with a 0.2 ms pulse width at a frequency of 3 Hz and 5 sec stimulation duration was applied with a stimulator (DS3, Digitimer, UK) via stainless steel bipolar subdermal needle electrodes inserted into the rat's left palmar forepaws (contralateral to the targeted occlusion) [11, 12]. The experimental protocol constituted resting-state ECoG and SSEP recordings. The resting-state ECoG was recorded for 1 min followed by 5 sec of stimulation to evoke neural activity for SSEP recording.

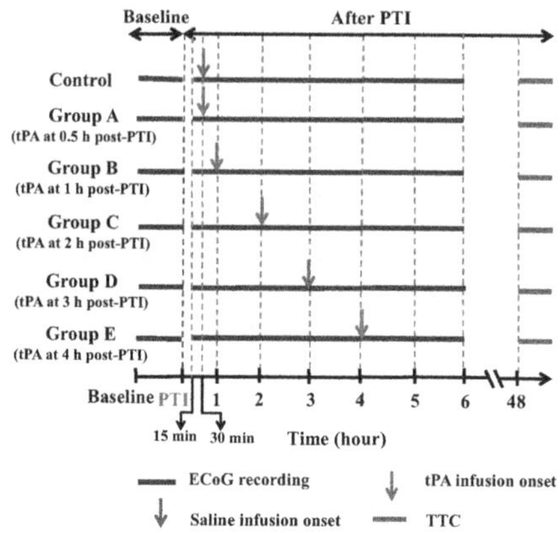

Fig. 2 Experimental groups for determining the effective thrombolysis time window.

D. rt-PA Induced Thrombolysis

To determine the effective therapeutic window of thrombolysis, rt-PA (10 mg/kg, Actilyse®, Boehringer Ingelheim) was administered intravenously (tail vein, 10% bolus, 90% infusion over 30 minutes), initiated at different times (i.e., 30 min, 1, 2, 3 and 4 hours post-PTI, as shown in Figure 2). The control group received the same dose of saline under identical conditions.

E. Data Analysis of Functional SSEP, Inter-hemispheric Coherence, and Alpha-Delta Ratio

The SSEPs evoked by sensory stimulation were sampled at 1 kHz, pre-amplified, band-pass filtered and recorded pre- and post-PTI. A SSEP extraction window was created within 100 ms of each stimulation onset and SSEPs were averaged to acquire proper evoked potential signals for analysis. Afterward, P1 and N1 components of the averaged SSEPs were extracted. The peak-amplitude changes of P1 and N1 were used to evaluate the neural activity changes after PTI.

We used a multivariate autoregressive (MVAR) model for spectral analysis and inter-hemispheric coherence (i.e., a measure of the linear relationship between two signals at a specific frequency) analysis. Once the raw data had been fitted to the MVAR model, inter-hemispheric coherence was calculated for analysis. Since delta and alpha bands have been reported to be strong indicators for both injury and recovery, inter-hemispheric coherence was calculated for only these two frequency bands. Alpha-delta ratio (ADR) was defined as the ratio between alpha power and delta power. For details on the calculations please refer to our earlier work [13].

F. Quantification of the Infarct Volume by TTC Staining

The extent of infarct was measured at 48 h following ischemia onset using 2, 3, 5-triphenyl-tetrazolium chloride (TTC), as detailed in earlier work [13].

III. RESULTS

A. Functional changes in SSEP, inter-hemispheric coherence, ADR with rt-PA thrombolysis at different onset timing post-PTI, and infarct volume assessment.

The SSEP parameters of P1, N1 and peak-to-peak amplitude were assessed in this study, and the peak amplitude changes of SSEP components in the different groups are shown in Figure 3A. All the evaluations were based on Ch4, because it is located in the S1FL of ischemic hemisphere (iS1FL) – in close proximity to the targeted PTI location. The contralateral left-forepaw stimulation was chosen as a reference to elicit an evoked response. The P1 amplitudes of the five experimental groups approximately decreased at least 40% at PTI onset compared to baseline, as shown in Figure 3B. After treatment, the P1 amplitude significantly increased to the baseline following rt-PA infusion in groups A - D. Unfortunately, the P1 amplitudes dropped in group E with rt-PA administered at 4 h post-PTI (i.e., decreased to 5% of the baseline amplitude). The N1 amplitude, similar to the P1 amplitude, decreased after PTI onset to approximately 60% of the baseline in the six groups, as shown in Figure 3C. An increase in the N1 amplitude was observed at end of treatment in groups A - D while a deteriorative trend was observed following group E treatment similar to the control group. The peak-to-peak amplitude followed the same trend as the P1 and N1 amplitudes. An initial decrease of 60% lower than baseline was observed in the peak-to-peak amplitude in all five experimental groups at PTI onset, as shown in Figure 3D. Substantial improvement in peak-to-peak amplitude values to approximately baseline was observed in groups A - D, respectively. On the other hand there was a decrease in values in control group and group E (i.e., decreased to 13% of baseline amplitude) at end of treatment.

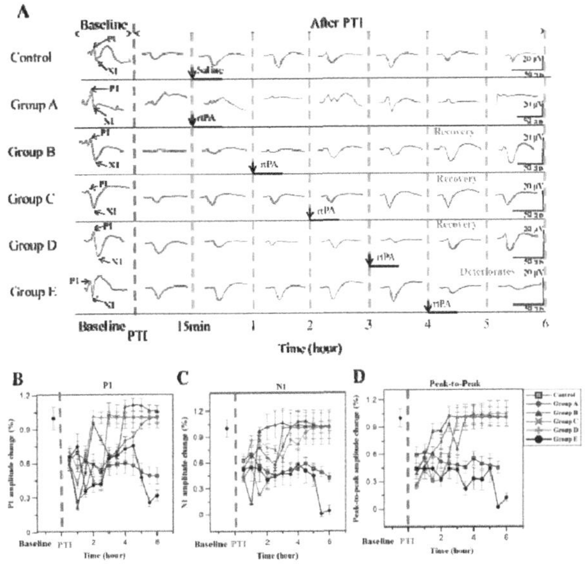

Fig. 3 Illustration of SSEP-related parameters and experimental results. (A) The SSEP waveform changes of different groups prior to and following PTI. (B - D) The corresponding parameter changes of SSEP components over the iS1FL region following PTI induction, with different treatments applied.

Inter-hemispheric coherence changes were evaluated across the bilateral S1FL regions (Ch3 - Ch4) pre- and post-PTI induction, as shown in Figure 4A-B. It was observed that the alpha coherence values dropped below baseline values following ischemic onset. A significant increase (to 93% of baseline) in the alpha coherence was observed after rt-PA treatment in group A – D. Also, a decrease (80% of baseline) in alpha coherence values was observed after group E treatment. The coherence changes in the delta band pre- and post-PTI were similar to the alpha coherence. Delta coherence decreased, among all groups, to at least 60% of baseline immediately after PTI onset, as shown in Figure 4B. We observed notable recovery in the delta coherence values only in group A – D. It is noteworthy that in group E, the delta coherence values increased at the beginning of treatment, but decreased with onset of rt-PA infusion delivered 4 hr post-PTI induction (i.e., decreased to 52% of baseline). The iS1FL ADR (Ch4) decreased approximately 53% after PTI induction, as shown in Figure 4C, compared to baseline. A moderate recovery of ADR (to 74% of baseline) followed group A treatment, a significant increase in ADR values at the iS1FL region was observed in group B - D following rt-PA treatment. The ADR of group E showed a deteriorative trend with the onset of rt-PA treatment at 4h post-PTI.

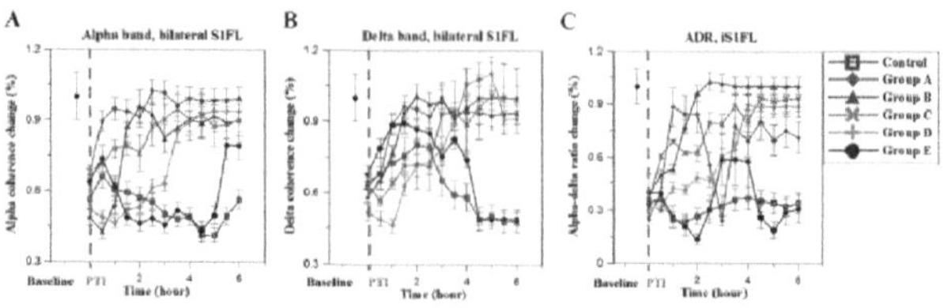

The infarct areas in coronal sections from each group were compared using TTC staining. The infarcts were pale (unstained) regions in the somatosensory cortex. Group B exhibited a significant reduction in the volume of the infarct (2% of lesioned hemisphere), while group E (13% infarct volume), similar to the control group (21% infarct volume), displayed a larger infarct.

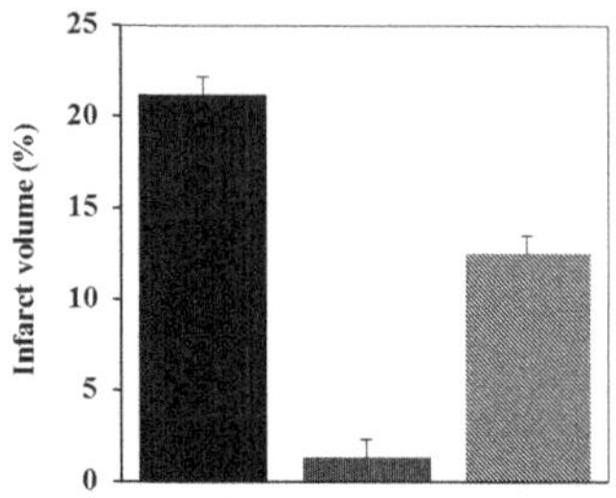

IV. Conclusions

The effective treatment time window for rt-PA thrombolysis has been established in this study as 1 - 3 hours post ischemic onset in a rat photothrombotic ischemic model. This correlates with the universally agreed time window in humans. The ECoG system was employed to evaluate the SSEP changes and resting-state ECoG changes in the bilateral S1FL regions pre- and post-PTI. Results indicate that the initial 1 to 3 hours post-ischemia is the time window suitable for effective thrombolysis, beyond which administration of rt-PA does not facilitate recovery. Also, recovered SSEP did not strictly correspond to reduced infarct, emphasizing the importance of multimodal imaging for holistic assessment of therapeutic efficacy. Further, this ECoG setup will be integrated with the functional photoacoustic microscopy (fPAM) system to probe neurovascular function changes effective with thrombolysis.

Conflict of Interest

The authors declare that they have no conflict of interest.

References

[1] "Tissue plasminogen activator for acute ischemic stroke. The national institute of neurological disorders and stroke rt-PA stroke study group," *New England Journal of Medicine,* vol. 333, pp. 1581-7, Dec 1995.

[2] R. Abu Fanne, T. Nassar, S. Yarovoi, A. Rayan, I. Lamensdorf, M. Karakoveski, P. Vadim, M. Jammal, D. B. Cines, and A. A. Higazi, "Blood-brain barrier permeability and tPA-mediated neurotoxicity," *Neuropharmacology,* vol. 58, pp. 972-980, Jun 2010.

[3] I. A. Tiebosch, B. J. Crielaard, M. J. Bouts, R. Zwartbol, A. Salas-Perdomo, T. Lammers, A. M. Planas, G. Storm, and R. M. Dijkhuizen, "Combined treatment with recombinant tissue plasminogen activator and dexamethasone phosphate-containing liposomes improves neurological outcome and restricts lesion progression after embolic stroke in rats," *Journal of neurochemistry,* vol. 123, pp. 65-74, Nov 2012.

[4] H. Zhu, X. Fan, Z. Yu, J. Liu, Y. Murata, J. Lu, S. Zhao, K. A. Hajjar, E. H. Lo, and X. Wang, "Annexin A2 combined with low-dose tPA improves thrombolytic therapy in a rat model of focal embolic stroke," *Journal of Cerebral Blood Flow & Metabolism,* vol. 30, pp. 1137-1146, Jan 2010.

[5] W. Zhang, K. Sato, T. Hayashi, N. Omori, I. Nagano, S. Kato, S. Horiuchi, and K. Abe, "Extension of ischemic therapeutic time window by a free radical scavenger, Edaravone, reperfused with tPA in rat brain," *Neurological research,* vol. 26, pp. 342-348, Apr 2004.

[6] H. Y. Kim, A. B. Singhal, and E. H. Lo, "Normobaric hyperoxia extends the reperfusion window in focal cerebral ischemia," *Annals of neurology,* vol. 57, pp. 571-575, Apr 2005.

[7] L. Jia, M. Chopp, L. Zhang, M. Lu, and Z. Zhang, "Erythropoietin in combination of tissue plasminogen activator exacerbates brain hemorrhage when treatment is initiated 6 hours after stroke," *Stroke,* vol. 41, pp. 2071-2076, Sep 2010.

[8] Y. Murata, A. Rosell, R. H. Scannevin, K. J. Rhodes, X. Wang, and E. H. Lo, "Extension of the thrombolytic time window with minocycline in experimental stroke," *Stroke,* vol. 39, pp. 3372-3377, Dec 2008.

[9] B. D. Watson, W. D. Dietrich, R. Busto, M. S. Wachtel, and M. D. Ginsberg, "Induction of reproducible brain infarction by photochemically initiated thrombosis," *Annals of neurology,* vol. 17, pp. 497-504, May 1985.

[10] L.-D. Liao, M.-L. Li, H.-Y. Lai, Y.-Y. I. Shih, Y.-C. Lo, S. Tsang, P. C.-P. Chao, C.-T. Lin, F.-S. Jaw, and Y.-Y. Chen, "Imaging brain hemodynamic changes during rat forepaw electrical stimulation using functional photoacoustic microscopy," *Neuroimage,* vol. 52, pp. 562-570, Aug 2010.

[11] L.-D. Liao, C.-T. Lin, Y.-Y. I. Shih, H.-Y. Lai, W.-T. Zhao, T. Q. Duong, J.-Y. Chang, Y.-Y. Chen, and M.-L. Li, "Investigation of the cerebral hemodynamic response function in single blood vessels by functional photoacoustic microscopy," *Journal of biomedical optics,* vol. 17, pp. 061210-10, Jun 2012.

[12] L. D. Liao, C. T. Lin, Y. Y. Shih, T. Q. Duong, H. Y. Lai, P. H. Wang, R. Wu, S. Tsang, J. Y. Chang, M. L. Li, and Y. Y. Chen, "Transcranial imaging of functional cerebral hemodynamic changes in single blood vessels using in vivo photoacoustic microscopy," *Journal of cerebral blood flow and metabolism,* vol. 32, pp. 938-951, Apr 2012.

[13] L.-D. Liao, A. Bandla, J. M. Ling, Y.-H. Liu, and N. Thakor, "Improving Neurovascular Outcomes with Bilateral Forepaw Stimulation in a Rat Photothrombotic Ischemic Stroke Model," *Neurophotonics,* vol. 1, 2014.

Using Radio Frequency Electrical Stimulation to Block External Urethral Sphincter Contraction and Improved Voiding Efficiency

E. Jen[1], Y.T. Lin[1], C.W. Peng[2], T.S. Kuo[1,3,4], S.T. Young[5], W.T. Lin[1], and C.W. Lin[1,3]

[1] The Institute of Biomedical Electronics and Bioinformatics, National Taiwan University, Taiwan
[2] Department of Physical Medicine and Rehabilitation, Taipei Medical University, Taiwan
[3] The Institute of Biomedical Engineering, National Taiwan University, Taiwan
[4] Department of Electrical Engineering, National Taiwan University, Taiwan
[5] Department of Health and Beauty Business Administration, Taiwan ShouFu University, Taiwan

Abstract— **Block of the external urethral sphincter contractions by using high frequency electrical stimulation of the pudendal nerves is a potential method for inhibiting detrusor sphincter dyssynergia. Most researchers use high frequency electrical stimulation at frequencies between 2kHz to 20kHz, but the parameters and mechanism of this block are not well understood. This paper demonstrated the use of radio frequency electrical stimulation (500kHz) as a method to block the external urethral sphincter contractions and improved voiding efficiency by electrical stimulation of unilateral pudendal nerve efferent axons. The most efficient waveform for conduction was 500kHz (with 0.2 to 1mA) constant-current biphasic sinusoidal, voiding efficiency increased from 53 to 71-92%. These results raise the possibility that using radio frequency electrical stimulation to block external urethral sphincter contraction may provide a new approach for improving voiding in spinal cord injured patients.**

Keywords— **Radio frequency, Electrical stimulation, Nerve block, Pudendal nerve, Voiding efficiency.**

I. Introduction

During normal micturition, the functions of bladder controls are mainly for storage and intermittent elimination of urine called voiding. Voiding relies on the coordinated behaviors of the external urethral sphincter (EUS) and bladder controlled by lumbosacral spinal cord. During voiding, the EUS relaxes and the bladder contracts and while during storage the bladder is relaxed and the EUS contracts [1]. The pudendal nerve (PN) is the primary conduit for somatic afferent and efferent nerve axons between the sacral spinal cord and urethra. PN plays an important role to modulate contraction of EUS [2]. However, after spinal cord injury and some neurological disorders, bladder and EUS contractions become uncoordinated and result in bladder and EUS contract simultaneously during voiding, which is termed detrusor sphincter dyssynergia (DSD) and could cause serious medical complications, such as high bladder pressures, urinary tract infections, renal failure, autonomic dysreflexia, and hydronephrosis [3]. Residual urine in the bladder can also lead to lower urinary tract infection. The conventional treatment of DSD is clean intermittent self-catheterization (CISC) by using balloon dilation of the EUS or intraurethral stent placement combined with anti-muscarinic drugs. One alternative approach to replace CISC is Sphincterotomy, which providesan effective surgical method to lower bladder pressure and increase voiding efficiency. However, the surgical process may have risks of complications, such as permanent incontinence, loss of reflex defecation, and loss of sexual function, for long term DSD patients [4]. High frequency alternating current (HFAC) stimulation has been used for blocking nerve conductions or briefly denervation of targeted muscles. HFAC is a reversible and immediate method to improve voiding efficiency [5]. Normally, HFAC stimulation waveform is in the kHz range for exhaustive blockage of nerve conduction [6]. Changfeng's research demonstrated that use 2 waveforms stimulation frequencies between 6 and 10 kHz were most effective in blocking EUS activation [7]. A review of the investigation indicates that bilateral HFAC block of the PN can generate effective voiding [8]. In our group, pulsed radio-frequency (PRF) stimulation has been successfully used to inhibit C-fiber excitatory responses and block the signal of pain conduction [9]. To the best of our knowledge, there is no report on using PRF electrical stimulation to block external urethral sphincter contraction yet.

The purpose of this study is to establish an in vitro experimental setup for the measurement of the effectiveness of PRF electrical stimulation of pudendal nerve to block the efferent pathway to the EUS offeasible current range from 0.2 to 1mA. The target of this investigation would be to relax EUS during voiding and the block can be reversible to maintain the function of EUS and continence during voiding periods.

II. Materials and Methods

All protocols involving the use of animals in this study were approved by the animal care and use committee at Taipei Medical University and Hospital. Four female Sprague-Dawley rats weighing 275~320 g were used in this study. Figure 1 shows the experimental setup. Four normal

I. Lackovic (ed.), *1st Global Conference on Biomedical Engineering & 9th Asian-Pacific Conference on Medical and Biological Engineering*,
IFMBE Proceedings 47, DOI: 10.1007/978-3-319-12262-5_65

rats were used in an experiment to record intravesical pressure (IVP) and EUS electromyograms (EMGs). IVP is the major biosignal that reflects the state of bladder condition and EUS EMG can quantify the power of EUS during contraction. Rats were anesthetized with urethane (1.2 g/kg, s.c, supplemented as needed). The temperature of the rat was maintained at 36~39°C with a recirculating water blanket, and the tail vein was catheterized for fluid and drug administration. A PE-50 tube was inserted into the bladder lumen for IVP measurements. Two insulated silver wire electrodes (0.05 mm in diameter) were inserted into the lateral aspects of the mid-urethra to measure the EMG from EUS. To record the IVP, the PE tube was connected via a three-way stopcock to an infusion pump and a pressure transducer (P23XL-1, Becton Dickinson, Franklin Lakes, NJ, USA). The bladder was infused continuously with physiological saline at the rate of 0.2ml per minute via the superpublic catheter until voiding occurred. The IVP and EUS EMG were simultaneously recorded for computational characterization.

In this experiment, the data of IVP and EUS EMG sampled via an analog-to-digital coverter at 5kHz (Biopac MP36, Biopac Systems) during continuous-infusion cystometry and saved to the computer system, the IVP signal was filtered by a 1kHz low-pass filter, and the EUS EKG signal was filtered by a 10-3k Hz band-pass filter. The tripolar electrode with a cuff was placed on unilateral pudendal nerve efferent axons, usually on the left side, and tripolar electrode was connected to the pulse electrical stimulator (A-M systems 2100). The high frequency biphasic rectangular waveform (500kHz) was generated by stimulator and was tested with current of 0.1 to 1mA to search for the effective current range at 500kHz to block EUS contractions during voiding. The data analysis, the following cystometric variables were measured to quantify the effects of pudendal nerve efferent axons stimulation during voiding: micturition volume threshold (VT) defined as the infused volume of saline sufficient to induce the first voiding contraction; bladder contraction duration (CD) during voiding; contraction amplitude (CA) defined as the maximum pressure during voiding; voiding efficient (VE), the ratio between the voided volume (VV) and the VT. The VV was obtained from the value of VT minus the residual volume (RV) of saline withdrawn through the intravesical catheter after the final voiding contraction. We use time-domain analysis to quantify the power of EUS EMG contraction, The Root Mean Square (RMS) value has been used to quantify the electric signal because it reflects the physiological activity in the motor unit during contraction. EUS EMG analysis was calculated with MATLAB.

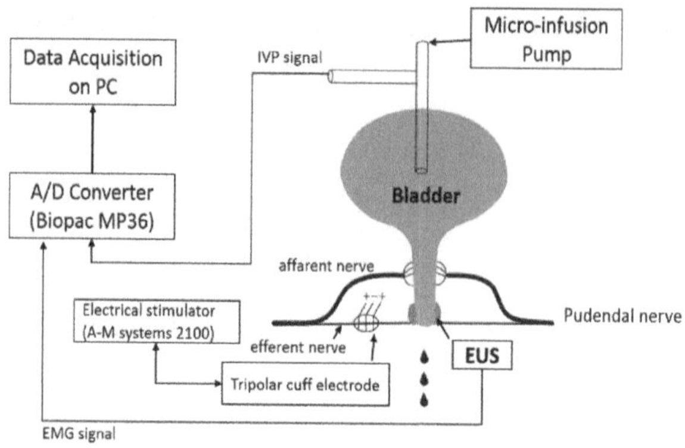

Fig. 1 The measurement system setup used to modulate pudendal nerve and record IVP and EUS EMG activities in rats

III. RESULTS AND DISCUSSION

A. EUS EMG RMS Value Comparison

The typical pattern of IVP and EUS EMG measurements in normal rats are shown in Fig.2. A single micturition contraction of the bladder can be separated into several phases of IVP and EUS EMG clearly showed a long bursting period (BP).

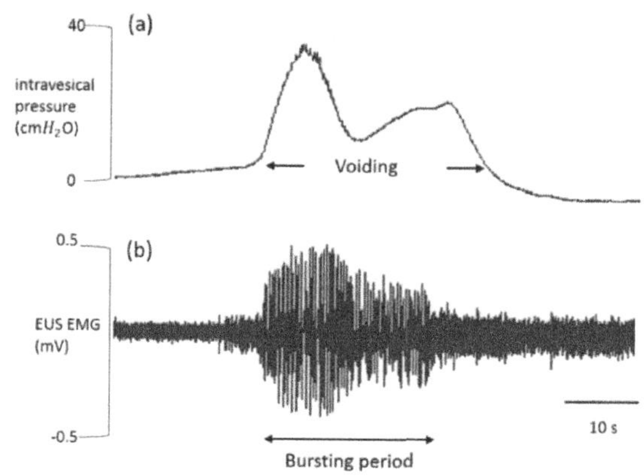

Fig. 2 Comparation of (a) intravesical pressure, (b) EUS EMG on the different phases during contraction

Pudendal nerve efferent axons were directly controlled EUS contractions. The objective of this experiment was that when effective block was happened, EUS can be relax and reflected on EUS EMG. To analysis EMG, we used RMS value to quantify the data, the RMS value is defined in (1),

$$\mathrm{RMS} = \sqrt{\frac{1}{N}\sum_{n=1}^{N} x_n{}^2} \tag{1}$$

Firstly, we recorded the normal rats (n=4) EUS EMG during voiding without stimulation. Secondly, gave radio

Table 1 Effects of conditional blocking electrical stimulation on cystometric parameters

Stimulation parameters	VT (c.c)	CA (cm-H_2O)	CD (s)	RV (c.c.)	VV(c.c)	VE
None-stimulaion	0.32±0.05	20.44±3.82	22±3.34	0.15±0.02	0.17±0.01	53%
500kHz, 0.2mA	0.26±0.03	24.87±5.23	19.2±1.96	0.02±0.01	0.24±0.01	92%
500kHz, 0.4mA	0.49±0.12	26.07±3.35	31.67±1.83	0.05±0.01	0.44±0.02	90%
500kHz, 0.6mA	0.17±0.01	26.47±2.76	43±4.82	0.05±0.02	0.12±0.01	71%
500kHz, 0.8mA	0.17±0.02	22.56±2.39	30.67±3.75	0.04±0.01	0.13±0.01	76%
500kHz, 1mA	0.4±0.02	21.09±3.32	23.17±1.83	0.038±0.01	0.36±0.02	90%

Values are mean ± SD, n=4

frequency stimulation on pudendal nerve efferent axons during voiding; this process was repeated until each trial included at least five voiding contractions. Figure 3 shows a clear and strong relationship that on normal voinding contractions, RMS values were between 4.67 to 6.2 , but start to stimulation (500kHz, 0.8mA), RMS values were decresed to 2.88 to 3.1.This results show a striking effect of radio frequency stimulation on pudendal nerve efferent axons during voiding contraction.

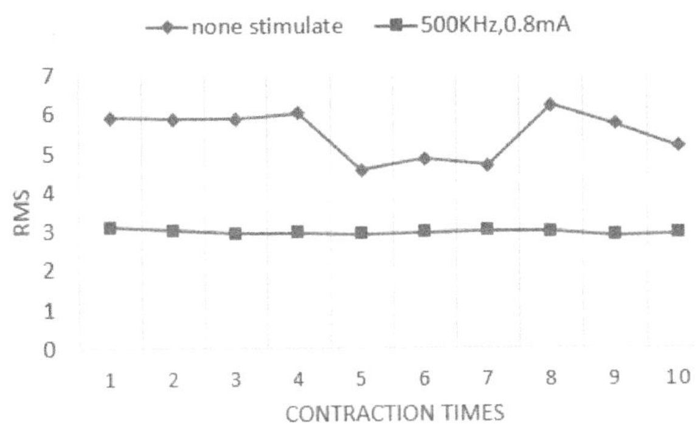

Fig. 3 Compariation of RMS values during voiding contractions

B. *Bursting Period Comparison*

EUS bursting activity happened on voiding period, we were compared the BP on different stimulation parameters (500 kHz with stimulation intensities at 0.2mA, 0.4mA, 0.6mA, 0.8mA, and 1mA). Interestingly,we found that the average bursting periods of stimulation on pudendal nerve efferent axons were longer than none stimulation, as shown in Figure 4.

C. *Urodynamic Measurement of Rats*

The results of urodynamic measurement are summarized in Table 1. All of the stimulation groups were better than none-stimulation groups. The VE were strongly positively correlated with blocking electrical stimulation on pudendal nerve efferent axons.

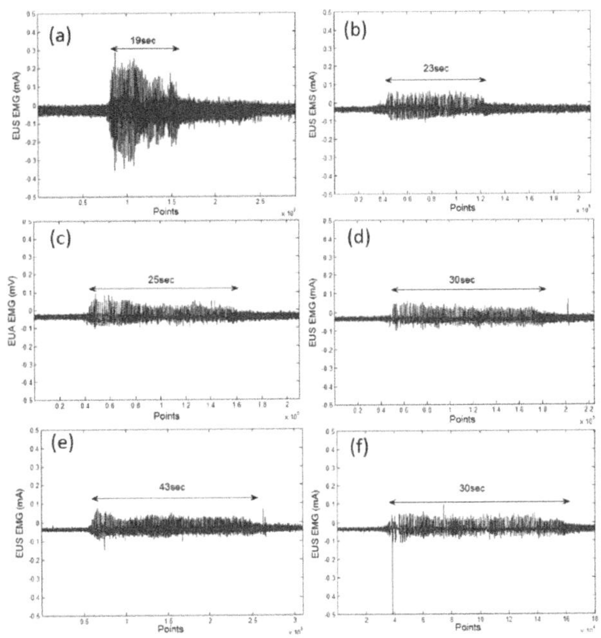

Fig. 4 Bursting periods on different stimulation parameters (500kHz), (a) none stimulation, (b) 0.2, (c) 0.4, (d) 0.6, (e) 0.8 (f) 1mA

IV. CONCLUSIONS

In this paper, we present the primary results of using radio frequency constant-current biphasic rectangular pulses to block the pudendal nerve efferent axons. The primary results demonstrated that the VE of normal rats were promoted by blocking electrical stimulation and the RMS of EUS EMG demonstrated stimulation can lead to EUS relax. However, the entire system should be used to spinal cord injured rats in the future and would also be expected to be successful. Thus, radio frequency electrical stimulation of the pudendal nerve efferent axons displays great potential for treating DSD and restoring normal function of the lower urinary tract after SCI.

ACKNOWLEDGMENT

We thank for the financially supporting from the R & D Foundation of Urological Medicine to Dr. T. S. Kuo.

REFERENCES

1. Shefchyk SJ (2002) Spinal cord neural organization controlling the urinary bladder and striated sphincter. Prog Brain Res 137:71–82
2. K. Akita, H. Sakamoto, T. Sato (2003) Origins and courses of the nervous branches to the male urethral sphincter. Surg Radiol Anat 25: 387-392
3. Burns, Anthony S. MD, Rivas, David A. MD, Ditunno, John F. MD (2001) The Management of Neurogenic Bladder and Sexual Dysfunction After Spinal Cord Injury. Spine 26:129-136
4. Vapnek JM, Couillard DR, Stone AR (1994) Is sphincterotomy the best management of the spinal cord injured bladder. The Journal of Urology 151: 961-964
5. J.D. Sweeney, J.T. Mortimer, and D.R. Bodner (1989) Acute Animal Studies on Electrically Induced Collision Block of Pudendal Nerve Motor Activity. 8: 521-536
6. K. L. Kilgore, N. Bhadra (2004) Nerve conduction block utilising high-frequency alternating current. Med. Biol. Eng. Comput 42: 394-406
7. Changfeng Tai, James R. roppolo, William C. de groat (2004) Block of External Urethral Sphincter Contraction by High Frequency Electrical Stimulation of Pudendal Nerve. The Journal of Urology 172: 2069-2072
8. Adam Boger, Narendra Bhadra, Kenneth J. Gustafson (2008) Bladder Voiding by Combined High Frequency Electrical Pudendal Nerve Block and Sacral Root Stimulation. Neurourology and Urodynamics 27: 435-439
9. Hung-Wei Chiu, Mu-Lien Lin, Chii-Wann Lin, I-Hsiu Ho, Wei-Tso Lin, Po-Hsiang Fang, Yi-Chin Lee, Yeong-Ray Wen, Shey-Shi Lu (2010) Pain Control on Demand Based on Pulsed Radio-Frequency Stimulation of the Dorsal Root Ganglion Using a Batteryless Implantable CMOS SoC. Ieee Transactions on Biomedical Circuits and Systems 4: 350-359

Author: Chii-Wann Lin
Institute: Institute of Biomedical Engineering,
National Taiwan University
Street: No.1, Sec.4, Roosevelt Road
City: Taipei
Country: 10617 Taiwan
Email: cwlinx@ntu.edu.tw

Effects of Eccentric Contraction Training with Neuromuscular Electrical Stimulation on Muscle Strength

J. Son and Y. Kim

Department of Biomedical Engineering, Yonsei University, Wonju, Republic of Korea
Institute for Convergence Study of Bio-Medical Wellness, Yonsei University, Wonju, Republic of Korea

Abstract— **In this study, a training system for an involuntary eccentric contraction of biceps brachii muscles was designed using a continuous passive movement and a commercial neuromuscular electrical stimulation devices. To investigate the effects of the involuntary eccentric contraction training by neuromuscular electrical stimulation on the enhancement of muscle strength, 7 healthy males participated, who were trained two times per week for 12 weeks. Each exercise session was performed for 30 minutes with no rest intervals. Isometric elbow flexion torque and biceps brachii muscle thickness were chosen as evaluation indices, and were measured at pre-/post-training. After the 12-week training, the isometric elbow flexion torques significantly increased by approximately 23% compared to the initial performance ($p < 0.01$). In addition, the biceps brachii muscle thicknesses significantly increased by around 8% at rest and 16% at MVC ($p < 0.01$). The developed system and the technique show promising results, suggesting that it has the potential to be used to increase the muscle strength in patients with neuromuscular disease and to be implemented in design rehabilitative protocols.**

Keywords— **Muscle strengthening, rehabilitation protocol.**

I. INTRODUCTION

Neuromuscular electrical stimulation (NMES) is widely used to improve impaired muscle functions in neuromuscular patients, but NMES-related studies have mostly focused on conditions that target muscles act as concentric contraction [1]. The eccentric training is well-known to be more beneficial to increase muscle strength than the concentric exercise [2]. From this point of view, Yanagi et al. [3] developed a hybrid strengthening technique that an agonist performs a volitional concentric contraction against an electrically stimulated antagonist. After 12-week training periods, there were significant increases in elbow extension torques and cross-sectional areas of each muscle. However, the hybrid exercise might not be adequate for patients severely affected with neuromuscular disease because they could not generate agonist muscle forces to overcome the resistance provided by electrically stimulated antagonist forces. In this study, we developed an involuntary eccentric contraction training system to enhance biceps brachii muscle strength, and evaluated our developed system and training for 7 health subjects.

II. METHODS

Our involuntary eccentric contraction system consists of a continuous passive movement (CPM) device for an elbow joint and a commercial NMES device. CPM device includes a DC motor (RE 40 with GP 42 C planetary gear head, Maxon Motor, Switzerland) to generate passive elbow joint movements with a constant angular velocity of 30°/s and exoskeleton to fix the arms. The exoskeleton allows the range of motion of the elbow joint from 0° (fully extended) to 90° (flexed). The commercial NMES device (Stim Plus DP-100, Cybermedic Co., Ltd., Korea) plays a role of stimulation to biceps brachii muscle only when the elbow joint was extending. In order to evaluate the developed system, 7 healthy male subjects with no neuromusuloskeletal injuries were recruited. Participants trained 2 times a week for 12 weeks. Each exercise session consists of passive elbow flexion and extension contractions during 30-minute with no rest interval. Using a commercial dynamometer (Biodex System 3 Pro, Biodex Medical Systems, USA), maximal isometric elbow flexion torques were measured at before the training (Pre) and after 12-week training (Post) each 3 times. The torque data were normalized by body weights of each subject. Moreover, muscle thicknesses of the biceps brachii muscle at Pre- and Post-training were obtained using ultrasonography (SonoAce pico, Samsung Medison Co., Ltd., Korea). Wilcoxon's signed-ranks was performed to evaluate paired differences. The significance level (p) was set to 0.05.

III. RESULTS AND DISCUSSION

Figure 1A shows the significantly increased mean maximum elbow joint torques from 0.63 ± 0.13 N-m/kg at Pre to 0.76 ± 0.14 N-m/kg at Post ($p < 0.01$). After the 12-week training, the maximum isometric flexion torque increased by approximately 23%. These results reveal that our involuntary eccentric contraction training system might be meaningful to enhance the muscle strength.

During the 12-week training, the biceps brachii muscle thickness was changed from 15.97 ± 4.86 mm to 16.23 ± 5.56 mm at rest, and from 21.37 ± 9.67 mm to 24.85 ± 11.32 mm at MVC (Figure 1B). The thickness significantly

I. Lackovic (ed.), *1st Global Conference on Biomedical Engineering & 9th Asian-Pacific Conference on Medical and Biological Engineering*,
IFMBE Proceedings 47, DOI: 10.1007/978-3-319-12262-5_66

increased by approximately 8% at rest and 16% at MVC ($p < 0.01$). These results imply that the increase in maximum torque may be attributed to the change in biceps brachii muscle thickness.

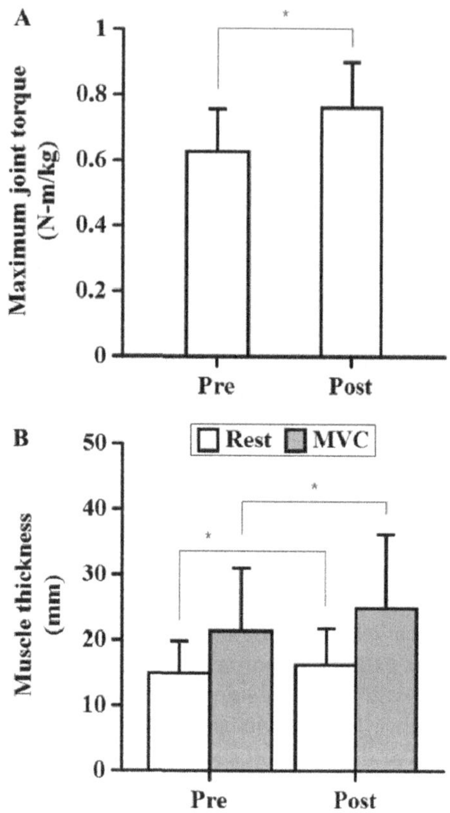

Fig. 1 Effects of an involuntary eccentric contraction training on maximum joint torque (A) and muscle thickness (B).

This study did not compare the involuntary eccentric contraction group with a control group undergoing either a sham therapy or a conventional treatment. Despite the lack of control group comparison, we could expect that involuntary eccentric contraction training is at least more beneficial to enhancing muscle strength than doing no exercise. This study does not answer the highly relevant clinical question of whether our training could be beneficial to enhance muscle strengths in acute, sub-acute, or chronic neuromuscular patients, and if so what amount of recovery could be expected. Also, the optimum therapy protocol such as stimulation intensity or treatment intensity is important, but unknown. In addition, it is yet to be determined whether involuntary eccentric contraction training can yield promising results on other muscles. We plan to perform further studies of the short- and long-term effects to answer to these questions.

IV. Conclusion

In this study, we developed an involuntary eccentric contraction training system, and evaluated its clinical relevance in terms of the enhancement of muscle strength. The developed system and technique showed promising results. Thus, we believe that it has the potential to be used to increase the muscle strength in patients with neuromuscular disease and to be implemented in design rehabilitative protocols.

Acknowledgment

This research was financially supported by the Ministry of Education (MOE) and National Research Foundation of Korea (NRF) through the Human Resource Training Project for Regional Innovation (No. 2013H1B8A2032194), and supported by the Quality of Life Technology R&D program (No. 10047956) of Ministry of Trade, Industry & Energy (MOTIE) and Korea Evaluation Institute of Industrial Technology (KEIT).

Conflict of Interest

The authors declare that they have no conflict of interest.

References

1. Bax L, Staes F, Verhagen A (2005) Does neuromuscular electrical stimulation strengthen the quadriceps femoris? Sports Med 35:191-212
2. Hortobágyi T, Maffiuletti NA (2011) Neural adaptations to electrical stimulation strength training. Euro. J Appl Physio 111:2439-2449
3. Yanagi T, Shiba N, Maeda T et al. (2003) Agonist contractions against electrically stimulated antagonists. Arch Phys Med Rehabil 84:843–848

Author: Youngho Kim
Institute: Yonsei University
Street: 1 Yonseidae-gil
City: Wonju-si
Country: Republic of Korea
Email: younghokim@yonsei.ac.kr

Study the Impact of the SH-SY5Y Cells under the Magnetic Stimulation with Different Frequency and Duration

H.Y. Chen and Y. Chang

Institute of Biomedical Engineering, National Yang-Ming University, Taipei, Taiwan

Abstract— **Repetitive transcranial magnetic stimulation (rTMS), which is produced by strong non-static magnetic fields, is an non-invasive means to stimulate the cerebral cortex. The recent studies show that rTMS affects treatment parkinson's dieses and improves motor symptoms in patients. However, the relationship between the clinical efficacy of rTMS and mechanism is still obscure. In this study we have investigated the effects of different stimulation frequencies and number of treatments on dopamine secretion and neural functions in SH-SY5Y cell cultures. A repetitive session of magnetic stimulation with no matter high or low frequency, intracellular ROS were decreased. In the same time, neurons after magnetic stimulation will release neurotransmitters. These results suggest a possible use of this particular physical stimulation to improve the functional capability of the cells to face oxidative stress. Based on our study we can more understand that the effect of repetitive transcranial magnetic stimulations (rTMS) on Parkinson's disease.**

Keywords— **repetitive transcranial magnetic stimulations, human neuroblastoma SH-SY5Y cells, magnetic stimulation, dopamine (DA), reactive oxygen species (ROS).**

I. INTRODUCTION

Parkinson's disease (PD) is an age-related progressive neurodegenerative disorder with a prevalence of 1%–2% in people over the age of 50[1]. The main symptoms associated with Parkinson's disease, namely hypokinesia, bradykinesia, rigidity and rest tremor. Pathologically, PD is characterized by the loss of mesencephalic dopaminergic neurons lead to nigrostriatal pathway dysfunction. Recent reports indicate that mitochondrial dysfunction、reactive oxidative stress increase、abnormal protein aggregation and dysfunction of the ubiquitin-proteasome pathway are pivotal to PD pathogenesis[2.3] . Because of the prevalence and lack of effective treatment, repetitive transcranial magnetic stimulations (rTMS) is one of the way to treat the disease[4.5]. In this study, we use SH-SY5Y cell line as an in vitro cell model of dopaminergic neurons for Parkinson's disease. Because it can perform many characteristics of DAergic neurons after differentiation. The aim of this study is to investigate the effects of the SH-SY5Y cells under the exposed of magnetic fields with different frequency and intensity.

II. MATERIALS AND METHODS

A. Parkinson's Disease Cell Model

(a)Cell line SH-SY5Y

Human neuroblastoma SH-SY5Y cells, were grown in Dulbecco's Modified Eagle's Medium/ F12 (DMEM/F12) supplemented with 10% fetal calf serum, 100 IU/ml penicillin at 37°C in a 5% CO_2 humidified incubator.

(b)RA induce SH-SY5Y differentiation

After sub-cultured Human neuroblastoma (SH-SY5Y) seeding at 6cm round dish cells were treated with retinoic acid (RA) in 1 μM concentration in 2% FBS for three days and replenishing with fresh medium containing 1μM RA in 0.5% FBS for another three days, after 7 days accompany with gradually decrease fetal bovine serum (FBS), the cell will differentiated into a functionally mature DAergic neuronal.

(c) MPP^+ neurotoxic mimic Parkinson's disease

After differentiated, cell line SH-SY5Y was treated by MPP^+ 24h with different concentrations of 0~1.5 mM and apply MTT assay for cell viability test.

B. Repetitive Magnetic Stimulation Construction

We apply a cheap TI555 as processor to construction the repetitive magnetic stimulation, to generate a 10Hz、1Hz frequency pulse current through the coil we build to made repetitive magnetic stimulation environment (Fig. 1).

The electromagnetic bioreactor was placed into the cell-culture incubator and exposed cells were continuousl stimulated for 6, 12 and 24h (the maximum culture period without the need of medium change). intensity of the magnetic field equal to 56 ± 2 Gs, amplitude of the induced electric tension equal to 5 ± 1 mV, signal frequency of 10 Hz and 1Hz, and pulse duration of about 1sec.

C. Observations

(a)magnetic field

FW Bell 5180 Gaussmeter to measurement magnetic field where the cell exposed (Fig. 3).

I. Lackovic (ed.), *1st Global Conference on Biomedical Engineering & 9th Asian-Pacific Conference on Medical and Biological Engineering*,
IFMBE Proceedings 47, DOI: 10.1007/978-3-319-12262-5_67

(b) 2',7'-dichlorofluorescin diacetate (DCF-DA)

Intracellular ROS production was measured by flow cytometry using *2',7'-dichlorofluorescin* diacetate as a probe (Fig. 5).

(c) Tetramethyl rhodamine methyl ester (TMRM)

Mitochondrial membranes potential was measured by flow cytometry using Tetramethyl rhodamine methyl ester as a probe (Fig. 6).

(d)neurotransmitter analysis

Concentrations of dopamine (DA), dihydroxyphenylacetic acid (DOPAC) and homovanillic acid (HVA), were determined by HPLC with a column of 5 mm spherical C-18. The mobile phase consisted of A solvent 50 mM KH_2PO_4 B solvent 50mM KH_2PO_4 /AeCN (90/10) (pH 3.1).

(e) morphology image were show by Fig. 1

III. RESULTS

A. RA-Induced Neurite Outgrowth in SH-SY5Y Cells

Seven days after RA treatment, further changes in morphology including the shrinkage of cell body and extensive elongation of neurites with secondary or tertiary branches can be observed (Fig. 1).

B. Cell Viability

After treated MPP^+ 24h in different concentrations respectively 0mM, 0.3mM, 0.5mM, 0.7mM, 1mM, 1.5mM, and cell viability was quantitated by MTT assay (Fig. 2).

C. Electromagnetic Bioreactor

The repetitive magnetic stimulation machine applied to the cells with the following characteristics: intensity of the magnetic field equal to 56 ± 2 Gs, amplitude of the induced electric tension equal to 5 ± 1 mV, signal frequency of 10 Hz and 1Hz, and pulse duration of about 1s (Fig. 3).

D. Neurotransmitters Analysis

Measurement the medium which after magnetic stimulation, Comparison to catecholamine standards, dopamine、DOPAC and homovanillic acid. And use capsaicin as positive control. Find that after 24h magnetic stimulation have a HVA substance (Fig. 4)

E. Intracellular Reactive Oxygen Species

Respectively investigate high frequency and low frequency, there is no significant different ; In different stimulation duration can observe the ROS progressively decreased when stimulation time increase. On the other hand, whether high frequency or low frequency in different intensity of the magnetic field, 56Gs、42Gs、27Gs, there is no significant change in ROS level.

F. Mitochondria Membrane Potential

Fluorescence images of TMRM loaded SH-SY5Y cells in 10 μM for 30mins. After repetitive magnetic stimulation 24hr, mitochondrial membranes potential was decreased (Fig. 6).

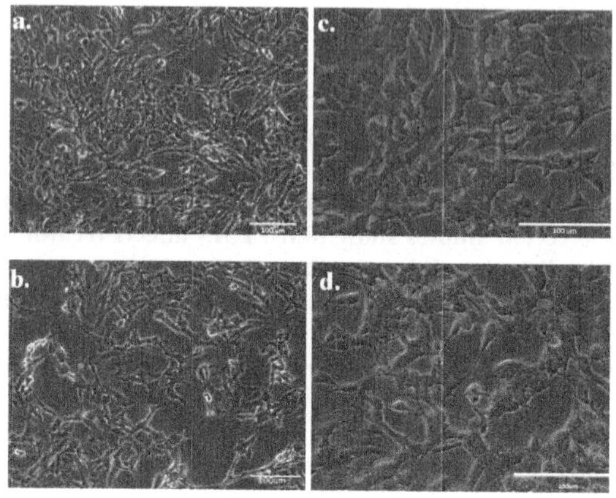

Fig. 1 Effect of RA on morphology of SHSY5Y cells.
After 7 days treatment the induce process cells morphology show different between RA group and control group. (a、c) Untreated cells (Leica DM6000B Phase contrast -X10、X20); (b、d) RA-treated cells (Leica DM6000B Phase contrast -X10、X20).

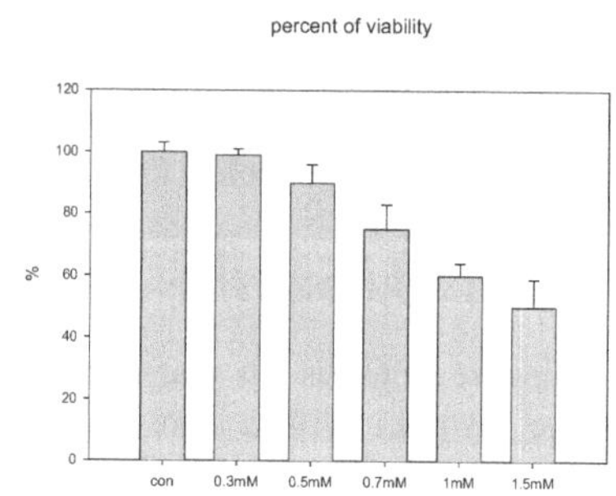

Fig. 2 Effects of MPP^+ on SH-SY5Y cell viability measured by MTT assay.
The cells were incubated 24hr with 0.3mM, 0.5mM, 0.7mM, 1mM, 1.5mM MPP^+. The viability of SH-SY5Y cell is significantly affected by the existence of MPP+ and is also concentration dependent.

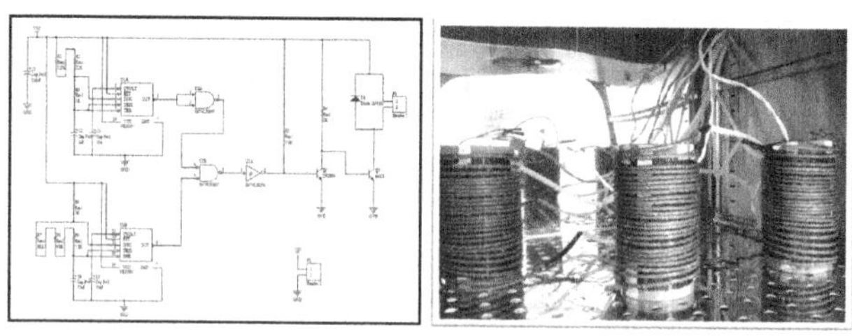

Fig. 3 Repetitive magnetic stimulation construction
Solenoid coil Machine in this experimental setup the magnetic field and the induced electric field were perpendicular and parallel to the seeded cells, respectively. (a) Cheap of the repetitive magnetic stimulation machine design, (b) The final completion set up in incubator

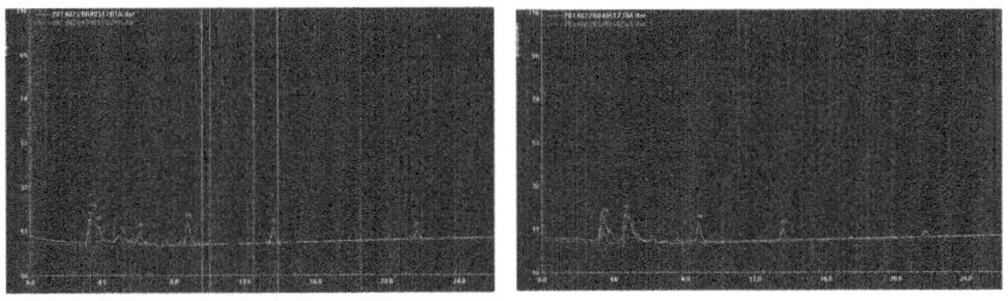

Fig. 4 Neurotransmitters released measurement by HPLC.
(a) Yellow light was analysis from cell medium, collected supernatant medium after Magnetic stimulation 24h, pink was homovanillic acid (HVA) standard. (b) A positive control, added capsaicin in SH-SY5Y cells in 10 μM for 3.5mins. The yellow light was cell medium, pink was homovanillic acid (HVA) standard. HVA is metabolites from dopamine. In fig. a、b result, we can confirm that, neuron after magnetic stimulation will release neurotransmitters.

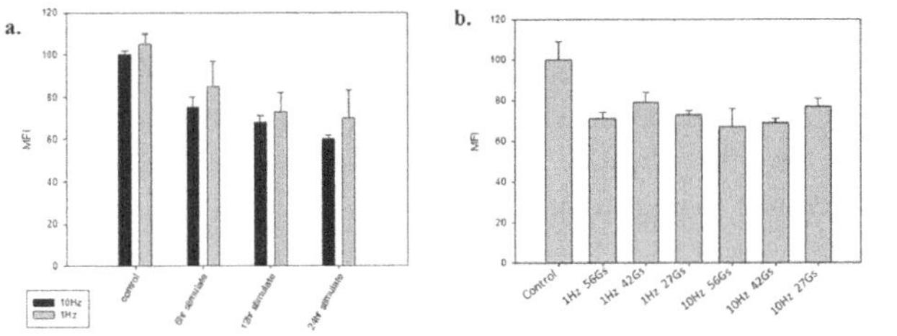

Fig. 5 Oxidative stress in SH-SY5Y cells after magnetic stimulation. Formation of reactive oxygen species was detected by dichlorofluorescein (DCF) fluorescence (n = 3). (a)With the different magnetic stimulation times, respectively 6hr、12hr、 24hr, the DCF signal progressively decreased, whereas the frequency had no significant effect. (b) In the same time, whether high frequency or low frequency in different intensity of the magnetic field, 56Gs、42Gs、27Gs, there is no significant change in ROS level.

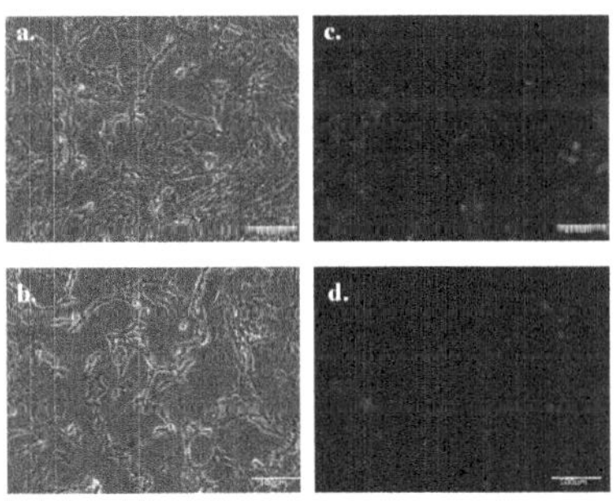

Fig. 6 Mitochondrial membranes potential using TMRM as the indicator dye in SH-SY5Y cells.
(a) Phase contrast images RA-treated cells. (b) fluorescence images of TMRM loaded SH-SY5Y cells in 10 μM for 30mins. (c) Phase contrast images after repetitive magnetic stimulation 24h. (d) fluorescence images of TMRM loaded SH-SY5Y cells after repeats magnetic stimulation 24h in 10 μM for 30mins. After repetitive magnetic stimulation, mitochondrial membranes potential was decreased.

IV. CONCLUSIONS

This study provides a chance to understand the effect of repeat magnetic stimulation on neural cells in different frequency、intensity and stimulation time. Fig. 7 clearly indicates that after magnetic stimulate, intracellular ROS were decreased. In the same time, neurons after magnetic stimulation will release neurotransmitters. These results suggest a possible use of this particular physical stimulation to improve the functional capability of the cells to face oxidative stress. Based on our study we can more understand that the effect of repetitive transcranial magnetic stimulations (rTMS) on Parkinson's disease.

REFERENCES

1. Xie H.R, HU L.S, LI G.Y (2010) SH-SY5Y human neuroblastoma cell line: in vitro cell model of dopaminergic neurons in Parkinson's disease. Chin Med J 123(8):1086-1092
2. Cheung YT, Way KW, Yu MS (2009) Effects of all-transretinoic acid on human SH-SY5Y neuroblastoma as in vitro model in neurotoxicity research., NeuroToxicology, 30(1): 127–135,
3. Giordano S, Lee J, Victor M. (2012) Distinct Effects of Rotnone,1-methyl-4-phenylpyridinium and 6-hydroxydopamine on Cellular Bioenergetics and Cell Death, Samantha Giordano, Bioenergetic Response to Neurotoxins, 7 (9): 1-11.
4. Kim JY, Chung EJ, Lee WY (2008) Therapeutic Effect of Rpetitive Transcranial Magnetic Stimulation in Parkinson's Disease: Analysis of [11C] raclopride PET Study. Mov Disord. 23(2): 207-211.
5. Osera C, Fassina L, Amadio M (2011) Cytoprotective Response Induced by Electromagnetic Stimulation on SH-SY5Y Human Neuroblastoma Cell Line, Cecilia Osera, Tissue Eng Part A 17(19 20): 2573 2582.

Immediate Effect of Exercise on Executive Function in Youth Group

Chia Yeh Hsieh, Pei Yin Tu, Jia Hong Sie, and Woei Chyn Chu*

Institute of Biomedical Engineering, National Yang-Ming University, Taipei, Taiwan

Abstract— **The benefit of physical activity and exercise is protecting against the deterioration of brain tissue with age. Previous studies have suggested that exercises have positive effects on cognition, but gender difference is still unclear. Therefore, we focus on the gender difference in cognitive ability, which is an important component for daily living and quality of life, before and after exercise. However, executive function is a higher-order cognitive function for daily life, including planning, scheduling, inhibiting, and working memory. We measure the executive function by tasks of psychology, including Wisconsin Card Sorting Test (WCST), Tower of Hanoi and N-back test. Fifty-six participants were recruited with the mean age of twenty-three years. Participants were asked to complete the WCST, Tower of Hanoi and N-back test before and after the exercise which be executed at least thirty minutes. Finally, we calculated the scores of tasks before and after exercise. The results indicated that there was a significant positive exercise effect on the WCST, Tower of Hanoi and N-back test in executive function and also found the light gender differences in the three tasks of psychology.**

Keywords— **Cognitive function, Executive function, Wisconsin Card Sorting Test, Tower of Hanoi, N-back test.**

I. INTRODUCTION

Cognitive ability is an important component for daily living, quality of life and even the ability to live independently [1]. Executive function is a higher-order cognitive function, including planning, scheduling, inhibition, and working memory [2]. However, brain volume shrinks with advancing age, often preceding or leading to cognitive impairment. Previous studies proposed several interventions that may retard or reverse age-related cognitive declines, and exercise is one of the interventions [3]. There is an inverted-U relationship between exercise intensity and cognitive performance by result of several studies [3-5]. Based on the inverted-U relationship, we design the exercise protocol in this study, including warm up five minutes, exercise twenty minutes and cold down five minutes.

This study evaluates the executive function by tasks of psychology, including Wisconsin card sorting test (WCST), Tower of Hanoi and N-back test. When participant finished WCST completely, software of WCST may extract seventeen parameters. This study adopts two parameters of those seventeen parameters, perseverative responses (PR) and non-perseverative errors (NPE), according to which is associated with executive function or not. PR represents planning of executive function, and NPR represents inhibition of executive function. Others, Tower of Hanoi represents scheduling and N-back test represents working memory.

Finally, previous studies have suggested that exercises have positive effects on cognition [5, 6], but gender difference is still unclear. Therefore, we focus on the gender difference in cognitive ability.

II. METHODS

A. Experimental

Fifty-six people (twenty-five females, age = 23.29 ± 1.52 years) were recruited. Table 1 presents participant demographic. First, we use the Physical Activity Readiness Questionnaire (PAR-Q) to ensure that doing exercise is safety for participant in this program. Then, we will calculate the metabolic equivalent (MET) of physical activity in the last seven days by International Physical Activity Questionnaire (IPAQ). Finally, participants were asked to complete the WCST, Tower of Hanoi and N-back test before and after the exercise which had to exercise least thirty minutes, including exercise twenty minutes and five minutes of warm up and cold down. Fig. 1 presents the flow chart of experiment. This protocol of experiment was approved by National Yang Ming University Institutional Review Board.

Table 1 Participant demographics

Measure	All	Males	Females
N	56	31	25
Age (year)	23.29(1.52)	23.39(1.58)	23.16(1.46)
Height (cm)	166.71(8.46)	172.44(9.24)	159.60(5.31)
Weight (kg)	59.89(9.86)	65.73(9.24)	52.66(4.20)
BMI (kg/m^2)	21.41(2.12)	22.04(2.33)	20.63(1.53)
IPAQ (MET)	1907.43(1453.22)	1939.87(1243.20)	1867(1704.30)
Education (year)	17.93(0.83)	18(0.86)	17.84(0.80)

* Corresponding author.

I. Lackovic (ed.), *1st Global Conference on Biomedical Engineering & 9th Asian-Pacific Conference on Medical and Biological Engineering*,
IFMBE Proceedings 47, DOI: 10.1007/978-3-319-12262-5_68

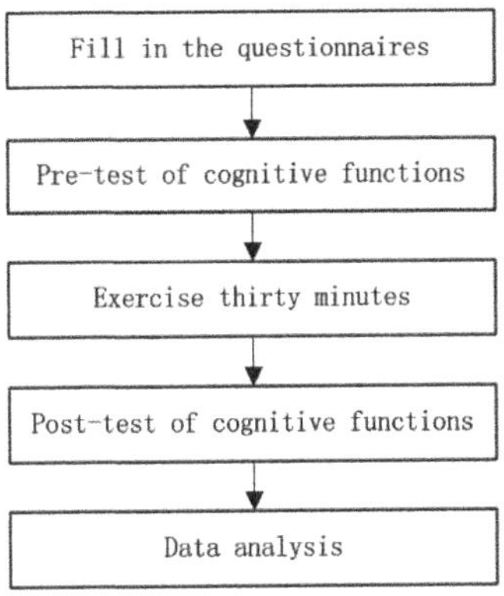

Fig. 1 Flow chart of experiment

B. Tools

a) Physical Activity Readiness Questionnaire (PAR-Q):

The PAR-Q is a screening tool and suitable for aged between fifteen and sixty-nine to ensure that doing exercise is safety for participant in this program.

b) International Physical Activity Questionnaire (IPAQ):

The purpose of the questionnaire is to provide common instruments that can be used to obtain internationally comparable data on health–related physical activity [7]. By this questionnaire, we find out the types of physical activities that people do during the last seven days. Therefore, the average MET score was derived for each of activity by compendium. Finally, we calculate the total METs of exercise last seven days.

c) Wisconsin card sorting test (WCST):

This test has four stimulus cards which combine three stimulus parameters (color, form, and number) and one hundred twenty-eight response cards. Participants need to sort the response cards according to different rules and to modify their approach during test [8].

d) Tower of Hanoi:

Tower of Hanoi is often used in psychological research that consists of three rods and many disks of different sizes following the level. The principles of test are [9]:

- All disks are slid from the leftest to the rightest rod.
- Only one disk can be moved at one time.
- Disk cann't placed on the top of a smaller disk.

e) N-back test:

Flash-based variant of the N-back test using visual and auditory paradigm. We take 2-back test in this study, which presents a series of stimuli at a constant rate. Test has to find the match between the current position and voice to the shown two steps earlier. However, if there is position or voice match press the corresponding match key.

III. RESULTS

A. Tower of Hanoi

Result from ANOVA revealed that there were main effect between pre-test and post-test (male in 5-layers: $F(1,61) = 63.673$ and 6-layers: $F(1,62) = 35.183$; female in 5-layers: $F(1,50) = 29.223$ and 6-layers: $F(1,50) = 14.745$). And, results also got $p < .01$ by paired T test, no matter in male or female. Table 2, Fig.2 and Fig.3 show the difference between pre-test and post-test.

Table 2 Results of Tower of Hanoi

Measure	Per-test	Post-test	p-value
Male_5 layers (time/steps)	2.08±0.76	1.10±0.37*	0.000*
Male_6 layers (time/steps)	1.66±0.46	1.18±0.35*	0.000*
Female_5 layers (time/steps)	1.78±0.48	0.96±0.28*	0.000*
Female_6 layers (time/steps)	1.59±0.36	1.09±0.28*	0.000*

*p value<0.01

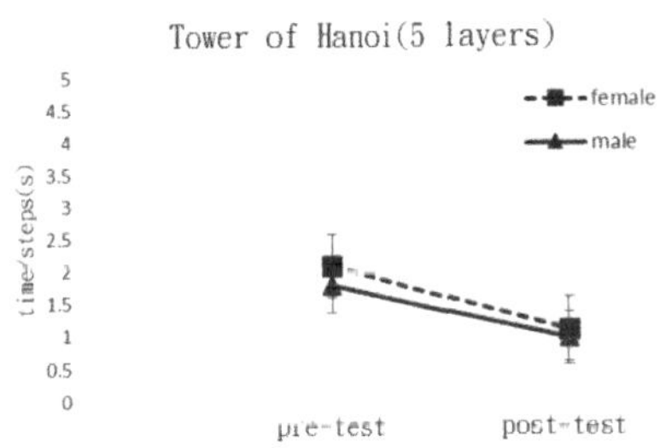

Fig. 2 Task performance of 5 layers Tower of Hanoi between male and female

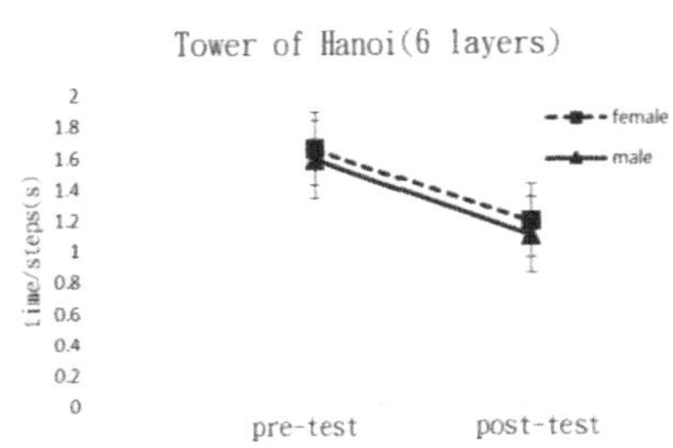

Fig. 3 Task performance of 6 layers Tower of Hanoi between male and female.

B. 2-Back Test

Based on the result of ANOVA between pre-test and post-test, male was $F(1,62)=40.299$, and female was

F(1,50)=30.125. According to the results from paired T test that effect on working memory have significant difference (p<.01) between pre-test and post-test. On the other hand, the result of two sample T test didn't have obvious difference. The results of 2-back test were shown in Table 2 and Fig.4.

Table 3 Results of 2-back test

Measure	Per-test	Post-test	p-value
Male_2-back test (%)	59.00±16.84	84.46±13.55	0.000*
Female_2-back test (%)	58.26±16.18	83.96±14.80	0.000*

*p value<0.01

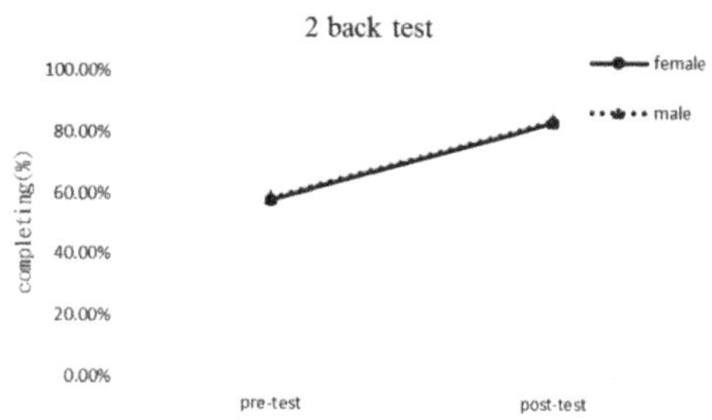

Fig. 4 Task performance of 2-back test between male and female.

C. *Wisconsin Card Sorting Test (WCST)*

The result of WCST would be corrected by Age & Education Demographically, and also found obvious various between pre-test and post-test (p<.01). However, we couldn't found obvious various in gender. In result of NPE, no matter pre-test or post-test male's completion were higher than female. Female's completion was higher at beginning in the result of PR, but PR values of male and female were almost same after doing exercise. Results of WCST were shown in Table 4, Table 5, Fig.5 and Fig.6.

Table 4 Results of NPE in WCST

Measure	Per-test	Post-test	p-value
Male_raw score	9.31±6.35	4.52±3.16	0.000*
Male_standard score	97.76±8.67	105.72±5.7	0.000*
Male_T score	48.38±5.9	53.90±3.76	0.000*
Male_percentile range	58.26±16.18	83.96±14.80	0.000*
Female_raw score	10.39±7.76	4.06±3.52	0.000*
Female_standard score	96.89±11.28	107.22±6.99	0.000*
Female_T score	47.94±7.51	54.94±4.69	0.000*
Female_percentile range	44.39±24.05	67.06±16.01	0.000*

*p value<0.01

Table 5 Results of PR in WCST

Measure	Per-test	Post-test	p-value
Male_raw score	13.07±8.09	5.73±3.68	0.000*
Male_standard score	90.63±11.66	105.2±8.23	0.000*
Male_T score	43.8±7.73	53.37±5.44	0.000*
Male_percentile range	31.77±21.74	62.5±18.94	0.000*
Female_raw score	9.39±5.94	5±2.09	0.000*
Female_standard score	97.44±10.99	107.83±10.59	0.000*
Female_T score	51.67±12.56	55.11±7.13	0.000*
Female_percentile range	45.44±23.66	65.56±17.08	0.000*

*p value<0.01

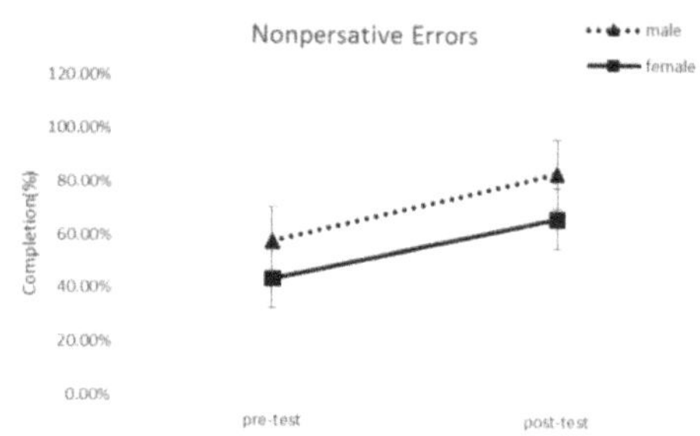

Fig. 5 Task performance of NPE in WCST between male and female.

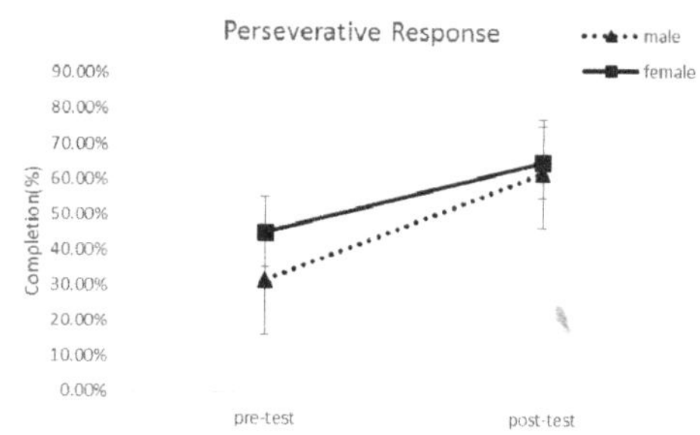

Fig. 6 Task performance of PR in WCST between male and female.

IV. Conclusions

This study has extended the literature by providing evidence that moderate-intensity aerobic exercise benefits planning, inhibition, scheduling and working memory. These finding supports Charles H. Hillman(2008) that aerobic exercise can improve brain cognition and performance.

References

1. Erickson, K. I., Raji, C. A., Lopez, O. L., Becker, J. T., Rosano, C., Newman, A. B., ... & Kuller, L. H. (2010). Physical activity predicts gray matter volume in late adulthood The Cardiovascular Health Study. *Neurology*, *75*(16), 1415-1422.

2. Chang, Y. K., Tsai, C. L., Huang, C. C., Wang, C. C., & Chu, I. H. (2014). Effects of acute resistance exercise on cognition in late middle-aged adults: General or specific cognitive improvement?. *Journal of Science and Medicine in Sport*, *17*(1), 51-55.
3. Salthouse, T. A. (2004). What and when of cognitive aging. *Current Directions in Psychological Science*, *13*(4), 140-144.
4. Hillman, C. H., Erickson, K. I., & Kramer, A. F. (2008). Be smart, exercise your heart: exercise effects on brain and cognition. *Nature Reviews Neuroscience*,*9*(1), 58-65.
5. Colcombe, S., & Kramer, A. F. (2003). Fitness effects on the cognitive function of older adults a meta-analytic study. *Psychological science*, *14*(2), 125-130.
6. Chang, Y. K., & Etnier, J. L. (2009). Exploring the dose-response relationship between resistance exercise intensity and cognitive function. *Journal of sport & exercise psychology*, *31*(5), 640.
7. Hagströmer, M., Oja, P., & Sjöström, M. (2006). The International Physical Activity Questionnaire (IPAQ): a study of concurrent and construct validity.*Public health nutrition*, *9*(06), 755-762.
8. Heaton, R. K., Chelune, G. J., Talley, J. L., Kay, G. G., & Curtiss, G. (1993). Wisconsin card sort test manual: Revised and expanded. *Odessa, FL: Psychological Assessment Resources*.
9. Zook, N. A., Davalos, D. B., DeLosh, E. L., & Davis, H. P. (2004). Working memory, inhibition, and fluid intelligence as predictors of performance on Tower of Hanoi and London tasks. *Brain and cognition*, *56*(3), 286-292.

Author: Woei Chyn Chu
Institute: Institute of Biomedical Engineering
Street: No.155, Sec.2, Linong Street
City: Taipei
Country: Taiwan
Email: wchu@ym.edu.tw

Real Time Measurement of Dopamine Releasing under Optogenetic Stimulation

Cho-Han Hsieh, Chun-Wei Wu, Meng-Chun Liu, and Jia-Jin Jason Chen

Institute of Biomedical Engineering, National Cheng-Kung University, Tainan, Taiwan

Abstract— **Dopamine (DA) is a neurotransmitter involved in controlling of fine movement, which is deficient in Parkinson's disease (PD). Measurement of DA is an urgent need concerning the development of PD therapy. We've developed a fast-scan cyclic voltammetry (FSCV) for real time measurement of dopamine releasing in dopaminergic SH-SY5Y cells under tissue-specific optogenetic stimulation. With the novel cellular optical-induced DA-releasing model, the performance of FSCV will be validated under various stimulating parameters.**

Keywords— **Dopamine, optogenetics, fast-scan cyclic voltammetry (FSCV), Parkinson's disease.**

I. INTRODUCTION

Dopamine is a neurotransmitter in the dopaminergic projections such as striatum, substantia nigra and ventral tegmental area (VTA). It is critically involved in voluntary motor control, attention, learning, perception and processing of rewarding and aversive stimuli [1]. Parkinson's disease is caused by the death of dopaminergic neuron. The deficient in dopamine releasing cause the abnormal motor symptom include muscular rigidity, tremor, bradykinesia and gait disturbance. In pharmacological treatment of Parkinson's disease, the levodopa is most used in clinical patients. For many years the role of dopamine transmission in different physiological and pathological processes was studied using electrical or chemical stimulation. And a novel technology, optogenetics has provided the field of neuroscience a new way to stimulate specific neuron precisely [2] (Figure 1).

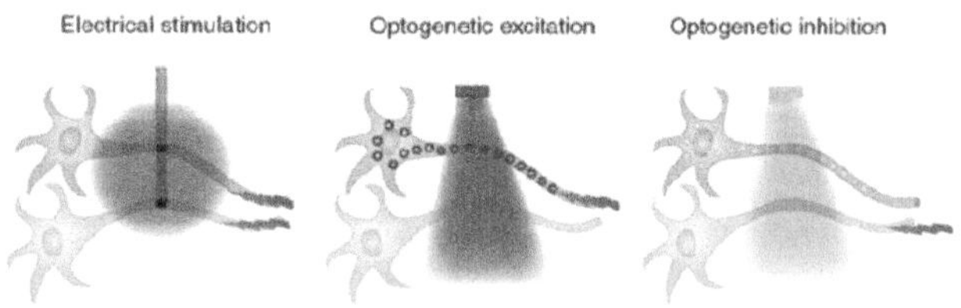

Fig. 1 Principle of optogenetics in neuroscience.

For real-time measurement of dopamine, several research groups began to combine optogenetics with fast-scan cyclic voltammetry (FSCV) to examine optically induced dopamine dynamics [3]. For ensure the best stimulus parameter for dopamine releasing, we used a dopaminergic neuron SH-SY5Y expressed channelrhodopsin-2 (ChR2) by lentivirus transduction. Simultaneously measurement of dopamine releasing using FSCV system, and recording of multi-unit activity from multi-electrode array system had been conducted under optical stimulation. Laser light power, pulse width and frequency will be determined for the references of future *in vivo* test.

II. MATERIAL AND METHODS

A. Viral Production

Second generation packaging system is used for virus transfection, psPAX2 is packaging plasmid and pMD2.G is envelope plasmid. The insert gene used are pLenti-EF1a-GFP, pLenti-CaMKIIa-ChR2(H134R) and pLenti-EF1a-ChR2(H134R). The plasmids were acquired from a nonprofit organization: addgene (www.addgene.com). For producing lentiviral particles, the 293FT cells were used for transfection using calcium chloride ($CaCl_2$) method. 10μl DNA contain 5 μg insert gene, 1.75μg pMD2.G and 3.25μg psPAX2 mix with 215 μl ddH_2O. And mixd with 250 μl calcium chloride. And the mixed solution was added in 500μl HeBS buffer (pH7.05) with vortex. Stand for 30 mins, the 500 μl mix solution will add to 6 cm dish contain 293FT cell. The medium was collected after 16 to 24 hours, and concentrate the viral solution by ultracentrifuge.

B. Viral Titration Test

For assessing the efficiency of transduction, the titration test was carried out by using SH-SY5Y. Before titration test, polybrene was added in the viral solution to enhance the efficiency. After the virus added in the medium, the expression of insert gene is observed everyday by fluorescence microscope for long-term monitoring of expression for 18 days.

C. Virus Transduction

In titration test, we find the best concentration of virus and polybrene for virus transduction. We directly add virus and polybrene in the 10 cm dish contain SH-SY5Y. 15 μl virus were added and the final concentration of polybrene was 1.0μl/ml. Avoid the cytotoxicity of polybrene, the medium were changed after one day transduction.

I. Lackovic (ed.), *1st Global Conference on Biomedical Engineering & 9th Asian-Pacific Conference on Medical and Biological Engineering*,
IFMBE Proceedings 47, DOI: 10.1007/978-3-319-12262-5_69

D. Measure Dopamine Releasing

To estimate the effect of different simulation schemes including light power, stimulation frequency and pulse width on the dopamine releasing from ChR2-expressing SH-SY5Y cells. Two different promoter were used, EF1a is a general promoter. CaMKIIa is a promoter specific expressed in the glutamatergic neuron. The calcium is necessary for dopamine releasing [4]. And the EF1a-GFP was used for control group. For comparison, continuous illumination (CI) and pulse of blue light with frequencies of 10, 20 and 30 Hz, Durations of 10, 20 and 30 ms were applied for 10 seconds. The LED is controlled by LabVIEW program. And the measurement of dopamine-releasing using FSCV by applying a triangular waveform (-0.3 to 1.4V versus Ag/AgCl electrode, 340 V/s). Data were sampled at 80 kHz via the ADC (DAQ pad-6221, National Instruments). The electrophysiology signals recording via microelectrode array (MEA) and recorded by LABView. (Figure. 3)

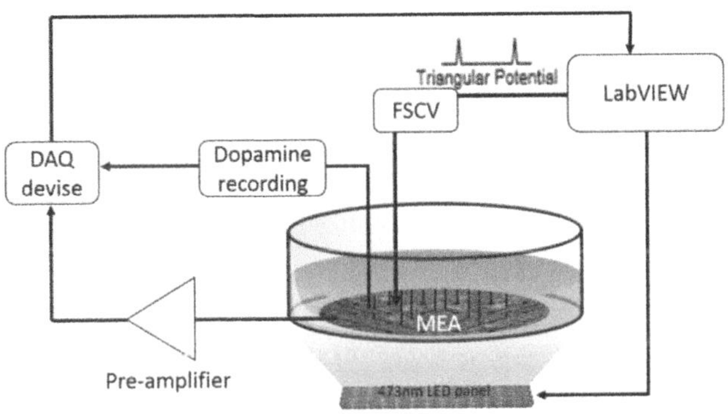

Fig. 2 Block diagrams of the *in vitro* measurement of dopamine and electrophysiology signals by optical stimulation

III. RESULT AND DISCUSSION

For in-vitro transduction in the SH-SY5Y cell, the expression of the pLenti-EF1a-GFP is strong and pLenti-CaMKIIa-ChR2(H134R)-EYFP-WPRE is relatively weaker. We observed the expression every day in 4 different concentrations of polybrene at 5 μg/ml, 1 μg/ml, 0.2 μg/ml and no polybrene control (Figure.3). The expression of 1 μg/ml has showns the best results. It might reflects that high concentration of polybrene has cytocoxity and could affects the growth of cell.

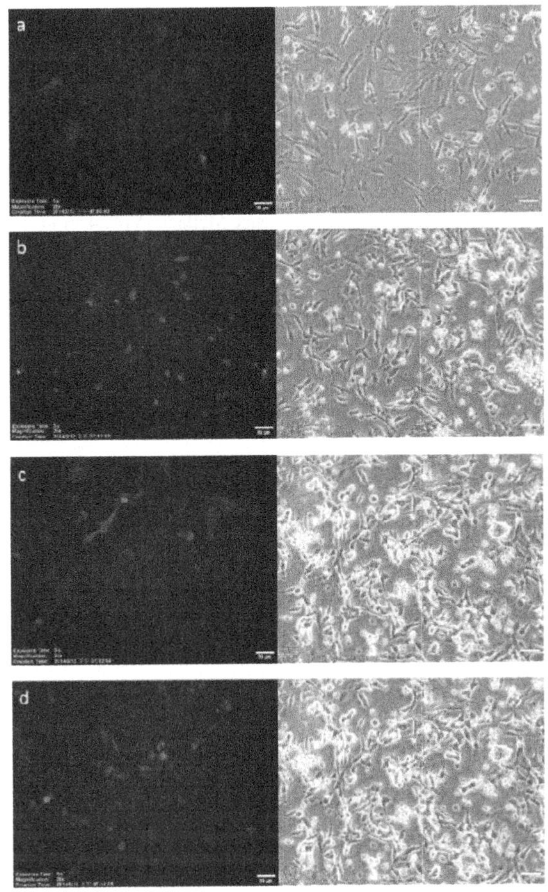

Fig. 3 ChR2-EYFP expression in the SH-SY5Y at 17 days. The concentrations of polybrene are (a) 5 μg/ml (b) 1 μg/ml (c) 0.2μg/ml (d)no control

IV. CONCLUSIONS

From *in vitro* virus transduction study, our results show that the promoter of EF1a and CaMKIIa can be expressed in the SH SY5Y. Participation of appropriate polybrene can enhance the efficiency for transduction. For comparing the dopamine releasing after different stimulation protocols including different frequency and theta burst stimulation. The measurement of electrophysiology will carry out for verifying those stimulation elicit neural plasticity or not. To evaluate the neural plasticity will affect the dopamine releasing or not, we will use those cell for long term treatment via different stimulation schemes. And detect the level exchange of dopamine releasing after treatment.

ACKNOWLEDGMENT

The authors would like to thank the Ministry of Science and Technology of R.O.C. for financially supporting this research under contract No. NSC 101-2221-E-006 -006 -MY3.

REFERENCES

1. Bass CE, Grinevich VP, Kulikova AD, Bonin KD and Budygin EA (2013) "Terminal effects of optogenetic stimulation on dopamine dynamics in rat striatum." J Neuroscience Methods. Vol 241:149–155.
2. Disseroth K (2011) "Optogenetics" Nature Methods. Vo.8, NO. 1:26–29.
3. Bass CE, Grinevich VP, Vance ZB, Sullivan RP, Bonin KD and Budygin EA (2010) "Optogenetic control of striatal dopamine release in rats" J Neurochemistry Vol 144:1344–1352
4. Chiu WT, Lin CM, Tsai TC, Wu CW, Tsai CL, Lin SH and Chen JJJ, "Real-Time Electrochemical Recording of Dopamine Release under Optogenetic Stimulation." PLOS ONE, Vol 9

Author: Cho-Han Hsieh
Institute: Biomedical Engineering, National Cheng-Kung University
Street: No.1, University Road
City: Tainan City 701
Country: Taiwan (R.O.C.)
Email: hank.jasonbiolab@gmail.com

Signal Conversion from Attention Signals to Light Emitting Diodes as an Attention Level Indicator

D.P.X. Kan, V.W.W. Lim, and P.F. Lee

Mechatronics & Biomedical Department, University of Tunku Abdul Rahman, Faculty of Engineering & Science, Malaysia

Abstract— **With the advancement of Brain-Computer Interface (BCI), human mind control devices is getting common in the medical field. In this paper, an attention level indicator was proposed in aid to monitor one's attention level especially for Attention Deficient Disorder (ADD) patient. It was designed to activate the number of lightening LED lights by monitoring of the human attention level. NeuroSky Mindwave mobile headset was used to acquire the brain wave attention signals. A MATLAB programme was developed to perform signal processing, included data extraction, error detection and command setting. The extracted attention level parameters from NeuroSky ThinkGear software were set as an input command for activating the LED lights. These programs and commands were delivered to a microcontroller board, the Arduino UNO, to regulate the input and output systems. The LEDs attention level indicator can be used to monitor attention level from time to time. Finally, an experiment was carried out to investigate which type of activities would generate the highest undergraduate engineering students' attention level. The results found out that female students obtained better focus on paying attention compared to male students. Also, female students shows result that able to focus better during visual based activity whereas male students were good at hands on based activity. However, in general, our group of samples of undergraduates students tend to pay higher attention on visual based activity than audio or hands on activities.**

Keywords— **Elecencephalogram (EEG), Brain-Controlled Interface(BCI), Attention, Indicator, NeuroSky.**

I. INTRODUCTION

BCI is an interfacing system that uses electrical signals from the brain (EEG) as an input to control other devices (Astiyani, Asadi & Birgani, 2008). It is a communication system that recognizes user's command only from his or her brain waves and reacts according to them (Teplan, 2002). Originally, BCI is developed for medical purposes, it allows the patients with severe motor disorder to control wheelchairs, prosthetics and even spell words on the computer screen by only using their thoughts (Long et al., 2012; Lopes, Pires, & Nunes, 2011; Murguialday et al., 2007). The main objective of this paper is to develop an attention level indicator from the EEG brain wave signal. This is a fundamental concept of BCI which involved the signal conversion from brain wave to an external device. With this indicator, the attention level of people can be monitored easily. It also can be acted as a diagnostic device to diagnose attention deficit disorder (ADD). According to statistic, ADD is affecting 3% to 10% of children and approximate 4% of the adult population in United State (Sohn et al., 2010). Thus, with this prototype, the attention level of patients can be monitored in a more convenient way. Besides that, an attention level indicator can be a device for parental monitoring on the attention level of children.

EEG system is a non-invasive method and technique which is easy and safely to use for brain electrical activity detection and measurement. The human brain waves were categorizes into different frequency band. Generally, delta waves (0.1 ~ 3 Hz) relate to deep sleep, theta waves (4 ~ 7 Hz) relate to drowsiness or early sleep, alpha waves (8 ~ 12 Hz) correlate with relaxation or rest state, while beta waves (13 ~ 30 Hz) correlate with mental concentration and active thinking (Baskaran, Milev, & Mcintyre, 2012). The compositions of frequency bands change depending on mental and emotional states and the locations of the electrodes. The NeuroSky had developed the attention and meditation algorithms based on these brainwaves components to monitor the mental attention and relaxation levels. The attention algorithm represents overall mental and visual attentions. It is sensitive to mental attention and visual focusing. The meditation algorithm shows sensitivity to eye open and close, and mental relaxation (Lee, 2009).

The aim of this project was to convert the attention signals from the NeuroSky MindWave electroencephalogram (EEG) as a command to activate an external device as an attention level indicator. The system architecture will be discussed in the following session followed by the result of experiment. An experiment was conducted using this device to investigate the effect of four activities based on audio, hands on, visual without sound and visual with annoying sounds in enhancing the attention level.

II. SYSTEM ARCHITECTURE OVERVIEW

In short, this project can be expressed into three stages. The first stage was the input acquisition procedure. Brain wave signals were detected and measured using EEG

I. Lackovic (ed.), *1st Global Conference on Biomedical Engineering & 9th Asian-Pacific Conference on Medical and Biological Engineering*,
IFMBE Proceedings 47, DOI: 10.1007/978-3-319-12262-5_70

headset. These EEG signals would then be displayed in the personal computer. The signal conversion process took place in the second stage. A MATLAB code was developed to perform the programming part, including EEG signals display, setting of system command and transmit commands to the external hardware. At the final output stage, LEDs were chosen as the monitoring device to monitor the real time attention level of a subject. An Arduino UNO was used to receive commands from MATLAB for controlling the LEDs. Nine colourful LEDs were functioning as the attention level indicator. LEDs would light up based on the subject's attention level. The number of LEDs lightens up increased when the attention level increased. This can be a device to monitor one's attention level from time to time. The connection between EEG system, computer and LEDs attention level indicator was showed in Fig.1. In this paper, the signal conversion from EEG attention level into LED monitoring device will further discuss in the following session.

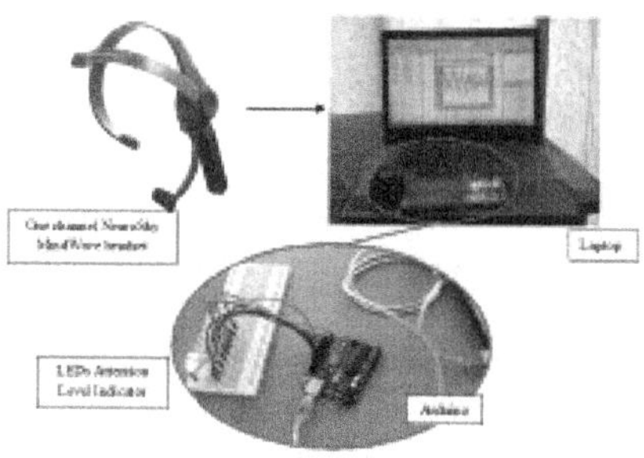

Fig. 1 EEG attention signals were transmitted from NeuroSky MindWave headset to MATLAB at computer via Bluetooth and connected to LEDs attention level indicator through Arduino.

III. Methods

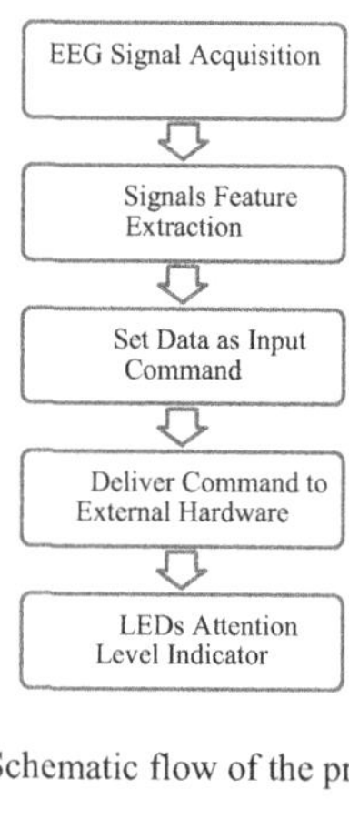

Fig. 2 Schematic flow of the project design

Fig. 2 showed the schematic flow of the project design. A single channel wearable NeuroSky Mindwave headset and NeuroSky ThinkGear software (NeuroSky Inc., U.S.A.) were used in this research. The Neurosky EEG headset was used to record and store the brain wave signals into the computer. The dry type EEG system used active electrode to record the EEG data at left prefrontal, FP1 with reference to the ear lobe. The EEG signals were filtered with a notch and band pass (0.5-30 hz) filters and converted to digital data at 128 Hz sampling rate. Noise and abnormal EEG signals which amplitudes exceed 100 microvolt were eliminated. The raw brain wave signals and attention and meditation levels were displayed by the NeuroSky Brainwave Visualizer on the computer monitor.

However, the attention signal was the main focus on this project to be extracted out as activation of external hardware. The level of attention was presented as a score from 0 to 100 indicating the intensity of a user's level of mental "focus" or "attention". The attention level was extracted out from the ThinkGear software by NeuroSky which would be used as the command to activate the LEDs attention level indicator. The function of the on-screen data displayed was to ensure the correct categorization of the LEDs attention level, in response to the commands.

A connecting device was used to transmit the attention signals from computer to LEDs attention level indicator. In this project, Arduino UNO was used as the connecting device which received the command from MATLAB and lightens the LEDs according to the output command. Arduino is a single-board microcontroller intended to make interaction between objects of environment more accessible. Arduino can sense the environment by receiving input from a variety of sensors, and can affect its surrounding objects by controlling lights, motors, and other actuators. Here, Arduino was receiving the attention signals from MATLAB and control the mode of LEDs.

The attention level was categorized into five levels which were "poor attention" (1-19), "less attention" (20-39), "neutral" (40-59), "good attention" (60-79) and "great attention" (80-100) (NeuroSky, 2011). This categorization of attention level was summarized in Table 1 below.

Table 1 Five category of attention levels

Attention Level	Category
80 – 100	Great Attention
60 -79	Good Attention
40 – 59	Neutral
20 -39	Less Attention
1 – 19	Poor Attention

Nine LEDs were used as the attention level indicator. Five red LEDs are used to represent level lower than 60.

Two green LEDs are used to indicate the "Good Attention" level, which range from 60 to 80, and two blue LEDs are represented "Great Attention" concentration level, range between 80 and 100. Therefore, the LEDs would light up based on the subject's attention level. The number of LEDs lightens up increased when the attention level increased. Fig. 3 showed the LEDs attention level indicator during different range of attention level. This can be a device to monitor one's attention level from time to time.

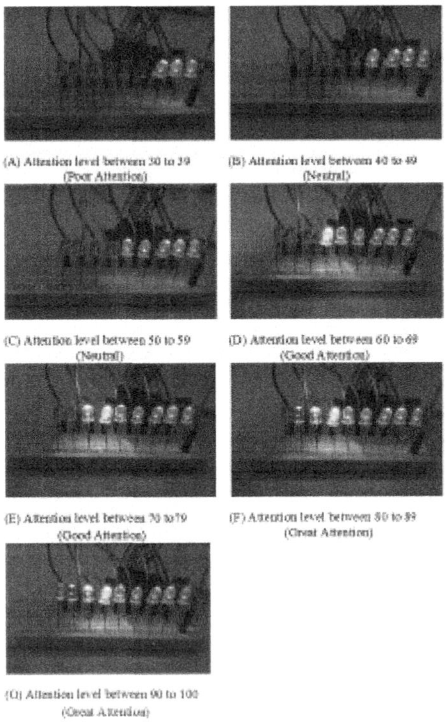

Fig. 3 LEDs attention level indicator for different range of attention level

IV. EXPERIMENTAL STUDY

Experiment was designed and conducted using the LEDs attention indicator to investigate the activities that enhance the attention level of undergraduate students. A total of ten students with 5 males and 5 females, aged from 23 to 25 with a mean age of 23.38 participated in this study. They were the undergraduate students from the University of Tunku Abdul Rahman, Malaysia. Their participation was voluntary and participant consent was obtained before the study began.

The experiment was carried out in a controlled environment. Distractions, wandering thoughts, lack of focus, or anxiety may lower the attention level of the subject. The test subject was required to wear a pair of earplug earphone throughout the whole experiment procedures. Four activities were carried out in this experiment, which included audio, hands on, visual without sound, and visual with annoying sound. The duration for each activity is 5 minutes. Before each activity, there would be 2 minutes relaxing time, with closed eyes but conscious, to serve as the refractory period for the subject's mind. This was to avoid brain wave being affected by previous activities.

The first activity was the audio based attention level test. The test subject was required to listen to 5 minutes of Mozart's Sonata for Two Pianos in D Major (K. 448). Researcher believed that listening to Mozart's music can enhance human concentration, commonly known as the Mozart effect (Bangerter & Heath, 2004). For the second activity, hands on based activity, the test subject was asked to perform simple paper art. The subject was required to cut paper into strips, and use the paper strips to fold star's origami. The whole process was repeated until 5 minutes were over. The third activity was a vision based activity. A list of word search game was given to the subject to play for 5 minutes. For the final activity, visual with annoying sound, the subject was required to listen to a restaurant sound recording and at the same time, the subject had to continue the word search game given in the third activity for another 5 minute period. The total times of subject's attention level remained at "Good Attention" and "Great Attention" level were recorded, which are between 60 to 79 and 80 to 100 respectively.

ANOVA analysis was used to evaluate the significant differences in attention level between gender and types of activities. The level of significant values was set at $p<0.005$. Data were analysed with Statistical Package for the Social Science (SPSS), ver 11.5. (SPSS Inc., Chicago, IL, USA).

V. RESULTS AND DISCUSSION

Comparison of Attention Level Based on Gender

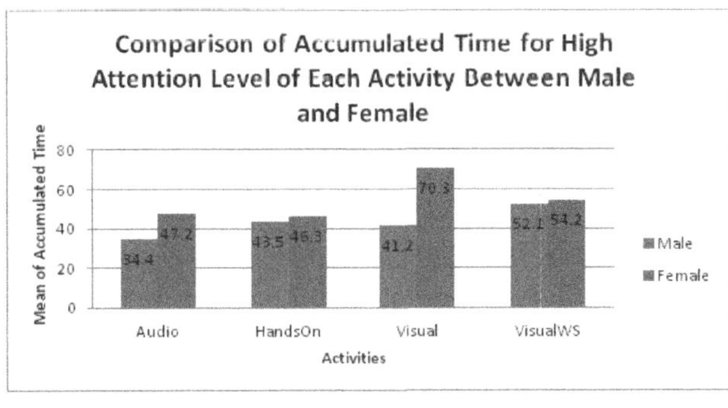

Fig. 4 Comparison of mean accumulated time during high attention level on each activities based on gender

The mean accumulated time of the 10 subjects was obtained and plotted in Fig. 4. The graph described the average of the total time during high attention level (good and great attention) for different type of activities. These results were compared between male and female. From the figure, the mean accumulated time of female during high attention level was higher than male for all types of activities. ANOVA analysis also showed that there was a significant difference in periods of high attention level between gender ($f(1) = 4.227$, $p<0.05$). Female in this experiment tended to pay more attention during the experiments compared to male. This finding was corresponding to the latest study that indicating male subjects were less able to pay attention to learning stimuli than their female counterparts (Chua, 2014).

Chief & Shallcross (1992) suggested that males and females have different paying attention abilities. Form the experiment, male subjects paid the longest attention on "visual with annoying sound" activity. This result showed that male would like to pay more attention under noisy environment. Two of the test subjects had responded on this condition. They stated that, under noisy environment, they tended to pay more attention to the activity – word search game, in order to complete their task under disturbance. The second activity that male had longer high attention time is the "hands on" activity. This can be explained by the concepts of male preference task. Male prefers physical task such as sports, circuit designs and driving, instead of paperwork. Nevertheless, for male students, the high attention time for each activity has not much significant different if compared to female student's results, the highest mean time was 52.1s and the lowest was 34.4s, the difference was 17.7s.

Whereas, for female students, the two activities that had the longest attention time were both visual based activities, "visual without noisy sound" activity followed by and "visual with annoying sound" activity. One of the reasons lead to this result was the NeuroSky Attention meter can be controlled through visual focus (NeuroSky, 2011). For example like staring at a point on the screen or imagine the action that trying to accomplish. In this experiment, word search game was used to test visual based attention. The test subjects would tend to search the listed words from rows of alphabet. Different from male, female prefers paperwork instead of physical tasks. However, there were large differences between the highest and lowest results of the female students, which the difference was 24s. The female was good in attention ability test, such as word search or alphabet search, whereas male can pay more attention in creative thinking test, which was not included in this study (Piaw, 2014). Although some researches on attention in literature point out there are no relation between subjects' gender and attention level (Mehmet & Gülsüm, 2010). Furthermore, female more likely to multitask especially during communication and audio activities compared to male (Cotten, Shank, & Anderson, 2014).

Comparison of Attention Level Based on Activities

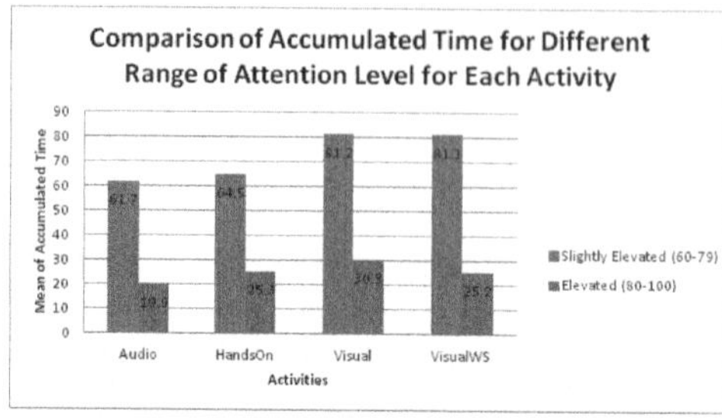

Fig. 5 Comparison of mean accumulated time between two ranges of attention level for each activity

Fig. 5 described the average of the total time during good and great attention level for different type of activities. Attention level range from 60 to 79 was categorized as "good attention", and range from 80 and above was "great attention" level. Audio activity had the lowest concentration period among the four activities for both good and great attention levels. Study had find out that listening to Mozart Sonata K.488 will increase human involuntary attention but decreased the voluntary attention (Zhu, Zhao, Zhang, & Ding, 2008). Visual without noisy sound has the highest period of concentration time for both attention levels. This indicated that visual activity may help in increasing one's attention level. By comparing both visual activities with audio and hands on activities, visual activities had higher concentration time than the remaining activities. ANOVA analysis revealed that there was no significant difference between the concentration time with activities ($f(3) = 1.506$, $p=0.221$). Thus, the type of activities may not affect the concentration time. However, in fact, both the visual based activities had the highest concentration time compared to the others. This may due to as mentioned earlier, the NeuroSky attention level of ThinkGear algorithm can be controlled through visual focus (NeuroSky, 2011).

VI. CONCLUSIONS

In conclusion, an attention level indicator was developed using light emitting diodes (LED). The numbers of LEDs light up were based on the subject's attention level. It was proposed as a real time attention level monitoring device. The development process of this prototype can be divided into three phases. The first phase was the brain wave signals acquisition phase, where NeuroSky Mindwave Mobile EEG headset was used to detect brain wave and transmit them into user's computer. Followed by the signal processing phase, where the attention level parameter was extracted out from the NeuroSky ThinkGear software and transferred to MATLAB for the command setting. For the final phase, the command was delivered to the external environment to activate the LED lights indicating the attention level of the subjects occasionally.

Based on the results of the experiment, female students had better ability to pay high attention compared to male students. Male students were good at hands on based or physical activity, whilst female students had a better attention span on visual based activity. The results were also compared between the activities. The overall result showed that visual based activity will lead to a longer high attention period compared to other activities. This indicated that the visual based activity can enhance one's attention level.

ACKNOWLEDGMENT

This research was funded by University of Tunku Abdul Rahman's Research Funding. We would like to thank to all the students who participated in this research.

CONFLICT OF INTEREST

The authors declare that they have no conflict of interest.

REFERENCES

1. Ashtiyani, M., Asadi, S., & Birgani, P. M. (2008). "EEG Classification using Neural networks and Independent component analysis", Biomed 2008,Proceedings 21,pp. 179-182.
2. Bangerter, A., & Heath, C. (2004). The Mozart effect: Tracking the evolution of a scientific legend. *British Journal of Social Psychology*, *43*, 605–623.
3. Baskaran, A., Milev, R., & Mcintyre, R. S. (2012). Neuropharmacology The neurobiology of the EEG biomarker as a predictor of treatment response in depression. *Neuropharmacology*, *63*(4), 507–513. doi:10.1016/j.neuropharm.2012.04.021
4. Cotten, S. R., Shank, D. B., & Anderson, W. a. (2014). Gender, technology use and ownership, and media-based multitasking among middle school students. *Computers in Human Behavior*, *35*, 99–106. doi:10.1016/j.chb.2014.02.041
5. Lee, K. (2009). Evaluation of Attention and Relaxation Levels of Archers in Shooting Process using Brain Wave Signal Analysis Algorithms Evaluation of Attention and Relaxation Levels of Archers in Shooting Process using Brain Wave Signal Analysis Algorithms NeuroSky Inc .*, *12*(3), 341–350.
6. Long, J., Li, Y., Wang, H., Yu, T., Pan, J., & Li, F. (2012). A Hybrid Brain Computer Interface to Control the Direction and Speed of a Simulated or Real Wheelchair. *IEEE TRANSACTIONS ON NEURAL SYSTEMS AND REHABILITATION ENGINEERING*, *20*(5), 720–729.
7. Lopes, A. C., Pires, G., & Nunes, U. (2011). Wheelchair Navigation Assisted by Human-Machine Shared-control and a P300-based Brain Computer Interface. In *Proceedings of the 2007 IEEE 10th International Conference on Rehabilitation Robotics* (pp. 2438–2444).
8. Mehmet, K., & Gülsüm, B. A. Ş. T. U. Ğ. (2010). Ovidius University Annals, Series Physical Education and Sport / SCIENCE, MOVEMENT AND HEALTH ., Issue 2 suppl. 2010 Our JOURNAL is nationally acknowledged by C.N.C.S.I.S., being included in the B+ category publications, 2008-2010. Indexed in: INDEX COPER. *Ovidius University Annals, Series Physical Education and Sport / SCIENCE, MOVEMENT AND HEALTH.*, (2), 2008–2010.
9. Murguialday, A. R., Aggarwal, V., Chatterjee, A., Cho, Y., Rasmussen, R., Rourke, B. O., … Thakor, N. V. (2007). Brain-Computer Interface for a Prosthetic Hand Using Local Machine Control and Haptic Feedback. In *Proceedings of the 2007 IEEE 10th International Conference on Rehabilitation Robotics* (Vol. 00, pp. 609–613).
10. Piaw, C. Y. (2014). Relationship between Thinking Styles and Ability to Pay Attention of Malaysian Male and Female Student Teachers. *Procedia - Social and Behavioral Sciences*, *116*, 4839–4843. doi:10.1016/j.sbspro.2014.01.1035
11. Teplan, M. (2002). FUNDAMENTALS OF EEG MEASUREMENT. *Measurement Science Review*, *2*, 1–11.
12. Zhu, W., Zhao, L., Zhang, J., & Ding, X. (2008). The influence of Mozart ' s sonata K . 448 on visual attention: An ERPs study. *Neuroscience Letters*, *434*, 35–40. doi:10.1016/j.neulet.2008.01.043

Sensory Stimulation-Induced Neuroprotection in Hyperacute Phase of Ischemic Stroke – A Multimodal Imaging Study

Lun-De Liao[1,*], Yu-Hang Liu[1,2], Aishwarya Bandla[1,3], Ji Min Ling[1], Hsin-Yi Lai[4], You-Yin Chen[5], and Nitish V. Thakor[1,6]

[1] Singapore Institute for Neurotechnology (SiNAPSE), Singapore
[2] Department of Electrical and Computer Engineering, National University of Singapore, Singapore
[3] Department of Biomedical Engineering, National University of Singapore, Singapore
[4] Department of Physical Medicine and Rehabilitation, Chang Gung University, Taiwan
[5] Department of Biomedical Engineering, National Yang Ming University, Taiwan
[6] Department of Biomedical Engineering, Johns Hopkins University, USA

Abstract— **Study of cerebral cortical functions affected by ischemic stroke explicates post-stroke brain plasticity. We report an innovative combination of electrocorticography (ECoG) recordings and functional photoacoustic microscopy (fPAM) imaging to investigate cortical functions after photothrombotic ischemia (PTI) in rat brain, with electrical forepaw stimulation applied as treatment. The cortical functions were assessed over a chosen ischemic region via somatosensory-evoked potential (SSEP), resting-state ECoG signals and evoked hemodynamic response. Two-phased experimental protocols based on sensory stimulation treatment are proposed and performed in this study. In the phase 1, the treatment is applied to the left forepaw, contralateral to the ischemic hemisphere, with 2 mA pulses initiated 0, 1, or 2 hours post-ischemia to determine optimal onset timing. After determining the optimal time window, in the phase 2, the treatment was delivered unilaterally or bilaterally using 2 or 4 mA pulses for validating if bilateral peripheral electrical stimulation with different current intensities could improve cerebral perfusion and restore cortical neurovascular response. Overall, the results demonstrated that our treatment administered bilaterally at 2 mA within 2 hours of ischemia can promote neuroprotection significantly via reversed cortical functions, suggesting effective recovery.**

Keywords— **ECoG, fPAM, Neuroprotection, Photothrombotic ischemia (PTI), Sensory stimulation.**

I. INTRODUCTION

Ischemic stroke occurs when a clot blocks the blood vessel interrupting blood flow to the brain area, which is a leading cause of death and disability, globally. It often results in irreversible brain damage where the neurons are subject to necrosis. Timely redistribution of blood flow into the ischemic penumbra could markedly improve final outcomes. To date, the most well-known therapeutic agent for stroke recovery in hyperacute phase is recombinant tissue plasminogen activator (rTPA), which acts by breaking down clots and reintroducing blood flow into the ischemic brain regions. Unfortunately, rTPA is suitable for only a small portion of stroke patients and may cause a larger degree of tissue damage by weakening vessel walls. Hence, a better neuroprotective therapy is necessary for ameliorating ischemic insult. Previous studies have shown that functional sensory stimulation can increase regional cerebral blood flow (CBF) in activated brain regions. In addition, whisker stimulation has been proven effective for stroke recovery in a rat model, by evoked blood flow and collateral circulation [2, 3].

Here, we propose a potential clinically translatable treatment method for enhancing cortical function recovery with forepaw electrical stimulation. An *in vivo* photothrombotic ischemic (PTI) model was used to study the effect of the proposed treatment in two phases. In the phase 1, for determining the optimal time window, we designed experiments employing unilateral sensory stimulation with fixed current intensity as a 120-min treatment at different onset timings post-PTI. Afterward, stimulation was delivered either unilaterally or bilaterally using 2 or 4 mA pulses based on the optimal onset time window for effective recovery. A multimodal imaging system integrating electrocorticography (ECoG) recordings and functional photoacoustic microscopy (fPAM) imaging (i.e., ECoG-fPAM) was introduced to investigate the neurovascular functions (simultaneous assessment of neural activity and hemodynamic functions) down to single-cerebral-blood-vessel level in rat brain [1]. Cerebral blood volume (CBV), somatosensory-evoked potential (SSEP) and alpha-to-delta ratio (ADR) were acquired by our system pre- and post-PTI for evaluating the proposed treatment method. Also, histology study was performed to assess the infarct volume following different treatment strategies in this study.

II. MATERIALS AND METHODS

A. Electrocorticography-Functional Photoacoustic Microscopy System (ECoG-fPAM)

The experimental structure of the integrated ECoG-fPAM system includes fPAM imaging and ECoG recordings. The 50-MHz dark field confocal fPAM system was used to image functional changes in selected cortical blood

* Corresponding author.

I. Lackovic (ed.), *1st Global Conference on Biomedical Engineering & 9th Asian-Pacific Conference on Medical and Biological Engineering*, IFMBE Proceedings 47, DOI: 10.1007/978-3-319-12262-5_71

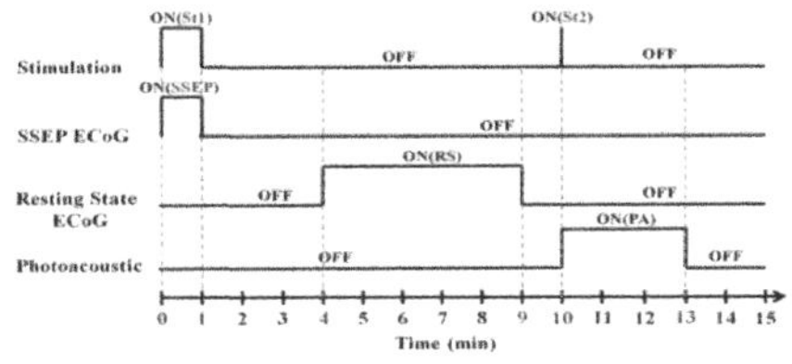

Fig. 1 Experimental protocol for stimulation treatment including blocks for SSEP, resting-state ECoG recording and PA imaging.

vessels offering an axial resolution of 32 μm and a lateral resolution of 61 μm [2]. Two visible wavelengths of the laser pulses, 560 and 570 nm (λ_{560} and λ_{570}), were employed for PA wave excitation [3, 4]. Seven stainless steel epidural electrodes (including one reference electrode) were secured on the skull to acquire SSEP and resting-state ECoG signals, which were pre-amplified (PZ2-32, Tucker-Davis Technologies, USA) and recorded by a signal acquisition system (RZ5D bio-amp processor, Tucker-Davis Technologies, USA) simultaneously with the stimulation treatment.

A. Animal Preparation

Totally 30 male Wistar rats for phase 1 and 38 male Wistar rats for phase 2 experiments, weighing 200–250 g (InVivos Pte Ltd, Singapore) were used in this study. All experimental procedures were approved by the Institutional Animal Care and Use Committee of the National University of Singapore. The animals were anesthetized with pentobarbital. The anesthetized rats were mounted on a stereotaxic head holder to reduce motion artifacts. The skin over the skull was then excised to expose the bregma landmark. Resting-state ECoG and SSEP recordings were obtained by securing six stainless steel epidural electrodes in the skull over the bilateral motor and primary somatosensory cortex forelimb region (S1FL) cortical regions. A reference electrode was positioned 3 mm to the right of the lambda landmark. To facilitate PA imaging and PTI stroke induction, a cranial window of approximately 3 mm × 8 mm was made with a high-speed drill, while keeping the dura intact.

B. Photothrombosis Technique for Focal Ischemic Stroke Induction

The photothrombosis technique was used to induce a focal ischemic stroke in a targeted cerebral arteriole located in the right S1FL. The photosensitizer Rose Bengal was infused over 2 minutes via tail vein injection. The cerebral arteriole targeted for occlusion was then illuminated with 10 mW, 532 nm CW laser light (MGM-20; Beta Electronics). The CW laser light was coupled into the designed dark-field optical path of the ECoG-fPAM system, and was focused on the selected arteriole located in the right S1FL region for 20 min until a stable clot formed.

C. Forepaw Electrical Stimulation Treatment Protocol

Forepaw electrical stimulation was delivered to facilitate adequate perfusion into the ischemic region and evoke hemodynamic response. Electrical stimulation treatment was applied with a stimulator (DS3, Digitimer, UK) via stainless steel bipolar subdermal needle electrodes inserted into the rat's palmar forepaws (either unilaterally or bilaterally). The experimental protocol consisted of a 15-min treatment block for ECoG recordings and PA imaging, with 8 blocks for each experimental group, as shown in *Figure 1*. Each block consisted of 1 min of stimulation for treatment and SSEP recording. The resting-state ECoG was then recorded for 5 min. The 2nd 5-sec stimulation was administered to evoke hemodynamic responses and was followed by a 3-min PA imaging. The PA B-scan images at λ_{560} or λ_{570} were acquired in each block at S1FL region. Treatment schema of the two phases (i.e. different onset timing and different method, current intensity) is shown in *Figure 2A-B*.

D. Data Analysis of Functional Changes in CBV, SSEP, ADR and Infarct Volume

To monitor functional changes in CBV, two optimized wavelengths (λ_{560} and λ_{570}) were employed. Please refer to previous studies for details on data analysis of the functional changes in single blood vessels [4, 5].

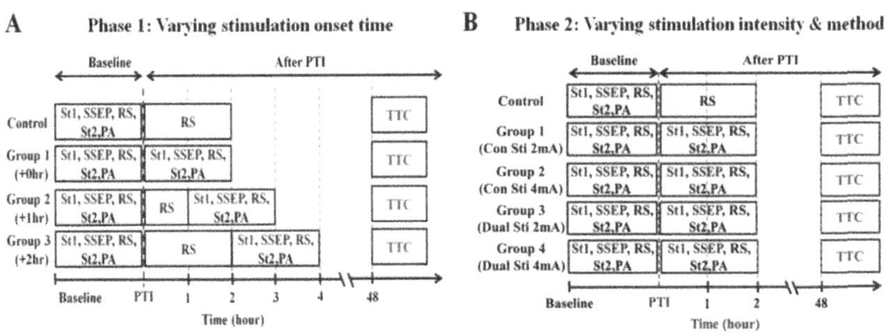

Fig. 2 Timings of stimulus administrations and recordings of SSEP, resting-state μECoG (RS) and PA imaging for every 30 min block.

The SSEPs induced by sensory stimulation were sampled at 1 kHz, pre-amplified, band-pass filtered and recorded pre- and post-PTI stroke. A SSEP extraction window was created within 100 ms of each stimulation onset. Since 3 Hz stimulation for 1 min was applied in each treatment block, 180 SSEPs were averaged to acquire proper evoked potential signals for analysis. Afterward, P1 and N1 components of the averaged SSEPs were extracted. The peak-to-peak amplitude changes of P1 and N1 were used to evaluate the neural activity changes after PTI stroke. ADR was defined as the ratio between alpha power and delta power. Fast Fourier transform (FFT) is used to calculate the mean power over each electrode channel for the signal located within the delta and alpha frequency bands. In this study, the percentage change in ADR was computed with respect to the baseline ADR for each channel. Also, volume of infarct was determined using 2, 3, 5-triphenyltetrazolium chloride (TTC) staining. The sectioned brain slices were incubated in 2 % TTC at 37 °C for 20 min in the dark and evaluated for the degree of stroke via the pale-white region of slices.

III. RESULTS

A. Functional Changes in CBV, SSEP and ADR at +0h, +1h and +2h post-PTI Stroke, and Infarct Volume Assessment (Phase 1)

Figure 3A shows the PAM-measured CBV (i.e., R_{CBV}) changes pre- and post-PTI stroke for group 1 from the region of interest (ischemic region). On comparing the results of CBV changes after treatment in each group, we saw that immediate treatment (group 1) could maximally restore perfusion level in the penumbra, than other groups (Figure 3A).

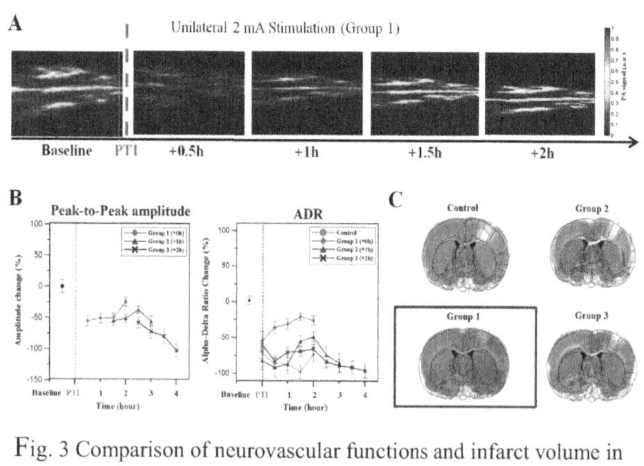

Fig. 3 Comparison of neurovascular functions and infarct volume in phase 1. (A) fPAM images of CBV changes before and after photothrombotic ischemic stroke. (B) Changes of peak-to-peak amplitude and ADR over different treatment groups. (C) TTC staining of infarct volume

The SSEP peak-to-peak amplitudes of P1 and N1 continually recovered to the baseline during group 1 treatment. Peak-to-peak amplitude of the other three experimental groups decreased about 56% after PTI induction, comparing to the baseline. Then, it continually increased to 89% of baseline after implementation of the 2-h treatment in group 1. Increases in the peak-to-peak amplitude were also significant observed in both group 2 and 3, in 2.5 and 3 h following PTI stroke onset, respectively. However, the peak-to-peak amplitude decreased when the forepaw electrical stimulation was continually delivered beyond 2.5 and 3 h following the stroke onset. ADR showed similar trends of results that both values decreased after PTI induction, and only group 1 treatment can help significantly recovery of neural activity, while other groups exhibited deteriorative performance when the treatments were delivered in inappropriate timings (Figure 3B).

Also, we compared the infarct areas from each group using TTC staining (Figure 3C). The infarcts were pale (unstained) regions in the somatosensory cortex. Group 1 exhibited a significant reduction in the volume of the infarct and group 2 slightly reduced the infarct area in comparison to the control group. In contrast, a reduction of the infarction was not observed in group 3. According to the above results, neural activity recovery effected when electrical stimulation was delivered within the first 2.5 h to 3 h following stroke onset, while sustained administration of the stimulation beyond the mentioned time window could deteriorate the activities and enlarge infarct volume.

B. Changes of Neurovascular Functions and Infarct Volume After Different Stimulation Method Delivered at +0h post-PTI (Phase 2)

Based on the phase 1 results, when the stimulation treatment was delivered within the optimal time window, neurovascular functions could largely recover. Therefore, we chose the group 1 method from phase 1 by integrating other strategies for evaluating if different stimulation method (either unilateral or bilateral) or current intensities could improve the performance of recovery. The animals of all groups in phase 2 were administered sensory stimulation immediately (at +0h) post-PTI stroke. As shown in Figure 4A, after PTI induction, an absence of CBV can be observed in the targeted arteriole located in the ischemic region. The PA image at +0h in Figure 4A represents the transcallosal pathway activation due to transcallosal disinhibition, in addition to the strengthened ipsilateral and weakened contralateral pathways. After delivering bilateral stimulation treatment with 2 mA, the activations of both ipsilateral and contralateral pathways could be enhanced, confirmed by the PA image with a increase in relative CBV changes.

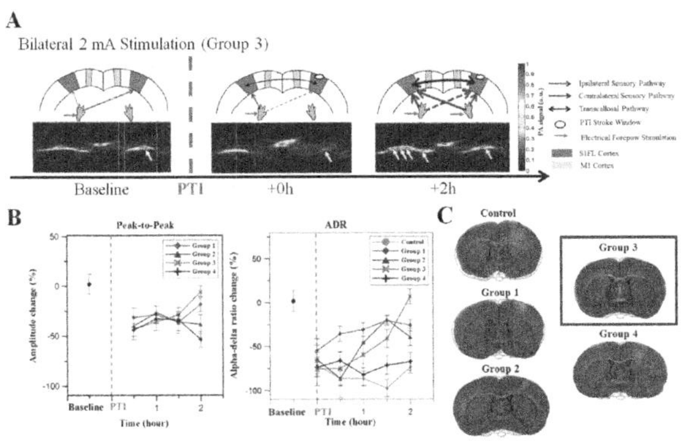

Fig. 4 Comparison of neurovascular functions and infarct volume based on different simulation method and intensity (phase 2).

There was a steady increase in peak-to-peak amplitudes in groups 1 and 3 with forepaw electrical stimulation at 2 mA intensity, indicating significant recovery of neural activity (Figure 4B). On the other hand, the SSEP amplitude values decreased in both groups 2 and 4 at end of the treatment. ADR values followed the same trend as SSEP with recovery of ADR in group 3 being significantly better than any other experimental group at end of treatment (Figure 4B).

Infarct volume detected by TTC staining in phase 2 is also presented in this study. Figure 4C shows the representative coronal sections of the control group and experimental groups that received contralateral forepaw electrical stimulation with 2 mA and 4 mA, bilateral forepaw electrical stimulation with 2 mA and 4 mA post-PTI and treatment, respectively. A reduction in infarct region was found in all treated groups that involved unilateral or bilateral forepaw electrical stimulation compared to the controls. Bilateral 2 mA stimulation in group 3 showed significant reduction in infarct volume than unilateral 2 mA stimulation in group 1. Above results validated that bilateral stimulation with 2 mA can enhance the performance of neurovascular function recovery when administered immediately post-PTI, while 4 mA is not as beneficial.

IV. CONCLUSIONS

The ECoG-fPAM system was employed to evaluate the evoked functional CBV changes, SSEP changes and resting-state ECoG changes in the bilateral S1FL regions pre- and post-PTI stroke. Results of phase 1 of the present study validated that unilateral forepaw electrical stimulation treatment administered within the first 2.5 to 3h optimal window following PTI onset is effective for PTI stroke recovery in rats. We inferred that forepaw electrical stimulation treatment initiated at appropriate timing facilitated recovery of neurovascular function in the PTI stroke region, whereas treatment delivered at an inappropriate time window could exacerbate stroke damage. Based on the conclusions from phase 1, we aimed to enhance the performance of our sensory stimulation treatment by investigating the best stimulation method and intensity. The results of phase 2 indicated that bilateral electrical forepaw stimulation at low electrical intensity (i.e. 2 mA) improved perfusion and restored neuronal integrity in the penumbra and thereby reduced the infarct volume in the hyperacute phase in a PTI model. This could be attributed to increase perfusion from collateral circulation due to neuronal excitation in the penumbra. Further studies will be required to properly titrate both the stimulus strength and rate to obtain the most beneficial regime for facilitating stroke recovery. In the future, post-treatment comparison of neurovascular functions among different experimental groups will be conducted to examine the efficacy of our treatment. Also, chronic PTI experiments will be conducted for evaluating the effect of stimulation treatment in behavioral improvement. This ECoG-fPAM technique will be valuable in studies related to cortical functions and may provide a unique opportunity to evaluate specific disease diagnoses, such as diabetes and epilepsy, in small animal models.

CONFLICT OF INTEREST

The authors declare that they have no conflict of interest.

REFERENCES

[1] L. D. Liao, C. T. Lin, Y. Y. I. Shih, T. Q. Duong, H. Y. Lai, P. H. Wang, R. Wu, S. Tsang, J. Y. Chang, and M. L. Li, "Transcranial imaging of functional cerebral hemodynamic changes in single blood vessels using in vivo photoacoustic microscopy," *J Cereb Blood Flow Metab*, vol. 32, pp. 938-951, 2012.

[2] L. D. Liao, V. Tsytsarev, I. Delgado-Martinez, M. L. Li, R. Erzurumlu, A. Vipin, J. Orellana, Y. R. Lin, H. Y. Lai, Y. Y. Chen, and N. V. Thakor, "Neurovascular coupling: in vivo optical techniques for functional brain imaging," *Biomedical Engineering Online*, vol. 12, p. 38, Apr 30 2013.

[3] L. D. Liao, C. T. Lin, Y. Y. I. Shih, H. Y. Lai, W. T. Zhao, T. Q. Duong, J. Y. Chang, Y. Y. Chen, and M. L. Li, "Investigation of the cerebral hemodynamic response function in single blood vessels by functional photoacoustic microscopy," *J Biomed Opt*, vol. 17, pp. 061210-1-061210-10, 2012.

[4] L.-D. Liao, M.-L. Li, H.-Y. Lai, Y.-Y. I. Shih, Y.-C. Lo, S. Tsang, P. C.-P. Chao, C.-T. Lin, F.-S. Jaw, and Y.-Y. Chen, "Imaging brain hemodynamic changes during rat forepaw electrical stimulation using functional photoacoustic microscopy," *NeuroImage*, vol. 52, pp. 562-570, 2010.

[5] V. Tsytsarev, C. Bernardelli, and K. I. Maslov, "Living brain optical imaging: technology, methods and applications," *J Neurosci Neuroeng*, vol. 1, 2012.

Author: Lun-De Liao*
Institute: Singapore Institute for Neurotechnology
Street: 28 Medical Drive, #05-COR
City: Singapore
Country: Singapore
Email: gs336.tw@gmail.com*

Optogenetic Deconstructing the Mechanism of Neuroplasticity Modulated by Repetitive Cortical Stimulation

Chun-Wei Wu, Cho-Han Hsieh, and Jia-Jin Jason Chen

Department of Biomedical Engineering, National Cheng-Kung University, Tainan, Taiwan

Abstract— **Cortical Theta burst stimulation (TBS) may modulate dopamine-dependent corticostriatal plasticity via long-term potentiation / depression (LTP/LTD) -like mechanism. This gives TBS a therapeutic potential for Parkinson's disease (PD) and other neural disorder. To unravel the mechanism beneath TBS-induced neuroplasticity, a novel optogenetic simulating method will be applied. CaMKII promoter-driven channelrhodopsin-2 (ChR2) will be delivered into glutamatergic pyramidal neuron in motor cortex by lentivirus. Under emitting of precisely controlled blue laser guided by fiber optics, the excitatory circuit in layer V will be elicited with TBS paradigm. Cortical excitabilities were examined by measuring optogenetic simulation-evoked potential and motor-evoked potential (MEP). In summary, we proposed a novel optical-TBS rodent model, which revealed the function role of glutamatergic circuit in motor plasticity.**

Keywords— **Theta burst stimulation, optogenctics, channel-rhodopsin, neuroplasticity, brain stimulation.**

I. INTRODUCTION

Repetitive transcranial magnetic stimulation (rTMS) is capable of modulating motor cortical excitability through long-term potentiation (LTP) and depression (LTD)-like mechanisms [1]. This non-invasive cerebral stimulation technique has been used to investigate dopamine (DA)-dependent motor plasticity in Parkinson's disease (PD). rTMS-induced motor plasticity was impaired in chronic and early PD patients, and was restored by dopaminergic medications [2]. Animal studies also showed that LTP and LTD were both depressed in 6-OHDA-induced DA-denervated rats [3, 4]. Recently, our study demonstrated that theta burst stimulation (TBS; 3 rTMS-pulses at 50 Hz repeated at 5 Hz)-induced motor plasticity was reduced in early 6-OHDA-lesioned PD and absent in chronic PD. Such reduction in plasticity strongly correlated with dopaminergic neuron loss [5]. Relevant to PD, rTMS over the primary motor cortex (M1) has been found to induce DA release in subcortical areas [6]. Similarly, in experimental animals, cortical rTMS is able to increase DA level in subcortical regions [7] and, in particular, increase in DA content of the dorsolateral striatum [8]. In spite of dopaminergic neurons in SNc were required for iTBS-induced motor plasticity, an NMDA-receptor dependent cortical excitation in M1 by iTBS was also observed [9]. It implicated that plasticity of glutamatergic synapses was modulated in M1 by TBS. In summary, we hypothesize that TBS can modulate corticostriatal plasticity via elevating excitability in cortex and DA content in striatum. In order to test the effects of LTP/LTD on glutamatergic connection from M1 to substantial nigra pars compacta (SNc), we plan to introduce a tissue-specific, optogenetic stimulation on glutamatergic neuron in M1 and on dopaminergic neuron in SNc. CaMKII promoter-driven channelrhodopsin-2 (ChR2) will be delivered into glutamatergic pyramidal neuron in motor cortex by lentivirus. TBS paradigms will be conducted by optical stimulation in M1. Motor evoked potential (MEP) in peripheral, excitatory post-synaptic potential (EPSP) and action potential in M1 and SNc will be recorded before and after TBS to assess motor plasticity. *In vivo* striatal DA-level will be monitored using an electrochemical-sensing system we had recently developed [10]. The fast-scan cyclic voltammetry (FSCV) provide excellent temporal resolution to detect single-pulse evoked DA releasing and recycling on a subsecond time scale. Compare to rTMS, optogenetic TBS provide a non-electromagnetic stimulation in cerebral cortex without any electromagnetic interference to neuro-electrical recording and to electrochemical DA-sensing. By applying optogenetic stimulation scheme, it will be feasible to trigger a specific neural pathway in the brain, unravel the mechanism of TBS-induced motor plasticity, and to deconstruct specific neuronal circuit involved in Parkinson's disease (Fig. 1).

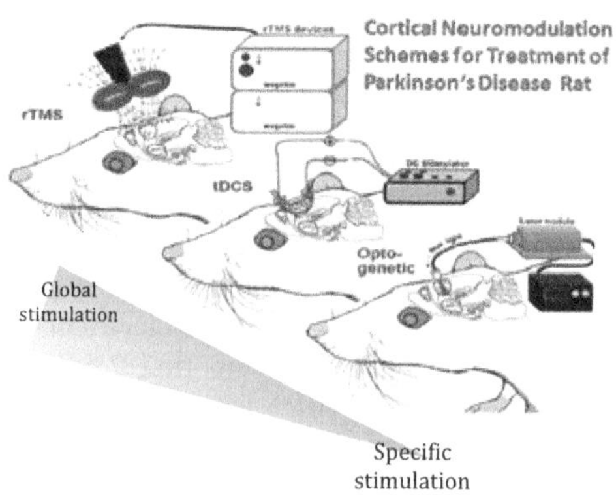

Fig. 1 Cortical neuromodulation schemes to unravel neural pathway of Parkinson's disease

I. Lackovic (ed.), *1st Global Conference on Biomedical Engineering & 9th Asian-Pacific Conference on Medical and Biological Engineering*,
IFMBE Proceedings 47, DOI: 10.1007/978-3-319-12262-5_72

II. MATERIAL AND METHODS

A. Lentivirus Production and ChR2 Expression

A second-generation lentivirus system was used for transduction of ChR2. The packaging plasmid psPAX2 and envelope plasmid pMD2.G were transfected into HEK293FT cell with ChR2 expressing plasmid: pLenti-CaMKIIa-ChR2(H134R)-EYFP-WPRE (addgene). The medium was collected and concentrated to harvest virus particle in 1,000 folds concentrated solution.

An anesthetized rat was fixed on the stereotactic apparatus. Skull was exposed to locate bregma. A hole was drilled over M1 corresponding to right forelimb (AP: +1.5 mm, ML: -3.0 mm). Viral solution was injected in M1 at two different depth: 2.0 mm and 2.5 mm. 200 μm-optical fiber was inserted in stainless steel cannula, which served as an electrocorticogram (ECoG) electrode, and implate into M1. After implantation, the optotrode and electrode were coverd with dental cement (Fig. 2).

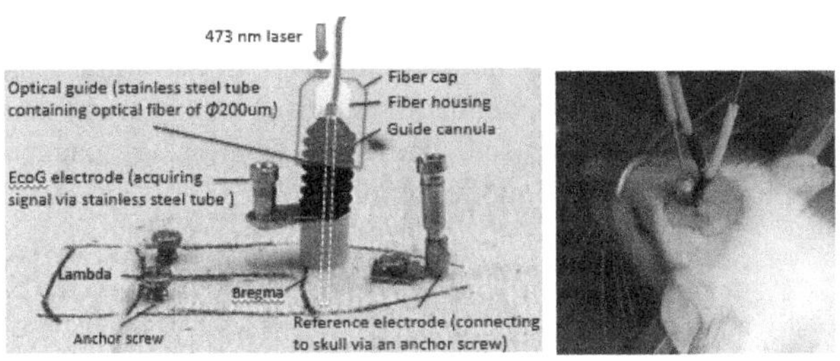

Fig. 2 Cortical fiber-optics stimulation and ECoG recording electrode

B. Optogenetic Stimulation and Recording of Electrophysiological Signals

To verify the function of ChR2 under optogenetics stimulation, the rat were anesthetized and fixed on the stereotactic apparatus, the event-related signals of the optical stimulation were recorded under a Labview controlled system (Fig. 3). The laser driver was triggered by LabVIEW program under TTL controlling manner. Optical-induced local field potential (LFP) and MEP signals were amplified and bandpass-filtered before be acquired by LabVIEW program. Averaging calculation was conducted using MATLAB functions. 473 nm laser power delivered by fiber-optics was measured at the end of the cannula. The amplitude responses under various laser output setting were plot (Fig. 4).

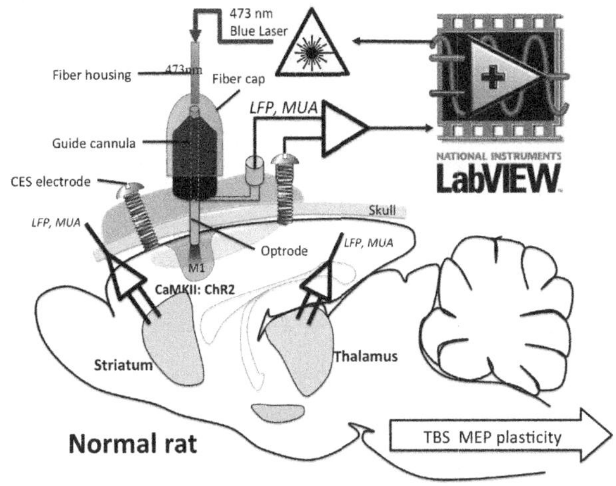

Fig. 3 Optogenetics stimulation and electrophysiological recording system

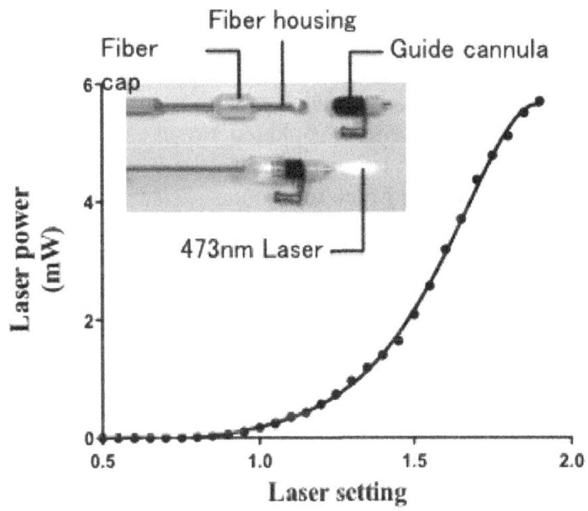

Fig. 4 Laser delivering from implantable optrode under various laser output setting

III. RESULTS

A. ChR2 Expression

Lentivirus containing pLenti-CaMKIIa-ChR2(H134R)-EYFP-WPRE was transduced in primary motor cortex for four weeks. Rats were sacrificed and brain tissues were sliced. Under the fluorescence microscopy, the expression of ChR2-EYFP fusion protein in motor cortex was observed under the excitation of blue light (Fig. 5).

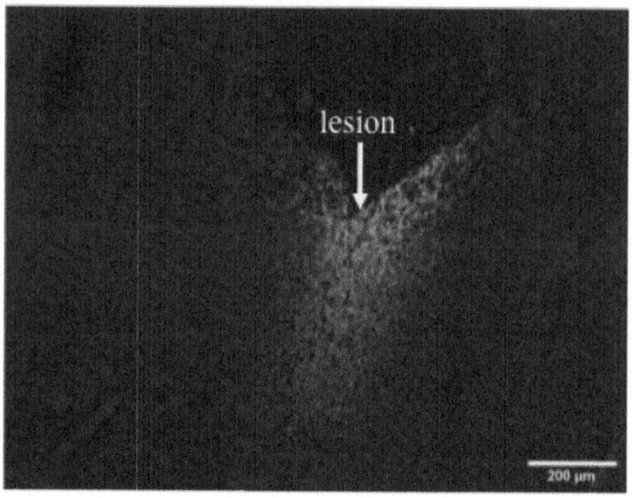

Fig. 5 Expression of ChR2 (H134R)-EYFP fusion protein in glutamatergic neurons in motor cortex (scale bar: 200 µm)

B. Optogenetic Evoked Potential (OEP) and Motor Evoked Potential under Laser Stimulation

After viral infection for 4-weeks, the activity of ChR2 was examined by laser stimulation with various parameters. The classic waveform of optogenetic evoked potentials were recorded under 1 ms laser pulse for 100 trials (Fig 6). The values of pick-to-pick amplitude varied from 23.6 uV to 57.7 uV. Typical latency of P1 and N1 were 17.0 and 34.4 ms. After averaging calculation, the pick-to-pick amplitudes were ploted with various laser power (Fig. 7). A significant correlation was observed between OEP amplitude and laser stimulation intensities.

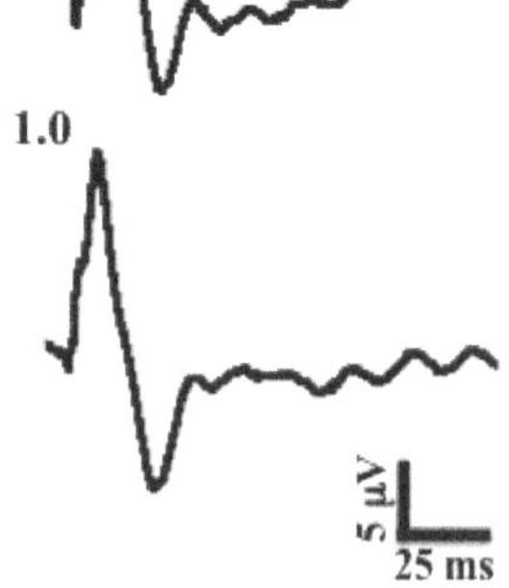

Fig. 6 Classic waveform of optogenetic evoked potential

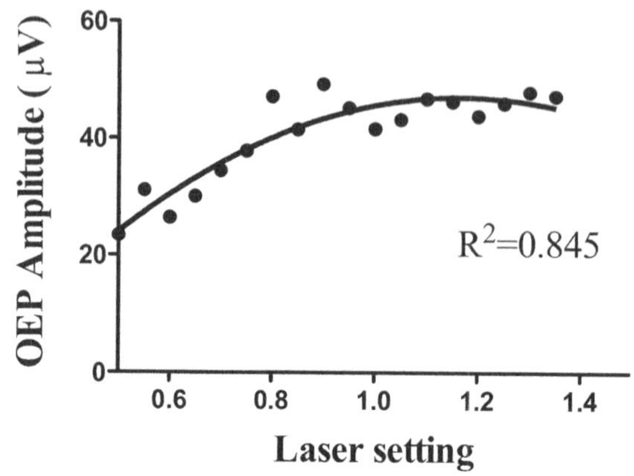

Fig. 7 Relation between laser power and amplitude of OEP

IV. DISCUSSION

Optogenetic animal model was build by transducing the tissue-specific expressed ChR2 (H134R)-EYFP in M1 glutamatergic neuron. The expression pattern of ChR2 (H134R)-EYFP was confirmed using immunofluorescence microscopy. The assessment of OEP indicated the activation of ChR2 expressed neuron in M1 under blue laser stimulation. A dose-dependent response was observed while laser power was increased. These results indicates a success in optogenetic animal model preparation.

V. CONCLUSIONS

We hypothesize that motor plasticity induced by M1 modulation (such as rTMS or optogenetic stimulation) is SNc-dopaminergic neuron dependent. Therefore, after the excitability is elevated by TBS in M1, activation in SNc will be observed accompanied by DA-releasing in CPu. The dependency shall be revealed when inhibiting SNc with eNpHR3.0-mediated hyper-polarization.

In the current study, we have successfully expressed ChR2 in motor cortex, and the optogenetic-evoked potential were recorded by our home-made optrode. The amplitude of OEP was highly correlated with laser power. In future work, the inhibitory opsin, eNpHR3.0, will be expressed in SNc to test the hypothesis that DA-releasing controlled by SNc activity will modulate corticalstriatal plasticity under optogenetic-TBS paradigm.

ACKNOWLEDGMENTS

The authors would like to thank the Ministry of Science and Technology of R.O.C. for financially supporting this research under contract No. NSC-101-2320-B-006-018-MY3.

Conflict of Interest

The authors declare that they have no conflict of interest.

References

1. Huang YZ, Chen RS, Rothwell JC et al. (2007) The after-effect of human theta burst stimulation is NMDA receptor dependent. Clin Neurophysiol 118:1028-1032.
2. Huang YZ, Rothwell JC, Lu CS et al. (2011) Abnormal bidirectional plasticity-like effects in Parkinson's disease. Brain 134:2312-2320.
3. Calabresi P, Pisani A, Centonze D et al. (1997) Synaptic plasticity and physiological interactions between dopamine and glutamate in the striatum. Neurosci Biobehav Rev 21:519-523.
4. Picconi B, Centonze D, Håkansson K et al. (2003) Loss of bidirectional striatal synaptic plasticity in L-DOPA-induced dyskinesia. Nat Neurosci 6:501-506.
5. Hsieh TH, Huang YZ, Rotenberg A et al. (2014) Functional Dopaminergic Neurons in Substantia Nigra are Required for Transcranial Magnetic Stimulation-Induced Motor Plasticity. Cerebral Cortex (in press)
6. Strafella AP, Paus T, Fraraccio M et al. (2003) Striatal dopamine release induced by repetitive transcranial magnetic stimulation of the human motor cortex. Brain 126:2609-2615.
7. Keck ME, Welt T, Müller MB et al. (2002) Repetitive transcranial magnetic stimulation increases the release of dopamine in the mesolimbic and mesostriatal system. Neuropharmacology 43:101-109.
8. Kanno M, Matsumoto M, Togashi H et al. (2004) Effects of acute repetitive transcranial magnetic stimulation on dopamine release in the rat dorsolateral striatum. J Neurol Sci 217:73-81.
9. Labedi A, Benali A, Mix A et al. (2014) Modulation of inhibitory activity markers by intermittent theta-burst stimulation in rat cortex is NMDA-receptor dependent. BRS 7:394-400.
10. Li YT, Wickens JR, Huang YL et al. (2013) Integrated wireless fast-scan cyclic voltammetry recording and electrical stimulation for reward-predictive learning in awake, freely moving rats. J Neural Eng 10:046007.

Author: Chun-Wei Wu
Institute: Department of Biomedical Engineering, National Cheng-Kung University
Street: No.1, University Road
City: Tainan City 701
Country: Taiwan (R.O.C.)
Email: chunwei0521@gmail.com

Integration of the Chemistry Analyzer and the Medical Information System

T. Chou[1], M.H. Yang[1], M.M. Lo[1], A.J. Lee[2], M.H. Tsai[3], J.H. Lin[4], and S.T. Tang[1]

[1] Department of Biomedical Engineering, Ming Chuan University, Taoyuan, Taiwan
[2] Department of Healthcare Information and Management, Ming Chuan University, Taoyuan, Taiwan
[3] Marketing Department, Sheng-He Hospital Management Consultation Co., Ltd., Taoyuan, Taiwan
[4] Department of Electronic Engineering, Kun Shan University, Tainan, Taiwan

Abstract— **In modern society, people are often suffered the nervous tension for a long time, and results in inevitably internal injury of bodily functions. The periodic and comprehensive medical examinations are necessary, makes the chemistry analyzer to play an important role. Although the chemistry analyzer is operating automatically, different manufacturer defines distinctive specifications. That causes the interoperability problems in the chemistry analyzers, and the analyzed results could not share and integrating. Therefore, this study proposed to solve the problem, which was basing on the international standard protocols of ISO/IEEE 11073 and Health Level Seven (HL7) to develop a software application. The developed application could control the different brands of chemistry analyzers according to the ISO/IEEE 11073 standards. The data will be further compiled into HL7 format and save as an XML (eXtensible Markup Language) text file. Finally, the data are uploaded to the current hospital information systems. In order to achieve an interoperability platform that supports a variety of instruments at the same time. Not only enable the messages' exchange in the healthcare systems, but also have high degree of sharing between the hospitals.**

Keywords— ***Chemistry Analyzer, ISO/IEEE 11073, HL7.***

I. INTRODUCTION

The rapid development of modern technology enables medical equipment automatically. But there are many different specifications in interfaces and data formats, which lead to the interoperability problems. Besides the inconvenient situation occur during the usage. It's also difficult to the medical laboratory in system development. This would increase the cost and time for laboratory development. In addition, if the inter-hospital referral is necessary, the patients usually need to repeat a series of examination procedure.

The Continua Health Alliance (CHA) established the ISO/IEEE 11073 international standards that are for solving the closed proprietary problems in different manufactures, and also to improve the interoperability between different instruments. But now it mainly focused on the integration of the information coming from the elder's home healthcare devices. Up to now, the ISO/IEEE 11073 international standards have not regulated the chemistry analyzer. The chemistry analyzer is also facing the same problem in the medical laboratory. There are too much manufactures, so that it's very hard to regulate the chemistry analyzers and their data formats. Our research is to introduce the international standards, and then interfacing and integrating the various chemistry analyzers.

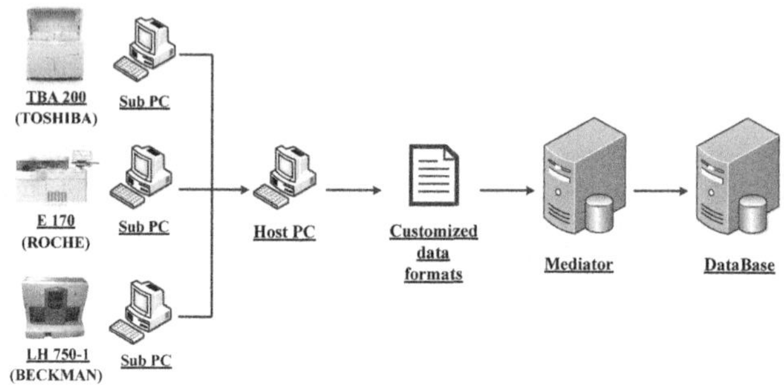

Fig. 1 The traditional instrument operating flowchart

A. *ISO/IEEE 11073 Standards*

ISO/IEEE 11073 standards are currently mainly in personalized healthcare for the system architecture, which establishs the communications interoperability. So that the elderly people or chronic disease patient can be supported by today's technology and services, further to reach the home care and achieve improved personal health management [1]. The standards of ISO/IEEE 11073 series enable the communication between the personal medical devices and application data servers So that it can enable the server end and personal medical devices to exchange messages with each other, to achieve the data integration [2, 3].

B. *Health Level Seven International (HL7)*

HL7 is the seven-layer communication model for open systems interconnection-application, which is a standard for exchanging information between medical applications. HL7 version3.0 use XML as a method for message encoding. This version obviously has normative and readability that make the HL7 interface have good performance and easy to popularize [4].

The main purpose of HL7 is to develop the protocols and standards between data message transmission, which is also regulated the clinical and managed message formats. And as well allows the data to be exchanged in various medical institutions by different systems. It can decrease the cost of the interconnection of information systems and improve the data sharing between hospital information systems (Fig. 2). Thus, achieving inter platform application on clinical and

I. Lackovic (ed.), *1st Global Conference on Biomedical Engineering & 9th Asian-Pacific Conference on Medical and Biological Engineering*,
IFMBE Proceedings 47, DOI: 10.1007/978-3-319-12262-5_73

have higher availability, security and more expandable. HL7 supported the services and management of clinical care so as to improve the quality of clinical care and patient safety [5]. HL7 standards provide a detailed protocol of text transferring. So that the original data is first converted into a standard HL7 message format, and then sent to the receiving end system [3].

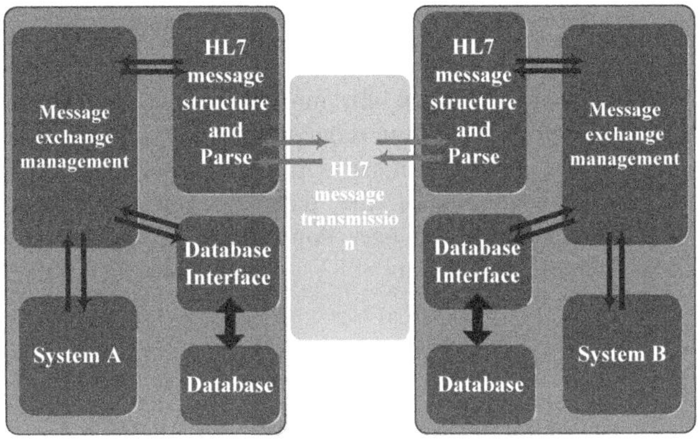

Fig. 2 Medical information exchange system block diagram

II. METHOD

We used the international standard protocols of ISO/IEEE 11073 and HL7 to resolve the problem of interoperability, and we developed an application by NI LabVIEW for the chemistry analyzers. The data will be firstly compiled into HL7 format and save as an XML text file. Finally, the data are uploaded to the database for archiving [6].

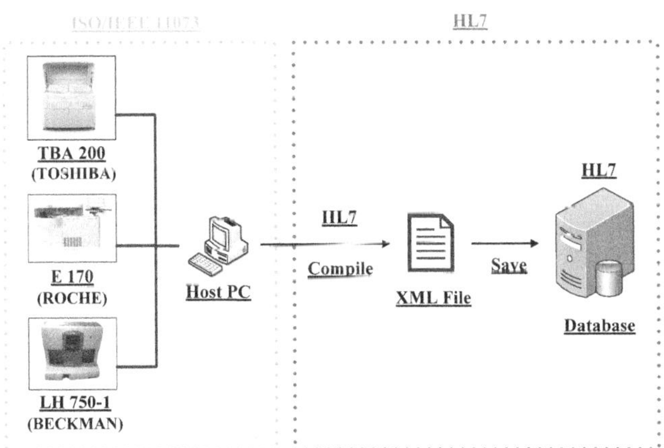

Fig. 3 Instrument operating flowchart (Target)

A. *Instruments Interoperability*

The traditional medical devices always lack interoperability, so it's important to explore the synergistic value. Value propositions of synergistic are including integrity of data, automatic electronic health records, increase flexibility of institutions, which are able to access information from the patient. They are expected to promote the development in the medical field.

We use CHA proposed ISO/IEEE 11073 DIM (Domain Information Model) to develop the central message tools and achieve synergistic and message exchange between medical devices. In this paper, we use ISO/IEEE 11073 and RS232 as a communication between consoles PC and instruments [7].

B. *Human Machine Interface*

LabVIEW is not only to optimize the measurement applications, but also develop the control program. It provides a powerful environment, which can be easily reached seamless integration, and user can focus on the development without spending too much time to verify. There are possibilities of test, control and design applications with LabVIEW Real-Time Systems. Most of hardware controls, measurements and operations are required with the software. When it comes to software integration, the compatibility is the main problem, and the hardware required driver which can communicate effectively, command and operate to the instrument [8].

In the paper, the development process of driver is shown in figure 4. There are four parts. First part is connecting hardware (Open). Second part is system initialization (Initialize). Third part is hardware setup (Setting). The fourth is back and forth to read and write data from the hardware (Data Dump). Finally it released the hardware connections.

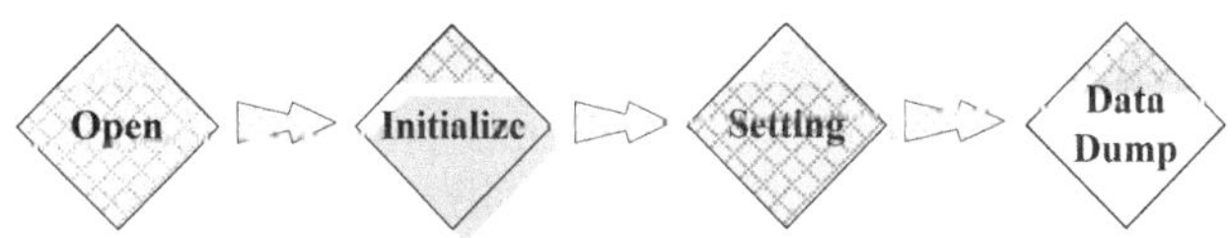

Fig 4 LabVIEW hardware driver's design process

Figure 5 is a message exchange flowchart with the chemistry analyzer and the console PC. When the chemistry analyzer tries to connect to the major PC, the chemistry analyzer will propose the association request message, but console PC could not distinguish the configuration of analyzer (configuration) so it responses to accept this requirement and request to offer messages of configuration (accepted-unknown-config) at the same time. Next, the analyzer transfer configuration information to the console PC. After the console PC is recognized and received an acceptable message (accepted-config) from the console PC's reply, the chemistry analyzer requests system to initialize. Next, user enters date and SID code of health check project before confirming, and the chemistry analyzer will begin to read and write the data. When the data transfer is complete, the chemistry analyzer requires to cut links automatically. If there is no error report, the console PC will response accepted [9].

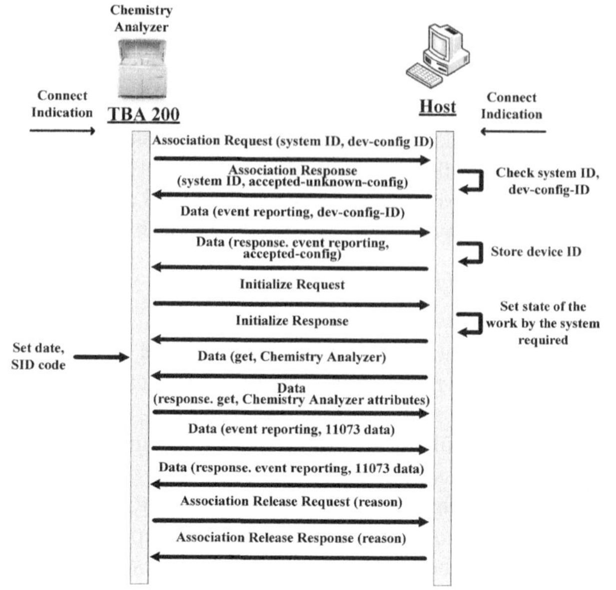

Fig. 5 Chemistry analyzer and console PC connecting for exchange message

III. RESULT

We developed the proposed system in the Taipei Veterans General Hospital, Taoyuan branch of medical examination centers. We have implemented the main management system interface by using the LabVIEW. In the future, we will use a computer as a host, through the driver to conform the ISO / IEEE 11073 and HL7 standards between platforms. We expect this program can control nearly 2/3 sets of chemistry analyzers in the medical laboratory center, so as to solve the problem about the compatibility and data integration, also achieve interoperability between instruments. Moreover, we will optimize the user interface, and then user can easily operate in a situation of non-standardized.

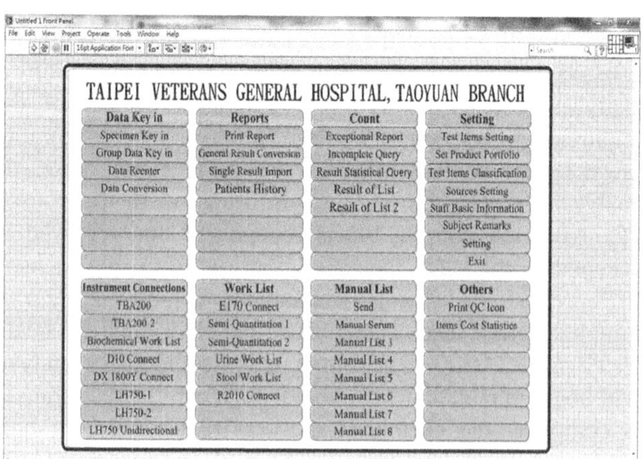

Fig. 6 Main Management System

IV. CONCLUSION

The developed software application has been able to integrate between hardware, and user used the application to control several and different brands of instruments. The problem of compatibility has been solved. The application output the data that are conforming HL7 format, which could reach the interoperability in the instruments and improve the integration of the data. User uses the application can operate different kinds of medical instruments, and it is not only more convenient on learning and operating, but also can reduce the human resources and time. On the other way, it can improve work's efficiency. In addition, integration of the data is more perfect for healthcare system, and user don't think to choose some specific brand instruments.

REFERENCES

Jianchu Y. and Steve W., APPLYING THE ISO/IEEE 11073 STANDARDS TO WEARABLE HOME HEALTH MONITORING SYSTEMS, (2005) Daegu, Korea, pp427–436.

Clarke M., Bogia D., Hassing K., Steubesand L., Chan T., and Ayyagari D., Developing a Standard for Personal Health Devices based on 11073, (2007) Lyon, France,pp 6174–6176.

Yuksel M. and Dogac A., Interoperability of Medical Device Information and the Clinical Applications: An HL7 RMIM based on the ISO/IEEE 11073 DIM, Vol. 15, pp 740–741.

Tung T., Hwa-Sun K. and Hune C., A Development of HL7 Middleware for Medical Device Communication, (2007) Korea, pp.485–492.

Ean-Wen H., Sheng-Hsiung H. and Der-Ming L., Peitou. Design and implementation of a web-based HL7 message generation and validation system, (2003) Taipei, Taiwan, pp49–58.

Schmitt L., Falck T., Wartena F. and Simons D., Novel ISO/IEEE 11073 Standards for Personal Telehealth Systems Interoperability, (2007) Europe, pp146–148 .

John JG., Martinez S., Rivello R. and Cherkaoui M., Moving Toward Semantic Interoperability of Medical Devices, Paper presented at: 2007 Joint Workshop on High Confidence Medical Devices, Software, and Systems and Medical Device Plug-and-Play Interoperability, (2007) Boston MA, pp13–19.

Bell I., Falcon J., LimrotJ. h and Robinson K., Bath, Integration of hardware into the labview environment for rapid prototyping and the development of control design applications, Paper presented at: UKACC Control 2004 Mini Symposia, (2004) pp79–81.

Yuan-Fa L., Personal Medical Monitoring System Based on x73-PHD Standards, (2012) Tainan, Taiwan.

Author: Shih-Tsang Tang
Institute:Yang Ming University
Street: 5 De Ming Rd., Gui Shan District
City: Taoyuan
Country: Taiwan
Email: sttang@mail.mcu.edu.tw

Prostate Cancer Detection Using a Combination of Raman Spectroscopy and Stiffness Sensing

O.A. Lindahl[1,2,4], M. Nyberg[1,2], V. Jalkanen[2,3], and K. Ramser[1,2]

[1] Department of engineering sciences and mathematics, Luleå University of Technology, Luleå, Sweden
[2] Centre for Biomedical Engineering and Physics (CMTF) Luleå, Umeå, Sweden
[3] Department of Applied Physics and Electronics, Umeå University, Umeå, Sweden
[4] Department of Radiation Sciences, Umeå University, Umeå, Sweden

Abstract— **Prostate cancer (PCa) is the most common cancer form for men in Europe. A sensor system combining Raman spectroscopy and stiffness sensing with a resonance sensor has recently been developed by us for prostate cancer detection. In this study the sensor system has been used for measurements on two slices of fresh human prostate tissue. The stiffness sensor could detect locations slices with significantly different stiffness contrasts ($p < 0.05$). Raman spectroscopic measurements could be performed with the dual-modality probe for tissue classification. The findings are important for the continued development of a combination probe for prostate cancer detection.**

Keywords— **Fiber optical Raman spectroscopy, tactile resonance sensor technology, histopathology, prostate cancer detection, radical.**

I. INTRODUCTION

Prostate cancer (PCa) is the most common cancer form for men in Europe with 382 300 men receiving a PCa diagnose in 2008. In the USA 192 000 men were diagnosed in 2009 [1, 2]. The treatment for PCa is usually radical prostatectomy (RP.

Current standard procedure after RP is to have the resected prostate examined by permanent section analysis after surgery. There is a risk of PCa re-occurrence if a positive surgical margin (PSM) is found, which indicates that some cancerous cells might have been left behind. Approximately 20% of RP procedures results in a PSM [3]. Frozen section analysis, during surgery, have a low sensitivity for detecting PSM[4]. Consequently, it would be beneficial for the patient to have an accurate and specific method of detecting possible PSM during surgery.

A sensor system combining Raman spectroscopy and stiffness sensing has recently been developed for prostate cancer detection [5]. It combines a tactile resonance sensor that assesses the tissue stiffness and fiber optical Raman spectroscopy that gives detailed information about the tissue biochemical content. One application of this instrument is to use it during radical prostatectomy (RP) to examine the surgical margin.

Tactile resonance sensors usually consist of piezoelectric transducers made from PZT (Lead Zirconate, Titanium). They have a mechanical resonance frequency or relative phase of oscillation that is dependent on the measured parameter. The sensors are used to develop measurement systems in industry as well as in medicine. Sensor systems have been developed for detection of breast cancer, for measuring muscular elasticity, for measuring stiffness of human ovum and for modeling micturition characteristics based on prostate stiffness.

Raman spectroscopy using fibre optic probes is another promising technique for prostate cancer detection. Already in 2004 it was shown by Crow et al. that an endoscopic Raman probe has high prospects to be used in clinical settings for prostate cancer detection [6]. The group had developed a prostate algorithm that was able to differentiate benign samples (benign prostatic hyperplasia and prostatitis) from malignant prostate cancer with an overall accuracy of 86 %. However, the method shows a low yield and therefore measurements are often carried out under dark circumstances to avoid background scattering. Furthermore, Raman spectroscopy on fresh tissue may suffers from a high intrinsic fluorescent background. Hence, it is good to combine the method with another technique.

Combining the two methods are the basis for a probe intended for detecting PSM during radical prostatectomy. The prostate surgical margin is to be scanned to locate stiffer areas using the tactile resonance sensor and harder nodules are an indication of tumor presence. Raman spectroscopy will then be applied at these locations to determine the boundaries between cancerous and non-cancerous stiff tissue.

The aim of this study was to investigate the ability of the combined probe to differentiate between different tissue types in prostate slices. To do so, measurements with both techniques were performed on some pre-chosen points on fresh prostate tissue directly after surgery.

II. MATERIAL AND METHODS

A. Measurement System

The stiffness sensor of the combined probe consisted of a resonance sensor attached to a strain gauge force transducer.

I. Lackovic (ed.), *1st Global Conference on Biomedical Engineering & 9th Asian-Pacific Conference on Medical and Biological Engineering*,
IFMBE Proceedings 47, DOI: 10.1007/978-3-319-12262-5_74

The resonance sensor was a hollow, cylindrical (5 mm outer diameter, 3 mm inner diameter, 15 mm length) PZT ceramic (Morgan Electro Ceramics, Bedford, OH, USA) with a hemispherical plastic tip (2.5 mm 70 radius). A 1.5 mm hole was drilled through the plastic tip which was covered by a thin hemispherical glass window (microscope cover slip Nr 1, Menzel-Gläser, Portsmouth, NH, USA). The resonance sensor was set to operate with a commercially available pick-up and driving electronics (P&M Co., Ltd., Aizuwa-kamatsu, Fukushima, Japan). The fiber optical Raman probe (Machida Endoscope Co., Tokyo, Japan) was connected to a RXN1 Raman spectroscope (RXN1/0002134, Kaiser Optical Systems (KOSI), Ann Arbor, MI, USA). The 0.8-mm pure silica Raman probe consists of one delivery fibre and eight collecting fibres and ends with a 10 cm long steel pipe of 0.8-mm diameter. The laser power was set to 140 mW and the integration time was 3x10s. The combined probe was mounted to an xyz-positioning stage (NRT150P1, three NRT100, BSC103, Thorlabs, Newton, NJ, USA). An in-house developed software controlled the movement of the positioning stage and the setting of the measurement grid.

B. Human Prostate and Measurements

Ethical approval was given by the ethics committee of Umeå University (Dnr 03-423, Dnr 2013-94-32M). The first prostate was resected from a 73 year old man with a PCa Gleason score 8 stage pT3b. The second was from a 59 year old man with a Gleason score 7 stage pT2c PCa.

The resected prostate was immediately brought to the pathology department where the prostate exterior was stained with tissue marking dye (Triangle biomedical sciences, Inc. Durham, NC, USA). Yellow ink was used at the prostate posterior, green at the right front side and red at the front left side. The prostate was transversally cut in approx. 5-6 mm thick slices.. One prostate slice was immediately put on ice after it was prepared by the pathologist, and brought to the experimental setup.

At the experimental setup the prostate slice was pinned to a Styrofoam bed. Nine measurement points were chosen for the first prostate from a 3x5 rectangular grid with 15 grid points by excluding points near or on a needle or the urethra. For the second prostate, 10 measurement points were chosen. The grid was set to include measurements at the posterior part of the prostate because it is more likely to find a PCa tumour there.

The Kolmogorov-Smirnoff test was used to test for data normality. Hierarchical cluster analysis (HCA), using were used to form groups. The non-parametric Kruskal-Wallis multiple comparison test was used to test for differences between hard and soft locations. Test results with $p < 0.05$ were considered statistically significant.

III. RESULTS AND DISCUSSION

A total of 19 measurements were performed on the two prostates. Each measurement series was performed within one hour after the prostates arrived at the pathology department.

Both prostate slices developed swellings that distorted the otherwise flat surface.

A. Histopathological Investigation of the Prostate Samples

A region with PCa was found above and to the right of point 1 on the first prostate and near and at point 6 on the second prostate (Fig. 1).

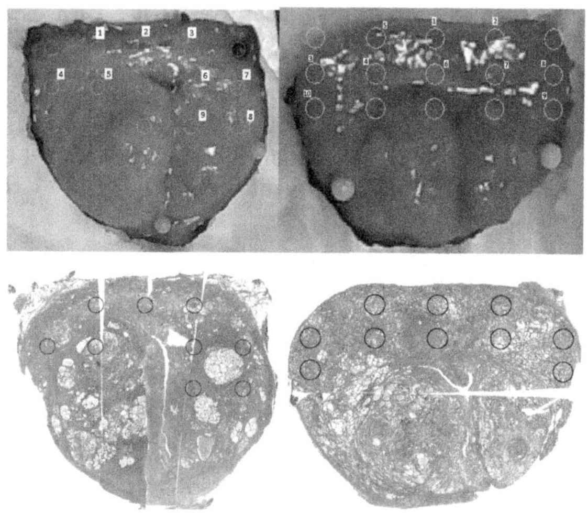

Fig 1. To the left, prostate nr. 1. Prostate slice (upper left picture), note the swelled tissue areas visible on and below the lower measurement points in the measurement grid and (lower left picture) histological image with measurement locations overlaid. Upper picture to the right prostate nr. 2. Note the swelled tissue areas visible on and below the bottom measurement points in the measurement grid. Lower picture to the right, histological image with measurement locations overlaid.

The histopathological analysis revealed that measurements mainly had been performed on tissue containing predominantly stroma on the first prostate and mainly on epithelial tissue on the second prostate. High grade PIN (prostate interepithelial neoplasia) was found in both prostate slices.

B. Prostate Stiffness

Stiffness sensor frequency (f) and impression force (F) were recorded during a 1 mm impression. This impression depth was chosen to avoid reaching the edge of the covering glass of the sensor tip. The tactile sensor's stiffness parameter, $dF/d\Delta f$ [5], was calculated by a linear fit to 26 data points corresponding to the first 0.5 mm impression.

The stiffness parameter was normalized by calculating a stiffness contrast parameter (SC) as the ratio between perceived stiffness differences from the average stiffness, ⟨dF/dΔf⟩, of each prostate to account for general inter-prostate differences (Eq1).

$$SC = \frac{dF/d\Delta f - \langle dF/d\Delta f \rangle}{\langle dF/d\Delta f \rangle} \qquad (Eq. 1)$$

The stiffness contrast (SC) of the two prostates yielded two distinct groups with different stiffness, one group with SC > 0 and a second with SC < 0 (Fig. 2e 3). These groups were confirmed by the HCA. The multiple comparison tests on the groups formed by the HCA revealed that they were significantly different ($p < 0.05$).

The average stiffness of the first prostate was 9.6 ± 7.7 μN/Hz and 3.0 ± 2.3 μN/Hz for the second. The two prostates had significantly different stiffness ($p < 0.05$).

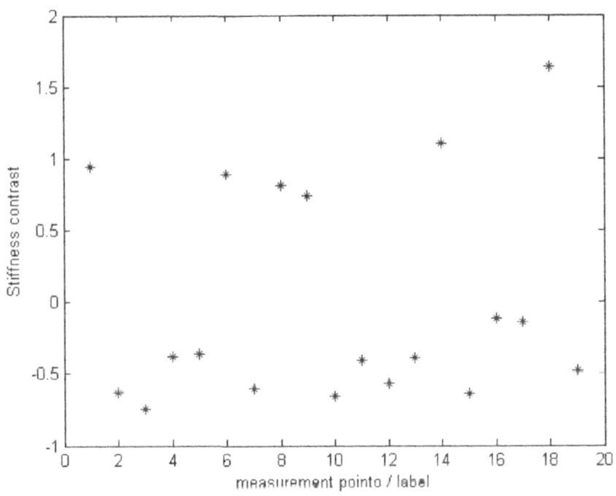

Fig. 2. Stiffness contrast for measurement on prostate 2 (labelled 1-10) and measurement on prostate 1 (labelled 11-19). The stiffness contrast of zero corresponds to the average tissue stiffness in respective prostate slice.

C. Raman Spectroscopy

The Raman spectra were afflicted with a high fluorescent background, therefore only the high wavenumber region (2700 cm^{-1} to 3200 cm^{-1})was investigated. The Raman spectroscopic datasets of each prostate were analyzed separately. The pre-processed Raman spectra in the high-wavenumber region of 2700 cm^{-1} to 3200 cm^{-1} were separated into four groups by the HCA (Fig. 3).

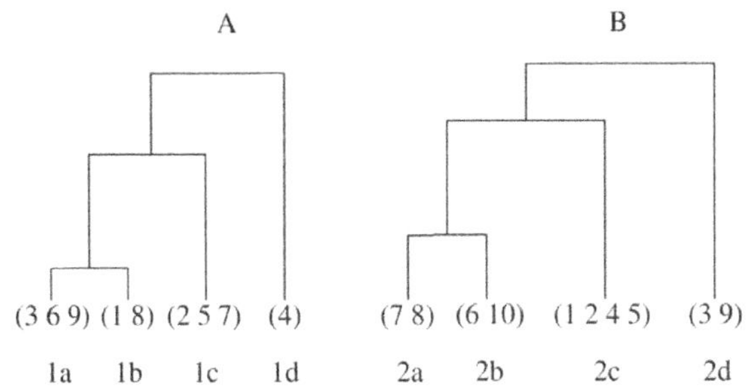

Fig. 3. HCA of the pre-processed Raman spectroscopic data in the high-wavenumber region. (A) Prostate nr.1 with groups 1a-d. (B) Prostate nr. 2 with groups 2a-d.

The most separated group on the first prostate consisted of the single measurement point 4 obtained at a location where a seminal vesicle duct was embedded in stroma afflicted with lots of prostatitis. Points 2, 5, 7 formed a group and consisted of tissue of mixed content. The two least separated groups, consisting of points 1, 6, 9 and 3, 8 consisted mostly of stroma with little or no prostatitis. The histopathological analysis of the second prostate revealed that all measurements except the one on PCa had been performed on epithelial tissue; the groups could thus not be explained by different tissue content.

IV. CONCLUSIONS

An in-house designed probe combining optic fibre Raman spectroscopy and a tactile resonance sensor has been used for measurements on slices of fresh human prostate tissue.

The tactile resonance sensor modality could be used for assessing tissue stiffness. The stiffness contrast parameter was used for classifying tissue by HCA. The stiffness sensor could detect locations on fresh human prostate tissue slices with significantly different stiffness contrasts ($p < 0.05$). The stiffness sensor discriminated between prostate slices consisting of mostly stroma or mostly epithelial tissue with significantly different stiffness ($p < 0.05$).

Raman spectroscopic measurements could be performed with the dual-modality probe for tissue classification. Though, the tissue classification could not fully be explained by the tissue content yet. The tissue fluorescence of fresh human prostate was high. Therefore, a high-wavenumber region was used for analysis.

In order to achieve the full clinical value and understanding of the data, more measurements are needed.

V. Acknowledgment

The study has received grants from the Kempe foundation and the EU structural fund Norra Norrland Objective II.

VI. Conflict of Interest

The authors declare that they have no conflict of interest.

References

1. Ferlay J, Steliarova-Foucher E, Lortet-Tieulent J et al. (2013), "Cancer incidence and mortality patterns in Europe: Estimates for 40 countries in 2012, Euro J of Cancer. 49: (6) 1374–1777 at http://www.sciencedirect.com/science/article/pii/S0959804913000075
2. Wolf A M D et al. (2010) American Cancer Society Guideline for the Early Detection of Prostate Cancer: Update 2010. CA: A Cancer J for Clinicians 60: (2) 70-98 DOI:10.3322/caac.20066
3. Djavan B, Ravery V, Rocco B et al. (2007) European study of radical prostatectomy: time trends in europe, 19932005 BJU International 100: 22–27 at http://dx.doi.org/10.1111/j.1464-410X.2007.06948.x
4. Tsuboi T Ohori M Kuroiwa K et al.(2005) Is intraoperative frozen section analysis an efficient way to reduce positive surgical margins? Urology 66:(6) 1287–1378
5. Nyberg M, Ramser K, Lindahl O (2013) Optical fibre probe NIR Raman measurements in ambient light and in combination with a tactile resonance sensor for possible cancer detection. Analyst 138: 4029-4063
6. Crow P, Molckovsky P, Stone N et al. (2005) Assessment of fiberoptic near-infrared Raman spectroscopy for diagnosis of bladder and prostate cancer Urology 65: (6) 1126–1156

Author: Olof Lindahl
Institute: Centre for Biomedical Engineering and Physics (CMTF)
Street: Umeå University
City: Umeå
Country: Sweden
Email: olof.lindahl@umu.se

Erratum: Prostate Cancer Detection Using a Combination of Raman Spectroscopy and Stiffness Sensing

O.A. Lindahl[1,2,4], M. Nyberg[1,2], V. Jalkanen[2,3], and K. Ramser[1,2]

[1] Department of engineering sciences and mathematics, Luleå University of Technology, Luleå, Sweden
[2] Centre for Biomedical Engineering and Physics (CMTF) Luleå, Umeå, Sweden
[3] Department of Applied Physics and Electronics, Umeå University, Umeå, Sweden
[4] Department of Radiation Sciences, Umeå University, Umeå, Sweden

I. Lackovic (ed.), 1st Global Conference on Biomedical Engineering & 9th Asian-Pacific Conference on Medical and Biological Engineering, IFMBE Proceedings 47, DOI: 10.1007/978-3-319-12262-5_74

DOI 10.1007/978-3-319-12262-5_75

"IFMBE Proceedings Vol. 47: "1st Global Conference on Biomedical Engineering & 9th Asian-Pacific Conference on Medical and Biological Engineering" missed the contribution "Prostate cancer detection using a combination of Raman spectroscopy and stiffness sensing" written by Olof Lindahl for technical reasons. The editors apologize for the mistake.

The original online version for this chapter can be found at
http://dx.doi.org/10.1007/978-3-319-12262-5_74

Author Index

Lee, Gi-Da 12
Lee, H.P. 80

Keyword Index

The manufacturer's authorised representative in the EU is Springer Nature Customer Service Centre GmbH, Europaplatz 3, 69115 Heidelberg, Germany. If you have any concerns regarding our products, please contact ProductSafety@springernature.com

Printed and bound by CPI Group (UK) Ltd, Croydon, CR0 4YY
02/10/2026
02226684-0001